Springer-Verlag Italia Srl.

A. Gullo (Ed.)

Anaesthesia, Pain, Intensive Care and Emergency Medicine - A.P.I.C.E.

Proceedings of the

16th Postgraduate Course in Critical Care Medicine
Trieste, Italy - November 16-20, 2001

Springer

Prof. Antonino Gullo, M.D.
Head, Department of Clinical Sciences
Section of Anaesthesia, Intensive Care and Pain Clinic
Trieste University School of Medicine
Trieste, Italy

Originally published by Springer-Verlag Italia, Milano in 2002

http://www.springer.de

ISBN 978-88-470-0176-3 ISBN 978-88-470-2099-3 (eBook)
DOI 10.1007/978-88-470-2099-3

SPIN 10858730

Table of Contents

Authors Index

Ajmone Cat C.
Department of Anaesthesia and Intensive Care, S. Camillo-Forlanini Hospital, Rome (Italy)

Alexander R.
Department of Anaesthesia and Intensive Care, Worcester Acute Hospitals NHS Trust, The Worcester Royal Infirmary, Worcester (U.K.)

Allaria B.
Intensive Care Unit, National Institute for the Study and Treatment of Tumours, Milan (Italy)

Almeida de Oliveira S.
Heart Thoracic Division, Heart Institute, FMUSP Clinical Hospital, São Paulo (Brazil)

Auler J.O.C.
Department of Anaesthesiology, Heart Institute, FMUSP Clinical Hospital, São Paulo (Brazil)

Banti S.
Department of Anaesthesia and Intensive Care, IRCCS Burlo Garofolo Hospital, Trieste (Italy)

Baumgartner C.
Department of Anaesthesia and General Intensive Care Medicine, University of Vienna, Vienna (Austria)

Berlot G.
Department of Clinical Sciences, Section of Anaesthesia, Intensive Care and Pain Clinic, Trieste University School of Medicine, Trieste (Italy)

Bigatello L.M.
Department of Anaesthesia and Critical Care, Massachusetts General Hospital, Harvard Medical School, Boston, Massachusetts (U.S.A.)

Biolo G.
Department of Clinical, Morphological and Technological Sciences, Division of Internal Medicine, University of Trieste, Trieste (Italy)

Bird F.M.
Bird Institute of Biomedical Technology, Sandpoint, Idaho (U.S.A.)

Blanch L.
Critical Care Centre, Sabadell Hospital, Parc Taulí University Institute, Sabadell (Spain)

Boezeman H.
Department of Clinical Neurophysiology, St. Antonius Hospital, Nieuwegein (The Netherlands)

Boyd O.F.
Department of Intensive Care, The Royal Sussex County Hospital, Brighton (U.K.)

Brandolese R.
Intensive Care Unit, Multidisciplinary Rehabilitation Centre, Padua City Hospital, Padua (Italy)

Brett S.J.
Department of Anaesthesia and Intensive Care, Hammersmith and Queen Charlotte's Hospital, London (U.K.)

Brisinda G.
Department of Surgery, Division of Organ Transplantation, Catholic University, University Hospital "A. Gemelli" and CNR, Rome (Italy)

Busoni P.
Department of Anaesthesia and Intensive Care, A. Meyer Hospital, Florence (Italy)

Caironi P.
Department of Anaesthesia and Intensive Care, Milan University, Maggiore Hospital, Milan (Italy)

Camorcia M.
Department of Anaesthesia, AfaR – CRCCS Fatebenefratelli General Hospital, Rome (Italy)

Candiani A.
Institute of Anaestehsiology and Intensive Care, University of Brescia, Spedali Civili, Brescia (Italy)

Capogna G.
Department of Anaesthesia, AfaR – CRCCS Fatebenefratelli General Hospital, Rome (Italy)

Carli F.
Department of Anaesthesia, McGill University Health Centre, Montreal, Quebec (Canada)

Castagneto M.
Department of Surgery, Division of Organ Transplantation, Catholic University, University Hospital "A. Gemelli" and CNR, Rome (Italy)

Cavaglià M.
Department of Anaesthesiology and Intensive Care, University "A. Avogadro" of Eastern Piedmont, Novara (Italy)

Cerchiari E.
Department of Anaesthesia and Intensive Care, S. Camillo-Forlanini Hospital, Rome (Italy)

Chierego M.L.
Department of Clinical Sciences, Section of Anaesthesia, Intensive Care and Pain Clinic, Trieste University School of Medicine, Trieste (Italy)

Colombo G.
Department of Clinical and Biologic Sciences, Insubria University, Varese (Italy)

Crowhurst J.A.
Department of Anaesthesia and Intensive Care, Hammersmith and Queen Charlotte's Hospital, London (U.K.)

D'Amato L.
Department of Surgical, Anaesthesiological and Emergency Sciences, Naples University "Federico II", Naples (Italy)

Dallan L.A.
Heart Thoracic Division, Heart Institute, FMUSP Clinical Hospital, São Paulo (Brazil)

De Blasio E.
Intensive Care Unit "Marchiafava", Emergency Department, S. Camillo-Forlanini Hospital, Rome (Italy)

de Haan P.
Department of Anaesthesiology, Onze Lieve Vrouwe Gasthuis, Amsterdam (The Netherlands)

De Robertis E.
Department of Anaesthesia and Intensive Care, Naples University "Federico II", Naples (Italy)

Della Corte F.
Department of Anaesthesiology and Intensive Care, University "A. Avogadro" of Eastern Piedmont, Novara (Italy)

Douglas J.
Department of Anaesthesia, British Columbia's Women's Hospital and University of British Columbia, Vancouver, British Columbia (Canada)

Drakulovic M.
Respiratory Intensive Care Unit, Department of Pneumology, Clinical Institute of Pneumology and Thoracic Surgery, Clinical Hospital, Institute of Biomedical Investigation Augusti Pi i Sunyer, University of Barcelona, Barcelona (Spain)

Fernandes C.R.
Department of Anaesthesiology, Heart Institute, FMUSP Clinical Hospital, São Paulo (Brazil)

Finsterer U.
Department of Anaesthesiology, Ludwig-Maximilians University, Munich (Germany)

Flabouris A.
Intensive Care Unit, Liverpool Hospital, University of New South Wales, Sydney (Australia)

Fontanesi L.
Department of Clinical Sciences, Section of Anaesthesia, Intensive Care and Pain Clinic, Trieste University School of Medicine, Trieste (Italy)

Frova G.
Department of Anaesthesia and Intensive Care, "Spedali Civili" Hospital, Brescia (Italy)

Galimberti G.
Department of Clinical Sciences, Section of Anaesthesia, Intensive Care and Pain Clinic, Trieste University School of Medicine, Trieste (Italy)

Gamberoni C.
Department of Anaesthesiology and Intensive Care, Insubria University, Varese (Italy)

Gattinoni L.
Department of Anaesthesia and Intensive Care, Milan University, Maggiore Hospital, Milan (Italy)

Giarratano A.
Department of Anaesthesiology and Intensive Care, Palermo University, Palermo (Italy)

Girardis M.
Department of Anaesthesia and Intensive Care, Modena General Hospital, Modena (Italy)

Giunta F.
Department of Anaesthesiology and Intensive Care, Pisa University, Pisa (Italy)

Gordini G.
Department of Intensive Care, 118 – Maggiore Hospital, Bologna (Italy)

Grocott M.
Surgical Outcomes Research Centre, University College, London (U.K.)

Gullo A.
Department of Clinical Sciences, Section of Anaesthesia, Intensive Care and Pain Clinic, Trieste University School of Medicine, Trieste (Italy)

Gurman G.M.
Division of Anaesthesiology, Soroka Medical Centre and Faculty of Health Sciences, Ben Gurion University of the Negev, Beer Sheva (Israel)

Hamilton M.
Centre for Anaesthesia, University College, London (U.K.)

Hammerle A.F.
Department of Anaesthesia and General Intensive Care Medicine, University of Vienna, Vienna (Austria)

Hedenstierna G.
Department of Clinical Physiology, University Hospital, Uppsala (Sweden)

Illievich U.M.
Department of Anaesthesiology and General Intensive Care, University of Vienna, Vienna (Austria)

Jakob S.M.
Department of Intensive Care Medicine, University Hospital, Bern (Switzerland)

Jonson B.
Department of Clinical Physiology, University Hospital, Lund (Sweden)

Josten C.
Department of Traumatology, University of Leipzig, Leipzig (Germany)

Kalkman C.J.
Department of Anaesthesiology, University Hospital, Utrecht (The Netherlands)

Kaplan L.J.
Departments of Surgery and Emergency Medicine, Medical College of Pennsylvania-Hahnemann University, Philadelphia, Pennsylvania (U.S.A.)

Kellum J.A.
Department of Critical Care Medicine, University of Pittsburgh Medical Center, Pittsburgh, Pennsylvania (U.S.A.)

Kesecioglu J.
Department of Intensive Care, University of Amsterdam, Academic Medical Centre, Amsterdam (The Netherlands)

Kovachev I.
Department of Anaesthesia and Intensive Care, University Hospital of Obstetrics and Gynaecology, Medical University, Sofia (Bulgaria)

Lachmann B.
Department of Anaesthesiology, Erasmus University Rotterdam, Rotterdam (The Netherlands)

Lapinsky S.E.
Intensive Care and Division of Respirology, Mount Sinai Hospital, Toronto, Ontario (Canada)

Latronico N.
Institute of Anaesthesiology and Intensive Care, University of Brescia, Spedali Civili, Brescia (Italy)

Lavoie J.-P.
School of Veterinary Medicine, University of Montreal, Ste Hyacinthe, Quebec (Canada)

Lingnau W.
Department of Anaesthesia and Critical Care Medicine, Leopold-Franzens-University, Innsbruck (Austria)

Lips J.
Department of Anaesthesiology, Academic Medical Centre, University of Amsterdam, Amsterdam (The Netherlands)

Lombardini C.
Department of Anaesthesia and Intensive Care, Modena General Hospital, Modena (Italy)

Lucangelo U.
Department of Clinical Sciences, Section of Anaesthesia, Intensive Care and Pain Clinic, Trieste University School of Medicine, Trieste (Italy)

Lumb P.D.
Department of Anaesthesiology, Keck School of Medicine at USC, Los Angeles, California (U.S.A.)

Lyons G.
Obstetric Anaesthesia, St. James' University Hospital, Leeds (U.K.)

Machata A.-M.
Department of Anaesthesiology and General Intensive Care, University of Vienna, Vienna (Austria)

Magder S.
Department of Medicine and Physiology, McGill University Hospital Centre, Montreal, Quebec (Canada)

Mangione S.
Department of Anaesthesiology and Intensive Care, Palermo University, Palermo (Italy)

Maria G.
Department of Surgery, Division of Organ Transplantation, Catholic University, University Hospital "A. Gemelli" and CNR, Rome (Italy)

Martin J.G.
Meakins-Christie Laboratories, Department of Medicine, McGill University, Montreal, Quebec (Canada)

McKeating E.G.
Department of Neuroanaesthesia and Critical Care, The Royal Preston Hospital, Preston (U.K.)

Melloni C.
Department of Anaesthesia and Intensive Care, Faenza Hospital, Faenza (Italy)

Menarini M.
Department of Intensive Care, 118 – Maggiore Hospital, Bologna (Italy)

Messeri A.
Department of Anaesthesia and Intensive Care, A. Meyer Hospital, Florence (Italy)

Minucci S.
Interventional Radiology, Department of Radiology, S. Camillo Forlanini Hospital, Rome (Italy)

Morgan T.J.
Intensive Care Facility, Royal Brisbane Hospital, Brisbane, Queensland (Australia)

Muchada R.
Department of Anaesthesia and Intensive Care, Eugène André Hospital, Lyon (France)

Muggia-Sullam M.
Department of Surgery, Hadassah Hebrew University Medical Centre, Jerusalem (Israel)

Murias G.
Critical Care Centre, Sabadell Hospital, Parc Taulí University Institute, Sabadell (Spain)

Mythen M.G.
Centre for Anaesthesia, University College, London (U.K.)

Nardi G.
Intensive Care Unit "Marchiafava", Emergency Department, S. Camillo-Forlanini Hospital, Rome (Italy)

Novak-Jankovic V.
Clinical Department of Anaesthesiology and Intensive Care, University Medical Centre, Ljubljana (Slovenia)

Paolicchi A.
Department of Anaesthesia and Intensive Care, Pisa Hospital, Pisa (Italy)

Parr M.J.A.
Intensive Care Unit, Liverpool Hospital, University of New South Wales, Sydney (Australia)

Pasetto A.
Department of Anaesthesia and Intensive Care, Modena General Hospital, Modena (Italy)

Paver Eržen V.
Clinical Department of Anaesthesiology and Intensive Care, University Medical Centre, Ljubljana (Slovenia)

Pellis T.
Department of Clinical Sciences, Section of Anaesthesia, Intensive Care and Pain Clinic, and The Institute of Critical Care Medicine, Palm Springs, California (U.S.A.)

Pelosi P.
Department of Anaesthesiology and Intensive Care, Insubria University, Varese (Italy)

Penney D.J.
Intensive Care Unit, Liverpool Hospital, University of New South Wales, Sydney (Australia)

Pino G.P.
Diagnostic Cardiology, Department of Cardiology, S. Camillo Forlanini Hospital, Rome (Italy)

Pittarello D.
Department of Pharmacology and Anaesthesiology, Padua General Hospital, Padua (Italy)

Poelma D.L.H.
Department of Anaesthesiology, Erasmus University Rotterdam, Rotterdam (The Netherlands)

Pozzi Mucelli F.
Radiology Department, University of Trieste, Trieste (Italy)

Primadei M.
Department of Pharmacology and Anaesthesiology, Padua General Hospital, Padua (Italy)

Rasmussen L.S.
Department of Anaesthesia, Copenhagen University Hospital, Rigshospitalet, Copenhagen (Denmark)

Rawal N.
Department of Anaesthesiology and Intensive Care, Örebro Medical Centre Hospital, Örebro (Sweden)

Rehm M.
Department of Anaesthesiology, Ludwig-Maximilians University, Munich (Germany)

Resta M.
Intensive Care Unit, National Institute for the Study and Treatment of Tumours, Milan (Italy)

Ricci Z.
Department of Nephrology, St. Bortolo Hospital, Vicenza (Italy)

Riccioni L.
Intensive Care Unit "Marchiafava", Emergency Department, S. Camillo-Forlanini Hospital, Rome (Italy)

Robson V.
Department of Anaesthesia and Intensive Care, Hammersmith and Queen Charlotte's Hospital, London (U.K.)

Rocco P.R.M.
Laboratory of Respiration Physiology, Carlos Chagas Filho Biophysics Institute, Federal University of Rio de Janeiro, Centre for Health Sciences, Rio de Janeiro (Brazil)

Ronco C.
Department of Nephrology, St. Bortolo Hospital, Vicenza (Italy)

Rupreht J.
Department of Anaesthesiology, University Hospital Rotterdam, Rotterdam (The Netherlands)

Russell I.F.
Department of Anaesthesia, Hull Royal Infirmary, Hull (U.K.)

Sarti A.
Department of Anaesthesia and Intensive Care, IRCCS Burlo Garofolo Hospital, Trieste (Italy)

Scarpa R.
Department of Anaesthesia and Intensive Care, IRCCS Burlo Garofolo Hospital, Trieste (Italy)

Scheibner L.
Intensive Care Unit, University of Leipzig, Leipzig (Germany)

Schepens M.A.
Department of Cardiothoracic Surgery, St. Antonius Hospital, Nieuwegein (The Netherlands)

Schmidt G.A.
Department of Clinical Medicine and Anaesthesia/Critical Care, University of Chicago, Chicago, Illinois (U.S.A.)

Schreiter D.
Intensive Care Unit, University of Leipzig, Leipzig (Germany)

Servillo G.
Department of Anaesthesia and Intensive Care, Naples University "Federico II", Naples (Italy)

Sganga G.
Department of Surgery, Division of Organ Transplantation, Catholic University, University Hospital "A. Gemelli" and CNR, Rome (Italy)

Silverstein J.H.
Department of Anaesthesiology, Mount Sinai School of Medicine, New York (U.S.A.)

Smilov I.
Department of Anaesthesia and Intensive Care, University Hospital of Obstetrics and Gynaecology, Medical University, Sofia (Bulgaria)

Sorbara C.
Department of Pharmacology and Anaesthesiology, Padua General Hospital, Padua (Italy)

Spiss C.K.
Department of Anaesthesiology and General Intensive Care, University of Vienna, Vienna (Austria)

Stefini R.
Institute of Neurosurgery, University of Brescia, Spedali Civili, Brescia (Italy)

Story D.A.
Department of Anaesthesia, Austin and Repatriation Medical Centre, Heidelberg, Victoria (Australia)

Sutcliffe A.J.
Department of Anaesthesia and Intensive Care, Queen Elizabeth Hospital, Birmingham (U.K.)

Tabor T.
Advisor to Florida Community College, Respiratory Physiology Programme, Jacksonville, Florida (U.S.A.)

Tang W.
The University of Southern California, Keck School of Medicine, Los Angeles, California (U.S.A.)

Tatschl C.
Department of Anaesthesia and General Intensive Care Medicine, University of Vienna, Vienna (Austria)

Tomasini A.
Department of Clinical Sciences, Section of Anaesthesia, Intensive Care and Pain Clinic, Trieste University School of Medicine, Trieste (Italy)

Torres A.
Respiratory Intensive Care Unit, Department of Pneumology, Clinical Institute of Pneumology and Thoracic Surgery, Clinical Hospital, Institute of Biomedical Investigation Augusti Pi i Sunyer, University of Barcelona, Barcelona (Spain)

Torri G.
Department of Anaesthesia and Intensive Care, University of San Raffaele, Milan (Italy)

Trayanov I.
Department of Anaesthesia and Intensive Care, University Hospital of Obstetrics and Gynaecology, Medical University, Sofia (Bulgaria)

Trevisanuto D.
Department of Paediatrics, Padua University Medical School, Padua (Italy)

Tufano R.
Department of Anaesthesia and Intensive Care, Naples University "Federico II", Naples (Italy)

van Dongen E.P.
Department of Anaesthesiology and Intensive Care, St. Antonius Hospital, Nieuwegein (The Netherlands)

Ventafridda V.
Floriani Foundation, Milan (Italy)

Vignazia G.L.
Department of Anaesthesiology and Intensive Care, University "A. Avogadro" of Eastern Piedmont, Novara (Italy)

Villagra A.
Critical Care Centre, Sabadell Hospital, Parc Taulí University Institute, Sabadell (Spain)

Volpe N.G.
Department of Anaesthesia and Intensive Care, Worcester Acute Hospitals NHS Trust, The Worcester Royal Infirmary, Worcester (U.K.)

Weksler N.
Division of Anaesthesiology, Soroka Medical Centre and Faculty of Health Sciences, Ben Gurion University of the Negev, Beer Sheva (Israel)

Zacchello F.
Department of Paediatrics, Padua University Medical School, Padua (Italy)

Zin W.A.
Laboratory of Respiration Physiology, Carlos Chagas Filho Biophysics Institute, Federal University of Rio de Janeiro, Centre for Health Sciences, Rio de Janeiro (Brazil)

Abbreviations

γ, surface tension

γGT, gamma-gluamyltranspeptidase

AAST, American Association for the Surgery of Trauma

ABF, aortic blood flow

ABS, apparent bicarbonate space

ACEIs, angiotensin-converting enzyme inhibitors

ACOG, American College of Obstetricians Gynecologists

ACTH, adrenocortitrophic hormone

ADH, antidiuretic hormone

ADL, activities of daily living

AED, automatic external defibrillator

AFE, amniotic fluid embolism

AG, anion gap

AIDS, acquired immunodeficiency syndrome

AIS, abbreviated injury scale

ALI, acute lung injury

ALS, advances life support

AMPA, alpha-amino-3-hydroxy-5-methyl-4-isoxazoleproprionate

ANH, acute normovolemic haemodilution

ANS, autonomic nervous system

AP, alkaline phosphatase

AP, arterial pressure

APACHE-II, Acute Physiology And Chronic Health Evaluation II

APOE, apolipoprotein E

APRV, airway pressure release ventilation

APS, Acute Pain Service

ARDS, acute respiratory distress syndrome

ARF, acute respiratory failure

ASA, American Society of Anesthesiologists

ASPIDS, aspirate dead space gas from the trachea

AT, abdominal trauma

A_{TOT}, total weak acid concentration

ATS, American Thoracic Society

BAI, blunt aortic injury

BCI, blunt cardiac injury

BCT, blunt cardiac trauma

BD, base deficit

BE, base excess

BEua, base excess caused by unmeasured strong anions

BP, blood pressure

BPI, bactericidial/permeability increasing protein

BUN, blood urea nitrogen

C/S, caesarean section

CAGB, coronary artery bypass grafting

CBF, cerebral blood flow

CCS, Canadian Cardiovascular Society

CDC, Centres for Disease Control

CEGA, combined epidural-general anaesthesia

CEMD, Confidential Enquiries into Maternal Deaths

CEMDEW or **CEMDUK**, Confidential Enquiry into maternal deaths of England and Wales (later United Kingdom)

CFAM, cerebral function analysing monitor

Cl_{CR}, creatinine clearance

CMV, continuous mechanical ventilation

CO, cardiac output

COP, colloid osmotic pressure

COPA, cuffed oropharyngeal airway

COPD, chronic obstructive pulmonary disease

COX, cyclooxygenase

CPAP, continuous positive airway pressure

CPB, cardiopulmonary bypass

CPP, cerebral perfusion pressure

CPR, cardiopulmonary resuscitation

CPRI, cardiopulmonary risk index

CRF, corticothropin releasing factor

CSA, continuous spinal anaesthesia

CSE, combined spinal epidural

CSF, cerebrospinal fluid

Cst, static compliance

CT, computed tomography

CTC, computed tomography of the chest

CTD, Common Technical Document

c-Tnl, cardiac troponin I

CVI, ventilator/computer interface
CVP, central venous pressure
D/FRC, dynamic functional residual capacities
D, dialysance
DAP, diastolic arterial pressure
DCA, dichloroacetate
DCS, damage control surgery
DIC, disseminated intravascular coagulation
DKA, diabetic ketoacidosis
DO_2, oxygen delivery
DPL, diagnostic peritoneal lavage
DVDR, dynamic volumetric diffusive respiration
DVT, deep vein thrombosis
E, expiratory time
EAA, epidural anaesthesia and analgesia
EBM, evidence-based medicine
ECG, electrocardiogram
ECMO, extracorporeal membrane oxygenation
ECV, extracellular volume
ED, emergency department
EE, energy expenditure
EF, external fixation
EFPIA, European Federation of Pharmaceutical Industries and Associations
EFTA, European Free Trade Area
EKG, electrocardiogram
ELSO, Extracorporeal Life Support Organization
EMS, emergency medical services
ER, extraction ratio
ESBL, extended-spectrum beta-lactamase
ESG, endovascular stent-grafting
Est:cw, elastance of the chest wall
FAST, focussed abdominal sonogram for trauma
FDA, Food and Drug Administration
FF, filtration fraction
FiO_2, fraction inspired oxygen
FMH, foetomaternal haemorrhage
FRC, functional residual capacity
GA, general anaesthesia
GCS, Glasgow Coma Scale
GDM, gestational diabetes mellitus
GER, gastroesophageal reflux
GFR, glomerular filtration rate
GIT, gastrointestinal tract
GOS, Glasgow Outcome Scale
GOSE, Glasgow Outcome Scale Extended
H^+, hydrogen ions
HA-1A, human IgM monoclonal antibody
HARM, Harborview assessment for risk of mortality
HCMA, hyperchloraemic metabolic acidosis
HCO_3^-, bicarbonate ions
HDF, haemodiafiltration
HDU, High Dependency Units
HES, hydroxyethyl starch
HF, haemofiltration
HFPV, high frequency percussive ventilation
HFV, high frequency ventilation
HGH, human growth hormone
HICPAC, Hospital Infection Control Advisory Committee
HPT, haemopneumothorax
HPV, hypoxic pulmonary vasoconstriction
HR, heart rate
HT, haemothorax
HU, Hounsfield units
I:E, inspiration expiration ratio
IACS, intra-abdominal compartment syndrome
IADL, independent activities of daily living
IAP, intra-abdominal pressure
IASP, International Association for the Study of Pain
IBD, inflammatory bowel disease
ICD-9-CM, international classification of disease – 9th Rev.
ICH, International Conference on Harmonisation
ICISS, international classification disease-9 based injury severity score
ICP, intracranial pressure
ICU, intensive care unit
IFPMA, International Federation of Pharmaceutical Manufacturers Association
IL, interleukin
ILCOR, International Liaison Committee on Resuscitation
IMN, intramedullary nail fixation
IMV, intermittent mandatory ventilation

INCB, International Narcotics Control Board
ipH, intracellular pH
IPPB, intermittent positive pressure breathing
IPV®, intrapulmonary percussive ventilation
ISPOCD, International Study of Postoperative Cognitive Dysfunction
ISS, Injury Severity Score
IV, intravenous
JCAHO, Joint Commission on Accreditation of Healthcare Organizations
JHRCS, Johns Hopkins Risk Classification System
JPMA, Japan Pharmaceutical Manufacturers Association
LA, local anaesthetic
LAR, late allergic response
LIP, lower inflection point
LMA, laryngeal mask airway
LPS, lipopolysaccharide
LV, left ventricule
LVETi, left ventricular ejection time indexed to the HR
LVSWI, left ventricular stroke work index
MAC, minimum alveolar concentration
MAP, mean arterial pressure
MH, malignant hyperthermia
MHLW, Ministry of Health, Labor and Welfare, Japan
MHP, mentally handicapped patients
MI, myocardial infarction
MODS, multiple organ dysfunction syndrome
MOF, multiple organ failure
MRS, magnetic resonance spectroscopy
MRUPL, minimal required upper pressure limit
MT, major trauma
MTR, mass transfer rate
MV, mechanical ventilation
MVA, motor vehicle accidents
MVO_2, myocardial oxygen consumption
NACA-scale, National Advisory Committee of Aeronautics scale
NAIS, non adrenergic inhibitory system
NGT, nasogastric tube
NIBP, non-invasive blood pressure
NICO, non-invasive cardiac output
NICU, neuro-intensive care unit
NIH, National Institute of Health
NISS, new injury severity score
NMDA, N-methyl-D-aspartate
NNIS, National Nosocomial Infections Surveillance
NO, nitric oxide
NP, nosocomial pneumonia
NPE, neurogenic pulmonary oedema
NSAIDs, non-steroidal anti-inflammatory drugs
NTB, necrotising tracheo-bronchitis
OPS, Orthogonal Polarization Spectral
OR, operating room
P, pressure
PA, pulmonary artery
PACU, Postanaesthesia Care Unit
PAD, public access defibrillation
PAF, platelet-aggregating factor
PAFS, preoperative assessment of fitness score
PAI-1, plasminogen activator inhibitor-1
Paw, airway pressure
PAWP, peak airway pressure
PCA, patient-controlled analgesia
PCBF, pulmonary capillary blood flow
PCEA, patient-controlled epidural analgesia
PCV, packed cell volume
PCWP, pulmonary capillary wedge pressure
PDH, pyruvate dehydrogenase
PDPH, post dural puncture headache
PDSA, plan-do-study-act
PE, pulmonary embolism
PEA, pulseless electrical activity
PEEP, positive end expiratory pressure
PEEPi, intrinsic positive end-expiratory pressure
PEPi, pre-ejection period indexed to the HR
Pes, esophageal pressure
PET, positron emission tomography
PGE2, prostaglandin
pHi, intramucosal pH
PhRMA, Pharmaceutical Research and Manufacturers of America
PIE, pulmonary interstitial emphysema
PMN, polymorphonuclear granulocytes
POCD, postoperative cognitive dysfunction
POD, postoperative day

PONV, postoperative nausea and vomiting

POPC, paediatric overall performance category

PPF, plasma protein fraction

PPMs, potentially pathogenic micro-organisms

PPV, positive pressure ventilation

PRC, packet red cells

PRCO, partial rebreathing for cardiac output measurement

PRMD, post-resuscitation myocardial dysfunction

PT, percutaneous tracheostomy

PT, pneumothorax

PT, prothrombin time

PTA, post-traumatic amnesia

PTCA, percutaneous transluminal coronary angiography

PTS, Paediatric Trauma Score

PTT, partial thromboplastin time

P-V, pressure-volume

PVC, premature ventricular contraction

$PvCO_2$, venous carbon dioxide tension

PVE, plasma volume expansion

r, radius

RBC, red blood cell

RBF, renal blood flow

rBPI, recombinant bactercidal/permeability increasing protein

REACT, rapid early action for coronary treatment

rhGH, recombinant human growth hormone

Rmax,cw, contribution of total resistance of the chest wall

Rmax,L, increase in total resistance of the lung

Rmax,rs, increase in total resistance of the respiratory system

ROC, receiver operating characteristic curve

ROSC, return to spontaneous circulation

RPF, renal plasma flow

RR, respiration rate

rSO_2, regional oxygen saturation

r-tPA, recombinant tissue plasminogen activator

RTS, Revised Trauma Score

RVEDV, right ventricular end diastolic volume

RVSWI, right ventricular stroke work index

SA, status asthmaticus

SAP, systolic arterial pressure

$SBCO_2$, single breath CO_2

SCBF, spinal cord blood flow

SCPP, spinal cord perfusion pressure

SCUF, slow continuous ultra filtration

SDD, selective digestive decontamination

SEP, somatosensory evoked potentials

SGOT-SGTP, serum-glutamic-oxalacetic transaminase and serum glutamic-pyruvic transaminase

SID, strong ion difference

SIDa, "apparent" SID

SIDe, effective SID

SIG, strong ion gap

SIMV, synchronous inspiratory intermittent mandatory ventilation

SIRS, systemic inflammatory response syndrome

SjO_2, oxygen saturation in the jugular vein

SLTA, severe life-threatening asthma

SPECT, single photon emission tomography

SSA, single shot spinal anaesthesia

SSEP, somatosensory evoked potentials

STI, systolic time interval

STS, Society of Thoracic Surgery

SV, stroke volume

SVRI, systemic vascular resistance index

SW, stroke work

TAAA, thoracoabdominal aortic aneurysm

TAE, transcatheter arterial embolization

T-AT, thrombin-antithrombin III

TBI, traumatic brain injury

TBW, total body water

TCD, trans-cranial Doppler

TCI, target controlled infusion

tcMEP, transcranial electrical stimulation

TDCO, thermodilution cardiac output measurement

TED, transoesophageal echodoppler

TEE, transesophageal echocardiography

TFPI, tissue factor and pathway inhibitor

TGI, tracheal gas insufflation

THAM, Tris-hydroxymethyl aminomethane

TIVA, total intravenous anaesthesia
TLT, translaryngeal tracheostomy
TMRL, transmyocardial revascularization laser
TNF, tumour necrosis factor
TNFα, tumour necrosis factor-α
TPN, total parenteral nutrition
TPT, hypertensive pneumothorax
TRISS, trauma revised injury score
TS, Trauma Score
TSVR, total systemic vascular resistance
TTS, trauma thoracic severity score
TV, tidal volume
TX, thromboxane
UHDDS, Uniform Health Discharge Data Set
UI-D, uterine incision-delivery interval
UIP, upper inflection point
UNESCO, United Nations Educational, Scientific, and Cultural Organization
UOP, urine output
US, ultrasound
V/Q, ventilation/perfusion matching
VAP, ventilator associated pneumonia
VAS, visual analogue scale
Vc, central compartment
VCO_2, CO_2 production
$V_{D\ ALV}$, alveolar dead space
VD/VT, total dead space
VF, ventricular fibrillation
VILI, ventilatory-induced lung injury
VISA, vancomycin-intermediate *S. aureus*
VO_2, oxygen consumption
VPS, verbal pain scale
VRE, enterococci with resistance to vancomycin
VRSA, vancomycin-resistant *S. aureus*
V_T, tidal volume
VT, ventricular tachycardia
WBC, white blood cell count
WHO, World Health Organization
$W_{I,aw}$, work done to overcome the airway resistance
$W_{I,dyn,rs}$, dynamic components of lung and chest wall
$W_{I,PEEPi}$, work due to PEEPi
$W_{I,rs}$, inspiratory work done on the respiratory system
$W_{I,st,rs}$, static components of lung and chest wall
Δpes, difference in esophageal pressure
ΔPt, difference in tracheal pressure
$\Delta W_{I,rs}$, work due to the viscoelastic properties of the thoracic tissues and/or time constant inequality within the lungs

ACID-BASE DISORDERS

Homeostasis – Basics, Definitions, Clinical Evidence

A. GULLO, M.L. CHIEREGO

Homeostasis is the ability of the human body's organs and tissues to maintain stable biohumoral conditions within the body. Partial oxygen and carbon dioxide pressure, the concentration of nutrients and waste products, osmotic pressure, the concentrations of several cations and anions, and the volume of the internal fluid environment are all maintained within a certain range of values considered to be normal. The kidneys play a primary role in regulating the concentration of metabolic waste, osmotic pressure, and the volume and composition of the internal environment. The lungs supply the oxygen needed by the cells and eliminate carbon dioxide. The digestive system provides nutrients. Many regulatory mechanisms operate according to the "negative feedback" principle: any deviation from a certain set point is detected by specific receptors. These "detectors" are able to trigger mechanisms that promote compensatory responses and eventually restore conditions of normality.

Acid-base disorders

When we talk about regulating the acid-base balance we mean regulating the concentration of hydrogen ions $[H^+]$ in the body fluids [1]. Even slight alterations from the norm may have considerable effects on the kinetics of cellular chemical reactions, depressing some and accelerating others. The regulation of hydrogen ion concentration is therefore one the most-important aspects of homeostasis. The concentration of hydrogen ions in the extracellular fluid is normally maintained at a value of 4×10^{-8} Eq/l, although fluctuations from 1.0×10^{-8} to 1.0×10^{-7} are still compatible with life. The concentration of hydrogen ions in the extracellular fluid depends on the balance between partial carbon dioxide pressure (pCO_2) and the concentration of bicarbonate $[HCO_3^-]$ [2]:

$$[H^+] \text{ nEq} = 24 \times (pCO_2/[HCO_3^-])$$

Hydrogen ion concentration is indicated by the symbol pH. The relationship between hydrogen ion concentration and pH is expressed by the equation:

$$pH = -\log[H^+] = \log 1/[H^+]$$

The pH is inversely proportional to $[H^+]$. A low pH indicates a high $[H^+]$, or *acidosis*, while an elevated pH corresponds to a low concentration of hydrogen ions, or *alkalosis*. The normal $[H^+]$ of 40 nEq/l corresponds to a pH of 7.40.

The normal pH of arterial blood is between 7.36 and 7.44, while the pH of venous blood and interstitial fluids is about 7.32-7.38, due to the presence of larger amounts of carbon dioxide, which forms carbonic acid.

The body is equipped with a series of control systems for limiting metabolic acidosis or alkalosis [3, 4]. (1) The body fluids have acid-base buffer systems that can instantly combine with an acid or base radical to avoid excessive variations in the hydrogen ion concentration. (2) If the hydrogen ion concentration is significantly changed, the *respiratory centers* are stimulated to produce a variation in lung ventilation and within minutes ventilatory volume - rather than respiration frequency - will increase (Kussmaul respiration). (3) The kidneys excrete a greater quantity of acids or bases with the urine. The kidney responds to the rise in acids by increasing HCO_3^- reabsorption in the proximal tubule and in the loop of Henle; increased excretion of H^+ from the distal tubule and the collecting duct is associated with an increase in ammonium (NH_4^+) excretion and bicarbonate production. Under normal conditions NH_4^+ excretion is about 30 mmol, but it can reach 280 mmol if the acidosis persists for days.

Metabolic acidosis results from the accumulation of nonvolatile acids or from an important loss of bicarbonates in the extracellular compartment. The blood pH is below 7.35, associated with a reduction in HCO_3^- concentration (HCO_3^- 20 mEq/l) and a compensatory reduction of $paCO_2$ [5]. Several conditions may give rise acidosis (Table 1).

Table 1. Causes of metabolic acidosis

-	Diabetes mellitus type 1
-	Prolonged fasting
-	Lactic acidosis
-	Acidosis from reduced H^+ elimination (hypoaldosteronism, kidney disease)
-	Uremic acidosis
-	Tubular acidosis with damage to distal tubule
-	Tubular acidosis with damage to proximal tubule

Based on a pathophysiological classification, a distinction is made between (1) metabolic acidosis with elevated anion gap and (2) hyperchloremic metabolic acidosis with normal anion gap (Table 2).

Table 2. Correlation of anion gap with causes of acidosis

Increased anion gap:
ketoacidosis
lactic acidosis
renal failure
intake of toxic substances
Normal anion gap:
diarrhea
renal tubular acidosis
use of carbonic anhydrase inhibitors

Used for interpreting acidosis, the anion gap parameter helps to differentiate between acidosis due to the accumulation of H^+ and acidosis due to a loss of HCO_3^-. The anion gap provides a measure of the relative excess of unmeasured anions [6]:

$$Na^+ - (Cl^- + HCO_3^-) = ANM - CNM$$

where ANM = unmeasured anions and CNM = unmeasured cations

Normal anion gap values are between 3 and 11 mEq/l, and the gap derives primarily from the negative charges of albumin [7]. The anion gap is increased when organic anions (such as ketoacids or lactates) are metabolized by HCO_3^-, causing the plasma levels of to fall and the anion gap to increase. This means that metabolic acidosis associated with an increased anion gap is a likely indication of an accumulation of organic acids (ketoacidosis, lactic acidosis, renal failure with decreased H^+ excretion) or toxic substances (salicylates, methanol, etc.) [8].

A metabolic acidosis due to HCO_3^- loss gives rise to an increase in chloride ions, which maintain electric charges neutral and do not cause the anion gap value to deviate from the norm. A loss of HCO_3^- may be due to gastrointestinal tract disorders such as diarrhea or biliary fistula, renal wastage, or insufficient production of HCO_3^- by the kidney. Renal causes can be distinguished from non renal causes by measuring excreted [NH_4^+]. In hyperchloremic acidosis, a urinary excretion of NH_4^+ under 1 mmol/kg will indicate a primary involvemer of the kidney in generating the acidosis.

Metabolic alkalosis is characterized by a pH 7.45 and increased HCC This condition is the most-frequent alteration of the acid-base balance foun hospitalized patients (Table 3) [4, 9, 10].

Table 3. Causes of metabolic alkalosis

Loss of H+ ions:	
from the gastrointestinal tract	
-	Vomiting
-	Nasogastric suction
-	Use of antacids
at the kidney level	
-	Diuretics
-	Excess of mineralocorticoids
hypokalemia (with H+ movement into cells)	
Increase in HCO_3^-:	
-	Administration of bicarbonates
-	milk-alkali syndrome

The loss of H^+ due to vomiting, nasogastric suction, or protracted use of diuretics is the most-frequent cause of metabolic alkalosis [11]. Excessive vomiting of stomach content without losing intestinal material results in an important loss of hydrochloric acid secreted by the stomach mucosa. This involves a depletion of chloride ions and a prevalence of HCO_3^- in the extracellular fluid. Excess generation of alkali in the kidney collecting duct may represent a response to the sustained increase in pCO_2 values, or to the increase in mineralocorticoid activity. Excess suprarenal secretion of aldosterone enhances distal tubular reabsorption of Na^+; this situation is associated with an increased secretion of H^+ or increased collecting duct release of Na^+, or it may be a consequence of potassium deficiency [12]. Secretion of H^+ by the collecting duct is increased in response to hypercapnia, and may persist after normal pCO_2 values have been restored [1, 13]. Under normal conditions $paCO_2$ pressure is maintained by alveolar ventilation at values around 38-42 mmHg under the control the respiratory centers. Changes in CO_2 production are accompanied by corresponding changes in alveolar ventilation, which aim at maintaining steady $paCO_2$ values. Respiratory alkalosis and acidosis result from $paCO_2$ modifications. *Respiratory acidosis* may be an acute event or a chronic event with possible acute exacerbation. $paCO_2$ is > 45 mmHg and pH < 7.35 [1, 14]. A sharp rise in CO_2 levels induces the patient to compensate by modifying ventilation; at the same time the hemoglobin dissociation curve changes, while it takes a few days for the kidney to increase the concentration of plasma HCO_3^-. Acute hypercapnia is usually followed by hyperphosphatemia. There are different reasons for this (Table 4): airway obstruction, depression of the respiration centers, neuro-muscular disorders, restrictive lung diseases, inadequate artificial ventilation, severe circulation deficit. The patient manifests anxiety and shortness of breath, he may show delirium, signs of encephalopathy, and myoclonus; these signs may become more apparent as the hypercapnic state

worsens. Chronic respiratory acidosis involves renal compensation by increased reabsorption of HCO_3^-. In exacerbated chronic respiratory acidosis it is the hypoxic - rather than hypercapnic - stimulus which triggers a ventilatory response.

Table 4. Causes of respiratory acidosis

-	alteration of respiration center
-	chest wall or respiratory muscle pathology
-	airway obstruction
-	obstructive and restrictive lung diseases

Respiratory alkalosis is characterized by a pH > 7.45 and a $PaCO_2$ < 35 mmHg [14]. The causes of acute hypocapnia are listed in Table 5. Typical signs are hypoxia, anxiety, and pain. Hypocapnia may manifest during sepsis, liver failure, central nervous system and respiratory system disorders, in pregnancy, and following drug intake. A sharp fall in pCO_2 leads to a slight decrease in HCO_3^- levels due to the cellular exchange for chloride. In addition, acute hypocapnia induces cellular uptake of phosphate and potassium. Patients with acute hypocapnia may develop severe arrhythmia, cerebral vasoconstriction, paresthesias, etc. Within minutes or hours of sustained hypocapnia, reabsorption of HCO_3^- by the proximal tubule is inhibited and renal secretion of H^+ is reduced [5].

Table 5. Causes of respiratory alkalosis (ARDS = acute respiratory distress syndrome)

-	mechanical ventilation
-	voluntary or psychogenic hyperventilation
-	drugs, hormones, pregnancy
-	liver failure
-	sepsis
-	neurological disorders
-	hypoxemia (pneumonia, pulmonary embolism, ARDS, pulmonary edema, and interstitial fibrosis)

Osmolality

Every non diffusible molecule dissolved in water lowers the chemical potential of the water by a given value. As a consequence, the tendency of the water solution to diffuse through a membrane is reduced proportionately to the number of non diffusible molecules it contains. When a molecule is dissociated into two or more ions, each of these ions exerts an osmotic pressure. A gram-molecule of a dissolved non diffusible and non ionizable substance is equal to 1 osmole. For ion monovalents, the osmotic activity expressed in milliosmoles is equal to the concentration of the ions in milliequivalents, expressed in units of volume [15].

Osmolality is defined as the concentration in osmoles in a solution, when the concentration is expressed in osmoles per kilogram of water; *osmolarity*, on the other hand, is used when the concentration is expressed in osmoles per liter of solution. In highly diluted solutions, such as body fluids, the differences are so minute that the two terms are used interchangeably. The normal osmolarity of plasma (285-295 mosmol/l) is largely attributable to its inorganic salt content (electrolytes). Four-fifths of the total osmolality of interstitial fluid and plasma is accounted for by sodium and chloride ions, while about half of intracellular fluid osmolality is accounted for by potassium ions, and the rest by the many other cell constituents. Plasma has a slightly higher osmolality than interstitial and intracellular fluids, mainly on account of the plasma proteins.

Fluid osmolarity can be determined in the laboratory, using electrical devices that measure osmotic pressure based on the freezing point (osmometers). These devices are sensitive to even minute changes in the freezing point; a decrease of 0.00186°C relative to the freezing point of water (assumed to be 0°C) is equal to 1 mosmol of osmotic activity/l. An easier method for calculating osmolarity takes into account only the principal electrolytes dissolved in body fluids, of which sodium is the principal determinant of relative intra- and extracellular fluid volumes. Chlorine is taken into account by doubling the sodium concentration. Glucose and urea are the most-abundant nonionic osmolar solutes in the extracellular fluid, and normally account for only 3% of total osmolarity; urea has a modest effective osmotic pressure as it penetrates cells too easily to have any significant osmotic effects [16].

$$\text{Plasma osmolality} = (2 \times [Na^+]) + ([\text{Glucose}]/18) + ([\text{BUN}]/2.8) =$$
$$(2 \times 140) + (90/18) + (14/2.8) = 290 \text{ mOsm/Kg } H_2O$$

The factors 18 and 2.8 allow conversion of milligrams per deciliter into milliosmoles per kilogram H_2O. This system, which is useful in clinical practice, is undoubtedly less precise than measured osmolarity, and yields an osmolar gap that is estimated to be about 10 mosmol/kg H_2O. The presence of some substances (e.g., ethanol, methanol, etc.) in the blood increases the difference between calculated and measured osmolarity, and in these cases the difference can be used as a screening test to identify the presence of toxins in the extracellular fluids [17, 18].

Generally, "osmolarity control" refers to controlling the concentration of sodium ions. Three control systems come into play to regulate extracellular osmolarity and sodium concentration: (1) the osmoreceptor-antidiuretic hormone (ADH), (2) the thirst response, (3) the mechanism regulating salt requirements [15].

ADH secretion is regulated by three important areas within the hypothalamus: the supraoptic and paraventricular nuclei, the subfornical organ, and the organum vasculosum of the lamina terminalis. The latter are supplied by a vascular network that lacks a blood-brain barrier, which allows for an easy exchange of ions and other solutes between the blood and the local interstitial fluid, and therefore a rapid osmoreceptor response.

Increased sodium concentrations provoke an almost-parallel increase in osmolality, which in turn activates the hypothalamus osmoreceptors. These stimulate secretion of ADH, which increases tubular permeability to H_2O, so that while less water is lost with the urine, the urinary solutes continue to be excreted. Conversely, when the extracellular fluid becomes too diluted, smaller amounts of ADH are released, so that proportionately more water than solutes are eliminated and the concentration of body fluids increases and returns to normal.

Electrolyte quintet

Water constitutes about 50-60% of body weight, to a total of about 35-42 l; 55-75% of water is intracellular, while 24-45% is extracellular [19]. The extracellular compartment is divided into intravascular and extravascular (interstitial) in a 1:3 ratio. The intra- and extracellular compartments are separated by the cell membranes, while the intravascular and extravascular compartments are separated by the capillary endothelium. The cell and capillary membranes are permeable to water, so that the subdivision into compartments is only schematic. The movement of water molecules is a consequence of capillary hydrostatic pressure and colloidal osmotic pressure. The distribution of electrolytes within the various compartments is uneven (Table 6). Electrolytes move from one compartment to another through active and passive mechanisms. The main solutes of the extracellular compartment are Na^+, Cl^-, and HCO_3^-. K^+ and organic phosphate esters are mainly found in the intracellular compartment and are necessary for the normal functioning of cells. Solutes confined to one or other compartment account for the effective osmolarity of that compartment [20].

Constant volume and composition of body fluids are vital factors for life.

Table 6. Electrolyte distribution

Extracellular:		**mEq/l**	**Intracellular:m**		**Eq/l**
Cations			*Cations*		
-	Na^+	142	-	Na^+	12
-	K^+	4.3	-	K^+	150
-	Ca^{2+}	2.5	-	Ca^{2+}	4
-	Mg^{2+}	1.1	-	Mg^{2+}	34
Anions			*Anions*		
-	Cl	104	-	Cl	4
-	HCO_3^-	24	-	HCO_3^-	12
-	HPO_4^-	2	-	HPO_4^-	40
-	Proteins	14	-	Proteins	54
-	Others	5.9	-	Others	90

Sodium

Sodium is the main cation of the extracellular compartment (85-90% of total sodium) [21]. It is the electrolyte with the greatest influence on osmotic pressure and it is an index of extracellular fluid volume. Cell membranes are permeable to water, but not to sodium, which is transported by a pump mechanism (Na^+/K^+-ATPase). The body sodium content of an individual weighing 70 kg is around 4,200 mEq (135-142 mmol/l) [22]. Daily intake is 85-250 mEq, 85-240 mEq of which is excreted with urine, and 0-10 mEq with the feces. Physiological regulatory mechanisms ensure that Na^+ excretion matches intake. The main mechanism that regulates the excretion of sodium is tubular sodium reabsorption, and two-thirds of filtered ions are reabsorbed by the proximal convoluted tubule; 25-30% is reabsorbed in the ascending segment of the loop of Henle, due to the co-transporter $Na^+/K^+/2Cl^-$, and a further 5% is reabsorbed in the distal convoluted tubule due to co-transport with Na^+/Cl^-. Final reabsorption takes place in the collecting tubules. Under normal conditions, sodium is filtered in the glomerulus and reabsorbed, but not excreted, at the tubular level. Therefore, excretion of sodium depends on both the quantity filtered and the quantity reabsorbed, and is influenced by the volume of extracellular fluid rather than by extracellular sodium concentration. Volume variations are perceived by the pressure receptors located in the arteries (aortic arch and carotid sinus). The factors that regulate the concentration of sodium in the glomerular filtrate are sympathetic activity and the atrial natriuretic peptide, which intervene in tubular sodium reabsorption together with aldosterone and angiotensin II. Alterations in volume regulation should be distinguished from alterations in osmoregulation. Variations in sodium concentrations generally indicate an alteration in water homeostasis, while alterations in sodium content manifest as a contraction or expansion of the extracellular compartment. A deficit or excess of sodium involve a reduction or an increase of the effective circulating volume, which in turn causes parallel alterations in the glomerular filtration rate. In most cases, sodium depletion with extracellular volume contraction is due to increased sodium losses rather than reduced sodium intake. Sodium may be lost through the kidney or extrarenally.

Hyponatremia

Hyponatremia is defined as a decrease in plasma sodium concentration below 135 mEq/l. Based on plasma osmolarity, hyponatremia can be classified into hyponatremia with normal or increased plasma osmolarity and hyponatremia with reduced plasma osmolarity (Table 7). Hyper- or normo-osmolar hyponatremias are also known as *pseudohyponatremia* [23, 24]; 93% of plasma is water, the remaining 7% consists of plasmatic proteins and lipids. An increase in the nonaqueous phase of plasma reduces by an artifact the concentration of sodium measured per liter of plasma. The main causes are severe hyperlipidemia (for each 460 mg/dl increase of triglycerides or cholesterol the plasma sodium concentration falls by 1 mEq/l) and hyperproteinemia (>10 g/day). The quantity of sodium contained in the plasma and plasma osmolarity do not vary even if natremia is reduced. Hypertonic hyponatremia may be due to an increase of osmotically active solutes such as glucose and mannitol in the extracellular fluids. Sodium is reduced by 1.6 mEq/l for each 100 mg/dl increase of glucose in the plasma. The rise in plasma osmolarity causes fluids to move out of the cell into the extracellular spaces with dilution of extracellular sodium. ***Hyponatremias with low plasma osmolarity*** become clinically manifest when the plasma sodium concentration is < 120 mEq/l. The low plasmatic osmolarity causes water to shift into the cell and the resulting cellular hyperhydration is responsible for the clinical symptoms: agitation, nausea, anorexia, disorientation, lethargy, muscle cramps, coma, depression of tendon reflexes, hypothermia, seizures, and Cheyne-Stokes respiration. The symptoms are more evident following a sharp fall in plasma sodium concentration [25]. On the other hand, an excessively rapid correction may lead to neurological damage and pontine myelinolysis. Based on the extracellular volume there are three types of hyponatremias. *Hyponatremia with reduced extracellular volume* is caused by a loss of sodium that is disproportionate to the loss of water, or by a loss of sodium corrected with hypotonic solutions. These conditions occur as a result of both extrarenal losses (natriuria < 20 mEq/l) and renal losses of sodium and water (natriuria > 20 mEq/l; e.g., osmotic diuresis, salt-losing nephropathy, diuretics, renal tubular acidosis, hyperaldosteronism).

The prevailing clinical manifestations are those of dehydration. Treatment consists of administering isotonic saline solutions and correcting the underlying cause [26]. *Hyponatremia with normal extracellular volume* is caused by inadequate sodium replacement in Addison's disease, chronic renal failure, and diuretic therapy [27]. *Hyponatremia with increased extracellular volume* is due to sodium deficit or excess water (SIADH, drugs, increased intake of free water, hypothyroidism), or excess water and salt (congestive heart failure, cirrhosis, nephrotic syndrome) [28]. SIADH is characterized by natriuria > 20 mEq/l, increased total water and intravascular volume, urine osmolarity > 200 mo-

Table 7. Causes of hyponatremia

1. Pseudohyponatremia:
with normal plasma osmolarity:
- Hyperlipidemia
- Hyperprotidemia
with elevated plasma osmolarity:
- Hyperglycemia
- Mannitol
2. Hypo-osmolar Hyponatremia:
Hypovolemic (HO_2 and $Na^{\pm}$):
renal causes:
- Salt-losing nephropathy
- Hypoaldosteronism
- Diuretics
extrarenal causes:
- Gastrointestial losses
Isovolemic (HO_2 and secondary $Na^{\pm}$):
- SIADH
- Hypothyroidism
- Psychogenic polydipsia
Hypervolemic ($Na^{\pm}$ and H_2O):
- Heart failure
- Kidney failure
- Liver failure

smol/kg, normal cardiac, renal, thyroid, and adrenal cortex function, absence of drugs able to stimulate ADH (cyclophosphamide, diuretics, etc.). SIADH may be induced by malignancies, central nervous system disorders, drugs, etc. Severe symptomatic hyponatremia (natremia < 110-115 mEq/l) is treated by IV administration of furosemide and iso-hypertonic saline solutions (0.9-3%). Severe hypothyroidism may induce hyponatremia by reducing excretion of free water.

Hypernatremia

Hypernatremia is defined as an elevation in the plasma sodium concentration above 145 mEq/l [22]. It may be caused by a relative deficit of water or excess sodium. Water deficit may be due to either poor intake of free water (disordered consciousness, impaired thirst mechanism due to hypothalamus lesions) or to water losses (cutaneous, gastrointestinal, renal, respiratory losses). Hypernatremia due to excess sodium may be caused by primary hyperaldosteronism and Cushing's syndrome, or increased enteral or parenteral salt intake. Hypernatremia becomes symptomatic when the plasma sodium concentration is > 160 mEq/l. Hypernatremia is not as common as hyponatremia. The clinical manifestations of hypernatremia are essentially neurological: altered mental state, lethargy, irritability, seizures (mainly in children), muscle cramps, hyperreflexia and spasticity, but also fever, nausea, vomiting, etc. The morbidity and mortality rates of acute hypernatremia are high in children, and survivors suffer neurological sequelae [29]. Mortality in chronic hypernatremia is lower (10%). In adults, natremia > 160 mEq/l is associated with a 75% mortality, while the mortality rate in chronic hypernatremia is 65%. A distinction must be made among hypovolemic, normovolemic, and hypervolemic hypernatremia. *Hypovolemic hypernatremia* is sustained by a loss of sodium and a relatively greater loss of water. Clinically the patient shows signs of hypovolemia: orthostatic hypotension, tachycardia, dry mucosas, dry skin, and sometimes altered mental state. The major cause is a loss of fluids from the kidney or the gastrointestinal tract. In the latter case there is a low urinary concentration of sodium. *Hypervolemic hypoernatremia* is the least common. It results from the use of saline solutions at 3% NaCl and from the use of NaHCO3 in the treatment of metabolic acidosis and hyperkalemia; although this practice is controversial, it is still used in the treatment cardiac-respiratory arrest. *Normovolemic hypernatremia* is the most-common form. Patients with hypernatremia due to a loss of water appear to be normovolemic, with normal total body concentrations of sodium. Water loss does not lead to hypernatremia as long as it is accompanied by a compensatory intake of fluids. Extrarenal water losses occur via the skin or the respiratory tract in febrile states or in other hypermetabolic conditions. Urine osmolarity is very high, which indicates correct functioning of the ADH-osmoreceptor system. Urinary sodium concentration depends on fluid intake. Renal fluid losses that lead to normovolemic hypernatremia result from a defect in the production or release of vasopressin or from damage to the collecting duct which fails to respond to the hormone. Central [30] and nephrogenic diabetes insipidus [31, 32] are included in normovolemic hypernatremia. In both disorders the patient presents polyuria and polydipsia. The two disorders can be distinguished by measuring vasopressin and the renal response to ADH administration. About 50% of cases with central diabetes insipidus are idiopathic, while the rest are caused by tumors, traumas, and infectious diseases.

Potassium

Potassium is the most-abundant cation in the body, and of the 4,000 mmol only 2% is extracellular [33]. The ratio between the K^+ concentration in extracellular and intracellular fluids is given by the resting membrane potential. The normal plasma concentration is equal to 3.5-5.5 mmol/l. This ion is sequestered in cells by a Na+-K+ (3:2) ionic exchange pump [34]. An increase in intracellular [Na+] leads to an increase in pump activity. Several factors (e.g., hormones, osmolarity, acid-base balance, etc.) may affect the distribution of K+ [35]. Insulin and catecholamines are the two main hormones that promote the passage of K+ into the cells, and both, with different mechanisms, act by exchanging sodium for potassium. Insulin exchanges Na+ with H+, while catecholamines act through Na+/K+-ATPase [36]. β_2-Adrenergic agonists promote cellular uptake of K+, while a-agonists reduce K+ uptake. Adrenal secretion of aldosterone is regulated by the extracellular concentration of the ion; an increase in aldosterone secretion can increase urinary excretion of K+ threefold. In metabolic acidosis H^+ are exchanged for intracellular K+ causing hyperkalemia [37]. The reverse, that is the movement of K+ into the cell, occurs in metabolic alkalosis. Homeostasis is ensured by the kidney, large amounts of potassium being reabsorbed in co-transport with sodium in the proximal tubules and in the thick ascending limb of the loop of Henle (90% of the filtered ion is reabsorbed), and small amounts also in the distal tubules and in the collecting ducts. In the collecting ducts the "principal" cells are able to secrete large amounts of potassium ions into the tubular lumen, when the K+ extracellular concentration reaches critical levels. Control of extracellular potassium ion concentration is ensured by the activity of the main cells of the kidney and by aldosterone secretion. An increase in extracellular potassium increases the potassium concentration gradient between the renal interstitial fluid and the inside of the tubular epithelial cell, the increase of potassium in the cell increases the exchange of potassium for sodium through the cell's luminal surface.

The scarce presence of potassium in the extracellular compartment limits the value of plasma concentration as an index of body stores. Hypokalemia and hyperkalemia may be associated with important clinical pictures [38].

Hypokalemia

Hypokalemia is defined as a concentration of potassium ions below 3.5 mEq/l (Table 9). It may be due to increased intracellular exchange of potassium or decreased total body content [33, 39]. The shift of K+ into the cells temporarily reduces the plasma concentration of K+, maintaining the total body content unchanged. Insulin, respiratory or metabolic alkalosis, and hypothermia promote the shift of K+ into cells (Table 8) [40, 41]. An increase in renal excretion of K+ occurs in hyperaldosteronism and in patients receiving chronic diuretic therapy. Severe protracted diarrhea is the most-frequent cause of extrarenal hypokalemia. Hypomagnesemia blocks renal reabsorption of potassium [42, 43]. Hypokalemia reduces the resting membrane potential. Clinically, it may cause myalgia, muscular weakness, progressively worsening asthenia, and eventually paralysis. Detectable electrocardiography (ECG) alterations are non specific and are due to delayed ventricular repolarization. There may be T-wave inversion and flattening, prominent U waves, and protracted QT interval.

Table 8. Causes of hypokalemia:

a) Reduced intake: - Undernutrition
b) Redistribution within cells: - Metabolic alkalosis - Insulin - β_2-adrenergic agonists - a-adrenergic antagonists - Pseudohypokalemia - Hypothermia
c) Increased losses: - Gastrointestinal (diarrhea, nasogastric suction, etc.) - Primary and secondary hyperaldosteronism - Salt-losing nephropathy - Hypomagnesemia - Osmotic diuresis - Diuretics, amphotericin B

Table 9. Estimated K+ deficit (for an adult weighing 70 kg)

Serum [K+] (mEq/l):	Body K+ deficit:
3.0	175
2.5	350
2.0	470
1.5	700
1.0	875

Hyperkalemia

Hyperkalemia is defined as a concentration of potassium ions above 5,5 mEq/l [33]. It may be caused by release of K+ content from cells or by decreased renal excretion. K+ release from cells is observed in metabolic acidosis, insulin deficiency and hyperosmolarity. Reduced secretion of K+ in the collecting tubule is due to both decreased Na+ reabsorption and increased Cl^- reabsorbtion; these factors reduce the transepithelial electric potential difference in the main cells. Clinically, particular attention is paid to K+ plasma values in patients with renal failure [44] and primary or secondary hypoaldosteronism (Table 10). Cardiac toxicity of hyperkalemia is the greatest concern, and it is not directly related to K+ plasma levels. Hyperkalemia induces protracted depolarization with decreased membrane excitability. Peaked or widened T waves, prolonged PR interval, and prolonged QRS complex are the most frequent ECG alterations [45].

Table 10. Causes of hyperkalemia (NSAIDs = non-steroidal anti-infammatory drugs, ACE = angiotensin converting enzyme)

- Renal failure
- Primitive and secondary hypoaldosteronism
- Pseudohypoaldosteronism
- Drugs: K+-sparing diuretics, ß-blockers, digitalis, heparin, cyclosporin, NSAIDs, ACE inhibitors, succinylcholine, etc.

Magnesium

The function of Mg^{2+} in biological processes was unknown for many years. Its physiology has only recently been described, and its possible pharmacological applications are currently being investigated [46]. Mg^{2+} is the second most-abundant intracellular cation. It acts as a co-factor in over 300 enzymatic processes, it is involved in gating calcium channels, regulating transmenbrane ion flux, controlling adenylate cyclase, muscle contraction, neuronal activity, vasomotor tone control, cardiac excitability, and neurotransmitter release. In many of its actions it has often been considered as a physiological calcium antagonist; 53% is distributed in bone, 27% is contained in muscle, 13% in soft tissues, and only 0.3% of total body Mg^{2+} is contained in the plasma; 62% of plasma magnesium is ionized, 33% bound to protein, and 5% complexed to bivalent ions (such as citrate and phosphate). Daily Mg^{2+} requirements are estimated to be around 200-250 mg. Excretion depends on the glomerular filtration of the unbound fraction, 60% is reabsorbed in the ascending limb of the loop of Henle. Extracellular Mg^{2+} concentration is about 1.8-2.5 mEq/l. As with the other intracellular elements, there may be total body Mg^{2+} depletion even in the presence of normal blood levels. Mg^{2+} deficiency is thought to contribute to several disorders, and it has been reported in 10% of general-ward inpatients and in 65% of intensive care unit (ICU) patients (Tab. 11). Depletion is caused either by a lack of dietary intake or by a loss. In either case Mg^{2+} deficiency has been shown to be associated with a deficiency of other ions. The association with hypokalemia has already been discussed (40% of cases) [42], and it is necessary to replace Mg^{2+} to correct the K+ deficiency. Hypophosphatemia (30% of cases) is, on the other hand, a cause of hypomagnesemia, as the phosphate deficiency leads to increased renal excretion of Mg^{2+}. If it is true that a moderate Mg^{2+} deficiency results in increased parathormone (PTH) secretion, it is equally true that an excessive lack of the ion interferes with the normal secretion and peripheral response to PTH, leading to hypocalcemia and an altered response of calcemia to PTH. Like hypokalemia, hypocalcemia resolves after restoring normal Mg^{2+} levels. Mg^{2+} depletion may result from inadequate renal reabsorption or from intestinal losses. Protracted intestinal malabsorption or steatorrhea lead to a deficiency of all the major ions. At the renal level, Mg^{2+} reabsorption may be reduced by the action of diuretics (furosemide, acetazolamide, ethacrynic acid, etc.), which act on Mg^{2+} by inhibiting sodium reabsorption, antibiotics (amphotericin, aminoglycosides,etc.) or cyclosporine and cisplatin. A moderate Mg^{2+} deficiency occurs in hyperparathyroidism, hypoparathyroidism, hyperthyroidism, hyperaldosteronism, and in recovery from diabetic ketoacidosis [43]. Low concentrations of Mg^{2+} lead to overexcitability of the nervous system, peripheral vasodilation, and arrhythmias (refractory arrhythmias, torsades de pointes). Typical symptoms of deficiency are paresthesias, muscle cramps, irritability, impaired attention, and mental confusion. An increase in the extracellular concentration of Mg^{2+} can be observed in patients with chronic renal failure; clinically severe pictures are not frequent. Hypermagnesemia presents with nausea, sedation, depressed deep tendon reflexes, muscular depression due to inhibited nervous system activity, and skeletal muscle contractility; the last effect can be blocked by administering calcium. With plasma concentrations of 10 mEq/l there will be bradycardia, vasodilation, hypotension, and eventually disappearance of reflexes, coma, and respiratory paralysis.

Possible pharmacological applications of Mg^{2+} involve mainly the fields of obstetrics and cardiology. In obstetrics [47], Mg^{2+} sulfate is used to treat eclampsia, as it is more effective than diazepam and phenytoin in convulsions. More recent is the use of Mg^{2+} as a tocolytic. The role of magnesium in the treatment of myocardial infarction is not yet understood [48]. Administered in pharmacological doses [49], it is a powerful vasodilator, it has a mild negative inotropic effect, it is an adrenergic antagonist, it has an important anti-arrhythmic action, and it is able to inhibit platelet aggregation. It also protects against reperfusion damage by blocking the intracellular build-up of calcium. Mg^{2+} is recommended in the treatment of torsades de pointes and resistant ventricular arrhythmia, and it can be useful in the prevention and treatment of bupivacaine-induced arrhythmias [50]. In view of its anti-adrenergic effects it is also used during surgery for pheochromocytoma [51].

Table 11. Treatment plan for hypomagnesemia

Mild hypomagnesemia (total deficit of 1-2 mEq/kg)
1. 1 mEq/kg for first 24 h
2. 0.5 mEq/kg for 3-5 days (even orally if Mg>1 mEq/l)
Moderate hypomagnesemia (Mg<1mEq/l)
1. 6 g MgSO4 in 250 or 500 ml of 0.9% SF over 3 h
2. 5 g MgSO4 in 250 or 500 ml of 0.9% SF in the following 6 h
3. 5 g MgSO4 in continuous infusion, every 12 h for 5 days
Severe hypomagnesemia (associated with complications)
1. 2 g MgSO4 IV in 2 min.
2. 5 g MgSO4 in 250 or 500 ml of 0.9% SF in the following 6 h
3. 5 g MgSO4 in continuous infusion, every 12 h for 6 days

Calcium

Calcium regulates several functions in the cell, and it is present in the form of insoluble complexes [52]. The concentration of intracellular free calcium, needed for its regulatory function, is about 0.1 μmol/l. Normal plasma concentrations range between 8 and 10.5 mg/dl, while ionized calcium values range from 4 to 4.6 mg/dl. The concentration of ionized calcium influences neuromuscular excitability and other cell functions [53]. Over 98% of total body calcium is present in bone; 1% of bone calcium is freely exchangeable with the extracellular fluid. In the plasma, about 50% circulates in the ionized form, 40% is bound to albumin and globulins, and 10% is bound to anions such as HCO_3^-, citrate, sulfate, phosphate, and lactates. The maintenance of normal serum concentrations in extracellular fluids depends on an integrated regulation in the bone, kidney, and intestine. PTH maintains extracellular concentrations of calcium stable, it acts directly on the bone and kidney and indirectly on the intestine in order to increase calcemia. It stimulates renal hydroxylation of 25-hydroxyvitamin D_3 to 1,25$(OH)_2D_3$ and calcium reabsorption by the distal tubule. PTH and 1,25$(OH)_2D_3$ stimulate reabsorption of bone tissue by the osteoclasts, promoting release of calcium into the extracellular fluid. At the intestinal level, efficiency of absorption is inversely correlated to dietary intake, while stool calcium is constant and does not vary with absorption or dietary intake. 1,25$(OH)_2D_3$ stimulates intestinal transport of calcium from the small bowel lumen into the bloodstream and promotes bone resorption. PTH production is closely regulated by the plasma concentration of ionized calcium. Rapid changes in calcemia are due to the effects of the hormone on the bone and on renal calcium clearance, while maintenance of the calcium balance results from the effects of the hormone on vitamin D, and therefore on intestinal reabsorption. There is a daily movement of 500 mg of calcium between the extracellular fluid and bone. The homeostatic action of the hormone is aimed at preserving the normal plasma concentration of calcium at the expense of bone destruction and calcium release from the bone.

Hypocalcemia

Hypocalcemia results from a net calcium loss from the extracelluar fluid [54]. The losses are generally renal and are not compensated for by the bone or intestine. Low albumin levels should be excluded, as they could lead to overestimation of hypocalcemia. Only the ionized fraction should be measured. Ionized calcium may be determined directly by means of specific electrodes that are sensitive to the ion. Clinically there is a prevalence of symptoms due to neuromuscular irritability, namely: paresthesias of the extremities, perioral paresthesias, muscle cramps, laryngospasm, tetany, and seizures. The cardiac signs are prolonged QT, which may lead to cardiac fibrillation and cardiac arrest, hypotension, decreased cardiac output, and ectopic ventricular activity [55].

Critically ill patients [56] may present transient hypocalcemia in association with conditions such as sepsis [57], burns, and acute renal failure, or following massive transfusions of blood containing citrate (Table 12). The acute hypocalcemia that may follow the administration of certain drugs is often transitory and asymptomatic. Over 50% of ICU patients have calcium concentrations $<$ 8.5 mg/dl, while 10% have reduced levels of ionized calcium. Patients with severe sepsis may have decreased ionized calcium, but in other patients the cause is hypoalbuminemia. Alkalosis, on the other hand, tends to increase the binding of calcium to proteins and, if present, it should prompt a direct

Table 12. Causes of hypocalcemia

- Hypoparathyroidism
- Pseudohypoparathyroidism
- Neoplasias
- Rhabdomyolysis
- Renal failure
- Parathyroidectomy
- Hypomagnesemia
- Acute pancreatitis
- Sepsis
- Vitamin D deficiency
- Alkalosis
- Blood transfusions
- Extracorporeal circulation
- Drugs (heparin, cimetidine, aminoglycosides, etc.),
- Air embolism

measurement of ionized calcium. Drugs such as protamine, heparin and glucagon may cause transient hypocalcemia. These apparent or real forms of hypocalcemia are not usually associated with tetany. Even the transient hypocalcemia due to repeated transfusions of citrate-containing blood resolves rapidly. Patients with acute pancreatitis [58] have a hypocalcemia that persists during acute inflammation and varies with the severity of the pancreatitis. The etiology of hypocalcemia in pancreatitis is still unknown.

Chronic hypocalcemia manifests with a clear set of symptoms and requires treatment (Table 13). Neurological and muscular symptoms are frequent. They are characterized by spasms, irritability, and psychosis, abdominal cramps and chronic malabsorption.

Table 13. Treatment of symptomatic hypocalcemia

1. Infuse calcium preferably into a central vein, paying attention to the osmolarity of the infusion solution (calcium chloride 10% = 2000 mosmol/l, 27 mg/ml of calcium; calcium gluconate 10%= 680 mosmol/l, 9 mg/ml of calcium)
2. Infuse a 200-mg bolus of elemental calcium, in 100 ml of 0.9% SF over 10 min.
3. Continuous infusion of 1-2 mg/kg per hour for 6-12 h.
4. Maintenance with 2-4 g/day

Hypercalcemia

Hypercalcemia occurs when the calcium influx into the extracellular fluid from the intestine and/or bone exceeds the calcium efflux to the intestine, bone, and/or kidney. This usually occurs when the calcium influx from bone or intestine exceeds the calcium excretory capacity. The symptoms resulting from excess calcium are correlated with the magnitude and the rate at which the calcium blood levels rise [59]. An intermediate hypercalcemia (10-12 mg/dl) is often observed in primary hyperparathyroidism and is generally asymptomatic. More severe hypercalcemia (>12 mg/dl) is often associated with neurological, renal, gastrointestinal, and cardiovascular symptoms [60]. Neurological symptoms include mental confusion, depression, lethargy, stupor, and coma; gastrointestinal symptoms include constipation, nausea, vomiting, ileus, and pancreatitis. At the renal level, hypercalciuria is associated with nephrogenic diabetes insipidus, polyuria, extracellular fluid depletion, reduced glomerular filtration rate, and consequent worsening of hypercalcemia. In addition, hypercalcemia also causes nephrocalcinosis, and enhances digitalis toxicity. Cardiovascular manifestations include: hypotension, hypovolemia, and shortening of QT segment. Primary hyperparathyroidism is the main cause of hypercalcemia, accounting for over 50% of cases (Table 14). The patients are often young

Table 14. Causes of hypercalcemia

- Hyperparathyroidism
- Malignancy
- Thiazide diuretics
- Immobilization
- Granulomatosis
- Familial hypocalciuria
- Thyrotoxicosis
- Vitamin D intoxication
- Renal insufficiency
- Milk-alkali syndrome

women who have been diagnosed with benign parathyroid adenoma; parathyroid carcinoma is very rare. Excess PTH leads to increased renal reabsorption of calcium, increased gastrointestinal absorption mediated by the increase in $1,25(OH)_2D_3$, and increased bone turnover with bone resorption prevailing over formation. Primary hyperparathyroidism is generally diagnosed by the finding of increased PTH in the presence of moderately elevated calcemia and normal renal function. Of patients with kidney stones, 6% have hyperparathyroidism. In these patients the portion of filtered calcium exceeds reabsorbed calcium, resulting in hypercalciuria and the formation of kidney stones. The second cause of increased calcium is the presence of malignant cells that cause bone destruction. All tumors may metastasize to the bones; some tumors can produce PTH-related peptides that bind to the PTH receptor. Thiazide diuretics enhance calcium reabsorption. Depending on severity of the hypercalcemia, possible treatments include restoration of volume with saline solutions, use of loop diuretics and, in severe hypercalcemia, use of biphosphonates (Table 15).

Table 15. Treatment of hypercalcemia

- Isotonic saline solution = to restore volume
- Furosemide (40-80 mg IV every 2 h) = to maintain urinary flow
- Calcitonin (4 UI/kg IM every 12 h) = to inhibit bone resorption
- Pamidronate (90 mg IV for 24 h) = to inhibit bone resorption

Albumin

Albumin is the most-important plasma protein in quantitative terms (60%), with normal plasma values ranging from 3.5 to 5 g/dl. Albumin has a specific weight of 67,000-69,000 daltons and is composed of a single chain of 584 amino acids. Despite its small size, albumin is prevented from crossing capillary membranes by its specific weight. Albumin is a highly stable protein due to a high aspartic and glutamic acid content and a low leucine and tryptophan content. Albumin is synthesized by the liver, and its production is regulated by hormonal factors and by the oncotic pressure of interstitial fluids; about 165 g of albumin are produced and metabolized daily, and the median half life is 18 days; 60% of total body albumin is extravascular and 40% intravascular; 50% of extravascular albumin is located at the cutaneous level, which explains the rapid protein losses after burns. Albumin has a high water-binding capacity (about 18 ml/g of protein) and it regulates the distribution of volume between the intravascular and interstitial space, leading to a colloidal-osmotic pressure of 16-18 mmHg [61]. Another important function of albumin, related to its negative charge, involves the binding and transport of a large number of endogenous and exogenous molecules [62].

Over the past 10 years a number of preparations with different percentages of human albumin have become commercially available. Three formulations are currently available [63].

5% albumin (50 g/l) is an iso-oncotic solution (colloidal-osmotic pressure around 20 mmHg) that improves the microcirculation by reducing blood viscosity. Its oncotic effects last about 12-18 h, and about half of the volume infused remains in the vascular space.

20% albumin (200 g/l) is a hyperosmotic solution that produces a volume 4 times greater than the volume administered, which is fundamental in the treatment of hypoalbuminemia; it must be administered together with colloids and crystalloids in severe hypovolemias. It is the most commonly used albumin in restoring volemia.

25% albumin (250 g/l) is a solution with a colloidal-osmotic pressure of about 70 mmHg. This formulation is supplied in small 50- and 100-ml volumes. It has been calculated that 100 ml of 25% albumin increases plasma volume by about 400-500 ml, with considerable uptake in the interstitial space.

The plasma protein fraction, an albumin product with lower purity, is made up of 86% albumin, 17% globulin, and 1% γ-globulin. Less expensive than the pure preparations, it is also less effective, and its use has been associated with hypotensive episodes.

Human albumin is used to treat shock and other conditions that require urgent restoration of blood volume, in the acute management of burns, and other clinical situations associated with hypoprotidemia [64-66]. Human albumin solutions are very expensive and cost 30 times as much as crystalloids.

The use of human albumin in the treatment of critical patients was challenged by a Cochrane review in 1998 [67]. The study found no evidence of decreased mortality in critical patients treated with albumin; in contrast, it argued that albumin might increase mortality in patients with hypovolemia, burns, or hypoprotidemia. The Cochrane review reported a mortality 6% higher in the group of patients treated with albumin compared with those treated with other agents. The mechanisms underlying the negative effect of albumin in hypovolemic states are two: albumin is believed to have anticoagulative effects, to inhibit platelet aggregation and increase inhibition of factor X by antithrombin III. This anticoagulative activity may be particularly negative in patients with hemorrhagic shock. Furthermore, it has been demonstrated that albumin can cross the capillary membrane, a process that is accelerated in critical patients. An increase in extravascular albumin would lead to a decrease in intravascular colloidal-osmotic pressure and promote the development of edema. The current licensed indications for albumin are the emergency treatment of shock and burns, and clinical situations associated with hypoprotidemia. In the light of the considerations expressed in the Cochrane review, the role of albumin in clinical practice should be reviewed.

Blood lactate levels

In the past several studies [68, 69] demonstrated the role of lactate dosages in evaluating critical patients. Huckabee [70] found a correlation between elevated blood lactate levels and hypovolemic shock, demonstrating an increase in lactates in conditions of anaerobic metabolism. Broader and Weil [71] reported a correlation between blood lactate levels and mortality. Since then several authors [72] have found increased mortality rates in patients with hyperlactacidemia in conditions of cardiogenic, neurogenic, septic, and hypovolemic shock [73]. Wieskopf and Fairley [74] demonstrated a stoichiometric relation between lactate levels and base deficit, while Davis et al. [75] used the base deficit to guide volume resuscitation in hypovolemic shock [76]. Some consider lactate dosage to be an objective indicator of shock severity. Measurement of blood lactate levels may have important diagnostic and therapeutic implications in critically ill patients with or without the classic signs of shock. All the body tissues can produce lactate through anaerobic glycolysis, but most tissues only produce small quantities as complete oxidation of the pyruvate produced by glycolysis supplies larger amounts of ATP [77].

Pyruvate + NADH + H+ Lactate + NAD

However, when oxygenation is inadequate, all the body tissues respond by increasing lactate production. The lactate produced by the body is either completely metabolized to CO_2 and H_2O or converted back to glucose through gluconeogenesis. Both reactions require oxygen. The decreased availability of oxygen promotes the production of lactate and decreases its utilization. Reduced lactate utilization may be due to liver disease, alcohol intake, or the use of certain drugs. Tissues with intense metabolic activity (intestine, brain, skeletal muscle) greatly contribute to the daily production of lactate. The normal blood levels are 1.3 mmol/l [78, 79]; 50% of the lactate is metabolized by the liver, 25% by the kidney, and the remaining 25% by skeletal muscle and the heart. Lactate can only be metabolized by conversion to pyruvate. Therefore, blood lactate levels depend on pyruvate metabolism. Pyruvate is converted into acetyl coenzyme A (through pyruvate dehydrogenase), which is metabolized in the Krebs cycle and produces ATP, CO_2, and H_2O. Lactate is also used in gluconeogenesis through conversion to oxaloacetate (Cori cycle). The regeneration of glucose from lactate is an important mechanism in restoring glucose levels and removing these products of tissue hypoxia from the systemic circulation. Finally, pyruvate may be converted to alanine and α-ketoglutarate. We may conclude that lactate levels increase when, in the presence of stable oxidation-reduction and cell pH, the formation of pyruvate exceeds its utilization or when conversion of pyruvate into acetyl coenzyme A is limited. Dysfunctions of the pyruvate dehydrogenase complex may occur in sepsis, so that pyruvate levels - and consequently lactate levels - are increased. Clinically, the most-important cause of limited utilization of pyruvate is cellular hypoxia. Pyruvate oxidation and gluconeogenesis require oxygen; when oxygen concentrations are reduced, larger amounts of glucose are converted into lactate. Production of ATP continues but it is less efficient (2 molecules of ATP as against the 34 molecules produced by the Krebs cycle). Although hyperlactacidemia is frequently associated with the presence of metabolic acidosis, lactate production is not responsible for a net increase in H^+ as the ions are used to produce ATP from AMP and ADP [80]. The inability of cells to re-utilize the hydrogen produced by ATP hydrolysis in hypoxia is the underlying cause of metabolic acidosis. In 1976, Cohen and Woods [81] classified hyperlactacidemia due to cell hypoxia as type A and hyperlactacidemia due to other causes as type B (Table 16). Stacpoole

Table 16. Classification of hyperlactacidemias

From tissue hypoxia:
- Flow deficit
- Deficit of arterial oxygen content
Other causes:
- Disease-related (diabetes mellitus, pancreatitis, or sepsis)
- Due to toxins or drugs (salicylates, carbon monoxide)
- Due to hereditary defects (deficit of pyruvate dehydrogenase, glucose-6-phosphatase)

[82] later subdivided type A hyperlactacidemia into two subtypes: hyperlactacidemia associated with poor blood flow and hyperlactacidemia related to arterial oxygen content. Type B was subdivided into three subtypes: (B1) hyperlactacidemia related to disease, but not caused by tissue hypoxia (diabetes mellitis, pancreatitis, or sepsis); (B2) due to the intake of toxins or drugs (salicylates, carbon monoxide, etc.); (B3) due to a congenital metabolic anomaly (deficit of pyruvate dehydrogenase or glucose-6-phosphatase). In ICU patients, many factors can contribute to the excess production of lactates and H^+: increased glycolysis, lipolysis, a pyruvate dehydrogenase deficiency, kidney failure, liver failure, increased catecholamine levels, etc. Stacpoole et al. [69] recently demonstrated that the presence of elevated blood lactate levels (> 5 mmol/l) associated with metabolic acidosis with pH values < 7.35 is related to an 83% mortality rate. Measuring blood lactate levels may be useful for diagnosis and treatment planning in critical patients. Increased lactate levels may be an early indication (increase in 1 h) of myocardial infarction. Schmiechen et al. [83] found a high sensitivity (96%) and low specificity (37%) for lactates (positive if > 1.6 mmol/l) as an index of acute myocardial infarction. In acute myocardial infarction patients lactate levels are an index of the risk of developing cardiogenic shock and an index of survival [84, 85]. In trauma patients [86, 87] they have therapeutic and prognostic significance, as hypovolemia due to blood loss results in hypoxia and therefore in increased lactate levels, so that the level of hyperlactacidemia may be an index of the severity of hypoxia. In neurotraumas, lactates may be a better index of intracranial hypertension than are heart rate, blood pressure, and cardiac output [88]. Several clinical studies have shown that initial blood levels, duration of hyperlactacidemia, and changes in lactate levels after volume replacement are well correlated with prognosis. Persistent hyperlactacidemia in sepsis is correlated

with multiple organ failure and consequently with death [89, 90]. The treatment of choice in patients with increased blood lactate levels is improvement of tissue oxygen transport, which may be achieved by restoring volume, improving hemoglobin levels, and through the use of inotropic agents.

Regulation of blood glucose

In normal subjects blood glucose concentration is maintained within a narrow range, usually between 80-90 mg/dl, as measured on an empty stomach in the morning. This concentration increases to 120-140 mg/dl during the 1st hour after a meal, but the feedback mechanisms for the regulation of glycemia rapidly restore the initial levels, usually within 2 h of carbohydrate intake. Insulin and glucagon are responsible for two distinct feedback control systems. The feedback mechanism based on the action of insulin is more important than that of glucagon, but when dietary intake of glucose is decreased or when there is overutilization of glucose, the glucagon mechanism prevails. In hypoglycemia, owing to the direct effect of low glucose concentrations on the hypothalamus, the sympathetic system is stimulated. The adrenalin released causes a further release of glucose by the liver. Even this mechanism serves to protect the body from severe hypoglycemia. In protracted hypoglycemia, after hours or days, there is secretion of the growth hormone and cortisol, both of which reduce glucose utilization by most of the body's cells. It is important to maintain glycemia at constant levels, because glucose is the only nutritional factor that can be used by the brain, retina, and the germinal epithelium of the gonads. In fasting, liver gluconeogenesis supplies the glucose necessary to maintain glycemia at basal levels. Liver glucose derives mainly from glycogenolysis; only 25% of the glucose released by the liver derives from gluconeogenesis. The main gluconeogenesis substrates are lactate, pyruvate, glycerol, and alanine. Depletion of the liver glycogen stores starts after 20-24 h of fasting, and the ready removal of glucose from the blood stream produces a moderate well-tolerated hypoglycemia (60-80 mg/dl). The decrease in blood glucose levels inhibits insulin secretion, reducing glucose consumption by insulin-dependent tissues and promoting the utilization of lipid derivatives as precursors of gluconeogenesis and alternative sources of energy (as are glycerol and free fatty acids). The increased availability of fatty acids stimulates ketone body production by the liver cells. The concomitant increase in glucagon levels causes marked ketogenesis and gluconeogenesis. These hormonal adjustments reduce the consumption of glucose to about half the amount consumed in the post-absorptive state, and the source of glucose in these conditions becomes almost exclusively liver gluconeogenesis. Substrates other than glucose, including ketone bodies and free fatty acids, provide the rest of the calories required. In prolonged fasting, the brain continues to consume over 80% of total body glucose. If fasting lasts for days, renal gluconeogenesis is activated [91]. During prolonged fasting blood glucose levels are generally maintained (approximately 60 mg/dl) at higher values than those associated with cerebral dysfunction. The hormones that regulate glucose homeostasis are sensitive to body stresses, such as traumas [92], surgery, sepsis, etc. Stress related to surgery and anesthesia induces a hormonal and metabolic response characterized by hypermetabolism, altered glucose, lipid and protein homeostasis, and water and salt retention [93]. Catecholamines [94] rise immediately after anesthesia is induced, modifying heart rate, arterial pressure, and plasma glucose content. The insulin response is markedly reduced by volatile anesthetics. This leads to hyperglycemia associated with the simultaneous increase of all counter-regulatory hormones (catecholamines, cortisol, and glucagon) [95].

Hormonal activity

Homeostasis is maintained by substances secreted into the bloodstream under the control of the neuroendocrine system [96]. This system controls a variety of metabolic functions, it participates in regulating cell growth and protein synthesis, it allows various substances to enter the cells, it regulates the speed of several chemical reactions, etc. The hormonal system is not isolated but it acts in close concert with the nervous system. Hormone secretion is regulated by feedback systems, by the circadian rhythm, and by the sleep-wake cycle. The hypothalamus, which is where all the body's signals converge, is capable of releasing several substances. The hypothalamus produces many releasing and inhibiting factors, which once in the hypothalamus-pituitary portal system modulate the action of the hypophysis. All the main hormones of the anterior hypophysis, except for growth hormone (GH), exert their action by stimulating the target glands (thyroid, adrenal cortex, ovaries, testes, and mammary glands).

GH promotes tissue growth by inducing a hypertrophic and hyperplastic state in the cells. Somatomedins exert the action of GH at tissue level. GH increases protein synthesis in all the body cells, it mobilizes fatty acids and reduces glucose utilization throughout the body. The hormone supplies energy in the form of large amounts of fatty acids that act as "protein- and carbohydrate--sparing agents". GH is not the only hormone to increase glycemia. At least three other hormones have this action: adrenocorticotropin (ACTH), thyroid--stimulating hormone, and prolactin. ACTH enhances cortisol secretion by the adrenal cortex. Cortisol, in turn, causes glycemia to rise by enhancing gluconeogenesis. The magnitude of hormone secretion can increase and decrease within minutes, depending on the subject's nutritional status or possible stress situations, such as in fasting, hypoglycemia, traumas [97, 98], surgical stress, etc. Conditions affecting the hypothalamus, such as traumas or stress, may influence secretion of the hormone by the hypothalamus. Increases in the plasma GH concentration before and after surgery have been observed, which correlated to the type of surgery [96,99]. Somatostatin is the GH-release inhibiting factor, it is secreted also by the pancreatic cells, and it can inhibit secretion of insulin and glucagon. GH, however, has a secondary role in the metabolic response to stress, especially if compared with cortisol. Plasma cortisol concentration varies between 20 μg/100 ml and 5 μg/100 ml. Cortisol acts on protein, carbohydrate, and lipid metabolism and has anti-inflammatory effects. It is surprising to note that almost every type of stress, either physical or neurogenic, is capable of inducing an immediate sharp rise in corticotropin secretion, which is closely followed by a marked increase in cortisol secretion by the adrenal cortex [100, 101]. This causes a rapid mobilization of amino acids and lipid from cell deposits, making them available both as sources of energy and for the synthesis of other compounds, including glucose. Cortisol mobilizes mainly labile proteins, making amino acids available for the cells that need to synthesize vital substances of life. Cortisol increases liver gluconeogenesis by 6-10 times, boosting the transport of amino acids from the extracellular fluid into the liver cells, making amino acids available for conversion into glucose, causing a quantitative increase of all enzymes needed for converting amino acids into glucose, and inducing a mobilization of amino acids from extrahepatic tissues, above all muscle tissue. Overall, it raises glycemia; it reduces protein stores in cells (above all in muscle and lymphoid tissue cells), except for liver cells. In the presence of high cortisol levels, muscles may weaken and the immune functions of lymphoid tissue may be strongly impaired. Only protein production by the liver is enhanced with an increase of plasma proteins released into the blood stream by the liver. Cortisol promotes a moderate mobilization of fatty acids from adipose tissue, increasing their utilization for energy production. In the presence of large amounts of cortisol, even the anti-inflammatory effects of the hormone become apparent: the inflammatory process resolves rapidly, the lysosomal membranes stabilize, capillary permeability decreases, the capacity of leukocytes to digest the phagocitated materials is depressed, the activity of the immune system is reduced, and fever drops.

Antidiuretic hormone (ADH) and aldosterone are not dependent on releasing factors but on plasma osmolarity. When body fluids become too concentrated,

ADH increases collecting tubule water permeability, so that water is reabsorbed while the electrolytes continue to be eliminated. At medium-high concentrations, ADH has a powerful vasoconstrictive effect on arterioles, causing arterial pressure to rise. When the blood volume drops by 25%, ADH secretion increases to levels 50-100 times higher than normal. The increase in secretion is thought to depend on the decreased tension recorded by the stretch receptors in the atria. The carotid and aortic baroceptors, and those located in the pulmonary circulation, are also involved in regulating ADH secretion; pain, anxiety, trauma, and certain drugs [102] may increase ADH secretion.

Regulation of aldosterone secretion is closely related to the regulation of electrolyte concentration in extracellular fluids, as well as to blood volume, arterial pressure, and renal function. There are four factors regulating aldosterone secretion: the concentration of potassium in the extracellular fluid, the renin-angiotensin system, natremia levels, and ACTH levels. An increase in $[K+] < 1$ mEq/l is sufficient to treble aldosterone secretion. At the renal level, in the distal tubules and in the collecting ducts there will be absorption of sodium in exchange for potassium, which is paralleled by an increase in extracellular volume. The decrease in sodium leads to a decrease in extracellular fluid and a consequent decrease in cardiac output and renal blood flow; the result is increased renin-angiotensin formation, which stimulates the secretion of aldosterone.

The hypothalamus also secretes TRH, the thyrotropin-releasing hormone. Thyrotropin is a substance produced by the adenohypophysis, which stimulates the thyroid. The thyroid hormones [103] enhance the metabolism of most of the body's cellular districts, and an excess production causes basal metabolism to increase up to 100% over normal levels. Thyroid hormones also enhance cell uptake of glucose, and the magnitude of glycolysis, gluconeogenesis, and insulin secretion. They also stimulate lipid metabolism by enhancing lipolysis and fatty acid oxidation [104]. The increased metabolism leads to a greater consumption of oxygen, with an increase in the products of metabolism that cause vasodilation, increased blood flow, cardiac output and heart rate, and frequency and depth of respiration. To adjust thyroid secretion to metabolic requirements, a number of feedback systems are in place that act through the hypothalamus and hypophysis.

Oxygen transport

The respiration process may be broken down into four phases [105, 106]:

1. pulmonary ventilation
2. exchange and diffusion of O_2 and CO_2 between alveoli and blood

3. transport of O_2 and CO_2,
4. utilization of O_2 by the cells

O_2 diffuses from the alveoli to the pulmonary capillaries by a difference in pressure (alveolar PaO_2 = 104 mmHg; pulmonary capillary PaO_2. = 40 mmHg) (Table 17). After passing one-third of the way along the pulmonary capillaries the blood is already oxygenated; 98% of the blood reaching the left atrium has a paO_2 = 104 mmHg, the remaining 2% derives from the bronchial vessels and has a PO_2 = 40 mmHg, so that the paO_2 of arterial blood is about 95 mmHg; 97% of the O_2 is carried by hemoglobin (Hb), which has a labile reversible bond with O_2; 3% of the O_2 is transported in the plasma.

When completely saturated, 1 g of Hb transports 1.34 ml of O_2. Hb carries 97% of the O_2 into the arterial blood and 99.5% of the O_2 into the venous blood.

Table 17. Partial pressures of respiratory gases

	Atmospheric air (mmHg)	Alveolar air (mmHg)	Expired air (mmHg)
N_2	597 (78.62%)	569 (74.9%)	566 (74.5%)
O_2	159 (20.93%)	104 (13.6%)	120 (15.7%)
CO_2	0.3 (0.04%)	40 (5.3%)	27 (3.6%)
H_2O	3.7 (0.5%)	47 (6.2%)	47 (6.2%)
Total	760	760	760

A decrease in Hb concentration has a stronger impact on arterial oxygenation than does a decrease in arterial O_2 pressure. A 50% decrease in Hb results in a 50% decrease in the arterial concentration of O_2, while a 50% reduction in arterial O_2 pressure results in a 20% reduction in the arterial concentration of O_2. The sigmoid pattern of the Hb dissociation curve shows that Hb is almost completely saturated at a arterial O_2 pressure of 60 mmHg [105].

Aterial O_2 concentration is:

$CaO_2 = (1.34 \times Hb \times SaO_2) + (0.003 \times PaO_2)$

- SaO2 is not expressed in %
- 0.003 is the solubility constant of O_2 in plasma.

$CaO_2 = (1.34 \times 15 \times 0.98) + (0.003 \times 100) = 20$ ml/100 ml

The transport of O_2 to the tissues depends on the arterial O_2 concentration and cardiac output (or more precisely on the cardiac index).

$DO_2 = CaO_2 \times C.I. = 520\text{-}570$ ml/min per m^2

- DO_2 = O_2 transport
- VO_2 = O_2 consumption

O_2 extraction at the level of the microcirculation depends on the cardiac index and the difference between arterial and venous O_2 content.

$VO_2 = C.I. \times (CaO_2 - CvO_2) = C.I. \times 1.34 \times Hb \times (SaO_2 - SvO_2)$

Arterial oxygen consumption is usually 110-160 ml/min per m^2.

The extraction fraction is expressed by the VO_2/DO_2 ratio. Extraction is normally 25-30%. In a healthy subject at rest VO_2 and DO_2 are constant and oxygen transport (16 ml/kg per min) largely exceeds O_2 consumption (4 ml/kg per min), so that within a wide range VO_2 is independent of DO_2 [107].

In physical exercise [108], O_2 consumption increases, so that cardiac output is increased; at the respiratory level, we have vasodilation and recruitment of capillaries, and locally produced metabolites increase in O_2 release. It should be recalled that O_2 delivery by Hb may be altered in certain conditions (Table 19). Metabolic acidosis, increased erythrocyte concentration of 2,3 diphosphoglycerate (a physiological adjustment to hypoxia), and hyperpyrexia, shift the Hb dissociation curve to the right, so that Hb releases O_2 more easily; conversely, the curve will be shifted to the left, i.e., less O_2 is delivered to the tissues in metabolic alkalosis, drop in body temperature and 2,3 diphosphoglycerol. Some of the conditions that result in decreased oxygen transport are listed in Table 18.

Table 18. Conditions resulting in decreased oxygen transport (Hb = hemoglobin)

Decreased CaO_2
- Decrease in alveolar pressure
- Hypoventilation
- V/Q alteration
- Altered diffusion
- Decrease in Hb
- Decreased affinity of Hb for oxygen
Decreased cardiac output:
- Global hypoperfusion
- Rheological blood alterations
- Heart disease

Table 19. Causes of decreased oxygen delivery to tissues

- Altered microcirculation regulatory mechanisms
- Increased Hb affinity for oxygen (e.g., fetal Hb)

Effects of vasoactive drugs on O_2T and tissue oxygenation

Clinical evidence supports a pathological dependence of oxygen consumption (VO_2) on oxygen transport (DO_2) in critical patients [109]. Patients with low VO_2 generally have worse morbidity and mortality rates compared with patients with normal or elevated O_2 consumption [110]. However, increased O_2 consumption does not indicate whether tissue O_2 requirements are being met. Optimizing O_2 transport to the tissues can potentially improve tissue oxygenation if O_2 extraction is also improved. The use of VO_2 and DO_2 to optimize hemodynamics seems to be a reasonable goal of treatment with vasoactive drugs. O_2 transport above the norm may be arbitrarily defined as having values of DO_2 >600 ml/min per m^2 and VO_2 > 250 ml/min per m^2. A treatment aimed at achieving these values led to improved outcome due to better local tissue oxygenation and decreased anaerobic metabolism [111]. Shoemaker et al. [112] demonstrated that failure to reach supranormal DO_2 and VO_2 values is associated with increased mortality in surgical patients, trauma patients, and all ICU patients. Although there is a general tendency to use vasoactive and inotropic drugs to improve O_2 homeostasis in critical patients, the claimed benefits are controversial [113].

The reluctance to optimize hemodynamics with vasoactive drugs derives from the rooted conviction that these agents - because of their peripheral vasoconstrictive effects [114] - may produce side effects that outweigh the beneficial effects on the systemic circulation. Vasoconstrictive drugs can produce lactic acidosis due to excessive vasoconstriction of peripheral arterioles. The plasma lactate concentration can increase as a consequence of glycogenolysis. There have been several reports of patients with finger necrosis resulting from the use of these drugs [115]. Patients with coronary disease, arteriosclerosis, cardiomyopathy, left ventricular hypertrophy, or arrhythmias may not tolerate $ß_1$-adrenergic receptor stimulants, which increase cardiac output. In patients with congestive heart failure and heart disease the tachycardia response may reduce ventricular filling with consequent reduction in cardiac output and therefore in O_2 transport. In patients with a healthy heart the use of ß-adrenergic drugs is well tolerated and leads to increased cardiac output, thereby improving O_2 transport and peripheral perfusion.

Endogenous catecholamines are responsible for regulating vascular and bronchial muscle tone and myocardiac contractility [100]. These effects are mediated by the adrenergic receptors of the autonomic nervous system located at the vascular, cardiac, and bronchial level. These adrenergic receptors may be activated by endogenous or exogenous catecholamines. α-Adrenergic receptors are divided into types 1 and 2; ß-adrenergic receptors are of three types. In sepsis, dopamine is the preferred catecholamine by many authors [111]. Dopamine is an endogenous catecholamine. It acts both on dopaminergic and adrenergic receptors and its effects are dose dependent [116]. It raises arterial pressure by increasing myocardial contractility and peripheral vascular resistance. It also increases heart rate and may be responsible for tachyarrhythmias. In addition, it may raise the hydrostatic pressure of pulmonary capillaries by constricting the pulmonary arteries. The effects on systemic and pulmonary circulation are associated with the elevated doses of dopamine (> 7.5 μg/kg per min) used in the treatment of septic shock, cardiogenic shock, and in every circulatory shock syndrome with systemic vasodilation. Low-dose dopamine (< 3 μg/kg per min) acts selectively on the dopamine-specific receptors, leading to increased blood flow at the renal, splanchnic, and cerebral level. At intermediate doses (3-7.5 μg/kg per min) dopamine increases cardiac output by acting on cardiac and peripheral circulation [117, 118].

Dobutamine is a synthetic catecholamine. It has mainly β_1-agonistic effects, with stimulation of cardiac activity, and moderate β_2 effects that lead to vasodilatation. It produces a marked increase in cardiac output and it is less likely to cause arrhythmia than dopamine. It may be useful in patients with low cardiac output and high filling pressures. Clinically, the increase in myocardial contractility and the resulting sympathetic tone reduction in response to the increased systolic ejection volume lowers peripheral resistance. Arterial pressure is generally unaffected. Dobutamine is indicated in the treatment of severe left heart failure and right heart failure. It is also used in the treatment of septic shock and in multiorgan failure; in these situations of hypermetabolism, dobutamine increases availability of O_2 for the tissues by increasing cardiac output [119]. Dobutamine is often administered in combination with other catecholamines with more predominantly α or ß adrenergic effects.

Noradrenalin is an α agonist, ß adrenergic used in refractory hypotension. It may reduce cardiac output and O_2 transport as a result of increased afterload (generally in high doses). It gives rise to generalized vasoconstriction, including the renal circulation, and for this reason it is administered together with low-dose dopamine to guarantee renal perfusion. It is not considered to be a first-choice drug in the treatment of states of shock, and it is used as a second drug, in addition to dopamine, in refractory hypotension. Its effect on systemic vascular resistance is dose dependent and, as doses are increased, the cardiac inotropic effect is obscured by vasoconstriction.

Phenylephrine [111] is an α_1-adrenergic agonist that increases systemic vascular resistance and cardiac contractility, thereby increasing cardiac output. It is used in severe refractory hypotension.

Adrenalin has combined α and ß agonistic effects. Because of its powerful action, above all on the splanchnic and renal districts, it is generally used as a second-choice vasoconstrictor. It may lead to hypermetabolism with lactic acidosis, accumulation of ketoacids (due to lipolysis), hyperglycemia (increase of gluconeogenesis), and hypokalemia. Adrenalin may produce a marked increase in the rate of basal metabolism; the resulting increase in tissue O_2 requirements may give rise to problems in patients with precarious tissue oxygenation. The effects of high-dose adrenalin - increased systemic vascular resistance and arterial pressure - result from the activation of α-adrenergic receptors, while extremely low doses only activate the ß-adrenergic receptors.

Methods for estimation of blood volume

The aim of appropriate monitoring is to avoid overload or inadequate fluid infusion. The hemodynamic data derived from blood pressure and heart rate monitoring are often unreliable and of little use for revealing a volume deficit or guiding a therapy that aims to restore volume. Pulmonary artery catheterization is common practice today despite the number of literature reports that do not support its use [120]. Doubts on the use of cardiac pressures as an index of volemia stem from the consideration that these parameters may be affected by several factors (problems relating to cardiac performance, vascular compliance, and intrathoracic pressures). Transesophageal echocardiography is a specific monitoring technique, and experiences with this technique are promising. Some authors [121] have demonstrated that the intraoperative use of transesophageal Doppler imaging in surgery for femur fractures allows correct volume replacement, decreasing postoperative hospital stays. The importance of occult hypovolemia in the development of organ hypoperfusion has been supported by numerous studies [122, 123]. There is no optimal method for routine evaluation of hypoperfusion. Hemodynamic parameters such as cardiac index, VO2 and DO2 are not optimal measures of the adequacy of regional and microcirculatory perfusion. The hypovolemic patient is at risk for splanchnic hypoperfusion with secondary bacterial translocation and development of a systemic inflammatory response [124, 125]. Abnormal splanchnic perfusion may also be present in the absence of systemic signs of hemodynamic deficit [126]. Measuring the gastric intramucosal pH may assist in diagnosis and monitoring, and may be useful for predicting postoperative complications [122].

References

1. Gluck SL (1998) Acid-base. Lancet 352: 474-479
2. Gilfix BM, Bique M, Magder S (1993) A physical chemical approach to the analysis of acid-base balance in the clinical setting. J Crit Care 8: 187-197
3. Rose BD (1989) Introduction to simple and mixed acid-base disorders. In: Rose BD (ed) Clinical physiology of acid-base and electrolyte disorders, 3rd edn. McGraw-Hill, pp 464-477
4. Smith H, Lumb PD (1992) Acid-base balance. In: Barash PG, Cullen BF, Stoelting RK (eds) Clinical anesthesia 2nd edn. Lippincott, Philadelphia, pp 237-250
5. Narins RG, Emmett M (1980) Simple and mixed acid-base disorders: a practical approach. Medicine (Baltimore) 59: 161-187
6. Oster JR, Perez GO, Materson BJ (1977) Clinical use of the anion gap. Medicine (Baltimore) 56: 38-54
7. Winter SD, Pearson JR, Gabow PA, et al (1990) The fall of serum anion gap. Arch Intern Med 150: 311-313
8. Salem MM, Mujais SM (1992) Gaps in anion gap. Arch Intern Med 152: 1625-1629
9. Fencl V, Rossing TH (1989) Acid-base disorders in clinical care medicine. Annu Rev Med 40: 17-29
10. Friedman BS, Lumb PD (1990) Prevention and management of metabolic alkalosis. J Intensive Care Med 5 [Suppl]: S22-S27
11. Galla JH, Luke RG (1987) Pathophysiology of metabolic alkalosis. Hosp Pract 22: 123-146
12. Stone DK, Seldin DW, Kokko JP, Jacobson HR (1983) Mineralocorticoid modulation of rabbit medullary collecting duct acidification. A sodium-independent effect. J Clin Invest 72: 77-83
13. Jacobson HR (1984) Medullary collecting duct acidification. J Clin Invest 74: 2107-2114
14. Silvestri L, Viviani M, Berlot G, Gullo A (1995) Fisiologia dell'equilibrio acido-base. In: Aspetti di fisiopatologia, clinici e di monitoraggio in anestesiologia, vol.1. Trieste: APICE: 4-58
15. Guyton AC (1991) Textbook of medical physiology, 8th edn. Saunders, Philadelphia, pp 341-348
16. Marino PL (1998) Osmolalità plasmatica. ICU Book, 2nd edn. Williams and Wilkins, pp 632-633
17. Sklar AK, Linas SL (1983) The osmolar gap in renal failure. Ann Intern Med 98: 481-482
18. Geheb M (1987) Clinical approach to the hyperosmolar patient. Crit Care Clin 5: 797-815
19. Guyton AC (1991) Textbook of medical physiology, 8th edn. Saunders, Philadelphia, pp 303-306
20. Luzzani A, Dal Corso B, Bianciardi L, Mastropasqua D (1995) Fattori di regolazione dei fluidi dei compartimenti nel periodo perioperatorio. In: Aspetti di fisiopatologia, clinici e di monitoraggio in anestesiologia, vol.1. Trieste: APICE: 59-62
21. Oh MS, Carrol HJ (1992) Disorders of sodium metabolism: hypernatremia and hyponatremia. Crit Care Med 20: 94-103
22. Kumar S, Berl T (1998) Electrolyte quintet, sodium. Lancet 352: 220-228
23. Schrier RW, Briner VA (1990) The differential diagnosis of hyponatremia. Hosp Pract 25: 29-37
24. Weisberg LS (1988) Pseudohyponatremia: a reappraisal. Am J Med 86: 315-318
25. Ayus JC, Arieff AI (1990) Symptomatic hyponatremia: making the diagnostic rapidly. J Crit Illness; 5: 846-856
26. Zarinetchi F, Berl T (1996) Evaluation and management of severe hyponatremia. Adv Intern Med 41: 251
27. Linas S, Berl T, Robertson G, et al (1980) Role of vasopressin in the impaired water excretion of glucocorticoid deficiency. Kidney Int 18: 58
28. Marino PL (1998) Sindromi ipertoniche ed ipotoniche. ICU book, 2nd edn. Williams and Wilkins, pp 631-646
29. Macaulay D, Watson M (1967) Hypernatraemia as a cause of brain damage. Arch Dis Child 42: 485
30. Blevins LS, Wand GS (1992) Diabetes insipidus. Crit Care Med 20: 69-79
31. Tannen R, Regal E, Dunn M, et al (1969) Vasopressin resistant hyposthenuria in advanced chronic renal disease. N Engl J Med 280: 1135

32. Teitelbaum I, McGuinness S (1955) Vasopressin resistance in chronic renal failure. J Clin Invest 96: 378
33. Halperin ML, Kamel S (1998) Electrolyte quintet. Potassium. Lancet 352: 135-140
34. Clausen T, Everts ME (1989) Regulation of the Na/K-pump in skeletal muscle. Kidney Int 35: 1-13
35. Sterns RH, Cox M, Feig PU, Singer I (1981) Internal potassium balance and the control of the plasma potassium balance. Medicine (Baltimore) 60: 339-351
36. Williams ME, Gervino EV, Rosa RM et al (1985) Catecholamine modulation of rapid potassium shifts during exercise. N Engl J Med 312: 823-827
37. Burger GA, Howard R (1993) Acidosis and [K+]. Anesth Analg 76:680
38. Kamel KS, Quaggin S, Scheich A, Halperin ML (1994) Disorders of potassium homeostasis: an approach based on pathophysiology. Am J Kidney Dis 24: 597-613
39. Freedman BI, Burkhart JM (1991) Hypokalemia. Crit Care Clin 7: 143-153
40. Adroguè HJ, Madias NE (1981) Changes in plasma potassium concentration during acute acid-base disturbances. Am J Med 71: 456-466
41. Magner PO, Robinson L, Halperin RM, et al (1988) The plasma potassium concentration in metabolic acidosis: a re-evaluation. Am J Kidney Dis 11: 220-224
42. Whang R, Flink EB, Dyckner T. et al (1985) Mg depletion as a cause of refractory potassium depletion. Arch Intern Med 145: 1686-1689
43. Fawcett WJ, Haxby EJ, Male DA (1999) Magnesium: physiology and pharmacology. Br J Anaesth 83: 302-320
44. Allon M (1993) Treatment and prevention of hyperkalemia in end-stage renal disease. Kidney Int 43: 1197-1209
45. Williams ME, Rosa RM (1988) Hyperkalemia: disorders of internal and external potassium balance. J Intensive Care Med 3: 52-64
46. James MFM (1999) Magnesium: quo vadis?. Br J Anaesth 83: 202-203
47. The Eclampsia Trial Collaborative Group (1995) Which anticonvulsant for women with eclampsia? Evidence from the Collaborative Eclampsia Trial. Lancet 345: 1455-1463
48. Seelig MS, Elin RJ, Antman EM (1998) Magnesium in acute myocardial infarction : still an open question. Can J Cardiol 14: 745-749
49. McLean RM (1994) Magnesium and its therapeutic uses: a review. Am J Med 96: 63-76
50. Frakes MA, Richardson LE (1997) Magnesium sulfate therapy in certain emergency conditions. Am J Emerg Med 15: 182-187
51. O'Riordan JA (1997) Pheochromocytoma and anesthesia. Int Anesthesiol Clin 35: 99-127
52. Bushinsky DA, Monk RD (1998) Electrolyte quintet. Calcium. Lancet 352: 306-311
53. Foreman DT, Lorenzo L (1991) Ionized calcium: it's significance and clinical usefulness. Ann Clin Lab Sci 21: 297-304
54. Gary P, Zaloga MD (1992) Hypocalcemia in critically ill patients. Crit Care Med 20: 251-262
55. Reber PM, Heath H (1995) Hypocalcemic emergencies. Med Clin North Am 79: 93-106
56. Zaloga GP (1992) Hypocalcemia in critically ill patients. Crit Care Med 20: 251-262
57. Burchard KW, Simms H, Robinson A, et al (1992) Hypocalcemia during sepsis. Arch Surg 127: 265-272
58. Steinberg W, Tenner S (1994) Acute pancreatitis. N Engl J Med 330: 1198-1210
59. Mundy GR (1994) Evaluation and treatment of hypercalcemia. Hosp Pract 29: 79-86
60. Bilezikian JP (1993) Management of hypercalcemia. J Clin Endocrinol Metab 77: 1445-1449
61. Griffel MI, Kaufman BS (1992) Pharmacology of colloids and crystalloids. Crit Care Clin 8: 235-254
62. Kaminski MV, Haase TJ (1992) Albumin and colloid osmotic pressure: implications for fluid resuscitation. Crit Care Clin 8: 311-322
63. Mercuriali F, Inghilleri G (2000) Albumin in critical care - use, abuse or misuse. In: Gullo A (ed) APICE. Springer, Berlin Heidelberg New York, pp 883-890
64. Doweiko JP, Nompleggi DJ (1991) Role of albumin in human physiology and pathophysiology. J Parent Enter Nutr 15: 207-211

65. Guthrie RD Jr, Hines C Jr (1991) Use of albumin in the critically ill patient. Am J Gastroenterol 86: 255-63
66. Imm A, Carlson RW (1993) Fluid resuscitation in circulatory shock. Critl Care Clin 9: 313-333
67. Cochrane Injuries Group (1998) Human albumin administration in critically ill patients: systematic review of randomised controlled trials. BMJ 317:235-240
68. Madias NE (1986) Nephrology forum: lactic acidosis. Kidney Int 29: 752-774
69. Stacpoole PW, Wright EC, Baumgartner TG (1994) Natural history and course of acquired lactic acidosis in adults. Am J Med 97: 47-54
70. Huckabee WE (1958) Relationships of pyruvate and lactate during anaerobic metabolism. Effects of infusion of pyruvate or glucose and of hyperventilation. J Clin Invest 37: 244
71. Broader G, Weil MH (1964) Excess lactate: an index of reversibility of shock in human patients. Science 143: 1457
72. Kruse JA, Metha KC, Carlson RW (1987) Definition of clinically significant lactic acidosis. Chest 95[Suppl]: 100
73. Robertson R, Eidt J, Bitzer L, et al (1995) Severe acidosis alone does not predict mortality in the trauma patient. Am J Surg 170: 691-695
74. Weiskopf RB, Fairley HB (1982) Anaesthesia for major trauma. Surg Clin North Am; 62: 31
75. Davis JW, Shackford SR, Mackersie RC, Hoyt DB (1988) Base deficit as a guide to volume resuscitation. J Trauma 28: 1464
76. Falcone RE, Santanello SA, Schulz MA, et al (1993) Correlation of metabolic acidosis with outcome following injury and its value as a scoring tool. World J Surg 17: 575-579
77. Bakker J (1999) Blood lactate levels. Curr Opin Crit Care 5: 234-239
78. Aduen J, Bernstein WK, Khastgir T (1994) The use and clinical importance of a sub-strate specific electrode for rapid determination of blood lactate concentrations. JAMA 272: 1678-1685
79. Auler JOC Jr, Coppola Gimenez S, Mondeiro Abbelani D (1999) Perioperative management strategy for cardiac surgery in pediatric patients. In: Gullo A (ed) APICE. Springer, Berlin Heidelberg New York, p 255
80. Gutierrez G, Wulf ME (1996) Lactic acidosis in sepsis: a commentary. Intensive Care Med 22:6-16
81. Cohen RD, Woods HF (1976) The clinical presentation and classification of lactic acidosis. In: Cohen RD, Woods HF (eds) Blackwell Scientific, Oxford
82. Stacpoole PW (1993) Lactic acidosis. Endocrinol Metab Clin North Am 22:221-245
83. Schmiechen NJ, Han C, Milzman DP (1997) ED use of rapid lactate to evaluate patients with acute chest pain. Ann Emerg Med 30: 571-577
84. Mavric Z, Zaputovic L (1991) Usefulness of blood lactate as a predictor of shock development in acute myocardial infarction. Am J Cardiol 67: 565-68
85. Henning RJ, Weil MH, Weiner F (1982) Blood lactate as prognostic indicator of survival in patients with acute myocardial infarction Circ Shock 9: 307-315
86. Sauaia A, Moore FA (1998) Multiple organ failure can be predicted as early as 12 hours after injury. J Trauma 45: 291-301
87. Hutchinson PJ, al-Rawi PG (2000) On-line monitoring of substrate delivery and brain metabolism in head injury. Acta Neurochir [Suppl] 76 :431-35
88. Scalea TM, Maltz S (1994) Resuscitation of multiple trauma and head injury: role of crystalloid fluids and inotropes. Criti Care Med 22: 1610-1615
89. Vary TC (1996) Sepsis-induced alterations in pyruvate dehydrogenase complex activity in rat skeletal muscle. Shock 6: 89-94
90. Bakker J, Gris P (1996) Serial blood lactate levels can predict the development of multiple organ failure following septic shock. Am J Surg 171: 221-226
91. Adroguè JH (1992) Glucose homeostasis and the kidney. Kidney Int 42: 1266-1282.
92. Malayappa J, Petersen SC, Shamos RF (1993) Protein and glucose fuel kinetics and hormonal changes in elderly trauma patients. Metabolism 42: 1255-1262
93. Iscra F, Margarit O, Limback-Stanic C, Bedin F (1995) Interazioni tra metabolismo e anestesia.

In: Aspetti di fisiopatologia, clinici e di monitoraggio in anestesiologia, vol.1. APICE, Trieste, p 117
94. Chernow B, Alexander HR, Smallridge RC, et al (1987) Hormonal responses to graded surgical stress. Arch Intern Med 147: 1273-1278
95. Weissman C (1990) The metabolic response to stress: an overview and update. Anesthesiology 73: 308-326
96. Iscra F, Bedin F, Limback-Stanic C, Margarit O (1995) Fattori di regolazione del metabolismo e della funzione endocrina. In: Aspetti di fisiopatologia, clinici e di monitoraggio in anestesiologia, vol.2. APICE, Trieste, pp 173-188
97. Woolf PD (1992) Hormonal response to trauma. Crit Care Med 20: 216-226
98. Duggan M, Browne I, Flynn C (1998) Adrenal failure in the critically ill. Br J Anaesth 81: 467-469
99. Weissman C (1990) Response to stress: an overview and update. Anesthesiology 73: 308-327
100 Chernow B, Rainey TG, Lake CR (1982) Endogenous and exogenous catecholamines in critical care medicine. Crit Care Med 10: 409-416
101. Masterson GR, Mostafa SM (1998) Adrenocortical function in critical illness. Br J Anaesth 81: 308-310
102. Buckingham JC (1985) Hypothalamo-pituitary responses to trauma. Br Med Bull 41: 203-211
103. Oppenheimer JH, Schwartz HL, Strait KA (1994) Thyroid hormone action 1994: the plot thickens. Eur J Endocrinol 130: 15-24
104. Smallridge R (1992) Metabolic and anatomic thyroid emergencies: a review. Crit Care Med 20: 276-291
105. Brandolese R, Andreose U (1996) Scambio gassoso. In: Aspetti di fisiopatologia, clinici e di monitoraggio in anestesiologia, vol.2. APICE, Trieste, pp 43-44
106. Guyton AC (1991) Textbook of medical physiology. 8th edn., Saunders, Philadelphia, pp 464-466
107. Marino PL (1998) Oxygen transport. ICU Book, 2nd edn. Williams and Wilkins, pp 18-30
108. Assmussen E, Nielsen M (1960) Alveolo-arterial gas exchange at rest and during work at different O2 tensions. Acta Anesthesiol Scand 50: 153-166
109. Hayes MA, Timmins AC, Yau EHS, et al (1994) Elevation of systemic oxygen delivery in the treatment of critically ill patients. N Engl J Med 330:1717-1722
110. Yu M, Levy MM, Smith P, et al (1993) Effect of maximizing oxygen delivery on morbidity and mortality rates in critically ill patients: a prospective, randomized, controlled study. Crit Care Med 21: 830-838
111. Rudis MI, Pharm D, Basha MA, Zarowitz BJ (1996) Is it time to reposition vasopressors and inotropes in sepsis?. Crit Care Med 24: 525-537
112. Shoemaker WC, Appel PL, Kram HB, et al (1988) Prospective trial of supranormal values of survivors as therapeutic goals in high-risk surgical patients. Chest 94: 1176-1186
113. Russel JA, Phang PT (1994) The oxygen delivery/consumption controversy. Approaches to management of the critically ill. Am J Crit Care Med 149: 533-537
114. Chiolero R, Flatt J-P, Revelly J-P, Jequier E (1991) Effects of cathecolamines on oxygen consumption and oxygen delivery in critically ill patients. Chest 100: 1676-1684
115. Hayes MA, Yau EHS, Hinds CJ et al (1992) Symmetrical peripheral gangrene: association with noradrenaline administration. Intensive Care Med 18: 433-436
116. Shoemaker WC, Appel PL, Kram HB (1986) Hemodynamic and oxygen transport effects of dobutamine in critically ill general surgical patients. Crit Care Med 14: 1032-1037
117. Marino PL (1998) Vasoactive drugs. ICU Book, 2nd edn. Williams and Wilkins, pp 273-294
118. Trujillo MH, Arai K, Bellorin-Font E (1994) Practical guide for drug administration by intravenous infusion in intensive care units. Crit Care Med 22: 1049-1063
119. Klem C, Dasta JF, Reilley TE, Flancbaum LJ (1994) Variability in dobutamine pharmacokinetics in unstable critically ill surgical patients. Crit Care Med 22: 1926-1932
120. Connors AF Jr., Speroff T, Dawson NV, et al (1996) The effectiveness of right heart catheterization in the initial care of critically ill patients. JAMA 276: 889-897

121. Sinclair S, James S, Singer M (1997) Intraoperative intravascular volume optimisation and length of hospital stay after repair of proximal femoral fracture: randomised controlled trial. BMJ 315: 909-912
122. Mythen MG, Webb AR (1994) The role of gut mucosal hypoperfusion in the pathogenesis of postoperative organ dysfunction. Intensive Care Med 20: 203-209
123. Pittard AJ, Hawkins WJ, Webster NR (1994) The role of the microcirculation in the multi-organ dysfunction syndrome. Clin Intensive Care 5: 186-190
124. Takala J (1994) Splanchnic perfusion in shock. Intensive Care Med 20: 403-404
125. Mythen MG, Webb AR (1995) Perioperative plasma volume expansion reduce the incidence of gut mucosal hypoperfusion during cardiac surgery. Ann Surg 130: 423-429
126. Marik PE, Iglesias J, Marini B (1997) Gastric intramucosal pH changes after volume replacement with hydroxyethyl starch or crystalloid in patients undergoing elective abdominal aortic aneurism repair. J Crit Care 12: 51-55

Physical Chemistry and Clinical Acid-Base Physiology

J. A. KELLUM

Unlike most other areas of medicine, critical care does not confine itself to a specific organ or region of the body, or to a specific disease process. Rather, practitioners of critical care are concerned with the interaction of various organs and disease states. Indeed, our practice is often defined by the management of certain syndromes (e.g., sepsis, multi-organ failure) and pathophysiological conditions (e.g., shock) that do not fall neatly into the domain of a single subspecialty. Acid-base regulation is one of these "areas" of medicine that crosses organ-specific boundaries and the intensive care unit (ICU) is often the place where severe derangements in this area exist. For these reasons, intensivists, and others called upon to care for critically ill patients in the ICU, operating room, or emergency department are expected to diagnose and manage complicated disorders of acid-base balance. Accordingly, it is fundamental to the practice of critical care to have an advanced understanding of acid-base chemistry and physiology. Unfortunately, our "acid-base science" has not kept pace with advances in other areas germane to critical care (e.g., mechanisms of inflammation and oxygen delivery to the tissues) and as such, our clinical practice of diagnosis and management of acid-base disorders is far less advanced. Indeed, little has changed in this field in over 40 years.

Perhaps one reason for the lack of advance in the field of clinical acid-base physiology is the lack of advance in basic acid-base chemistry. Furthermore, we have generally been slow to adopt those advances that have occurred. More than 15 years ago Stewart [1, 2] published his revolutionary physical chemical analysis of acid-base physiology. Although this approach is based on the same physical chemical principles more-traditional methods are based on, this new approach is vastly different. The most important difference is the emphasis on mathematics and on independent and dependent variables. Using this approach, it is clear that neither hydrogen ions (H^+) nor bicarbonate ions (HCO_3^-) are independent variables, but are determined by other factors. Changes in H^+ concentration (and thus pH) are not the result of the generation or removal of these ions per se, but rather are the result of changes in the independent variables. This change in focus may seem merely semantic at first, but it has far-reaching implications. Indeed, the change has been compared with that of pre- and post-Copernican astronomy in its scope and significance to their respective fields [3, 4].

The physical-chemical approach to acid-base physiology has now been validated in a wide variety of patient types [5-11] and experimental conditions [12-16]. Recently, it has been shown that quantitatively this approach is compatible with more-traditional approaches [17-19]; the difference lies in the understanding of the mechanisms involved. The observation that metabolic acidosis is associated with a decrease in plasma bicarbonate and base excess remains valid. However, the implication that these changes cause the acidosis is not. Some might argue that such a change makes little difference. If one can measure the size and origin (respiratory vs. metabolic) of a change in acid-base status, does the average clinician really need to understand how it occurs? The obvious answer is this: only if we wish to know how acid-base derangements occur and how to treat them sensibly.

In this review, I will explain the fundamental aspects of the Stewart approach, review the implications for clinical medicine, particularly in the ICU, and consider some of the more-practical aspects of acid-base management from this prospective. Several more-detailed treatments of the Stewart approach are available in the literature [1, 2, 20, 21]. The purpose of this discussion is to provide the reader with a general understanding of the approach and its implications. However, the interested reader is advised to seek out these other sources as well.

Physical chemical principles of hydrogen ion regulation

Large living organisms seek to maintain plasma pH within strict tolerance limits. Indeed, H^+ concentration is maintained within the range of 36-43 nmol/l. In contrast, most other plasma ions are regulated in the mmol/L range. One reason H^+ concentration is so closely regulated is that these ions have very high charge densities and consequently very large electric fields. Furthermore, the strength of H^+ bonds (ubiquitous in biological systems) is very sensitive to local H^+ concentration. Biochemical reactions, as well as interactions of hormones and drugs with plasma proteins and cell surface receptors, are also influenced by changes in H^+ concentration. In addition, fluctuations in intracellular H^+ concentration have major effects on cellular performance, presumably by altering protein charge, thereby affecting structure and enzymatic function.

Obviously then, in order to understand how the body regulates plasma H^+ concentration, we must first understand the physical-chemical determinants of H^+ concentration.

Biochemistry of aqueous solutions

Virtually all solutions in human biology contain water and aqueous solutions provide a virtually inexhaustible source of H^+. In these solutions, H^+ concentration is determined by the dissociation of water into H^+ and OH^- ions. Said another way, changes in H^+ concentration occur not as a result of how much H^+ is added or removed, but as a consequence of water dissociation. The factors that determine the dissociation of water are the laws of physical chemistry. Two in particular apply here, electroneutrality (which dictates that in aqueous solutions the sum of all positively charged ions must equal the sum of all negatively charged ions) and conservation of mass (which means that the amount of a substance remains constant unless it is added or generated, or removed or destroyed). In pure water, according to the principle of electroneutrality, the concentration of H+ must always equal the concentration of OH-. In more-complex solutions, we have to consider other determinants of water dissociation, but still the source of H^+ remains water. Fortunately, even in a solution as complex as blood plasma, the determinants of H^+ concentration can be reduced to three. If we know the value of these three determinants, the H^+ concentration can be predicted under any condition. These three determinants are the strong ion difference (SID), PCO_2, and total weak acid concentration (A_{TOT}).

The SID is the net charge balance of all strong ions present where a "strong" ion is one that is completely (or near completely) dissociated. For practical purposes this means ($Na^+ + K^+ + Ca^{2+} + Mg^{2+}$) - ($Cl^-$ + lactate$^-$). This is often referred to as the "apparent" SID (SIDa), with the understanding that some "unmeasured" ions might also be present [12]. In healthy humans, this value is 40-42 mEq/l, although it is often quite different in critically ill patients. Of note, neither H^+ nor HCO_3^- are strong ions. The PCO_2 is an independent variable assuming that the system is open (i.e., ventilation is present). Finally, the weak acids (A^-), which are mostly proteins and phosphates, contribute the remaining charges to satisfy the principle of electroneutrality. A^-, however, is not an independent variable because it changes with alterations in SID and PCO_2. Instead, A_{TOT}, ($AH + A^-$) is the third independent variable. The essence of the physical-chemical approach (and indeed what is revolutionary) is the understanding that only these three variables are important. Neither H^+ nor HCO_3^- can change unless one or more of these three variables change. The principle of conservation of mass makes this point more than semantics. Strong ions cannot be created or destroyed to satisfy electroneutrality, but H^+ is generated or consumed by changes in water dissociation. Hence, in order to understand how the body regulates pH we need only ask how it regulates these three independent variables (SID, PCO_2 and A_{TOT}).

Clinical applications

This "new" approach changes nothing about the measurement or classification of acid-base disorders. All of the careful observations that have been made over the years are no less valid under this approach. What does change is the interpretation of these observations. While I will discuss some clinical examples of this, there are many others that will become obvious as one ponders the various aspects of this approach.

Quantification of acid-base disorders

While the understanding of how an acid-base disorder occurs is now quite different, it is important to emphasize that not only does the traditional approach to quantifying an acid-base disorder still "work", it is entirely complementary to this physical-chemical analysis. In fact the standard base excess (SBE) can be used to quantify the amount of change in SID from baseline [17, 18]. The SBE can be thought of as the amount of change in the SID that is required in order to restore the pH to 7.40, given a pCO_2 of 40 mmHg (a negative SBE refers to the amount the SID must increase). This is because the SID is essentially equal to the buffer base of Singer and Hastings [22] and BE quantifies the change in buffer base. SBE is superior to BE because the former has been "standardized" to account for the difference between CO_2 equilibration in vitro compared with in vivo. Although SBE is not strictly comparable to the change in SID because it deals with whole blood as opposed to plasma [23], the two are generally close enough for most clinical circumstances. Thus, SBE provides an estimate of the amount of strong anion that needs to be removed or strong cation added in order to normalize the pH. For example, in order to change the SBE from -20 to -10 mEq/l by adding $NaHCO_3$, the serum Na^+ concentration would need to be increased by 10 mEq/l.

Recently, Schlichtig et al. [23] described the changes in SBE that occur with acute and chronic disorders of $paCO_2$. The SBE does not change with acute changes in $paCO_2$. During chronic respiratory acidosis or alkalosis the change in the SBE is equal to 0.4 x ($paCO_2$ – 40). Similarly, the expected change in $paCO_2$ for a given abnormality in SBE is as follows: for acidosis, the decrease in $paCO_2$ is equal to the change in SBE; for alkalosis the increase in $paCO_2$ is equal to 0.6xSBE [23].

Hyper and hypochloremia

One of the most important implications of the physical-chemical analysis is the role of Cl^- in acid-base homeostasis. If the body is to alter the SID, its primary tools are Na^+ and Cl^-. An increase in Na^+ relative to Cl^- (or a decrease in Cl^- relative to Na^+) increases the SID and hence the pH. The opposite effects, a decrease in the SID and a fall in the pH, occur when Na^+ and Cl^- concentrations move closer together. Since Na^+ concentration is tightly regulated by the body to control tonicity, Cl^- emerges as the body's foremost tool for adjusting the SID and hence the plasma pH. Furthermore, acid-base abnormalities are frequently the result of disorders in chloride homoestasis. For example, a common form of metabolic alkalosis seen in the ICU is caused by the loss of gastric secretions. The loss of HCl from the stomach results in a hypochloremic metabolic alkalosis, sometimes severe enough to require therapy. Of course this is the loss of H^+, but H^+ is also lost with every molecule of water removed from the body. Moreover, gastric secretions may reach a pH of 1.0, or a H^+ concentration of 10^8 nmol/l. If 1 liter of gastric fluid is lost, this would mean that 10^8 nmol (0.1 mol) of H^+ would be removed. If one considers that plasma H^+ concentration is 40 nmol/l (or $4x10^{-8}$ mol/l), and if the majority of body fluids are at or near this concentration, one sees that the amount of total body free H^+ is only about $1.6x10^{-7}$ mol. If physiology were just simple accounting, a patient with a 200 ml emesis would entirely deplete the H^+ stores of the entire body and die of severe alkalemia in minutes. Of course this is not what happens, and in reality the H^+ concentration decreases by a much-smaller amount. The reason it decreases at all is because the plasma SID is increased and this is because Cl^- (a strong anion) is lost without loss of a strong cation. This increased SID forces a decrease in the amount of water dissociation and hence a decrease in the plasma H^+ concentration. When H^+ is "lost" as water rather than HCl, there is virtually no change in the SID and hence no change in the plasma H^+ concentration. Next, consider the treatment for a hypochloremic metabolic alkalosis. Aside from preventing further Cl^- loss, the therapy is to give back Cl^-. Saline works in this regard because even though one is giving equal amounts of Na^+ and Cl^-, the plasma Cl^- concentration is always much lower than the plasma Na^+ concentration, and thus Cl^- increases more than Na^+ when large amounts of saline are administered. KCl works better for this indication because, with a metabolic alkalosis, much of the K^+ goes into the cell, leaving much of the Cl^- in the plasma to decrease the SID.

From the example above, one can easily understand not only how administration of 0.9% saline can correct a hypochloremic metabolic alkalosis but also how massive amounts would lead to a decreased plasma SID and thus a hyperchloremic metabolic acidosis. This particular issue has been the focus of several recent studies. In the first study [16], we administered *Escherichia coli* endotoxin to dogs and then volume resuscitated with 0.9% saline. Over a 3-h period, each animal received an average of 1.8 l of saline and the pH decreased from 7.32 to 7.11 ($P<0.01$) while CO_2 and lactate were unchanged. Using the SID it was possible to calculate the amount of acidosis that was attributable to saline. Although the serum Na^+ concentration did not change, the serum Cl^- concentration increased by almost 10 mmol/l. It was concluded that saline alone was responsible for 42% of the total acid load experienced by these animals. In a second study, Scheingraber et al. [8] randomized patients undergoing major gynecological surgery to receive either 0.9% saline or lactated Ringer's solution. Patients receiving saline exhibited a decrease in their arterial pH from 7.41 to 7.28, while no change occurred in the lactated Ringer's group. These investigators also used the SID to calculate the expected change in pH with saline and found that the acidosis was entirely explained by Cl^- administration. More recently, a series of three studies published in the *Journal of Anesthesiology* provided conclusive evidence that the Cl^- content of volume-expanding solutions determines the degree of acidosis. In a study by Lisasker et al. [9], two types of pump-priming solutions for cardiopulmonary bypass were compared. A hyperchloremic solution and a solution with acetate and gluconate as metabolizable anions were used. As predicted, both caused an acute acidosis, but with the acetate/gluconate solution it resolved quickly, while the hyperchloremic solution caused a persistent hyperchloremic acidosis. The next two studies found that normovolumic hemodilution with hydroxyethyl starch or albumin in saline [10] produced similar amounts of acidosis, while albumin in a normo-chloremic solution [11] produced no acidosis at all. The accompanying editorial to these papers [24] seemed to have missed this point entirely. Finally, we have preliminarily shown that saline-induced acidosis decreased survival time in experimental sepsis in the rat compared with a solution of hydroxyethyl starch in a balanced electrolyte solution [25].

The clinical implication for management of patients in the ICU is that when large volumes of fluid are used for resuscitation they should be more physiological than saline. One alternative is lactated Ringer's solution. This fluid contains a more-physiological difference between Na^+ and Cl^- and thus the SID is closer to normal (roughly 28 mEq/l compared with the saline with a SID of 0 mEq/l). Of course this assumes that the lactate in lactated Ringer's is metabolized, which may take several minutes. Until the lactate is removed the effect of lactated Ringer's is identical to saline, since one strong anion (i.e., lactate) is as good as another (i.e., Cl^-). Therefore, massive doses of sodium lactate, for example given as replacement fluid for hemofiltration, may transiently result in acidosis as the SID decreases. The other problem with lactated Ringer's solution is that it is hypotonic and is therefore not as effective as a volume expander. More-modern solutions such as Hextend, hydroxyethyl starch in a balanced electrolyte solution, may be a better alternative when large volume resuscitation is needed.

Other Ions

When the SID decreases, metabolic acidosis ensues. When this occurs as a result of increased Cl^-, the anion gap (AG), which is a measure of missing charge, does not change. However, when other anions are present, the AG increases. Unfortunately, the accuracy of the AG is questionable in certain clinical situations [26], particularly in critically ill patients who are frequently hypoalbuminemic and acidotic. This has prompted some authors to adjust the "normal range" for the AG by the patient's albumin [27] or even phosphate [28] concentration. Each gram per deciliter of albumin has a charge of 2.8 mEq/l at pH 7.4 (2.3 mEq/l at 7.0 and 3.0 mEq/l at 7.6) and each milligram per deciliter of phosphate has a charge of 0.59 mEq/l at pH 7.4 (0.55 mEq/l at 7.0 and 0.61 mEq/l at 7.6). Except in cases of abnormal paraproteins, globulin does not contribute to the AG [12]. Thus a convenient way to estimate the "normal range" of the AG for a given patient is by use of the following formula:

"normal" AG = 2(albumin g/dl) + 0.5(phosphate mg/dl)

Or for international units:

"normal" AG = 0.2(albumin g/l) + 1.5(phosphate mmol/l)

Figge et al. [29] have shown that in the majority of critically ill, the "normal" AG can be estimated by using 2.5 times the albumin concentration in g/dl (or 0.25 for albumin in g/l). However, if the serum phosphate concentration is significantly abnormal, this estimate will be inaccurate.

The etiology of anions other than Cl^- varies depending on the population studied. Ketones, organic acids accumulating in renal failure, and toxins are important causes in appropriate patient groups. In critically ill patients, lactate is a particularly important cause. Lactate is a strong ion by virtue of the fact that at pH within the physiological range, it is almost completely dissociated (i.e., the pK of lactate is 3.9; at a pH of 7.4, 3,162 ions are dissociated for every 1 that is not). Because the body can produce and dispose of lactate rapidly, it functions as one of the most-dynamic components of the SID. Lactic acid therefore can produce significant acidemia. However, often critically ill patients have hyperlactatemia that is much greater than the extent of acidosis seen. Physical chemistry also allows us to understand how hyperlactatemia may exist without metabolic acidosis. First, acid is not being "generated" apart from lactate such as through "unreversed ATP hydrolysis", as some have suggested [30]. Phosphate is a weak acid and does not contribute substantially to metabolic acidosis even under extreme circumstances. Furthermore, the H^+ concentration is not determined by how much H^+ is produced or removed from the plasma but rather by changes in one of the three independent variables (SID, PCO_2, or A_{TOT}). Virtually anywhere in the body, pH is above 6.0 and lactate behaves as a strong ion. Its generation will then decrease the SID and result in increased water dissociation and thus increased H^+ concentration.

How then might the plasma lactate concentration be increased and the H^+ concentration not? There are two possible answers. First, if lactate is added to the plasma, not as lactic acid but rather as the salt of a strong acid (i.e., sodium lactate), there will be little change in the SID. This is because a strong cation (Na^+) is being added along with a strong anion. In fact, as lactate is then removed by metabolism, the remaining Na^+ will increase the SID, resulting in metabolic alkalosis. Hence it would be possible to give enough lactate to increase the plasma lactate concentration without any change in H^+ concentration. However, the amount of exogenous lactate required would be very large. This is because normal metabolism results in the turnover of approximately 1,500 - 4,500 mmol of lactic acid per day. Thus, only very large amounts of lactate infused rapidly will result in appreciable increases in the plasma lactate concentration. In this setting, a mild acidosis may occur until the lactate is metabolized (usually within several minutes). Levraut et al. [31] infused 1 mmol/kg of lactate over 15 min in ten patients with acute renal failure on continuous renal replacement therapy. Their mean plasma lactate concentration increased from 1.4 to 4.8 mmol/l after the infusion, but normalized rapidly. Under such conditions it is possible (if transiently) to produce hyperlactatemia without acidemia. Unfortunately, these authors do not report the acid-base status of their patients. However, in another recent study, Morgera et al. [32] showed that lactate-based hemofiltration resulted in increased plasma HCO_3^- concentration and pH as well as hyperlactatemia. A more-important mechanism whereby hyperlactatemia exists without acidemia (or with less acidemia than expected) is where the SID is corrected by the elimination of another strong anion from the plasma. This was demonstrated by Madias et al. [33]. In the setting of sustained lactic acidosis induced by lactic acid infusion, these investigators found that Cl^- moves out of the plasma space, normalizing the pH. Under these conditions, hyperlactatemia may persist but BE may be normalized by compensatory mechanisms to restore the SID. The meaning of hyperlacticemia is very different depending on the patient population being considered. Healthy humans can achieve plasma lactate concentrations with exercise in excess of 25 mmol/l without any long-term sequelae. In contrast, hyperlacticemia in the critically ill is an important predictor of mortality. However, the mechanisms responsible for hyperlacticemia are not as universal as once thought, and vary across patient types.

It is important to note that not all anions appearing in the blood of the critically ill can be explained. The SID can be used to detect unexplained anions because the apparent SID (SIDa) calculated from the measurable ions should be equal to the effective (SIDe) derived from the remaining charges attributable to CO_2 and A^- [12]. If a difference exists between the SIDa and SIDe, then unmeasured anions must be present. This difference has been termed the strong ion gap (SIG) to distinguish it from the anion gap (AG) [6]. Unlike the AG, the SIG is normally zero and does not change with changes in pH or albumin concentration, as does the AG. However, it should be noted that this "gap" need not be filled by strong ions. Weak acids may also play a role.

In recent years, unmeasured anions have been reported in the blood of patients with sepsis [5,34] and liver disease [6,35]. These anions may be the source of much of the unexplained acidosis seen in patients with critical illness. The presence of unexplained anions in the blood of both patients with sepsis and liver disease was investigated further in an animal model of sepsis using endotoxemia [14]. In this study, it was found that during control conditions, the liver cleared unmeasured anions from the circulation (mean flux -0.34 mEq/min). With early endotoxemia, however, the liver switched to release of anions (0.12 mEq/min, $P < 0.005$). These data suggest that the liver has a role in systemic acid-base balance by way of regulating anion fluxes apart from metabolism of lactate.

Effects of plasma proteins

Considerable controversy has developed over the past decade as to how to classify acid-base derangements occurring as a result of abnormalities in the weak acids, A_{TOT}. A sudden decrease in A_{TOT} produces alkalosis, while an increase is acidifying. Some have advocated a third classification for this effect, perhaps termed "proteinaceous acidosis or alkalosis", to be added to "metabolic" (SID) and "respiratory" (pCO_2) [36, 37]. Using observational data, Fencl et al. [37] argued for a re-classification of metabolic acid-base disorders into those that alter SID and those that affect A_{TOT}. The controversy arises when a low A_{TOT} and a low SID coexist with a normal pH and normal BE. This was a common occurrence in this study (1 of 6 patients) and the authors classify it a mixed disorder. However, other evidence [19, 28, 38] suggests that these changes in SID may be a compensatory response to a reduced A_{TOT}. When the SID of critically ill patients was compared with the SBE, the intercept for SBE=0 was 30-35 mEq/l rather than 40-42 mEq/l as for healthy individuals [28]. Thus, in these critically ill patients, many of whom had a decreased A_{TOT} secondary to hypoalbuminemia, the SID was reduced even when there was no apparent acid-base disorder. The reason for this is obvious from a physical chemical perspective. As a patient's albumin decreases so does A_{TOT} and thus A^-. This decrease in weak acid has a slightly alkalinizing effect. The body could adapt to this change by retaining CO_2, but it appears to reserve this adaptation for changes in SID. Instead, the body adapts to a decreased A_{TOT} by decreasing the SID. While Fencl et al. [37] classified this adaptation as a mixed acid-base disorder, a hypoalbuminemic alkalosis with a compensatory metabolic acidosis, it does not appear to be a disorder at all. Indeed, a patient who failed to reduce their SID in response to a decreased A_{TOT} would presumably be considered to have a metabolic alkalosis as a consequence of failed renal homeostatic mechanisms (e.g., secondary to hypovolemia), not a proteinacious alkalosis secondary to hypoalbumemia. The findings of Wilkes [38] in critically ill patients and Wooten [19] in mathematical simulations appear to support this assertion. Both authors have demonstrated that the "set point" for the SID to achieve a normal pH, given a normal PCO2, changes with changes in A_{TOT}. Furthermore, although the loss of weak acid from the plasma space is an alkalinizing process, there is no evidence that the body regulates A_{TOT} to maintain acid-base balance, and there is no evidence that clinicians should treat hypoalbuminemia as an acid-base disorder. However, this issue is by no means settled, and there is much still unknown about the role of the liver and gut in the control of acid-base balance. For example, the liver modifies its metabolism of nitrogen in response to pH, such that under alkalemic conditions (which should prevail under conditions of hypoalbumenia) more nitrogen is "packaged" as urea, making less glutamate available for the kidney to use for ammonia genesis [39]. Does the liver also modify albumin production in the setting of chronic acidosis? There is no direct evidence that it does but this area has not been fully explored.

Conclusion

In order understand the causes of the acid-base derangements, many of which are common in the ICU, we need only look at three independent variables (SID, PCO_2, and A_{TOT}). Metabolic acidemia results from a decrease in the plasma SID, usually brought about by the addition of strong anions (lactate, Cl^-, other "unknown" anions). Conversely, metabolic alkalemia occurs when the plasma SID is increased, either as a result of the addition of strong cations without strong anions (e.g., $NaHCO_3$) or by the removal of strong anions without strong cations (e.g., gastric suctioning).

This "new" understanding has considerable impact on how we think about gastric suction alkalosis, dilutional acidosis and lactic acidosis, as well as how we approach the treatment of these disorders. Our understanding of many other medical conditions (e.g., renal tubular acidosis) relies on a paradigm of acid -base regulation that is inconsistent with established physical-chemical principles. We will need to rethink our approach to these areas in the light of these data.

References

1. Stewart PA (1981) How to understand acid-base. In: Stewart PA (ed) A quantitative acid-base primer for biology and medicine. Edited by Stewart PA. Elsevier, New York, 1-286
2. Stewart PA (1983) Modern quantitative acid-base chemistry. Can J Physiol Pharmacol 61:1444 -1461
3. Magder S (1998) Pathophysiology of metabolic acid-base disturbances in patients with critical illness. In: Ronco C, Bellomo R (eds) Critical care nephrology Kluwer, Dordrecht, The Netherlands, 279-296
4. Kellum JA (1999) Acid-base physiology in the post-Copernican era. Curr Opin in Criti Care 5: 429-435
5. Gilfix BM, Bique M, Magder S (1993) A physical chemical approach to the analysis of acid-base balance in the clinical setting. J Crit Care 8:187-197
6. Kellum JA, Kramer DJ, Pinsky MR (1995) Strong ion gap: a methodology for exploring unexplained anions. J Crit Care 10:51-55
7. Alfaro V, Torras R, Ibanez J, Palacios L: (1996) A physical-chemical analysis of the acid-base response to chronic obstructive pulmonary disease. Can J Physiol Pharmacol 74:1229-1235
8. Scheingraber S, Rehm M, Sehmisch C, Finsterer U (1999) Rapid saline infusion produces hyperchloremic acidosis in patients undergoing gynecologic surgery. Anesthesiology 90:1265 -1270
9. Liskaser FJ, Bellomo R, Hayhoe M, et al (2000) Role of pump prime in the etiology and pathogenesis of cardiopulmonary bypass-associated acidosis. Anesthesiology 93:1170-1173
10. Rehm M, Orth V, Scheingraber S, et al (2000) Acid-base changes caused by 5% albumin versus 6% hydroxyethyl starch solution in patients undergoing acute normovolemic hemodilution: a randomized prospective study. Anesthesiology 93:1174-1183
11. Waters JH, Bernstein CA (2000) Dilutional acidosis following Hetastarch or albumin in healthy volunteers. Anesthesiology 93:1184-1187
12. Figge J, Mydosh T, Fencl V (1992) Serum proteins and acid-base equilibria: a follow-up. J Lab Clin Med 120:713-719

13. Rozenfeld RA, Dishart MK, Tonnessen TI, Schlichtig R (1996) Methods for detecting local intestinal ischemic anaerobic metabolic acidosis by PCO2. J Appl Physiol 81:1834-1842
14. Kellum JA, Bellomo R, Kramer DJ, Pinksy MR (1995) Hepatic anion flux during acute endotoxemia. J Appl Physiol 78:2212-2217
15. Lindinger MI, Heigenhauser GJF, McKelvie RS, Jones NL (1992) Blood ion regulation during repeated maximal exercise and recovery in humans. Am J Physiol 262:R126-136.
16. Kellum JA, Bellomo R, Kramer DJ, Pinsky MR (1998) Etiology of metabolic acidosis during saline resuscitation in endotoxemia. Shock 9: 364-368
17. Schlichtig R (1997) Base excess vs strong ion difference: which is more helpful? Adv Exp Med Biol 411:91-95
18. Kellum JA, Bellomo R, Kramer DJ, Pinsky MR (1997) Splanchnic buffering of metabolic acid during early endotoxemia. J Crit Care 12:7-12
19. Wooten EW (1999) Analytic calculation of physiological acid-base parameters. J Appl Physiol 86:326-334
20. Leblanc M, Kellum JA (1998) Biochemical and biophysical principles of hydrogen ion regulation. In: Ronco C, Bellomo R (eds) Critical care nephrology. Kluwer, Dordrecht, The Netherlands, 261-277
21. Kellum JA (2000) Determinants of blood pH in health and disease. Crit Care 4:6-14
22. Singer RB, Hastings AB: (1948) An improved clinical method for the estimation of disturbances of the acid-base balance of human blood. Medicine (Baltimore) 27:223-242
23. Schlichtig R, Grogono AW, Severinghaus JW (1998) Human $PaCO_2$ and standard base excess compensation for acid-base imbalance. Crit Care Med 26:1173-1179
24. Prough DS (2000) Acidosis associated with perioperative saline administration: dilution or delusion? Anesthesiology 93:1167-1169
25. Kellum JA, Schmigel J, Venkataraman S (2000) Fluid resuscitation and hyperchloremic acidosis in experimental sepsis: improved survival and acid-base balance with a synthetic colloid in a balanced electrolyte solution compared to saline. (abstract) Crit Care Med 28: A199
26. Salem MM, Mujais SK (1992) Gaps in the anion gap. Arch Intern Med 152:1625-1629
27. Gabow PA (1985) Disorders associated with an altered anion gap. Kidney Int 27:472-483
28. Kellum JA (1998) Recent advances in acid-base physiology applied to critical care. In: Vincent JL (ed) Yearbook of intensive care and emergency medicine. Springer Heidelberg Berlin New York, pp 579-587
29. Figge J, Jabor A, Kazda A, Fencl V (1998) Anion gap and hypoalbuminemia. Crit Care Med 26:1807-1810
30. Zilva JF (1978) The origin of acidosis in hyperlactatemia. Ann Clin Biochem 15:40-43
31. Levraut J, Ciebiera JP, Jambou P, et al (1997) Effect of continuous venovenous hemofiltration with dialysis on lactate clearance in critically ill patients. Crit Care Med 25:58-62
32. Morgera S, Heering P, Szentandrasi T, et al (1997) Comparison of a lactate-versus acetate-based hemofiltration replacement fluid in patients with acute renal failure. Ren Fail 19:155-164
33. Madias NE, Homer SM, Johns CA, Cohen JJ (1984) Hypochloremia as a consequence of anion gap metabolic acidosis. J Lab Clin Med 104:15-23
34. Mecher C, Rackow EC, Astiz ME, Weil MH (1991) Unaccounted for anion in metabolic acidosis during severe sepsis in humans. Crit Care Med 19:705-711
35. Kirschbaum B (1997) Increased anion gap after liver transplantation. Am J Med Sci 313:107-110
36. Fencl V, Leith DE (1993) Stewart's quantitative acid-base chemistry: applications in biology and medicine. Respir Physiol 91:1-16
37. Fencl V, Jabor A, Kazda A, Figge J (2000) Diagnosis of metabolic acid-base disturbances in critically ill patients. Am J Respir Crit Care Med 162:2246-2251
38. Wilkes P (1998) Hypoproteinemia, strong ion difference, and acid-base status in critically ill patients. J Appl Physiol 84:1740-1748
39. Oliver J, Bourke E (1975) Adaptations in urea and ammonium excretion in metabolic acidosis in the rat: a reinterpretation. Clin Sci Mol Med 48:515-520

A "Post-copernican" Analysis of Intracellular pH

S. Magder

Hydrogen ion concentration is one of the most-important regulated aspects of the intracellular environment, since changes in hydrogen ion concentration are associated with alterations in virtually all cell processes. Intracellular pH is typically more acidic than the pH of the extracellular space, and is in the range of 6.8-7.2 [1]. This represents the average pH in the cytoplasm and nucleus, but the pH of intracellular organelles can range from as low as 5.0 in lysosomes to as high as 8.0 in the mitochondria (Fig. 1).

As in all other physiological systems, intracellular acid-base balance traditionally has been analyzed with a specialized form of the Henderson-Hasselbalch equation which is based on the mass action equation of carbonic acid and bicarbonate and the solubility of CO_2 in water:

$$pH = pK'_a + \log \frac{[HCO_3^-]}{a \cdot P_{CO_2}}$$

Since this equation is based on basic chemical principles, it is internally consistent and valid. However, it does not give any insight into the mechanisms which regulate $[H^+]$ and $[HCO_3^-]$. For example the equation could be re-arranged to:

$$\log [a \cdot P_{CO_2}] = pK'_a + \log [HCO_3^-] - pH$$

but this would not mean that $[H^+]$ and $[HCO_3^-]$ actually determine pCO_2 in the body.

The fallacy of analyzing acid-base balance with just the Henderson-Hasselbalch equation for the CO_2/HCO_3^- relationship is that this system is only one of the many equilibrium relations that make up the solution of the intracellular environment. Furthermore, in an open system, i.e., one in which the cells are somehow connected to the circulatory system and the lungs, CO_2 is regulated

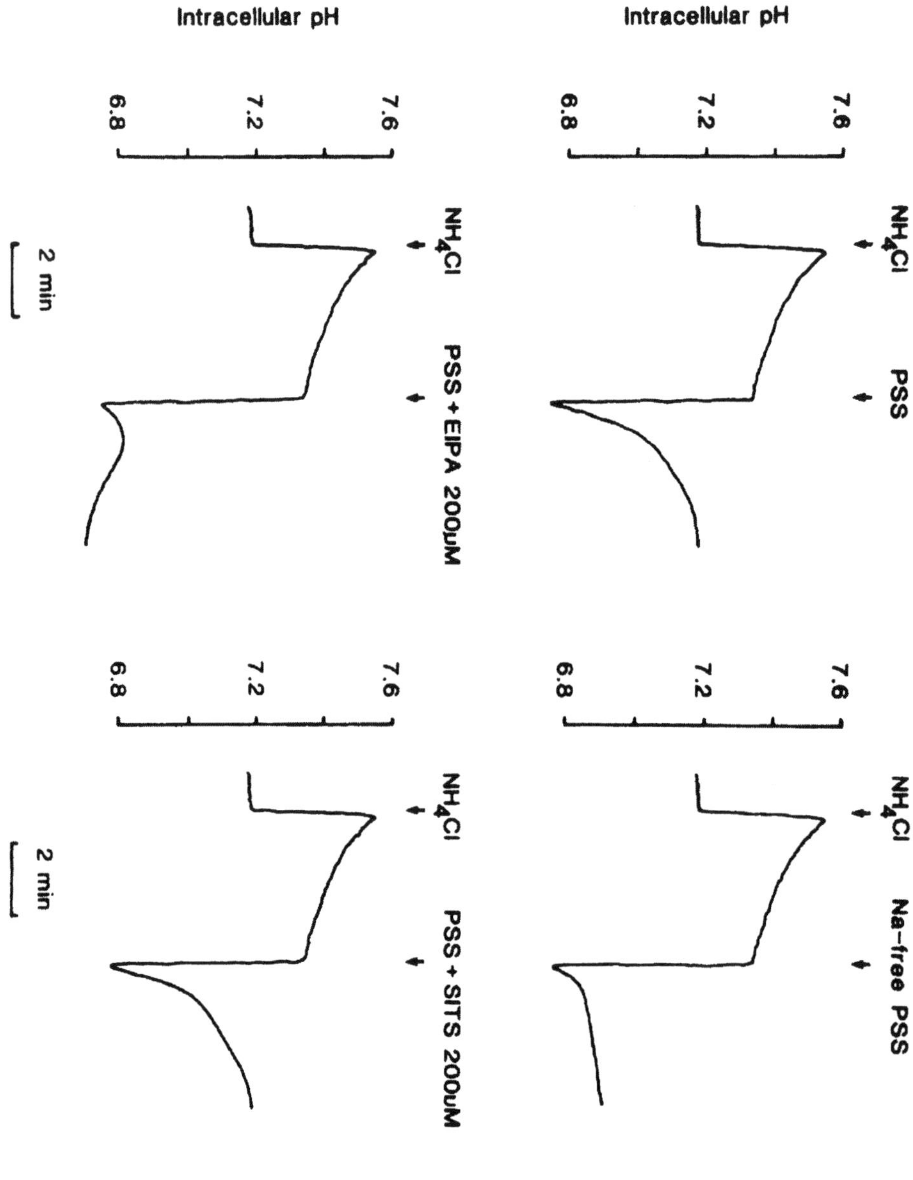

Fig. 1. An example of intracellular measurement of pH with a microelectrode. The addition of ammonium chloride NH_4Cl results in an initial increase in pH followed by a drift downward. When the NH_4Cl is washed out (PSS), there is an immediate fall in pH and gradual recovery. This was blocked by the exchange blocker, EIPA (*lower left*), or a Na-free solution (*upper right*). The blocker of a purported HCO_3^- exchanger, SITS, had no effect (*lower right*).
Reproduced with permission from [2]

by cellular metabolism and ventilation, and is thus the independent variable in the CO_2/HCO^- relationship. As argued by Stewart [3], $[H^+]$ and $[HCO_3^-]$ are dependent variables and their values are determined by the strong ion difference (SID), CO_2, and concentration of weak acids (A_{Total}). If the system is closed, i.e., not connected to the environment, then the total amount of CO_2 and its components is the independent variable. Stewart provided a physical-chemical analysis of biological solutions that is based on basic chemistry principles and the interaction of the many components of the solutions. It thus provides a strong scientific basis for acid-base analysis, rather than the simply empirical and limited analysis of the traditional approach. As I have discussed previously [4], the approach to acid-base analysis after Stewart can be thought of as comparing pre- and post-Copernican analysis of the heavenly bodies. Pre-Copernican astronomers could predict the position of the planets, but only with complex patterns and without any scientific basis. Post Copernicus, astronomers could use physics to truly understand the motions of the heavenly bodies.

There has been very little application of the physical chemical approach to the analysis of intracellular pH regulation [5-8] and there is no comprehensive analysis of the implications of this type of analysis for the overall mechanisms of acid production and regulation. Importantly, the evaluation of the regulatory mechanisms of intracelluar acid-base balance has been performed with the classical approach and $[H^{+}]$ as an independent variable. However, once one considers basic chemical principles and adapts a physical-chemical analysis, the result is extremely subversive, for it implies that there is a fundamental error throughout our current analysis of metabolic processes. The analysis thus raises questions about a huge number of currently accepted beliefs in cell biology and biochemistry. It also raises important questions about many of the experimental techniques used to study acid-base regulation in cells. The reader should be warned that the views presented in this paper are highly speculative and controversial. However, once one starts down this path, it raises the need for a re-evaluation of all intracellular functions with a physical-chemical approach.

General principle of the Stewart approach

Strong ion difference

The basis of the Stewart approach is given elsewhere, but some key elements need to be reviewed for this discussion of intracellular pH. A central element in the physical-chemical approach presented by Stewart is the concept of the SID. This is the difference in the equivalents of strong cations and strong anions.

Strong ions are ions that are almost completely dissociated in solution. In almost all biological fluids, the concentration of cations is greater than the concentration of anions. This difference in charge creates a strong electrical potential that must be balanced by negatively charged ions. In a solution of Na+ and Cl- with Na+ > Cl-, the only possible negatively charged ion to balance this charge difference is the OH- of water. The charge difference thus creates a force which alters the dissociation of water and the [SID] is the major determinant of hydrogen ion concentration ($[H^+]$). It is also important to appreciate that even in the solutions of the body with other substances besides strong ions, water is the major source of $[H^+]$ and [OH-], for the concentration of water is 55.3 M at 37° C. Furthermore, although there is only a very small dissociation of pure water (the ka at 37°C is 4.3×10^{-16} Eq/l), normal $[H^+]$ is very small, i.e., 4×10^{-8} Eq/l, and therefore only an order of magnitude below the normal equilibrium value. The neglect of the significant role played by water, and the role of the SID has created important and major misconceptions about the mechanisms involved in the control of acid-base balance.

What is a buffer?

Another concept that needs to be reviewed is that of a "buffer". Buffers have been considered traditionally as substances that reduce the change in pH or $[H^+]$ when a base or acid is added to a solution [1]. This is defined as:

$$\beta = \frac{dB}{dpH}$$

where β is the buffer strength, *d*B is the amount of base added, and *d*pH is the change in pH. A potentially confusing point that can lead to erroneous predictions is the standard definition of a base as a proton acceptor. Thus Cl- is defined as a base because it "accepts" a proton as an H^+. However, nothing of the sort happens. Cl- is a strong anion, which means that it does not bind with another ion in solution. In a solution with a negative [SID] and Cl- as the only anion, $[H^+]$ will always equal Cl-. This has led to the erroneous conclusion that $[H^+]$ is an independent variable. However, this is not the case in a solution with a positive [SID]. In a solution with a positive [SID], the addition of HCl will result in a smaller change in H^+ than the change in Cl-. This occurs even without a weak acid, or so-called buffer, being present. It is the change in [SID] that determines the change in $[H^+]$. Thus, what is really happening when buffer strength is tested is that the addition of a strong cation or anion changes the [SID] and that is what produces the change in pH.

In a solution with only strong electrolytes, a positive [SID] and essentially no non-volatile weak acids, such as interstitial fluid, the addition of a strong acid or base only produces a small change in pH, and would thus seem to be "buffered" (Fig. 2). The addition of non-volatile weak acids, as is the case in plasma and the intracellular environment, has some important consequences. There are now two important variables, the [SID] and [A_{Total}] where [A_{Total}] is the total concentration of weak acids that are classically viewed as "buffers". Over the [SID] from 0 to [A_{Total}], H^+ actually increases more rapidly than is the case where there is no weak acid, i.e., the opposite of what a buffer should do. What the weak acid does, though, is markedly lower the pH and thus lower the pH range that the solution experiences for a given change in [SID] values. If the dissociation constant of the weak acid is within an order of magnitude of 10^{-7} Eq/l (i.e., $\sqrt{K'_w}$, where K'_w is the association constant of water times the concentration of water molecules), which is the case for what are usually considered to be physiologically important buffers, and [SID] is increased, more negative ions are needed to balance the positive charge difference, and this drives the dissociation of the weak acid. When the SID equals [A_{Total}], the weak acid is almost completely dissociated.

The intracellular environment has a large concentration of weak acids and these take part in many of the cell's metabolic pathways. The failure to consider the chemical properties of these substances, and the effect of the [SID] on their dissociation, has led to many erroneous conclusions about the biochemistry of

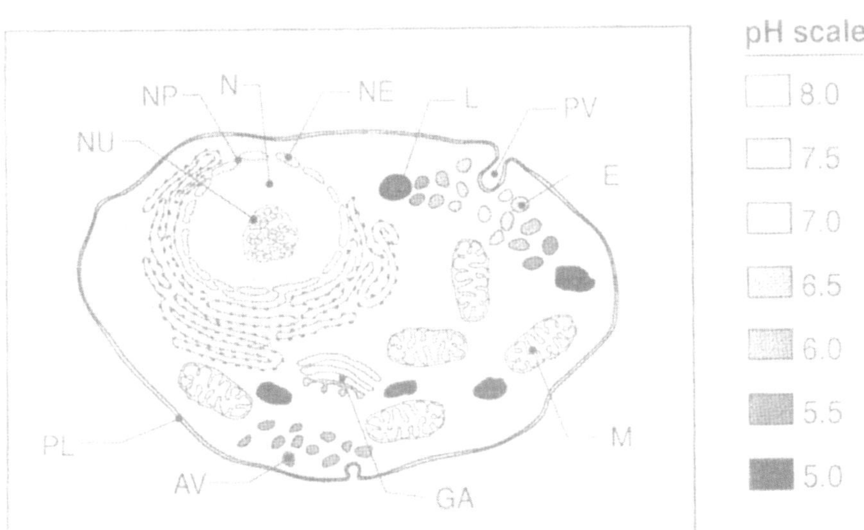

Fig. 2. Intracellular pH. Note that the pH ranges from 5.0 in lysosomes to 8.0 in the mitochondria. (Used with permission from [1])

the cell and the regulation of acid-base status. Most importantly it becomes clear that $[H^+]$ does not regulate the dissociation of weak acids in proteins, but rather the factors which regulate $[H^+]$ i.e., [SID], $[A_{Total}]$, and CO_2, regulate the dissociation of proteins. That is why in the opening paragraph I said that changes in $[H^+]$ are associated with alterations in virtually all cell processes; they do not necessarily determine them.

The intracellular environment

To analyze the intracellular regulation of acid-base balance with Stewart's principles, it is important to first know what are the components of the intracellular environment. I shall begin with Stewart's analysis of the intracellular environment of the red blood cell (RBC) [3]. RBCs are frequently used experimentally because they are easy to isolate and analyze, but the composition of the intracellular fluid (ICF) of the RBC is not the same as that of the "general" cell. However, the conclusions obtained from the RBC-ICF still can be applied to other cell types by substituting the appropriate values for parameters and the independent variables. The compositions of interstitial fluid, plasma, RBC-ICF, and the intracellular fluid of "general cells" are shown in Table 1. The RBC-ICF pCO_2 is the same as that in plasma, but lower than that in most cells. RBC-ICF Na+ is much lower than that in plasma, and the potassium ion (K+) is the major intracellular cation. The RBC-ICF intracellular magnesium ion is higher than that in the plasma and the RBC-ICF calcium ion is only at the concentration of $[H^+]$. RBC-ICF Cl- is only half that of plasma and there are more "other" strong

Table 1. Composition of body fluids

Quantity	Solution: Interstitial fluid	Blood plasma	RBC-ICF	General ICF
[Na+]	137	143	19	10
[K+]	3	4	95	155
[Mg2+]	2	2	5	10
[Ca2+]	1	1	–	35
[Cl-]	111	107	52	10
Other strong anions	1	1	10	35
pCO_2	50	40	40	50
[SID]	31	42	57	130
A_{Total}	–	20	60	200
HCO_3^-	31	25	15	16
pH	7.4	7.4	7.2	7.0

Adapted from reference [3]. All values are in mEq/l except pCO_2 which is mmHg and pH which has no units anions in the RBC-ICF. It is necessary to use a different *K*c for the CO_2, H^+, and [HCO_3^-] reaction than that used for plasma, because the high intracellular protein concentration effects CO_2 solubility, which is incorporated in *K*c. The A_{Total} of the RBC-ICF is almost three times that of plasma with contributions from hemoglobin and diphosphoglyceric acid. The strong ion difference is estimated to be 57 mEq/l, whereas that of plasma is 42 mEq/l. This results in a [HCO_3^-] of 15 mEq/l and a pH of 7.2. The gamblegram of the RBC is compared with that of plasma in Fig. 3. One should note that the total electrolyte

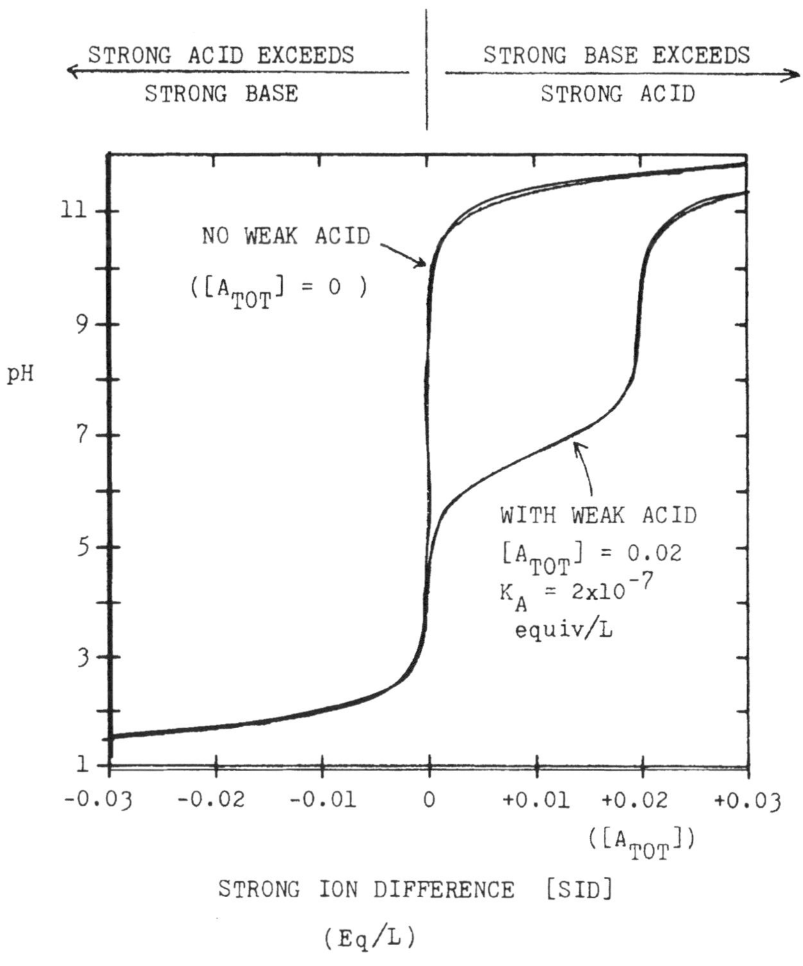

Fig. 3. "Buffering action" of a weak acid. When no weak acid is present, there is an abrupt change in pH when the [SID] changes from negative to positive. When a weak acid is present, there is another plateau around the range of [SID] of 0 to [A_{total}]. Note that in the range of [SID] of .01 Eq/ l, the pH actually rises faster with changes in SID than without the weak acid. Thus a "buffer" changes the range of the pH changes, but does not affect the degree of change for a given change in base used with permission from [3])

composition of the RBC is less, the [A-] is much larger, and [HCO_3] smaller than the values in the plasma. Since the osmolality of the cell must equal that of the interstitial space, and approximately that of plasma, there must be other osmoles that come from non-ionic substances.

Figure 4 compares the change in [H^+] and [HCO_3^-] in response to changes in [SID], and Fig. 5 the response to changes in CO_2 in RBC-ICF and plasma. [H^+] is both larger and less well regulated in the RBC than in plasma, although the directional changes are the same. [H^+] decreases with increasing [SID] and increases with increases in pCO_2. Despite the larger [SID], the intracellular [HCO_3^-] is smaller than plasma because [A-] is much larger. [HCO_3^-] is also more strongly dependent on pCO_2.

It is often said that hemoglobin in RBCs "buffers" the plasma. First of all, because hemoglobin is in the RBC-ICF environment, and surrounded by the RBC cell membrane, it cannot directly effect plasma [H^+]. Second, for the RBC-ICF to affect plasma [H^+], the effect must be distributed a throughout the total extracellular space and, since the RBC-ICF is relatively small compared with the total extracellular space, the RBC can have only a small effect on plasma [H+].

An interesting observation and application of Stewart's principles was recently made by Prange et al. [8] who showed that the decrease in pO_2 in venous blood increases binding of Cl- to hemoblobin, and this reduces oxyhemaglobin affinity, and thus partly explains the Haldane effect. It also reduces the increase in RBC-ICF Cl- that occurs in venous blood by what is known as the Cl^- shift. The binding of Cl- to hemoglobin means that there is less of a decrease in intracellular SID of venous blood than would otherwise occur, and this means that there is a decrease in the acidifying effect from the influx of Cl- The authors propose that this can explain why [H^+] is lower and [HCO_3^-] higher than predicted.

The ICF of the "general cell" of the body is compared with that of the RBC-ICF in Table 2. Na+ is lower but K+ is much higher and the Mg^{2+} double. Thus, even though the Cl- is higher, the [SID] is 2.5^- fold that of the RBC and the pH is higher. The [A_{Total}] is tenfold that of plasma, and thus plays a very important role in regulating [H^+].

Sources of intracellular H+

It is next worth considering where the H^+ comes from. Biochemical and physiological texts frequently refer to the production of H^+ by metabolic processes and do an accounting of the production and clearance of H^+. These analyses are based on the misconception that H^+ is an independent variable but this fails to take into account that [H^+] is determined by [SID], CO_2, and [A_{Total}].

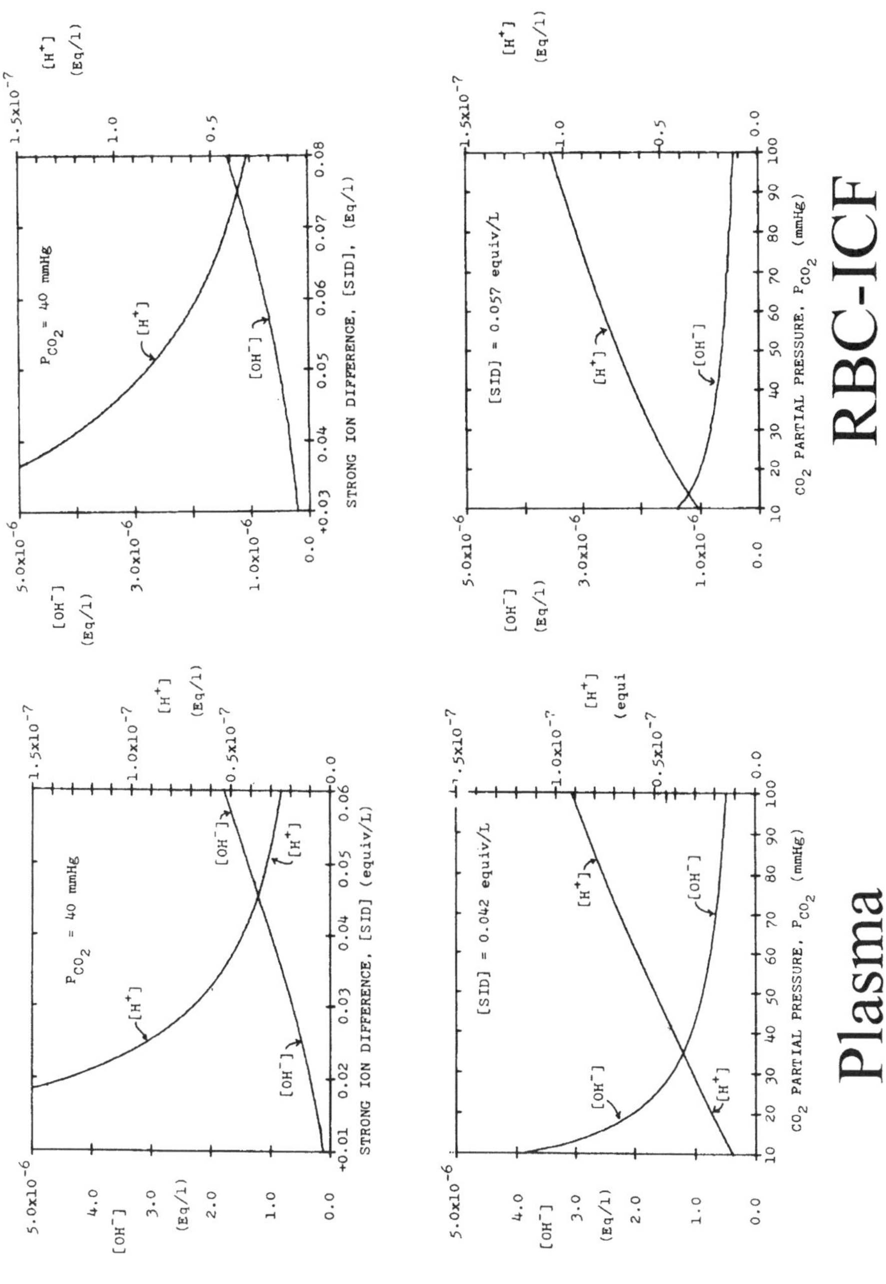

Fig. 4. Effect of changes in [SID] and CO_2 on H+ and OH- in plasma (*left side*) and red blood cell intracellular fluid (RBC-ICF, *right side*). The change in H+ is steeper in the RBC-ICF with changes in [SID] than in the plasma whereas the change in H+ for a change in pCO_2 is less (*lower panels*) (with permission from [3])

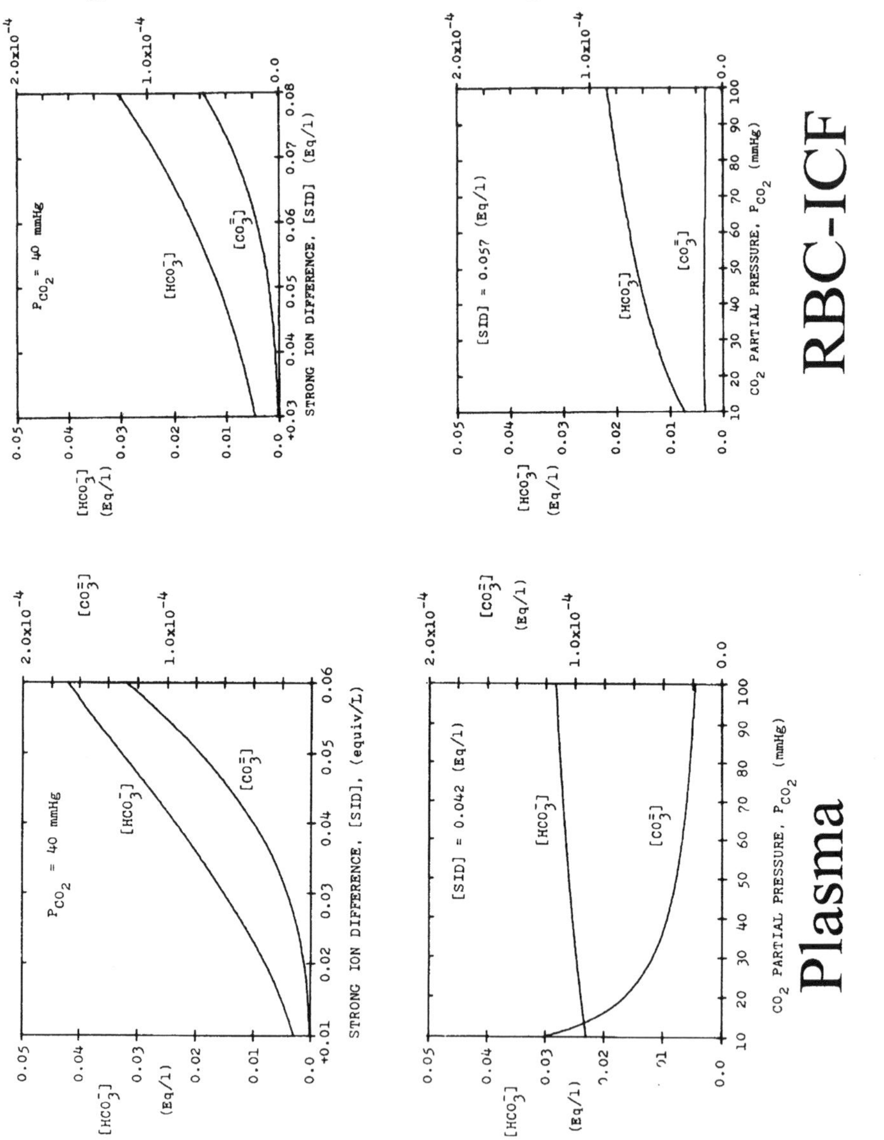

Fig. 5. Effect of changes in [SID] and CO_2 on HCO_3^- and CO_3^{2-} in plasma (*left side*) and RBC-ICF (*right side*). The change in HCO_3^- and CO_3^{2-} is much less steep in the RBC-ICF with changes in [SID] than in the plasma. The change in HCO_3^- for a change in pCO_2 is greater, whereas there is almost no change in CO_3^{2-} (*lower panels*) (with permission from [3])

This is partly because in solutions with only strong ions and a negative [SID], $[H^+]$ will equal the concentration of the anion and thus seems to be independent. However, in all cells [SID] is positive, and $[H^+]$ does not change in direct proportion to the change in [SID].

When examining the production of H^+ in a reaction, one needs to consider the pKa of the reaction. If the reaction has a low pKa, as is the case for lactate, the ion produced will be effectively a strong anion . If the pKa is high, it will act as a weak acid. If the pKa is within an order of magnitude of 7, then the concentration will be particularly important for it will contribute to A_{Total} of the solution. The magnitude of the effect will depend upon how much $[A_{Total}]$ is changed, and its dissociation will depend on the [SID] and CO_2 . An example is the hydrolysis of ATP. The pKa of $HATP^{3-}$X $H^+ + ATP^{4-}$ is 6.95 and the pKa of $HADP^{2-}$X $H^+ + ADP^{3-}$ 6.88, which are very close to normal intracellular pH. They therefore act as weak acids in much the same way that albumin does in the blood. Hydrolysis of ATP leads to the formation of $HADP^{3-}$ and orthophosphate. The equilibrium reaction of HPO_4^{2-} with $H_2PO_4^{1-}$ has a Pka of 6.8. The dissociation of this molecule and the free $[H^+]$ is thus very dependent upon the [SID] and pCO_2. At normal pH, a considerable amount of the H^+ produced in the reaction will combine with OH- to form water.

The consequences of partial dissociation of the products of normal metabolism of glucose and glycogen were reviewed in an often quoted paper by Hochachka and Mommsen [9]. They noted that: "The two main intracellular factors determining the amount of H^+ released during ATP hydrolysis again are Mg^{2+} and pH" and "over the range of pH 6.5 to 8.0, the lower the pH, the fewer the moles of H^+ formed per mole of ATP hydrolysed". They unfortunately formulate their analysis with H^+ as an independent variable that is produced by the reactions rather than considering it as a dependent variable. What happens during metabolism is that either the concentration of the weak acids, ATP and ADP as well as their pKa change, or there is production of a strong anion, such as lactate. The impact of the production of weak acids will depend on their percentage of the overall $[A_{Total}]$ and their pKa, whereas the production of a strong ion such as lactate will have major effects on the pH because of the change in [SID]. As noted by these investigators, Mg^{2+} plays a particularly important role in intracellular pH regulation. This is because its concentration is higher than in the extracellular space (approximately 4.4 mM, which could give up to 8.8 mEq/l) and it is therefore a significant contributor to the [SID]. It also interacts with ATP and ADP and markedly lowers their pKa (i.e., makes them stronger acids).

Much confusion arises when the reactions are considered alone and the three determinants of H^+, [SID], CO_2, and $[A_{Total}]$, are not considered. This is especially a problem when the reactions are studies in a test-tube without CO_2 or an [A_{Total}]. The analysis is further complicated if reactions are studied in intact cells, for shifts in electrolytes, either into or out of the cell, will alter the [SID] and thus have major effects on [H^+].

Regulation of intracellular [H^+]

Although cells walls are said to be highly permeable to H^+, the passive distribution of H^+ across the cell membrane based on the Nernst equation, an extracellular pH of 7.4, and a transmembrane potential of -60 mV relative to the outside would give an internal pH of only 6.4. This would impair most intracellular functions. Since intracellular pH is known to be in the range of 6.8-7.2, there has to be an active membrane transport mechanism to regulate intracellular pH. Although the permeability of the cell wall is high for H^+, it is the conductance of H^+ that determines the net flux. Conductance is a function of the concentration of the substance, which in the case of H^+ is very low, and the permeability, and thus the conductance is low. Another factor is that [H^+] is also affected by the rest of the solution, and in particular the [SID], which will have a greater impact than the charge from the transmembrane gradient difference.

Experimental measurement of control of intracellular pH

Before discussing the mechanisms which regulate intracellular [H^+], it is worthwhile reviewing how intracellular [H^+] is determined experimentally. A common experimental approach is to expose cells to ammonium chloride (NH_4Cl) and measure the intracellular pH by either an electrode or a dye [10]. An example is shown in Fig. 6. The addition of extracellular NH_4Cl produced an initially rapid increase in intracellular pH, which then gradually drifts back to baseline. When the NH_4Cl was washed out with physiological salt solution, there was a rapid fall in intracellular pH to below the baseline. This decrease in pH was rapidly corrected, indicating an intracellular exchange mechanism, for it could be totally blocked by amiloride (lower left panel of Fig. 6). Removing Na^+ also markedly reduced the recovery (upper right panel of Fig. 6) while the inhibitor SITS which inhibits a purported HCO_3^--dependent mechanism had little affect (right lower panel). The classic explanation for the changes in intracellular pH that occurs with the addition and then withdrawal of NH_4Cl is that the lipid-soluble ammonia (NH_3) moves freely across the cell membrane. In the cell, some of it binds H^+ to form NH_4 which decreases intracellular H^+ and thus increases intracellular pH. There is then said to be a slow influx of

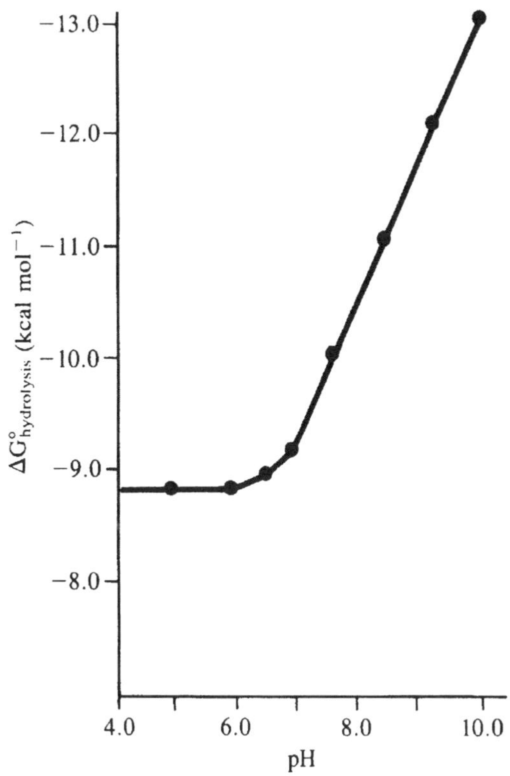

Fig. 6. The effect of pH on the free energy released from ATP. Increases in pH above 7.0 greatly increase the free energy release when ATP is hydrolyzed (with permission from [11])

NH_4 from the extracellular environment, which brings in H^+ and increases intracellular $[H^+]$ and decreases the pH. During the washout phase, NH_3 is removed from the cell; this reduces the pH and allows the acidification produced by the influx of NH_4 to be observed.

Based on a physical chemical analysis, the influx of NH_3 to the cell adds an add-on base that acts as a weak base with the opposite effect of a weak acid. Thus the same way that a weak acid decreases the pH (Fig. 2), the weak base raises pH. Also, just as occurs with a weak acid, the proportion that occurs as NH_4 versus that which occurs as NH_3, the equivalent of a conjugated acid such as H_2CO_3, is dependent upon the [SID], CO_2, and total of NH_3 and NH_4. Rather than there being a leak of NH_4 from the extracellular space into the cell, it is more likely that there is a change in a strong ion, which could be the influx of Cl- down the increased concentration gradient created by the extracellular NH_4Cl or the efflux of Na+. Both of these would decrease the intracellular [SID] and thus decrease pH. In the classic approach these are not looked for.

The role of Na+ in these experiments is studied by substituting a weak base. This changes the transmembrane Na+ gradient and presumably alters intracellular Na+, which will change the intracellular SID. If the intracellular pH is not changed from that observed when Na+ was present, there was likely movement of some other ion, such as influx of K+ or loss of Cl-, to maintain the [SID].

The other variable that is "controlled" in these studies is CO_2/HCO_3. This is done by producing a solution with HCO_3^- bubbled with CO_2. It is thought that the HCO_3 moves into the cell by a Na+ -dependent mechanism. First, the movement of Na+ into the cell by itself will result in an increase in HCO_3, which is a dependent variable, as well as a decrease in $[H^+]$. Furthermore, it is the CO_2 in the solution that freely crosses the cell membrane and increases the intracellular H^+ as well as HCO_3^-. The concentration of CO_2 is controlled in these experiments by bubbling CO_2 into the solution and then if necessary making the system air tight. If this is not done, the loss of CO_2 will decrease the HCO_3^- and appear as a HCO_3^- -dependent mechanism [12].

Another technique to study intracellular pH is to cannulate the cell with a micropipette and perform internal dialysis to alter the intracellular milieu [12]. This was performed in a classic paper which identified a Cl- transport mechanism [13]. A number of observations in this study that seemed puzzling to the investigators are easily explained by a physical-chemical analysis. The authors observed that when they added an ATP-containing solution there was a continued fall in pH in the presence of cyanide. This is likely because ATP is a weak acid and an increase in ATP will decrease pH (Fig. 2). Furthermore, there was most likely also a loss of Na+ (or gain of Cl-) that was not compensated when metabolism was inhibited by the cyanide. These investigators also found that Cl- efflux was enhanced by the addition of HCO_3/CO_2. Based on a physical-chemical analysis, the addition of the volatile weak acid, i.e., CO_2, would acidify the intracellular environment and enhance the removal of Cl- as an effective compensatory mechanism.

Active regulation of intracellular pH

A number of membrane proteins have been identified which regulate intracellular pH [1, 12]. I will use the classical description of them first but, as will be seen, there are major problems with the terminology if one uses a physical-chemical approach. They include the Na/H exchanger, HCO_3^- -dependent transporters, which include the Cl/HCO_3 exchange, $(Na + HCO_3)/Cl$ exchanger, and the $Na\text{-}HCO_3$ co-transporter, H^+-ATPases (proton pumps), Na+-organic anion transporters, and Cl/formate exchange. These various mechanisms are distinguished by the inhibitors used to block their actions and by the substrates used in the experiments.

The Na/H exchanger (NHE) is one of the best-described systems [2, 14]. These are a family of highly regulated phosphoproteins that are found in all mammalian tissues. They are found in both the plasma membrane and inner mitochondrial membrane. There are five well-characterized isoforms, and a sixth less well-characterized form has recently been identified. These are large molecules with 10 to 12 membrane-spanning domains. As the name indicates, these exchangers are purported to exchange Na+ for H^+ in a 1:1 ratio [2, 15, 16]. This seems to be a highly unlikely event considering the relative concentrations of H^+ and Na+. At pH 7.4, [H^+] is 40 x 10^{-9} Eq/l, whereas [Na+] is 140 x 10^{-3} Eq/l. It seems very strange that two molecules with a 10^6 -fold difference exchange 1:1. Even more so, based on the physical-chemical principle, which views [H^+] as a dependent variable, and given the extremely low concentration of H^+, it seems unlikely that H^+ is being transported across a cell. There has never been a study in which a radio labelled H^+ has been shown to cross the cell membrane. What is done instead is that the pH is measured on both sides of the membrane. Sometimes this is only done indirectly by measuring the dissociation of weak acids or bases, which are also affected by changes in the SID [16].

A far more-likely explanation for the change in intracellular pH by this pump is that the movement of Na+ into the cell changes the [SID] on both sides of the membrane, and this alters intra- and extracellular [H^+]. To appreciate the magnitude of the change, cells which were acid loaded to produce a pHi of 6.25 had an increase in [Na+] of 15.6 ± 2.3 mmol/l. This would produce a significant change in the [SID] if there were no other electrolyte shifts. The exchanger is thought to be electrically neutral [2], which is why the exchange was thought to be 1:1. However, this could occur by some water moving with the Na+ and the Na+ being matched by an OH- from the water.

The failure to consider the dependent nature of [H^+], and misconceptions about buffers, has resulted in numerous experimental problems in the literature on the theses exchangers, and the errors are far too many for this discussion. However, a few noteworthy ones are worth commenting on. A central point has been the argument that the exchange works with a 1:1 stoichiometry. This is based on the comparison of "a rate of H^+ efflux" and a net change in Na+. The rate of H^+ extrusion is based on a formula that uses the "change in pH" over time, some measure of membrane thickness, the buffer power of the solution. This resulted in one study with "rates of H^+ efflux" in the 7-10 mmol/l per min range [15]. To put this in perspective, assuming a pH in the whole body of 7.4, and a total volume of water of 40 l, the total body H^+ content would be 1.6 x

10^{-6} M; in other words, 1,000 times less than is argued exchanged per litre per minute in these isolated cells! The error in the stoichiometry arises from the comparison of a rate and a net value, the multiplication by a "buffer value", which is based on a calculation from a titration with a weak base, or sometimes even a weak base, and the normalization by a length term when the electrolytes are dissolved in solutions on either side. Of course the major error is the failure to appreciate that $[H^+]$ is a dependent variable, and its value is determined by the [SID], CO_2, and $[A_{Total}]$.

The purported HCO_3^- exchangers raise a number of important problems. Based on a physical-chemical principle, HCO_3^- is a dependent variable, and therefore even if it were transported from an extracellular environment with a given pH to the intracellular environment with a different [SID] and $[A_{Total}]$, this difference would change the actual concentration of HCO_3^-. More importantly, HCO_3^- is in equilibrium with CO_2, which in the body is controlled by a balance between production and ventilation, or in experiments is hopefully being controlled by the use of an air-tight container or continuous bubbling of CO_2 in the fluid bathing the extracellular space. I say hopefully, because this is not always done in experiments and will result in a steady loss of CO_2 and therefore of HCO_3,$^-$ which could then appear as a HCO_3^- -dependent mechanism. Since CO_2 rapidly diffuses across cell membranes, if CO_2 is controlled the extracellular CO_2 will very quickly equilibrate with intracellular CO_2, and the added HCO_3^- itself will have a negligible effect compared with the pCO_2 being bubbled into the solution. What is important when HCO_3^- is added is the accompanying cation, which is most commonly Na+. I therefore found it remarkable in reviewing a number of studies on this exchanger that the methods sections only refer to HCO_3^- and do not even identify the cation [15, 17]. In all the descriptions of HCO_3^- -dependent transporters, either Na+ or Cl-, both strong ions, are included. Based on the physical-chemical principle, it is the movement of these ions that is truly regulating intracellular pH.

In this discussion, pCO_2 has been viewed as an independent variable. This is only true if the system is open and the CO_2 can evaporate into the atmosphere or be regulated by ventilation. In a closed system, it is the total CO_2 in the solution, including dissolved gas, H_2CO_3, HCO_3^-, and $CO_3^{=}$. In this case, the CO_2 produced by cellular respiration is crucial, as well as any "added" CO_2 in the form of HCO_3^-.

An interesting group of proteins is the H^+ - ATP exchangers [18-20]. There are three types, but a characteristic of them all is that by catalyzing ATP hydrolysis they impose an electrochemical gradient across biomembranes. A well-recognized member is the P-type, which is characterized by the Na+/K+ P-ATPase that hydrolyzes ATP to generate the Na+ and K+ electrochemical gradient across the cell membrane. The gradient is essential for signaling, nutrient uptake, and other cellular functions. Because it changes the concentration of intracellular strong ions, it will also affect intracellular pH. Another type is the F-type, which is found in mitochondria and is purported to use a proton electrochemical gradient across the membranes of mitochondrial christae to make ATP. The third group are the V-ATPases. They are found in vacuolar membranes, other endomembranes, and some plasma membranes. They are thus responsible for the areas in the cell shown in Fig. 1 that have a pH lower than the pH of the cytoplasm. In contrast to the other two types of ATPases, the V-type only act as ATP hydrolases.

The physical-chemical principle requires some change in [SID], $[A_{Total}]$, or CO_2, the three independent variables that determine $[H^+]$, for this exchange to change $[H^+]$. It is unlikely that these exchangers alter CO_2. All three of the exchangers produce an electrochemical gradient. This must require the increase in a negative ion or the decrease in a cation. These could be strong or weak ions. Except for the Na+/K+ P-ATPase, there are no cations included in the usual description of the mechanism of acidification by these proteins, but based on the physical-chemical principle, it is very likely that a strong ion is associated. Indeed Cl- is known to "modulate" the process [19], and it is likely that it plays a role in the pH change. K+ is also associated with some of the exchangers, for example a P-type that is active in the kidney [1]. A P-type H^+ ATPase is said to be responsible for acidifying the stomach. The stomach fluid has a low pH because of the negative SID. It is essentially a solution with Cl- and very little Na+. Since most secreted fluids bare a resemblance to the composition of interstitial fluid, and stomach acid not always so acidic, this means that it is most likely that Na+ was removed, but this issue does not seem to have been investigated. A potential mechanism for these exchangers is that they could act by binding a strong cation such as Mg2+, which has a high enough intracellular concentration to produce changes in intracellular [SID]. For example, Mg2+ binds to ATP and alters its pKa. It is also possible that theses exchangers act by increasing the concentration of a weak acid intracellularly, including ATP, which has a pKa of 6.95. As shown in Fig. 2, the addition of 0.02 mEq/l of a weak acid with a pKa = 7 to a solution with only strong ions and an [SID] of .01 would decrease the pH of the solution from 11 to approximately 6.5.

A fourth group of regulators of intracellular pH are Na+-organic anion transporters. These transporters mediate the influx of Na+ with an organic ion such as acetate or lactate. The traditional explanation for the way this transporter works is an excellent example of the faulty reasoning that is rampant in this field. For example, in one text [1] it is argued that the lactate and acetate would act as weak bases and therefore bind intracellular H^+ which would alkalinize the intracellular environment. First of all, both lactate and acetate are strong ions, not weak ions, and therefore would remain dissociated and not bind H^+. If they are transported with equal amounts of Na+, there would be no change in the [SID], and thus no change in [H^+]. However, both lactate and acetate can be metabolized in the cell. This will decrease their concentration and increase the [SID], which would account for the alkalinization of the intracellular environment.

A fifth group of intracellular regulators are Cl- exchangers, which are believed to act by exchanging with an organic ion such as formate [1], as well as a yet poorly defined "pump 3" for Cl-. In this case, movements of Cl- would have important effects on the SID and thus pH on both sides of the membrane, and the associated organic acid formed could be easily metabolized, thus amplifying the change but maintaining electrical neutrality.

Importance of intracellular H+

Although the concentration of H^+ in bodly fluids is extremely low, [H^+] has important effects on the function of a multitude of cellular functions, including intracellular metabolism, cytoskeleton shape and mobility, muscle contraction, cell-cell coupling, membrane conductance, intracellular messengers, cell activation, growth, and proliferation, and regulation of cell volume [1]. This is partly because [H^+] is involved directly in so many chemical processes. Even more importantly, H^+ are very small, and therefore have a large charge density. This means that H^+ have very large electric field gradients that effect any of molecules in their neighborhood This affects macromolecular structures and configurations, which consequently affect protein function. Since [H^+] is a dependent variable and [H^+] is dependent on the concentrations of other parts of the intracellular solution, [H^+] is also a reflection of the balance of these forces in the solution, which will affect the function of any weak electrolytes with a pKa close to the pH of the normal solution in cells.

An important example of the effect of [H^+] on metabolism is its effect on the activity of phosphofructokinase, a key glycolytic enzyme that converts fructose 6-phosphate to fructose 1,6-diphosphate. Decreases in pH from 7.5 to 6.5 markedly decrease its activity [1]. Similarly decreases in pH markedly decrease the activation of a phosphorylase that catalyzes the breakdown of glycogen. Changes in pH also have a profound effect on the energy released upon hydrolysis of ATP (Fig. 6) [11]. This is because the pKa of ATP is 6.95 and as the pH increases more of the ATP is in the ATP^{4+} form, which has much less-electrostatic repulsion among the negatively charged oxgyens of the triphosphoanhydride group of ATP than occurs in the ATP^{2+} form.

Changes in pH affect cell shape and mobility, which could affect cells that have to move. An example is the pH dependence of the cross linking of actin filaments. Actin-binding proteins have different pH profiles, so that alkalinization increases cross linking in some cells, whereas it decreases it in others [1]. A likely explanation is differences in their pKa, which would affect their dissociation at different pH. It is important to remember that this in turn is affected by the [SID].

Changes in pH are known to affect muscle contraction. This could be because of the effects of pH on the various pumps that regulate intracellular Ca2+. Since the pKa of ATP and ADP are close to that of the intracellular environment, most associated and dissociated forms will be very sensitive to changes in intracellular pH. Similarly, changes in pH could affect the function of every channel involved in excitability of cells and cell-cell signaling.

It is well recognized that regulators of intracellular H^+ affect intracellular volume, and that changes in intracellular volume affect regulators of intracellular [H^+]. For example, the application a hypertonic solution to the extracellular environment will cause cell shrinkage and this is known to activate the Na^+/H^+ exchanger, although the mechanism is said to not be understood [1]. A physical -chemical analysis offers some important insights into the link between intracellular volume and pH. With no change in the amount of intracellular ions, a decrease in intracellular volume by an extracellular osmotic agent will result in an increase in the [SID], because both the cation and anion concentrations will increase by the same fraction. However, the cations start from a larger number. Thus the difference, i.e., the [SID], will increase and this will alkalinize the cell. There will also be an increase in [A_{Total}], which will increase H^+ and acidify the cell. The net effect will depend upon the relative concentrations of each, but the change in [SID] should predominate. This increase in [SID] will decrease intracellular H^+ or increase pH. Conversely, an increase in intracellular water will decrease the [SID], which will decrease pH. These effects of changes in intracellular volume on intracellular pH must be borne in mind when examining the effects of resuscitation with colloid versus crystalloid solutions.

The relationship between volume and pH is particularly important in proliferating and growing cells. For example, if cell volume through growth of a cell is associated with an increase in non-ionic molecules, this will increase the osmolality without changing the concentrations of electrolytes, and there would be a decrease in the [SID] and thus a decrease in the pH. On the other hand, if the increase in cell volume is associated with an increase in electrolyte concentrations, there would be an increase in the [SID] and thus an increase in the pH. This means that proteins regulating intracellular pH must appear early in the development of a cell.

Conclusions

When the physicochemical analysis of acid-base regulation is applied to the examination of clinical acid-base disorders questions related to its benefits are raised. The answer is that it allows a true understanding of the underlying mechanisms regulating $[H^+]$. The application of the analysis to the intracellular environment, however, opens up a whole new area of investigation, because it challenges a fundamental principle that is central in the analysis of biochemical pathways and the function of the cell transporters and exchangers that regulate intracellular pH. Traditional analyses are all based on the principle that $[H^+]$ is an independent variable that is added or removed from the system, rather than $[H^+]$ being a dependent variable with a concentration based on the other elements of a solution. I have only laid out the theoretical basis for analysis and touched on some of the implications. A comprehensive analysis of all the implications of this approach are well beyond the scope of this paper, but it becomes apparent that what is needed is a virtual revolution with a re-evaluation of all biochemical pathways and intracellular physiological mechanisms based on the realizations that $[H^+]$ and $[HCO_3^-]$ are dependent variable. In other words, a post-Copernican view of intracellular acid-base physiology is needed.

References

1. Putnam RW (1998) Intracellular pH regulation. In: Cell physiology source book, Sperelakis. Academic Press, Cincinnati pp 293-311
2. Orlowski J, Grinstein S (1997) Na+/H+ exchangers of mammalian cells. J Biol Chem 272: 22373-22376
3. Stewart PA (1981) How to Understand Acid-Base. A Quantitative Acid-Base Primer for Biology and Medicine. Elsevier New York
4. Magder S (1998) Pathophysiology of metabolic acid-base disturbances in patients with critical illness. In: Ronco C, Bellorno R (eds.) Crit Care Nephrol Kluwer Academic Publishers, Netherlands 279-296
5. Heigenhauser GJF, Lindinger MI (1988) Ion fluxes during tetanic stimulation in isolated perfused rat hindlimb. Am J Physiol 245:R117-R126
6. Kowalchuk JM, Heigenhauser GJF, Lindinger MI (1981) Factors influencing hydrogen ion concentration in muscle after intense exercise. J Appl Physiol. 65: 2080-2089
7. Lindinger MI (1995) Origins of [H+] changes in exercising skeletal muscle. Can J Appl Physiol 20:357-368
8. Prange HD, Shoemaker JLJ, Westen EA, et al (2001) Physiological consequences of oxygen-dependent chloride binding to hemoglobin. J Appl Physiol 91:33-38
9. Hochachka PW, Mommsen TP (1983) Protons and anaerobiosis. Science 219:1391-1397
10. Neylon CB, Little PJ, Cragoe EJ Jr, Bobik A (1990) Intracellular pH in human arterial smooth muscle: regulation by Na+/H+ exchange and a novel 5-(n-ethyl-n-isopropyl) amiloride-sensitive Na+ - and HCO3- - dependent mechanism. Circ Res 67:814-825
11. Rawn JD (1989) Bioenergetics: The significance of the hydrolysis of ATP and other energy-rich metabolites. In: Daisy L , Hodgin KC, O'QuinTL, Olsen S and Swan JA. Burlington: Patterson, pp 265-287

12. Roos A, Boron WF (1981) Intracellular pH. Physiol Rev 61: 296-434
13. Russell JM (1976) Role of chloride transport in regulation of intracellular pH. Nature 4: 73-74
14. Counillon L, Pouysségur J (2000) The expanding family of eucaryotic Na /H exchangers. BiolChem 275:1-4
15. Grinstein S, Cohen S, Rothstein A (1984) Cytoplasmic pH regulation in thymic lymphocytes by an amiloride-sensitive Na+/H+ Antiport. J Gen Physiol 83:341-369
16. Moolenaar WH, Boonstra J, Saag PT van der, de Laat SW (1981) Sodium/proton exchange in mouse neuroblastoma cells. J Biol Chem 256:12883-12887
17. Boron WF, Russel JM (1983) Stoichiometry and ion dependencies of the intracellular-pH-regulating mechanism in squid giant axons. J Gen Physiol 81:373-399
18. Stevens TH, Forgac M (1997) Structure, function and regulation of the vacuolar (H+)-ATPase. Annu Rev Cell Dev Biol 13: 779-808
19. Stone DK, Xie X-S (1988) Proton translocating ATPase: issues in structure and function. Kidney International 33: 767-774
20. Wieczorek H, Brown D, Grinstein S, et al (1999) Animal plasma membrane energization by proton-motive V-ATPases. Biol Essays 21: 637-648

Physiological Consequences of Acid-Base Disorders

D. A. STORY

The physiological consequences of acid-base disorders constitute a difficult topic for many reasons. The consequences of acid-base disorders that I will discuss are derived from in vitro, animal, and clinical work reviewed by experts in acid-base disorders [1-4]. Unfortunately these reviewers either ignore or downplay the acid-base approach of Peter Stewart [5].

Several factors complicate analysis of the clinical importance of acid-base disorders in critically ill patients. One complicating factor is separating the effects of the acid-base disorders and organ failure. Metabolic acidosis secondary to cardiogenic shock is one example. What is due to acidosis and what is due to tissue hypoxia? To further complicate the cardiogenic shock example the acidosis and myocardial failure will promote each other [1]. A second factor complicating analysis of acid-base disorders is that some effects may be indirect, particularly those effects due to acid-base disorders stimulating the sympathetic nervous system and effects on extracellular potassium. A third factor is effect of the acid-base disorder on intracellular and extracellular osmolality. A final factor is our limited ability to understand the intracellular events during acid-base disorders.

The Stewart approach

Several presenters at APICE 2001 will use the Stewart approach to acid-base regulation [5]. Briefly, in both the Stewart approach and the Henderson-Hasselbalch approach carbon dioxide plays an important role. On the metabolic side, however, in the Stewart approach bicarbonate is a dependent variable and the strong ion difference and total weak acid concentration are the independent factors. To analyze the effects on dependent factors, including hydrogen ions and bicarbonate ions, the Stewart approach requires analysis of the simultaneous effects of the three independent factors: carbon dioxide, strong ion difference, and total weak acid concentration. The major source of hydrogen ions is the dissociation of water. In plasma, albumin is the dominant variable in the total weak acid concentration. An important point is that the constants for the dissociation of water and the weak acids are temperature dependent.

The fundamental cause of acid-base effects

Albumin is a weak acid. The most-important site for weak acid activity is the imidazole group of the amino acid histidine. The pKa of a weak acid is the pH at which it is 50% dissociated. The pH (and therefore the hydrogen ion concentration) is changed by changes in the three independent factors. If independent factors change the pH in a range within 1 pH unit of the pKa of a weak acid, there can be considerable change in the proportion of the total weak acid that is dissociated into its dissociated form and a hydrogen ion. The ratio of the dissociated form to the total concentration of the weak acid is known as alpha, and we will return to this when discussing the alpha-stat approach to alkalemia during cardiopulmonary bypass.

Each albumin molecule has 16 imidazole groups associated with histidine. The imidazole groups of histidine have pKas within the physiological pH range at 37°C [6]. When independent factors change the pH at 37°C for a given change in pH, there will be marked changes in the dissociation of the imidazole groups. As with albumin, on other proteins (including enzymes, structural proteins, and receptors) the most important weak acid component is the imidazole group. When the dissociation of the imidazole (and other less important groups) changes, the structure and function of the protein changes. This is the fundamental cause of altered organ function in acid-base disorders.

Acidemia

Clinically important acidemia probably starts at around pH 7.20. This is a hydrogen ion concentration of about 65 nmol/l; pH 7.40 being a hydrogen ion concentration of 40 nmol/l. The important effects of acidemia are in Table 1 [1, 3, 4]. The overall pattern is of deteriorating cardiac and skeletal muscle function aggravated by neurological and metabolic effects. These effects occur whether the disorder is respiratory, metabolic, or mixed. The effects and the organ dysfunction can promote each other, and if severe enough can kill the patient.

Table 1. Adverse effects of acidemia

Respiratory	
	Hyperventilation
	Muscle fatigue
	Hemoglobin right shift
Cardiovascular	
	Reduced cardiac contractility
	Dilated arterioles, constricted veins
	Pulmonary vasoconstriction - V/Q mismatching
	Reduced hepatic and renal blood flow
	Increased myocardial irritability
Metabolic	
	Sympathetic stimulation
	Increased metabolic rate
	Hyperkalemia
	Insulin resistance
	Reduced ATP synthesis
	Impaired anaerobic glycolysis
	Altered protein drug binding
Neurological	
	Reduced metabolism and cell volume regulation
	Coma
	Enhanced neuromuscular blockade

Alkalemia

Clinically important alkalemia probably starts at round pH 7.60. This is a hydrogen ion concentration of about 25 nmol/l. Some of the important effects are shown in Table 2 [2, 4]. In head-injured patients, planned cerebral vasoconstriction from respiratory alkalosis may be detrimental if excessive. The hypoventilation from metabolic alkalosis can make weaning from mechanical ventilation difficult.

Table 2. Consequences of alkalemia

Respiratory	
	Decreased minute ventilation
	Hemoglobin left shift
Cardiovascular	
	Systemic arteriolar constriction.
	Decreased coronary blood flow
	Arrhythmias
Metabolic	
	Decreased potassium, ionized calcium, magnesium, and phosphate
	Increased anaerobic glycolysis
	Altered protein drug binding
Neurological	
	Decreased cerebral blood flow
	Fitting
	Tetany

Alpha-stat and pH-stat

One common cause of alkalemia in the operating room is the cooling of patients during cardiopulmonary bypass [7, 8]. The increase in plasma pH is about 0.15 pH units per 10°C drop in temperature. Thus at 30°C the pH is around 7.55.

There are two divergent clinical strategies to manage this alkalemia. The older strategy is based on the physiology of hibernating warm-blooded mammals. The blood gases are measured at 37°C and then corrected to the patient's temperature. The management is to produce a corrected pH of 7.40 by adding carbon dioxide to the bypass circuit. This strategy is called pH-stat.

A newer strategy is based on the physiology of cold-blooded animals as well as human blood passing from the warm body core to cooler extremities. The blood gases are measured at 37° C. The strategy is to accept the alkalemia and maintain a pH of 7.40 measured at 37°C. By doing this, the ratio of dissociated imidazole to total imidazole, alpha, is kept constant. Theoretically, by keeping alpha constant, there would be less change in protein function. This strategy is called alpha-stat.

Both alpha-stat and pH-stat strategies are still used. The major controversy is about the effects on cerebral blood flow. The supporters of alpha-stat suggest that this approach prevents excessive brain perfusion. The supporters of pH-stat, however, suggest that treating the alkalemia will prevent cerebral ischemia. Clinical studies of neurological outcome after cardiopulmonary bypass with the two strategies have been inconclusive [7, 8].

Traditionally, the complex explanation for cold-associated alkalemia has been the binary buffer system of carbon dioxide/bicarbonate and imidazole [9]. The Stewart approach, however, provides a more-straightforward explanation through altered dissociation constants for weak acids and water at lower temperatures. Researchers in this area, including Rahn et al. [9], working before Stewart published his work, noted that the temperature-related increase in pH ran in parallel with the temperature-related changes in the dissociation of water. Without knowing it, these workers produced data supporting the ideas of Peter Stewart.

References

1. Hindman BJ (1990) Sodium bicarbonate in the treatment of subtypes of acute lactic acidosis: physiologic considerations. Anesthesiology 72:1064-1076
2. Adrogue HJ, Madias NE (1998) Management of life-threatening acid-base disorders. II. N Engl J Med 338:107-111
3. Adrogue HJ, Madias NE (1998) Management of life-threatening acid-base disorders. I. N Engl J Med 338:26-34
4. Shangraw R (2000) Acid-base balance. In: Miller R (ed) Anesthesia. Churchill Livingstone, Philadelphia, pp 1390-1413

5. Stewart PA (1983) Modern quantitative acid-base chemistry. Can J Physiol Pharmacol 61: 1444-1461
6. Figge J, Mydosh T, Fencl V (1992) Serum proteins and acid-base equilibria: a follow-up. J Lab Clin Med 120:713-719
7. Burrows FA (1995) Con: pH-stat management of blood gases is preferable to alpha-stat in patients undergoing brain cooling for cardiac surgery. J Cardiothorac Vasc Anesth 9:219-221
8. Kern FH, Greeley WJ (1995) Pro: pH-stat management of blood gases is not preferable to alpha-stat in patients undergoing brain cooling for cardiac surgery. J Cardiothorac Vasc Anesth 9:215-218
9. Rahn H, Reeves RB, Howell BJ (1975) Hydrogen ion regulation, temperature, and evolution. Am Rev Respir Dis 112:165-172

Clinical Approach to Acid-Base Balance

S. MAGDER

The assessment of acid-base balance is one of the most-fundamental aspects of the management of critically ill patients. Traditional teaching has been based on the Henderson-Hasselbalch equation, which is the mass action equation written in the form of the equilibrium relationship of H+ to CO_2 and HCO_3^-. The equation is

$$pH=6.1+\log([HCO_3^-]/[0.0301 x PCO_2])$$

where 0.031 is the constant to account for the solubility of CO_2 in water, and 6.1 the negative log of the pKa of the dissociation of carbonic acid. Using this approach, one first determines if there is an acid-base disturbance by observing whether there is a deviation in the pH from the physiological neutral value of 7.4. Increases or decreases in the pCO_2 are used to determine if there is a respiratory component, and variations in HCO_3^- are used to determine if there is a metabolic component. A complex set of equations can then be used to determine if the changes are acute or chronic and compensated or uncompensated. This approach has by and large served clinicians adequately. However, it provides no insight into physiological mechanisms and potentially produces some very faulty reasoning.

The limitations of the conventional approach were pointed out by Peter Stewart [1] who presented a physical-chemical approach to acid-base balance. The details of this approach are given elsewhere in the chapter by Kellum, but a few key points need to be emphasized before explaining how these principles can be applied to clinical practice. The most-important point of Stewart's analysis is that in water solutions, H^+ and HCO_3^- are dependent variables and not independent variables, as they are traditionally treated in clinical biochemical analysis. This means that adding H^+ or HCO_3^- to a solution does not necessarily result in a change in the concentration of H^+ or HCO_3^- that is equal to the amount added. In fact, since all solutions in the body are actually alkaline, i.e., H^+ OH-, the addition of H^+ or HCO_3^- never produces a change in its concentration that is equal to that given. Stewart pointed out that the three independent variables that determine H^+ (and HCO_3^-) are the pCO_2, strong ion difference [SID], and the concentration of weak proteins [A_{Total}]. The significance of each of these will be discussed in the next sections.

Neutral pH

For clinical purposes we call pH 7.4 physiologically "normal". This is the value that is seen in the extracellular environment of most organisms, although intracellular pH is usually somewhat lower (see chapter by Magder). The pH is tightly regulated over a narrow range in all organisms, because the function of many enzymes, structural proteins, and signaling pathways are highly pH dependent. Just as with the traditional approach, with the physical-chemical approach, a pH in the blood below 7.4 is called acidemia and pH greater than 7.4 alkalemia. However, it is important to understand that a pH value below 7.4 does not mean that the solution is acidic. In chemical terms, an acid solution is defined as one in which the H^+ is greater than OH-, a neutral solution is one in which H^+ equals OH-, and an alkaline solution is one in which H^+ is less than OH- [1]. Pure water at body temperature of 37°C has a pH of 6.68, but is neutral because H^+ equals OH-. As noted above, all bodily fluids, with the exception of the stomach after fasting, are alkaline, i.e., H+ is less than OH-.

pCO_2

Stewart treated pCO_2 as an independent variable because CO_2- production is determined by metabolic activity and the pCO_2 in the blood is determined by ventilation, which is normally tightly controlled by the brain. As in the conventional approach, pCO_2 is an important determinant of H^+ and it defines the respiratory component of acid-base disorders. However, it should be appreciated that once the value of pCO_2 is fixed, then the dissociation of H_2CO_3 is determined by the pKa of the reaction and by other factors in the solution, including the [SID] and [A_{Total}]. Therefore, the products of this equilibrium reaction, H^+ and HCO_3^-, are dependent variables.

As in the traditional approach, a pCO_2 of 40 mmHg is called a respiratory acidosis and a pCO_2 of 40 mmHg, a respiratory alkalosis. Since the suffix "-osis" refers to a process, these definitions are even true if the pH is not acidemic or alkalemic. In the physical-chemical approach, compensated or uncompensated conditions are not considered under respiratory derangements because these really refer to metabolic processes, and are discussed under metabolic alterations. The physical-chemical approach allows a better understanding of the processes involved in metabolic acid-base disturbance.

Strong ion difference

The most important regulator of the metabolic component of acid-base balance is the strong ion difference [SID]. This is the difference in concentrations (measured in equivalence) of strong cations and strong ions. Examples of strong cation are Na^+, K^+, Mg^{2+}, and Ca^{2+}. Examples of strong anions are Cl^-, SO_4^{2+}, and lactate. The reason why [SID] is so important is that the difference in charge requires that another ion be available to maintain electrical neutrality or else a large charge will develop. In a solution with only strong electrolytes in water, the only other source of ions is water. The electrical charge from the [SID] thus affects the dissociation of water. It also affects the dissociation of weak acids.

The predominant strong ions in plasma are Na^+ and Cl^-, and the normal [SID] of plasma is about 42 mEq/l. The other ions in plasma, such as K^+, Mg^{2+} , Ca^{2+} and SO_4^{2+}, are found in much smaller quantities, i.e., 1 - 4 meq/l, and small deviations from their normal value have major physiological effects. Therefore they do not play a significant role in regulating the [SID]. Furthermore, Na^+ is very important for the regulation of plasma osmolality and the volume status of the extracellular space. Therefore, changing plasma and extracellular Na^+ is not a viable option for the maintenance of the normal [SID]. Thus, the only electrolyte that can readily be altered by the body to regulate the [SID] is Cl^-, and it becomes clear that regulation of Cl^- is critical for maintenance of the normal [SID] and normal acid-base balance.

Disorders of the SID

Principles

A useful way to think of the effect of changes in the SID is that an increase in Na^+ requires a negative ion to balance it, and this will tend to increase OH-. It thus acts like NaOH and has an alkalinizing effect. An increase in Cl^- requires a positive ion to balance it, and this will tend to increase H^+. It thus acts like HCl and has an acidifying effect. The SID can be altered by changes in the amount of water or by the gain or loss of a strong ion. Let us first consider changes in water.

Changes in water

Figure 1 shows a beaker with1 litre of water, Na^+ = 140x10^{-6}Eq/l and Cl^- = 100x10^{-6} Eq/l. The [SID] is thus 40x10^{-6} Eq/l and the solution has a pH of 10.6. If 1 l of water is added, the Na^+ is 0.70x10^{-6} Eq/l, the Cl^- is 0.50x10^{-6} Eq/l, and the [SID] is reduced to 0.20x10^{-6} Eq/l. This gives a pH of 10.1. Thus, just adding water will change the pH, and this explains dilutional acidosis. In contrast, a loss of water will result in an increase in the [SID], which has an alkalinizing effect.

Changes in Cl^-

As noted above, the two major ions in plasma are Na^+ and Cl^-. Changes in Na^+ are usually related to changes in water, although an interesting exception is the administration of $NaHCO_3$. As explained above, of the primary ions normally present in the plasma, Cl^- is the most-important for the regulation of acid-base balance. A common clinical abnormality is the metabolic acidemia seen after resuscitation with normal saline. This can be easily explained by the physical-

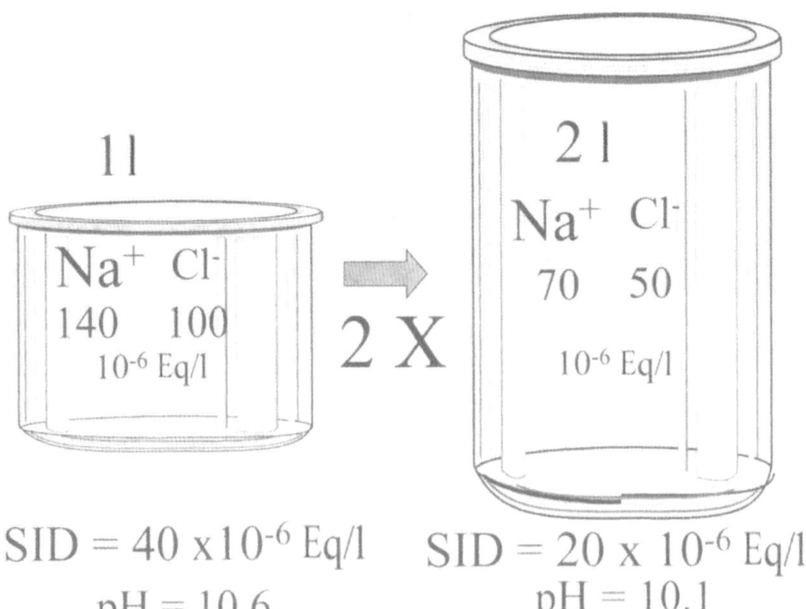

Fig. 1. The effect of changes in water on the strong ion difference [SID]. Doubling the amount of water without changing the amount of electrolytes reduces the [SID] by half. This decreases the pH

-chemical approach by considering the effect on the [SID]. Since the [SID] of normal saline is 0, the administration of this fluid narrows the [SID] in blood and thus produces an acidosis. Furthermore, the kidney tends to counter increases in Na^+ faster than it counters increases in Cl^-, so that the excretion of Cl^- lags behind the excretion of Na^+, which further narrows the [SID]. Consequently there is a hyperchloremic acidemia.

The failure to excrete Cl^- is common in renal disease. The traditional explanation for renal tubular acidosis is that there is a failure to re-absorb HCO3-, but this is a dependent variable and is determined by the pCO_2 and [SID]. Based on the physical-chemical approach, what really is happening is that there is a failure to excrete Cl^-. Part of the problem in these conditions is that a cation is needed to balance the Cl^- in the urine besides Na^+, or else there would be a steady decrease in the [SID] of blood which would produce an acidosis. Normally, the kidney does this by forming NH_3, which freely moves across the tubular membranes into the urine and forms NH_4^+, a weak base in the tubule. The diseased kidney is unable to make NH_3 and thus must use Na^+ to balance Cl^-.

Another situation where the [SID] is narrowed because of hyperchloremia is diarrhea. In the upper bowel, the normal fluid is alkaline with a low Cl^- and large [SID]. When diarrhea is present, the more-rapid transit in the bowel results in a failure to reabsorb Na^+ and loss of water (and possibly to excrete Cl^-) in the distal bowel. The loss of volume and decrease in Na^+ will have an acidifying effect by narrowing the [SID]. Retention of Cl^- would make this worse. The situation also is made worse when NaCl is used as the resuscitation fluid, for it will narrow the [SID].

The opposite occurs when there is gastric suction. In this situation there is a loss of Cl^- without Na^+, and thus the [SID] is widened and there is an alkalosis. It needs to be appreciated that this will only occur when the stomach contents are acidic, for otherwise the loss of Na^+ could be greater than the loss of Cl^-, in which case there could even be an acidosis.

Addition of "other" strong ions

Another way the [SID] can be changed is by the addition of a strong ion, which is usually an anion. Examples of strong anions that can accumulate in pathological conditions include lactate, formate, oxylate, β-hydroxybutyrate, acetoacetate, and salicylate. These will be recognized as the classical "wide anion gap" acidosis [2]. It is important to appreciate that for acid-base balance, the addition of a strong ion such as lactate has the same effect as the addition of Cl^-. The only difference is that lactate can be metabolized, whereas Cl^- has to be excreted.

The realization that these substances produce an acidosis by narrowing the

[SID] helps explain why $NaHCO_3$ cannot successfully treat these kinds of acidosis. The only way the addition of $NaHCO_3$ could correct the acidemia is by widening the [SID] by the addition of Na^+. The HCO_3^- is a dependent variable and in an open system plays no role. Thus to correct a lactic acidemia of 10 mmol/l, the Na^+ would have to increase by 10 mEq/l, which would produce severe hypernatremia with consequent effects on cellular volumes. Furthermore it is likely that this excess Na^+ will be excreted by the kidney or bowel and therefore the body will not even allow the Na^+ to increase.

Weak acids

Principles

Weak acids are substances that are only partially dissociated in a solution. The two important variables for determining their effect on H^+ are the total amount added (referred to as A_{Total}) and the pKa of the dissociation reaction, for this defines how much of the substance is dissociated at a given pH. Weak acids that are particularly important for acid-base balance have pKas within an order of magnitude of the $\sqrt{Kw'}$ of water which is in the range of 10^{-7} Eq/l. If the pKa is below this value, they will be mainly dissociated and function more like strong ions, and if the pKa is higher than this, they will be largely associated at normal pH.

Albumin

The most-important normal weak acid in plasma is albumin. The histidine side-chains have a pKa of close to normal pH, and therefore changes in [SID] in plasma have a major effect on their dissociation. These ions account for most of the normal "anion gap", so that a decrease in albumin is associated with a decrease in the anion gap [2]. As discussed elsewhere in this symposium (see chapter by Magder), this has traditionally been referred to as buffering, but what they really do is set a range over which there are small changes in pH for given changes in [SID]. A major problem with the application of the physical--chemical approach is assigning an "equivalence" value to the anion of albumin. This was performed empirically by Figge et al. [3, 4] who did titration curves of different albumin concentrations with different [SID] and provided a formula for the anion equivalence of albumin at different pH:

$$\text{Albumin effect} = (0.123 \times pH - 0.631) \times (42 - [\text{albumin}])$$

where albumin is in g/l.

Decreases in albumin concentration are very common in critically ill patients [5-7]. The reduction in this weak acid has an alkalinizing effect and an increase in the albumin concentration has an acidifying effect. For example, a decrease in albumin from 42 to 20 g/l has the same alkalinizing effect as a decrease in a strong anion of 6 mEq/l. This means that this decrease in albumin would have the same effect on H^+ as a decrease in lactate from 8 mEq/l to 2 mEq/l.

A decrease in water with dehydration can increase the albumin concentration. This can lead to a widening of the [SID] and an alkalinizing effect. However, the increase in albumin concentration would result in an acidifying effect that would counteract the change in [SID]. The final effect will depend upon how the normal regulatory mechanisms respond to the increase in Na^+ and Cl^- concentrations. Since Na^+ is normally well regulated, it is likely that the increase in Na^+ will be regulated first and that would narrow the [SID] and lead to an acidemia. Indeed, this has been observed during a cholera outbreak [8].

The second weak acid of potential clinical importance is phosphate (PO_4^{3+}). The dissociation of phosphoric acid to PO_4^{3+} has three steps with three pKas. At 37°C the first pKa is only 1.91 and therefore this component acts like a strong acid and is largely dissociated. The second pKa is 6.66 and is very much affected by the other components of plasma. The third pKa is very high, 11.8, and is therefore essentially not dissociated in the plasma [3]. Normal PO_4^{3+} in plasma is only around 1 mmol/l and therefore changes in its dissociation actually have little effect on H^+, but PO_4^{3+} can play a role when its concentration increases with disease. The relationship again from Figge et al. [3] is:

$$(Pi-) = (Pi) \times (0.309 \times pH - 0.469)$$

where Pi- is the ionized portion and Pi is the total phosphate.

Clinical approaches at the bedside

Stewart's original presentation

The physical-chemical analysis was first presented by Stewart and further developed by Figge et al. [3, 4] and Fencyl and Rossing [9], who gave a comprehensive analysis of the regulation of H^+ in the body. Stewart provided six equations that could be solved simultaneously by combining them into a quadratic equation to calculate H^+ [1]. He then did the calculations for changes in pCO_2 and changes in [SID] at a fixed A_{Total}. This is shown in Fig. 2. He then proposed that one could start by plotting the pH (or H+) and pCO_2 and determining the expected [SID]. For example, if a patient has an increased pCO_2 and pH and a normal [SID] of 42 mEq/l, then the problem is purely respiratory

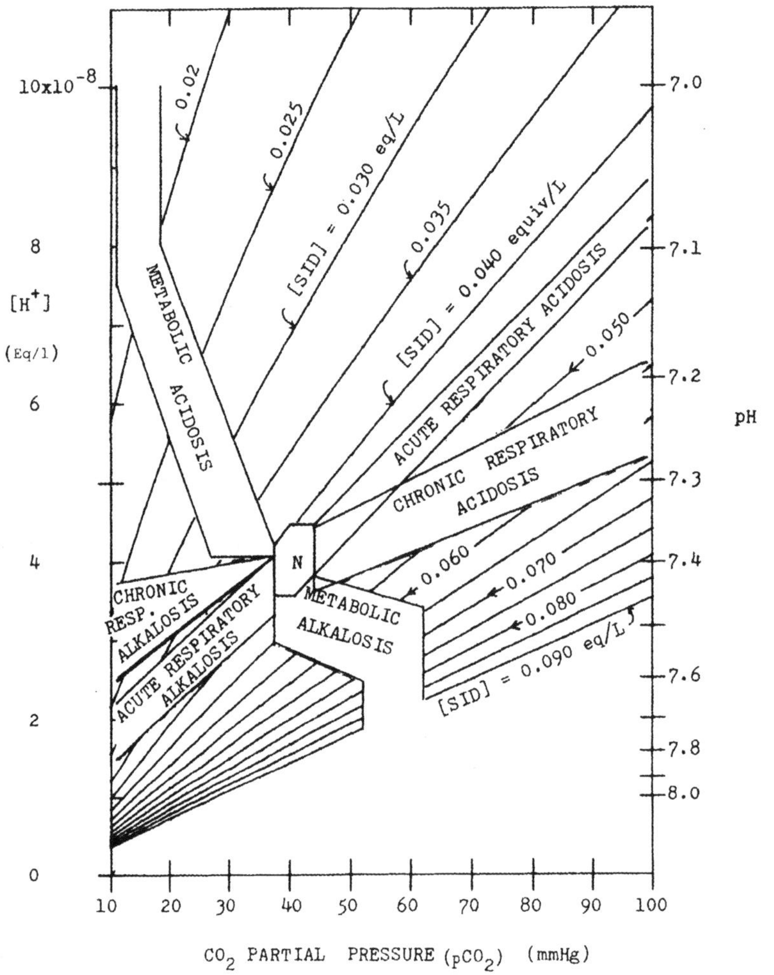

Fig. 2. Stewart's nomogram for effects of changes in CO_2 and strong ion difference ([SID]) on H^+ or pH. (Used with permission from [1])

and the solution is to treat the respiratory problem. In contrast, if there is a decrease in pH with a decrease in pCO_2 and a decrease in the SID, then there is a metabolic problem.

The next step is to determine why the [SID] is abnormal. This is done by determining the sum of [Na^+] + [K^+] - [Cl^-] , the common major strong ions in the plasma, for they give an indication of the inorganic [SID]. If this value is not the same as that given by the nomogram, then the next step is to determine whether this is because of an increase in [Cl^-] or a decrease in [Na^+]. If Na^+ or K^+ are normal, and the value differs from that predicted by the nomogram, then there must be other unidentified anions. These anions are the same as those that explain the traditional wide anion gap acidosis.

Stewart also pointed out that if the nomogram is not available, then the expected [SID] can be estimated by [SID] = HCO_3^- + A- and A- can be estimated from [Na^+]+ [K^+] - [Cl^-]- [HCO_3^-], i.e., the anion gap.

A weakness in the simple approach first presented by Stewart is that it did not take into account changes in [A_{Total}] and how to quantitatively analyze them. They thus do not show up on the nomogram in Fig. 2, for it assumes a constant [A_{Total}], which usually is not the case in critically ill patients.

Presentation by Jones

Norman Jones was an early advocate of the Stewart approach [10, 11]. He basically used the same approach as Stewart, but elaborated on the relationship of the measured and predicted [SID], and thus introduced the concept of a [SID] gap. Like Stewart he used the nomogram in Fig. 2 to predict the [SID], and compared it with that obtained by measuring the electrolytes in the plasma. He also pointed out that [SID] -[HCO_3]–[A-] = O, and this allows one to assess the role of each of these three factors in the acid-base disorder.

The concept of SIG

The concept of a strong ion difference was further elaborated by Kellum et al. [12]. They introduced the term SIG for the strong ion gap. It is a measure of the anion/cation balance, which is measured as [SID]a minus the [SID]e determined from the Stewart equation with the exclusion of strong measured anions and bicarbonate, as modified by Figge. Based on the work of Stewart [1] and Figge et al. [3], SIG is defined as the differences between the apparent strong ion difference [SID]a and the effective strong ion difference [SID]e where

[SID]a = [Na^+] + [K^+] + [Mg^{2+}] + [Ca^{2+}] - [Cl^-] - [lactate] - [urate]

(all ionized concentrations are in mEq/l) and

[SID]e = 1000 2.46E-11 pCO_2/(10-pH) + [albumin] (0.123 pH - 0.631) + [PO_4] (0.309 pH - 0.469)

([PO_4] is in mmol/l and albumin is in g/l). The formula for calculating all the components of the analysis are given at a web site created by J Kellum called The Acid Base Phorum: *http://www.anes.upmc.edu/mcctp/phorum.html.*

The SIG should normally be zero. If it is not, there are unexplained anions.

They found that there are large amounts of unknown anions in some patients with sepsis and liver disease. Thus they proposed that the SIG should be used instead of the anion gap for evaluating patients [12].

As shown by a number of investigators, this approach can be used to evaluate the abnormalities of various conditions [13-15], or the effect of interventions [16-18]. The basic approach is to first examine whether the [SID] deviates from the normal value of 40 mEq/l. If it is abnormal, the next question is what measured ions are abnormal to account for the abnormality. For example, is the lactate increased? If there is a SIG with a [SID]e less than the [SID]a, then there are unmeasured anions that are greater than the unmeasured cation, and if SIG is positive, there must be unexplained cations.

Base excess and base excess gap

Gilfix et al. [19] introduced an approach that classified the abnormalities into those of water, Cl^-, albumin, and "other" factors. The "other" factors were calculated by using the base excess (BE) rather than the SIG. This was based on an approach used at Harvard by V. Fencyl and D. Leith, but never published.

In this approach, and in all of the physical-chemical approaches, the first step in evaluating acid-base balance is to determine if there is an acidemia or alkalemia, and this is done by simply determining if there is a deviation in pH from the physiological normal value of 7.40. If the pH is greater than 7.40, there is an alkalemia, and if the pH is less than 7.40 there is an acidemia.

The next step is to evaluate the respiratory component. This is done by examining the deviation of the pCO_2 from the standard value of 40 mmHg. If the pCO_2 is greater than 40 mmHg there is a respiratory acidosis regardless of the pH, for the PCO_2 defines a process.

The metabolic components are examined next. First one examines the role of changes in the concentrations of electrolytes that are due to changes in "water". Since the amount of extracellular water is determined largely by the Na^+ concentration, $[Na^+]$ can be used to assess water effects. This is done by comparing the measured $[Na^+]$ with the [Na+] reference value, which is 140 mEq/l, and by assuming normal [SID] of 42 mEq/l as follows:

$$\text{Water effect (mEq/l)} = [(Na-140)/140] \times 42 = 0.3\,([Na+]-140)$$

The major mechanism the body has to regulate the [SID] is the regulation of $[Cl^-]$. Therefore, an important step is the evaluation of the changes in $[Cl^-]$. To do this, one must first account for the effect of changes in water on $[Cl^-]$, for this was already accounted for in the previous step. This is done by correcting the measured $[Cl^-]$ by the ratio of the standard value of $[Na^+]$ of 140 mEq/l and the measured $[Na^+]$:

$$[Cl^-]\text{-corrected (mEq/l)} = [Cl^{-}] \times 140/[Na^+].$$

The effect of the change in $[Cl^-]$ can then be calculated from:

$$\text{Chloride effect (mEq/l)} = 102 - \{ [Cl^-]\text{-corrected (mEq/l)} \}$$

where 102mEq/l is the standard $[Cl^-]$ value.

The third metabolic factor is the effect of changes in albumin, for it is the major determinant of the effect of weak acids. This is based on the anionic effect of albumin, which can be determined by an empirical formula developed by Figge et al. [3]:

$$\text{Albumin effect (mEq/l)} = 42- \{ [\text{albumin}] \times (0.123 \times \text{pH}- 0.631) \}$$

where albumin is in g/l and 42 represents the standard value of albumin.

Once the effect of these three factors, water, $[Cl^-]$, and albumin, are accounted for, the presence of any "other" factors can be determined by the use of the SIG. Alternatively we found that it is very convenient to use the BE measurement from the blood gas measurement. To this, one adds the value (in mEq/l) of the water effect, chloride effect, and albumin effect, and subtracts this sum from the calculated BE:

$$\text{"Other" (mEq/l)} = \text{BE-(Water effect + Chloride effect + Albumin effect)}$$

To understand the rationale for this last step it is necessary to understand the concept of BE. BE was a concept developed in the early part of the last century to account for the non-respiratory component of an acid-base disturbance. This was obtained by doing titration reactions with a strong base or strong acid and it therefore was essentially a titration of the [SID] to determine how much it needs to change to restore pH to 7.4 with a pCO_2 of 40 mmHg. It is thus an empirical assessment of the SIG. Indeed there is a tight relationship between measurements of "other" by this method (or the BE gap) and the SIG (Fig. 3).

The BE reported on blood gases today comes from the work of Siggaard-Andersen [20] who created a nomogram to determine the BE. Because the electrolytes in plasma are in equilibrium with the interstitial space, a titration in a test tube of blood is not the same as a titration on whole blood or, for that matter, on serum. This has often been viewed as being due to a greater "buffering effect" of hemoglobin in the test tube, and because of this BE is often given as "standard base excess" which is based on a hemoglobin value of 50 g/l, which takes into account the distribution of electrolytes throughout the

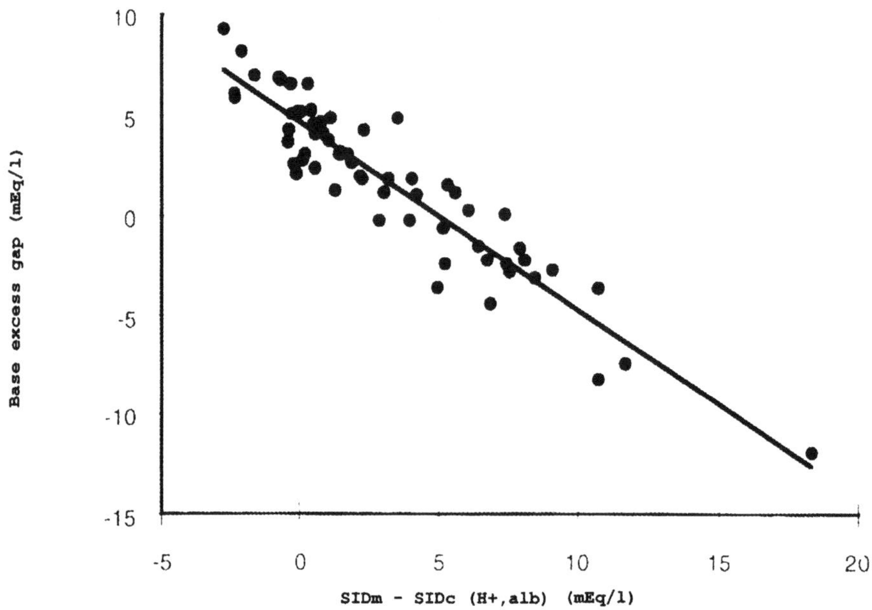

Fig. 3. Relationship of base excess gap to the strong ion gap (SIG). There is a tight relationship between these two measures. Used with permission from [6]

extracellular space [21, 22]. However, the differences are really quite small, and we have used the BE based on a hemoglobin of 150 g/l. The reason why the effect is small is that hemoglobin does not actually "buffer" the plasma because it is not in contact with it. The only way red cells in the plasma affect [H+] is by electrolyte shifts between the intracellular space and the plasma, which then can alter plasma [SID]. However, the red cell intracellular volume is small compared with the plasma. In the body, the intracellular compartment of the red blood cell interacts with the whole extracellular volume, and therefore has only a minimal effect on electrolyte concentrations.

The analysis based on the effects of water, chloride, albumin, and BE has the advantage of indicating which major regulator is causing the acid-base abnormality. It is also easier to calculate than the full equation for determining the apparent H^+. The disadvantage is that it introduces another empirical measurement, i.e., the BE, and therefore has the potential for other confounding factors that may not have been accounted for in the original titration experiments performed to obtain the BE. The effects of other factors, such as phosphate, also become more of a problem at the extremes of the range of pH values [23].

Conclusions

An appreciation of the physical-chemical factors that determine $[H^+]$ is essential for understanding the mechanisms behind acid-base disorders. Once one understands the basic processes, an examination of the electrolytes will give a quick but not quantitative insight into the basic mechanism. For example, a low $[Na^+]$ indicates a major water effect, a high $[Cl^-]$ indicates a "non-anion gap" metabolic acidosis, and a low albumin indicates a metabolic alkalosis. An abnormal BE in the absence of major $[Cl^-]$ abnormalities means that there are very likely abnormal anions present. When a more-quantitative analysis is desired, one can calculate the SIG or use the calculations given above to quantify the water effect, chloride effect, albumin effect, and "other".

References

1. Stewart PA (1981) How to understand acid-base. A quantitative acid-base primer for biology and medicine. Elsevier, New York
2. Emmett M, Narins RG (1977) Clinical use of the anion gap. Medicine (Baltimore) 56: 38-54
3. Figge J, Mydosh T, Fencl V (1992) Serum proteins and acid-base equilibria: a follow-up. J Lab Clin Med. 120: 713-719
4. Figge J, Rossing TH, Fencl V. (1991) The role of serum proteins in acid-base equilibria. J Lab Clin Med 117: 453-467
5. Rossing TH, Boixeda D, Maffeo N (1986) Hyperventilation with hypoproteinemia. J Lab Clin Med 117: 453-467
6. Rossing TH, Maffeo N, Fencl V (1986) Acid-base effects of altering plasma protein concentration in human blood in vitro. J Appl Physiol 61: 2260-2265
7. Wilkes P (1998) Hypoproteinemia, strong-ion difference, and acid-base status in critically ill patients. J Appl Physiol 84: 1740-17481998
8. Wang F, Butler T, Rabbani GH. (1986) The acidosis of cholera: contributions of hyperproteinemia, lactic acidemia and hyperphosphatemia to an increased serum anion gap. N Engl J Med 315: 1591-1595
9. Fencl V, Rossing TH (1989) Acid-base disorders in critical care medicine. Ann Rev Med 40: 17-29
10. Jones NL (1990) A quantitative physiochemical approach to acid-base physiology. Clin Biochem 23: 189-195
11. Jones NL (1990) Should we change our approach to acid-base physiology? Ann RCPSC 23: 235-240
12. Kellum JA, Kramer DJ, Pinsky MR (1995) Strong ion gap: a methodology for exploring unexplained anions. J Crit Care 10: 51-55
13. Fencl VJAKAFJ (2000) Diagnosis of metabolic acid-base disturbances in critically ill patients. Am J Respir Crit Care Med 162: 2246-2251
14. Kellum JA (1998) Metabolic acidosis in the critically ill: lessons from physical chemistry. Kidney Int 53: S-81-S-86
15. Kellum JA, Bellomo R, Kramer DJ, Pinksy MR (1995) Hepatic anion flux during acute endotoxemia. J Appl Physiol 78: 2212-2217
16. Hayhoe M, Bellomo R, Lui G, et al (1999) Role of the splanchnic circulation in acid-base balance during cardiopulmonary bypass. Crit Care Med 27: 2671-2677

17. Liskaser FJ, Bellomo R, Hayhoe M et al (2000) Role of pump prime in the etiology and pathogenesis of cardiopulmonary bypass - associated acidosis. Anesthesiology 93: 1170-1173
18. Rehm M, Orth V, Scheingraber S, et al (2000) Acid-base changes caused by 5% albumin versus 6% hydroxyethyl starch solution in patients undergoing acute normovolemic hemodilution. Anesthesiology 93: 1174-1187
19. Gilfix BM, Bique M, Magder SA (1993) A physiological approach to the analysis of acid-base balance in the clinical setting. J Crit Care 8: 187-197
20. Siggaard-Andersen O (1964) The acid-base status of the blood. Williams and Wilkins, Baltmore
21. Mizock BA (1998) Utility of standard base excess in acid-base analysis. Crit Care Med 26: 1146-1147
22. Schlichtig R, Grogono AW, Severinghaus JW (1998) Human Paco2 and standard base excess compensation for acid-base imbalance. Crit Care Med 26: 1173-1179
23. Waters JH, Scanlon TS, Howard RS, Leivers D (1995) Role of minor electrolytes when applied to Stewart's acid-base approach in an acidotic rabbit model. Anesth Analg 81: 1043-1051

Using Base Excess

T. J. MORGAN

Arterial blood gas analysis was part of everyday intensive care practice for much of the second half of the last century, yet in 2001 considerable differences of opinion and entrenched viewpoints still characterize the evaluation of acid-base disturbances. There are of course relatively non-controversial areas. All agree that in healthy people living near sea-level, the arterial pH will be close to 7.4, and the arterial pCO_2 ($paCO_2$) will be close to 40 mmHg. Most define acidemia as arterial pH < 7.35, and alkalemia as pH > 7.45, and agree that in isolated respiratory acidosis, $paCO_2$ exceeds 45 mmHg, and in isolated respiratory alkalosis, $paCO_2$ is less than 35 mmHg. It is also widely understood that metabolic (non-respiratory) acid-base abnormalities are those which manifest on blood gas analysis as a disturbed pH / $paCO_2$ relationship (Fig. 1).

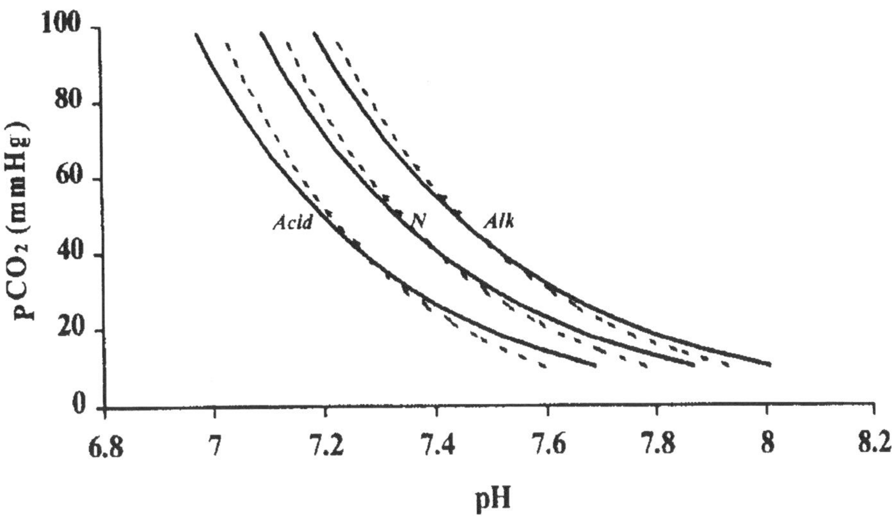

Fig. 1. $PaCO_2$ / pH relationships. Illustrated are the normal curve (n) and examples of metabolic acidosis (Acid) and metabolic alkalosis (Alk). *Solid curves* represent in vivo and interrupted curves in vitro relationships, respectively

Where disagreement arises is in the best way to identify and quantify these metabolic acid-base disturbances. In other words, at any given $paCO_2$ and pH, what is the best tool to delineate the separate respiratory and metabolic contributions to the overall acid-base status?

The ideal bedside metabolic acid-base index should fulfil three criteria:

1. It should be simple and 'user friendly'.
2. It should always be independent of $paCO_2$ (CO_2 invariant).
3. It should be stoichiometric. This means that the index should quantify the amount of strong acid or base required to correct any metabolic acid-base disturbance.

There are three contenders, which in the pages to follow I will evaluate by the above criteria:

1. The $paCO_2$/[HCO_3^-] 'rules' of the Boston school.
2. Strong ion difference (Stewart's physical-chemical approach).
3. Standard base excess (Copenhagen approach).

The contention of this author will be that, on evaluation, standard base excess is the most-practical working tool for the clinician. However, it is important to state at the outset that all three approaches can be reconciled, since in reality they are different ways of describing the same processes [1].

The Boston 'rules'

To overcome perceived deficiencies in the base excess concept of the Copenhagen school, a group led by Schwartz and Relman at Tufts University advanced a $paCO_2$/[HCO_3^-] - based approach [2,3]. Six equations were derived using genuine in vivo data, including data from human volunteers and patients (Table 1).

Table 1. The six paCO2 / [HCO3-] rules (paCO2 values are in mmHg, [HCO3-] in mmol/l)

1. The '1 for 10' rule of acute respiratory acidosis
Expected [HCO_3^-] = 24 + {($paCO_2$ – 40)}/10
2. The '4 for 10' rule of chronic respiratory acidosis
Expected [HCO_3^-] = 24 + 4_{($paCO_2$ – 40)}/10
3. The '2 for 10' rule of acute respiratory alkalosis
Expected [HCO_3^-] = 24 - 2_{(40 - $paCO_2$)}/10
4. The '5 for 10' rule of chronic respiratory alkalosis
Expected [HCO_3^-] = 24 - 5_{(40 - $paCO_2$)}/10
5. The '1.5 plus 8' rule of metabolic acidosis
Expected $paCO_2$ = 1.5 _ [HCO_3^-] + 8
6. The '0.9 plus 9' rule of metabolic alkalosis
Expected $paCO_2$ = 0.9 _ [HCO_3^-] + 8

The first observation that can be made is that the Boston 'rules' are neither simple nor user-friendly. In fact they require feats of memory and considerable bedside 'mental gymnastics' [1]. Many practitioners (including this author) find carrying these equations around in their heads quite burdensome. Mistakes and memory lapses can happen, perhaps with adverse clinical consequences. It is true that the equations apply throughout the normal 'working' range of $paCO_2$. CO_2 invariance therefore comes into operation once a decision is made as to whether any respiratory acid-base disturbance is acute or chronic. However, although a significant deviation from the normal $[HCO_3^-]$ for any given $paCO_2$ signals a metabolic acid-base disturbance, it does not quantify the amount of strong acid or base required to correct it [4]. This is because the impact of acid-base disturbances is spread across the entire 'buffer base', of which $[HCO_3^-]$ is only one component. Consequently, $[HCO_3^-]$ offsets are not stoichiometric.

Strong ion difference

Stewart's analysis of acid-base using the principles of physical chemistry has been a major conceptual advance [5]. In the Stewart approach, pH and $[HCO_3^-]$ are dependent variables determined by three independent variables, which are pCO_2, strong ion difference ([SID]), and the total concentration of non-volatile weak acid buffer ($[A_{TOT}]$). Strong ions such as Na^+, K^+, Cl^- and lactate are essentially fully ionized under all physiological acid-base conditions. [SID] = [strong cations] – [strong anions]. In whole blood, A_{TOT} is made up primarily of the histidine residues on hemoglobin, whereas A_{TOT} in plasma is comprised largely of albumin and inorganic phosphate.

In normal plasma, [SID] is approximately 40 mmol/l. [SID] in whole blood is harder to quantify, but it can be derived using expressions for intra-erythrocytic buffering and plasma/erythrocyte distribution equations [1]. To preserve electrical neutrality, the SID 'space' is filled passively by the buffer base anions. These consist of the weak ions HCO_3^- and non-volatile buffer anions (A^-), where $[A_{TOT}] = [HA] + [A^-]$. [SID] thus defines, controls and is numerically identical to the buffer base concentration [6]. In metabolic acidosis, [SID] and buffer base are decreased, whereas in metabolic alkalosis they are increased. On the other hand, uncompensated reductions in $[A_{TOT}]$ cause metabolic alkalosis, and elevations cause metabolic acidosis [7].

In the physical-chemical approach, [SID] is thus one of two determinants of metabolic acid-base status, the other being $[A_{TOT}]$. The focus of Stewart and his followers has always been on plasma [SID] rather than whole-blood [SID].

However, nomograms have been available since the late 1940s, which allow the calculation of whole-blood [SID]. They were developed by Singer and Hastings [8], who used the term 'buffer base' rather than [SID], since it was calculated as the sum of the weak buffer base anions ($[HCO_3^-] + [A^-]$). This is also the easiest way to calculate plasma [SID], rather than by the more-complex simultaneous equations approach or by laborious direct measurement of all strong anions and cations [9]. It has also been argued that although [SID] defines, controls, and is identical to the buffer base concentration, it is nevertheless buffer base which determines metabolic acid-base status by setting the relationship between pCO_2 and pH (Fig. 1) [6].

The strength of the Stewart approach lies in the conceptual insights it provides, but practical application at the bedside is not 'simple and user friendly' by any stretch of the imagination. [SID] certainly qualifies as CO_2 invariant, since it is an independent variable. However, its interpretation as an index of metabolic acid-base status is linked to the third independent variable $[A_{TOT}]$, which can be regarded as setting the normal range of [SID] in vivo. The only way that [SID] becomes a stoichiometric index of metabolic acid-base status is by conversion to SIDex, which is the change in whole-blood [SID] required to bring the pH to 7.4 after the pCO_2 is corrected to 40 mmHg [1]. SIDex, however, is virtually identical to base excess (Fig. 2), but has the disadvantage that unlike base excess it cannot be calculated from blood gas analysis alone.

Standard base excess

The evolution of the standard base excess concept makes interesting reading [10]. Jørgensen and Astrup [11] began by using tonometry to convert small volumes of blood to fully oxygenated specimens with a pCO_2 of 40 mmHg at 38°C. Measurement of pH on these equilibrated specimens allowed determination of the 'standard bicarbonate' concentration, by substituting pCO_2 (40 mmHg) and the measured pH value in the Henderson-Hasselbalch equation [11]. CO_2 invariance was thus ensured by physically returning the pCO_2 to 40 mmHg. However, there are two problems with this approach. The first is that [HCO3-] indices are not stoichiometric. The second is that the in vitro blood pH/pCO_2 equilibration curve differs from the in vivo curve (Fig. 1).

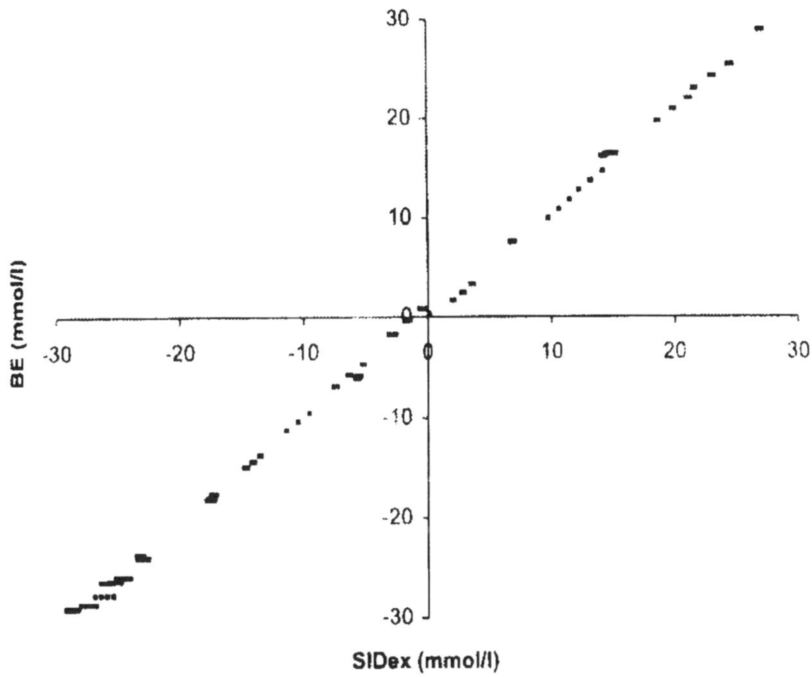

Fig. 2. Relationship between whole blood base excess (BE) and whole blood strong ion difference excess (SIDex). There are 216 data points, with [hemoglobin] ranging from 50 to 150 g/l, [albumin] from 20 to 40 g/l, $paCO_2$ from 10 to 60 mmHg, and pH from 6.9 to 7.6. By inspection, values are almost identical. $R^2 = 0.999$. By linear regression, BE = (1.0406 × SIDex) + 0.30

The answer to the stoichiometry problem

Siggaard-Andersen and Fogh-Andersen [12] solved the stoichiometry problem by introducing a new parameter called base excess (BE), defined as the concentration of titratable hydrogen ion required to return the pH of an in vitro specimen to 7.4, while maintaining pCO_2 at 40 mmHg at 37°C by equilibration. If pH is > 7.4 once the pCO_2 has been returned to 40 mmHg, BE is the mmol/l of strong acid that brings the pH to 7.4 (while pCO_2 continues to be maintained at 40 mmHg). BE then has a positive sign. If pH < 7.4, BE is quantified by the strong base required (BE then has a negative sign).

To circumvent the need for tedious bench-top tonometry and acid-base titrations on each specimen, a series of in vitro experiments was carried out. These recorded the effect on plasma pH of adding known amounts of acid or base to blood followed by tonometry to various known pCO_2 values at 37°C

[13,14]. The experiments were performed across a wide range of hemoglobin concentrations, which is a way of factoring in the effects of varying [A_{TOT}]. From the data, an 'alignment nomogram' was eventually created. This nomogram allowed BE determinations from one measurement of pH, pCO_2, and hemoglobin concentration at 37°C, without any tonometry or acid-base titrations. By the late 1960s, blood gas analyzers could be programmed with the nomogram in the form of look-up tables or equations.

However, in 1977 Siggaard-Andersen [15] went one step further by publishing the Van Slyke equation, which enables BE to be calculated from pH, $paCO_2$, and hemoglobin concentration using expressions for plasma and intra-erythrocytic buffering and Gibbs-Donnan distributions rather than empirical relationships. The equation for whole-blood BE can be written:

$$BE = \{[HCO_3^-] - 24.4 + (2.3 \times [Hb] + 7.7) \times (pH - 7.4)\} \times (1 - 0.023 \times [Hb])$$

where [HCO_3^-] and pH are plasma values and [Hb] is the blood hemoglobin concentration expressed in mmol/L. On publication, Siggaard-Andersen reported close agreement between this equation and its predecessor – the experimentally derived BE nomogram. We recently re-evaluated the in vitro accuracy of the Van Slyke equation, and were able to confirm that it quantifies metabolic acid-base change with acceptable degrees of precision and minimal bias [16]. We found that the accuracy was maintained at very low hemoglobin concentrations, and was little affected by large simultaneous alterations in pCO_2.

The in vivo versus in vitro buffering problem

In 1963, Schwarz and Relman [2] observed that BE is not CO_2 invariant in vivo. This is because for any specimen of arterial blood the in vitro blood pH / PCO_2 equilibration curve differs from the in vivo curve, since in vivo buffering occurs throughout the total extracellular compartment (Fig. 1). An isolated in vivo change in $paCO_2$ shifts BE in the opposite direction (although no overall extracellular metabolic acid-base alteration has occurred), due to differential buffering in the intravascular and interstitial compartments.

The answer to this problem was not long in forthcoming. If BE is calculated from the measured plasma pH and pCO_2 as originally described, but at a hemoglobin concentration of 50 g/l (the approximate mean extracellular hemoglobin concentration), total extracellular buffering is emulated successfully [6]. BE calculated in this way is termed standard BE (SBE). "Rules of thumb" equations derived by meta-analysis of published numerical and graphical data now describe the appropriate SBE responses to acute and chronic acid-base disturbances [17]. They are similar in nature to the Boston rules, and are set out in Table 2. Importantly, the meta-analysis showed SBE to be CO_2 invariant in vivo (Table 2, rule 1), confirming that although SBE is only an approximation of total extracellular buffering, it successfully emulates the in vivo situation.

Table 2. The four paCO2 / SBE rules (SBE in mmol/l, paCO2 in mmHg).

1.	Acute respiratory acidosis and alkalosis	Δ SBE = 0 × $\Delta paCO_2$
2.	Chronic respiratory acidosis and alkalosis	ΔSBE = 0.4 × $\Delta paCO_2$
3.	Metabolic acidosis	Δ $paCO_2$ = Δ SBE
4.	Metabolic alkalosis	Δ $paCO_2$ = 0.6 × Δ SBE

Clinical application of base excess

In most laboratories, the reference range for SBE is approximately -3 mmol/l to + 3 mmol/l. When examining blood gas data, the primary acid-base disturbance is first ascertained from the pH. For example, if the pH, $paCO_2$, and SBE are all elevated, the primary process is a metabolic alkalosis rather than a respiratory acidosis. The next step in this case is to determine whether the respiratory acidosis is purely compensatory. If so, the $paCO_2$ should be within a few mmHg of (40 + 0.6 × Δ SBE) mmHg. If this is not so, there are two primary acid-base disturbances (metabolic and respiratory). Another sign of a dual respiratory/metabolic acid-base disturbance is when the pH is normal but $paCO_2$, and thus SBE, are both abnormal.

In any analysis of metabolic acid-base status (not just metabolic acidosis), it is important to check the anion gap. This can change management. For example, a falling SBE during resuscitation from shock may actually be due to saline administration [18-20] (normal anion gap metabolic acidosis), rather than a lactic acidosis from ongoing tissue dysoxia (elevated anion gap metabolic acidosis). The anion gap in plasma is ($[Na^+] + [K^+]$) – ($[Cl^-] + [HCO_3^-]$), although $[K^+]$ is omitted in many laboratories. A metabolic acidosis with a raised anion gap means that [SID] and thus SBE have been reduced by the presence of unmeasured strong anions, important among which are lactate, ketoacids, uremic accumulation of phosphates, and sulfates, and the products of exogenous compounds, such as salicylic acid, ethylene glycol, or methanol. In a normal anion gap metabolic acidosis, [SID] and SBE reductions stem from a simple narrowing of the difference between $[Na^+]$ and $[Cl^-]$. Causes include exogenous fluids such as saline, or abnormal renal or gastro-intestinal Cl^- homeostasis [21]. However, the anion gap is limited by relatively low sensitivity, and consequently may fail to detect small elevations of unmeasured strong anions reliably [22,23]. This is mainly due to the fact that the normal anion gap in the absence of unmeasured anions is the same as $[A^-]$, which varies with $[A_{TOT}]$ and pH. Since hypoalbuminemia and acid-base disturbances are common in critical illness, the sensitivity of anion gap can be improved by correction for these plasma $[A^-]$ perturbations [24].

Two further parameters derived from Stewart's physical -chemical approach have been developed primarily to improve the diagnostic sensitivity and specificity for unmeasured strong anions. They are the strong ion gap [25] and BE caused by unmeasured anions (BEua) [26]. Both were designed to be independent of variations in plasma $[A^-]$, and BEua is also corrected for the effect of free water and for changes in $[Cl^-]$. In one study of critically ill pediatric patients, BEua was more strongly associated with mortality than BE, lactate, or anion gap [27]. However, in this small study BEua was no better than the anion gap in the identification of elevated lactate concentrations [27]. Nevertheless, some believe that BEua is sufficiently sensitive and specific to flag small concentrations of unknown and otherwise unsuspected cations [26].

It is important to understand that a normal SBE can still conceal complex metabolic acid-base disturbances. The example given by Schlichtig et al. [1] is of an acute lactic acidosis superimposed on chronic lung disease with CO_2 retention and metabolic compensation. In this case [SID], originally elevated by the compensatory metabolic alkalosis, is subsequently reduced acutely to normal by an increased concentration of strong anions in the form of lactate. SBE can thus be normal, and the appearance on blood gas analysis one of a simple acute respiratory acidosis with a normal pH / pCO_2 equilibration curve. Here the truth can only be revealed by attention to history and examination, supplemented by the anion gap (which is likely to be elevated) and a measured plasma lactate.

In vivo evaluation of SBE

The meta-analysis by Schlichtig et al. [17] provided good evidence of in vivo CO_2 invariance. What is more difficult to demonstrate is the accuracy with which SBE tracks changes in whole-blood metabolic acid-base status in vivo. For example, is an isolated in vivo elevation of whole-blood lactate accurately reflected by the accompanying reduction in SBE? The question is simple to pose but difficult to answer, and the study has never been performed. More indirect evidence of the clinical utility of SBE is all that is available at present. Furthermore, in virtually all published in vivo studies, it is BE rather than SBE that has been evaluated. The difference between BE and SBE is usually quite small.

Some animal studies

In 1991, Davis et al. [28] bled 16 pigs to 40% of their blood volumes over 30 min, waited a further 30 min, then resuscitated the animals with crystalloid and blood. With the onset of hypovolemia, mean arterial pressure and mixed venous oxygen saturations decreased promptly and arterio-venous oxygen extraction increased, but all began to improve from compensatory homeostasis before resuscitation was commenced. BE decreased just as promptly, but improvement was delayed until volume replacement. The authors commented that BE was more reflective of the true volume deficit in compensated hypovolemic shock. In a related study, BE correlated significantly with arterial lactate concentrations ($R = 0.81$) [29].

Another report in 1991 came from Dunham et al. [30], who subjected 63 dogs to hemorrhagic shock titrated to predetermined oxygen debts. Baseline oxygen consumption was measured prior to controlled bleeding over 1 h to oxygen debts ranging from 60 ml/kg to 120 ml/kg. At 60 min there was no statistically significant difference in shed blood volumes among the groups, and neither blood pressure nor cardiac output discriminated well between the degrees of oxygen debt. However lactate and BE were both highly significant discriminators of oxygen debt, with BE having the highest explained variability. The fall in BE prior to resuscitation was almost twice the rise in plasma lactate, perhaps reflecting additional dysoxic metabolites.

Some clinical studies

In a retrospective analysis, it was possible using the admission BE to stratify 209 patients with blunt or penetrating trauma into groups with very similar initial mean arterial pressures, trauma scores, blood and total fluid requirements [31]. A decreasing BE was associated with ongoing hemorrhage in 65% of cases. Another retrospective review of 3,223 blunt trauma patients revealed the admission BE as the single most- important predictor of the need for laparotomy (odds ratio 6.2) [32]. The less-successful predictors were admission hypotension (odds ratio 5.1), chest injury (odds ratio 4.8), pelvic fracture (odds ratio 3.3) and pre-hospital hypotension (odds ratio 3.1). The authors recommended that in cases of blunt abdominal trauma, an admission BE of < -6.0 mmol/l should be considered an indication for diagnostic peritoneal lavage or abdominal computed tomography. In burns, the admission BE predicts resuscitation volume requirements, and when ≤ -6.0 mmol/l it portends a greatly increased mortality rate (9% versus 72%, $P < 0.001$) [33].

Siegel et al. [34] studied admission data from 185 consecutive patients with hepatic trauma. By linear logistic modeling, BE predicted death as successfully as the 24-h blood transfusion requirement, and better than arterial lactate, the Glasgow Coma Score, and the Injury Severity Score. A predictive model incorporating BE and the Glasgow Coma Score was then tested successfully against 323 additional patients with pelvic fracture as their index injury. In one recent study of general medical/surgical intensive care patients, the admission BE was strongly linked with mortality [35]. By combining the admission BE with the admission plasma lactate concentration, it was possible to predict mortality with a sensitivity of 80.3% and a specificity of 58.7%. Failure to improve BE significantly over 24 h in this population was an adverse prognostic factor. In shocked trauma patients, failure to increase BE to > -6 mmol/l in the first 24 h predicted an increased frequency of acute respiratory distress syndrome, multiple organ failure, and death [36]. There are other similar studies [37, 38].

In summary, SBE is a CO_2-invariant index of extracellular metabolic acid-base status. It is stoichiometric on in vitro evaluation. It is simple and user friendly. From studies in shock, trauma, and in intensive care patients in general, BE appears to have clinical meaning. It can be a guide to the overall severity of shock and trauma, and is closely related to oxygen debt in experimental hemorrhagic shock. It tracks elevated plasma lactate concentrations, and at times adds information to lactate analysis. BE may have some utility as a guide to resuscitation or even surgical intervention. Importantly, it is quite consistent with the physical-chemical analysis of acid-base status, and complements rather than antagonizes the Stewart approach.

References

1. Schlichtig R, Grogono AW, Severinghaus JW (1998) Current status of acid-base quantitation in physiology and medicine. Anesthesiol Clin North Am 16:211-233.
2. Schwartz WB, Relman AS (1963) A critique of the parameters used in the evaluation of acid-base disorders. N Engl J Med 268:1382-1388
3. Narins RB, Emmett M (1980) Simple and mixed acid-base disorders: a practical approach. Medicine (Baltimore) 59:161-187
4. Severinghaus JW (1993) Siggaard-Andersen and the "Great Trans-Atlantic Acid-Base Debate". Scand J Clin Lab Invest 53 [Suppl] 214:99-104
5. Stewart PA (1983) Modern quantitative acid-base chemistry. Can J Physiol Pharmacol 61:1444 -1461
6. Siggaard-Andersen O, Fogh-Andersen N (1995) Base excess or buffer base (strong ion difference) as measure of a non-respiratory acid-base disturbance. Acta Anesthesiol Scand 39 [Suppl]: 107, 123-128
7. Rossing TH, Maffeo N, Fencl V (1986) Acid-base effects of altering plasma protein concentration in human blood in vitro. J Appl Physiol:2260-2265
8. Singer RB, Hastings AB (1948) An improved clinical method for the estimation of disturbances of the acid-base balance of human blood. Medicine (Baltimore) 27:223-242
9. Figge J, Mydosh T, Fencl V (1992) Serum proteins and acid-base equilibria: a follow-up. J Lab Clin Med 120:713-719
10. Severinghaus JW (1986) AHA! In: Astrup P, Severinghaus JW (eds.) The history of blood gases, acids and bases. Munksgaard, Copenhagen, pp 264-276
11. Jørgensen K, Astrup P (1957) Standard bicarbonate, its clinical significance, and a new method for its determination. Scand J Clin Lab Invest 9:122
12. Siggaard-Andersen O, Fogh-Andersen N (1995) Base excess or buffer base (strong ion difference) as measure of a non-respiratory acid-base disturbance. Acta Anesthiesol Scand 39 [Suppl]: 107, 123-128
13. Siggaard-Andersen O, Engel K (1960) A micro method for determination of pH, carbon dioxide tension, base excess and standard bicarbonate in capillary blood. Scand J Clin Lab Invest 12: 172-176
14. Astrup P, Jorgensen K, Siggaard-Andersen O, et al (1960) Acid-base metabolism: new approach. Lancet 1: 1035-1039
15. Siggaard-Andersen O (1977) The Van Slyke equation. Scand J Clin Lab Invest 37 [Suppl 146]:15-20
16. Morgan TJ, Clark C, Endre ZH (2000) The accuracy of base excess – an *in vitro* evaluation of the Van Slyke equation. Crit Care Med 28:2932-2936.
17. Schlichtig R, Grogono AW, Severinghaus JW (1988) Human $PaCO_2$ and standard base excess compensation for acid-base imbalance. Crit Care Med 26:1173-1179
18. Scheingraber S, Rehm M, Sehmisch C, et al (1999) Rapid saline infusion produces hyperchloremic acidosis in patients undergoing gynecologic surgery. Anesthesiology 90:1265-1270
19. McFarlane C, Lee A (1994) A comparison of Plasmalyte 148 and 0.9% saline for intra-operative fluid replacement. Anaesthesia 49:779-781
20. Prough DS, Bidani A (1999) Hyperchloremic metabolic acidosis is a predictable consequence of intraoperative infusion of 0.9% saline. Anesthesiology 90:1247-1249
21. Worthley LIG (1997) Acid-base balance and disorders In: Oh TE (ed.) Intensive care manual. Butterworth-Heinemann, Oxford, pp 689-699
22. Iberti TJ, Leibowitz AB, Papadakos PJ, et al (1991) Low sensitivity of the anion gap as a screen to detect hyperlactemia in critically ill patients. Crit Care Med 19:130-131
23. Salem MM, Mujais SK (1992) Gaps in the anion gap. Arch Intern Med 152:1625-1629
24. Fencl V, Jabor A, Kazda A, et al (2000) Diagnosis of metabolic acid-base disturbances in critically ill patients. Am J Respir Crit Care Med 162:2246-2251

25. Kellum JA, Kramer DJ, Pinsky MR (1995) Strong ion gap: a methodology for exploring unexplained anions. J Crit Care 10:51-55
26. Gilfix BM, Bique M, Magder S (1993) A physical chemical approach to the analysis of acid-base balance in the clinical setting. J Crit Care 8:187-197
27. Balasubramanyan N, Havens PL, Hoffman GM (1999) Unmeasured anions identified by the Fencl-Stewart method predict mortality better than base excess, anion gap, and lactate in patients in the pediatric intensive care unit. Crit Care Med 27:1577-1581
28. Davis JW, Shackford SR, Holbrook TL (1991) Base deficit as a sensitive indicator of compensated shock and tissue oxygen utilization. Surg Gynecol Obstet 173:473-476
29. Davis JW (1994) The relationship of base deficit to lactate in porcine hemorrhagic shock and resuscitation. J Trauma 36:168-172
30. Dunham CM, Siegel JH, Weireter L, et al (1991) Oxygen debt and metabolic acidemia as quantitative predictors of mortality and the severity of the ischemic insult in hemorrhagic shock. Crit Care Med 19:231-243
31. Davis JW, Shackford SR, Mackersie RC, et al (1988) Base deficit as a guide to volume resuscitation. J Trauma 28:1464-1467
32. Davis JW, Mackersie RC, Holbrook TL, et al (1991) Base deficit as an indicator of significant abdominal injury. Ann Emerg Med 20:842-844
33. Kaups KL, Davis JW, Dominic WJ (1998) Base deficit as an indicator of resuscitation needs in patients with burn injuries. J Burn Care Rehabil 19:346-348
34. Siegel JH, Rivkind AI, Dalal S, et al (1990) Early physiologic predictors of injury severity and death in blunt multiple trauma. Arch Surg 125:498-508
35. Smith I, Kumar P, Molloy S, et al (2001) Base excess and lactate as prognostic indicators for patients admitted to intensive care. Intensive Care Med 27:74-83
36. Davis JW, Kaups KL, Parks SN (1998) Base deficit is superior to pH in evaluating clearance of acidosis after traumatic shock. J Trauma 44:114-118
37. Davis JW, Parks SN, Kaups KL, et al (1996) Admission base deficit predicts transfusion requirements and risk of complications. J Trauma 41:769-774
38. Davis JW, Kaups KL (1998) Base deficit in the elderly: a marker of severe injury and death. J Trauma 45:873-877

Intraoperative Fluid Management

M. Rehm, U. Finsterer

In the perioperative period, large volumes of intravenous infusions (crystalloids and colloids) are often administered to compensate for major surgical blood losses. The occurrence of metabolic acidosis due to administered intravenous infusion solutions has been known since at least the 1940s [1, 2]. To date, however, there is an ongoing controversy about the causes for this acidosis. Advocates of the 'classical' approach, according to Siggaard-Andersen [3], favor the dilution hypothesis, which was originally proposed by Peters and van Slyke in 1946 [2]. This implies the dilution of the entire extracellular volume (ECV) with different electrolyte solutions that are free of bicarbonate. Since 1983, however, an alternative approach can be used to explain this form of a metabolic acidosis [4]. Stewart's quantitative approach [4], which is discussed in detail elsewhere [5], defines $paCO_2$, strong ion difference (SID), and the sum of all anionic charges of weak plasma acids ($[A_{TOT}]$) as independent pH-regulating variables, whereas pH and bicarbonate (Bic) are dependent variables [4]. Stewart's algorithms explain that a decrease in SID or an increase in $[Prot^-]$ will result in a decrease in pH (and vice versa) [4]. Recently, this approach has received much attention mainly because it explains the whole mystery of acid-base chemistry in a relatively simple quantitative manner [6-15]. Advocates of the Stewart approach argue that the reason for a metabolic acidosis after the administration of intravenous infusions is not the dilution of Bic but the infusion of strong anions. In the following section, data of two studies from our laboratory that were published recently are presented and reviewed in the light of the 'classical' Henderson-Hasselbalch approach and the 'modern' Stewart approach. Scheingraber et al. [16] (study 1) investigated acid-base changes during the intraoperative administration of colloid-free *crystalloid solutions* (0.9% saline or lactated Ringer's solution) in 24 patients undergoing major gynecological surgery. The effects of colloid infusions on acid-base equilibrium were evaluated by a randomized prospective study by Rehm et al. [17] (study 2), in which 5% albumin solution or 6% hetastarch solution were used for preoperative acute normovolemic hemodilution in 20 patients before major gynecological surgery.

In study 1, 24 female patients without apparent cardiac, pulmonary, or renal diseases (ASA class I or II) scheduled for elective gynecological lower abdominal surgery were studied. During study 1, no patient received colloids, plasma products, or blood transfusions. The patients were randomly assigned to receive either 0.9% saline (*saline group* N=12) or lactated Ringer's solution (*Ringer's group* N=12). The saline solution used contained 154 mmol/l of sodium and 154 mmol/l of chloride, the lactated Ringer's solution contained 130 mmol/l of sodium, 5.4 mmol/l of potassium, 1.8 mmol/l of calcium, 112 mmol/l of chloride, and 27 mmol/l of lactate.

After the induction of general anesthesia, mechanical ventilation was performed to maintain paO_2 at 250 - 300 mmHg and $paCO_2$ as close as possible to 40 mmHg. Under stable anesthetic conditions and at the time of surgical incision, the investigation was started and arterial blood was withdrawn to measure baseline values (= 0 min). The samples were analyzed for paO_2, pH, $paCO_2$ (standard electrodes), the concentrations of serum sodium $[Na^+]$, potassium $[K^+]$, chloride $[Cl^-]$ (ion-selective electrodes), and serum lactate $[Lac^-]$ (enzymatic method, quantification of H_2O_2), all integrated in a Radiometer analyzer (Radiometer ABL 620 GL, Radiometer Company, Copenhagen, Denmark). Additionally, serum total protein concentration was determined using the Biuret method. Subsequent to the baseline blood samples crystalloid infusion (0.9% saline vs. lactated Ringer's solution) was started. A common infusion device was used and the infusion rate was 30 ml/kg per hour in both groups. Every 30 min, new blood samples were taken, urine production was measured, and blood loss was estimated.

For each sample *strong ion difference* was calculated as: $SID = [Na^+] + [K^+] - [Cl^-] - [Lac^-]$. *The amount of weak plasma acid* $[Prot^-]$ was calculated as the product of serum total protein concentration (g/l) and the empirically derived factor 0.243 according to Van Slyke et al. [18]. Serum bicarbonate concentration $[Bic_{HH}]$ and base excess $[BE_{HH}]$ were taken from the blood gas analyzer, which uses the Henderson-Hasselbalch equation and the Siggaard-Andersen formula [3]. Additionally, serum bicarbonate concentration $[Bic_S]$ was calculated as the difference between SID and $[Prot^-]$ using the Stewart model.

As all measured and calculated data described above were normally distributed (tested by Kolmogorov-Smirnov tests), they are presented as mean values with standard deviations. For demographic data, T-tests for unpaired data were performed. Two-way repeated measures analysis of variance was performed comparing intragroup and intergroup differences at 30, 60, 90, and 120 min of crystalloid infusion with 0 min. Post hoc testing was performed by the Student-Newman-Keuls method for multiple comparisons. A p value of 0.05 was considered to be statistically significant.

Table 1. Patients characteristics (study 1)

Mean and standard deviation (SD). Intergroup differences are indicated (* $P < 0.05$.)

	Saline group (N=12)		Ringer group (N=12)	
		SD		SD
Age	46	14	53	5
Height (cm)	165	7.0	165	8.0
Weight (kg)	68	13	77	20
Body surface area (m²)	1.79.	0.20	1.89.	0.28
Crystalloid infusion after 120 min (ml/m²)	2,714	521	2,653	589
Estimated blood loss (ml)	962	332	704.	447
Urine production (ml)	717	459	1,075	799

Table 1 shows the demographic data, the volume of crystalloid infusion, estimated blood loss, and urine production after 120 min for both groups. There were no significant differences between both groups with respect to the volume of crystalloid infusion, estimated blood loss, and urine production, respectively, 120 min after the start of infusion. Hemoglobin concentration decreased from about 12 to 9 g/dl in both groups.

In Fig. 1, $paCO_2$, pH, $[Lac^-]$, $[BE_{HH}]$, $[Cl^-]$, and $[Na^+]$, as well as $[Prot^-]$, and SID are shown at the various points described above. In both groups, $paCO_2$ did not show major deviations from 40 mmHg. During the infusion of the crystalloid solution, there was a significant decrease in pH from 7.41 to 7.28 in the saline group. No major pH changes were observed in the Ringer's group. In the saline group, starting from a low level of 0.6 mmol/l, $[Lac^-]$ decreased to a mean of 0.4 mmol/l. During the infusion of lactated Ringer's solution, $[Lac^-]$ slightly rose to about 2 mmol/l. In the saline group, starting from a control value of -0.4 mmol/l, $[BE_{HH}]$ decreased to -6.7 mmol/l at 120 min. There were no major changes of $[BE_{HH}]$ in the Ringer's group. $[Cl^-]$ increased in both groups, but this increase was by far larger with 0.9% saline solution. Mean increase in $[Cl^-]$ during the administration of 0.9% saline was 11 mmol/l. Only a slight but significant increase in $[Cl^-]$ from 104 to 106 mmo/l was observed in the Ringer's group. The infusion of 0.9% saline solution led to a slow and continuous increase in $[Na^+]$. There was a slight but significant decrease in $[Na^+]$ in the Ringer's group, in which the infused solution contained only 130 mmol/l of Na^+. $[K^+]$ (not illustrated) was kept at a level of about 4 mmol/l by substituting K^+ as needed and did not show any intra- and intergroup differences.

Due to the dilution with crystalloids and surgical bleeding, serum total protein concentration decreased in both groups from a mean of about 6.2 to 4.3 g/dl and $[Prot^-]$ decreased from about 15 to 11mmol/l. SID initially decreased in both groups. With continuous 0.9 % saline infusion there was a significantly larger decrease to about 30 mmol/l than with lactated Ringer's solution.

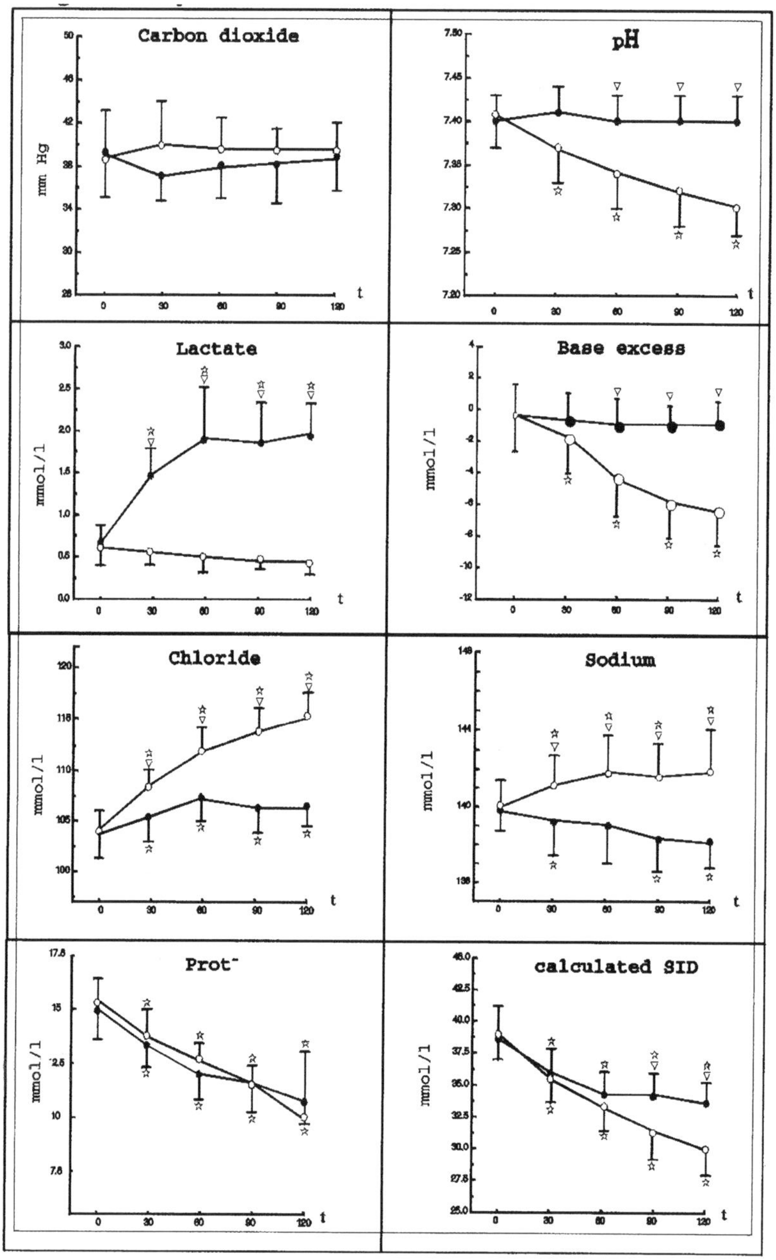

Fig. 1. Study 1. Measured and calculated values (mean±standard deviation) at the different measuring points. Saline group = white dots; Ringer's group = black dots.
☆ intragroup differences $P<0.05$; ∇ intergroup differences $P<0.05$. Modified according to Scheingraber et al. [16] (SID = strong ion difference)

The main finding of study 1 was a rather impressive, predictable, and dose-dependent acidosis (7.41 to 7.28) after a relatively brief interval (2 h) of 0.9% saline infusion, but not after lactated Ringer's solution infusion, at rates of about 30 ml/kg per hour under anesthesia and surgery. The conventional Henderson-Hasselbalch or Siggaard-Andersen approach [3] would indicate that in the saline group metabolic acidosis occurred due to constant $paCO_2$ and decreasing $[Bic_{HH}]$ and $[BE_{HH}]$, whereas in the Ringer's group the acid-base balance was largely unchanged. According to this "classical approach", the reason for the metabolic acidosis in the saline group should be the dilution of bicarbonate in the ECV, with concomitant hyperchloremia due to the infusion of a bicarbonate-free crystalloid solution that contains a high Cl^- concentration. In the Ringer's group, the infusion of a bicarbonate "precursor" in the form of lactate should explain the almost-constant $[Bic_{HH}]$ and pH.

Fig. 2 illustrates changes in $[Bic_{HH}]$ and $[Bic_S]$, and therefore in pH, in the context of SID and $[Prot^-]$ according to the Stewart model. Variables in Fig. 2 were calculated using mean values of the two groups after 120 min of crystalloid infusion compared with the corresponding baseline values. It should be noted that $[Bic_{HH}]$ was the result of the Henderson-Hasselbalch equation and $[Bic_S]$ was a function of $SID = [Na^+] + [K^+] - [Cl^-] - [Lac^-]$ and $[Prot^-]$. Under 0.9% saline infusion, changes in serum bicarbonate concentration were accompanied by a profound decrease in SID of about 9 mmol/l, and were probably attenuated by a simultaneous decrease in $[Prot^-]$. In the Ringer's group, SID and $[Prot^-]$ decreased almost by the same amount, and serum bicarbonate concentration was virtually unchanged under crystalloid infusion. As a result, in both groups the Stewart approach could explain sufficiently the changes in Bic in the context of changing SID and $[Prot^-]$.

In order to evaluate the changes in acid-base homeostasis during the infusion of almost isooncotic, bicarbonate-free colloid solutions, study 2 was performed. In this study, we used 5% albumin solution and 6% hydroxyethylstarch (HES) solution during acute preoperative normovolemic hemodilution (ANH). According to the Stewart model [4], two components will determine acid-base changes during the course of ANH: firstly, changes in cations and anions, the distribution space of which is the ECV, and, secondly, changes in the concentration of plasma proteins. Infusion solutions free of bicarbonate but containing high Cl- concentrations may lead to a dilution of the ECV and a change in SID. Additionally, using two different colloid solutions - one containing albumin at a supraphysiological concentration and one free of albumin - will produce reverse changes in plasma albumin concentration. Consequently, if colloid solutions are used, two different compartments, namely ECV, i.e., the distribution space of small ions, and plasma

Fig. 2 Study 1. Changes of serum bicarbonate concentration using the Henderson-Hasselblach equation [BicHH] or Stewart's formulae [BicS] and of SID and [Prot⁻] after 120 min of infusing 0.9% saline or Ringer's lactate
Modified according to Scheingraber et al. [16]

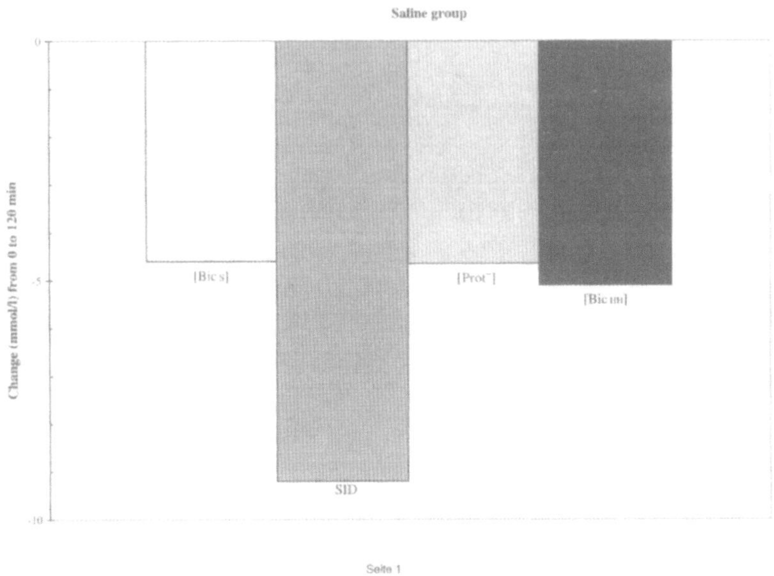

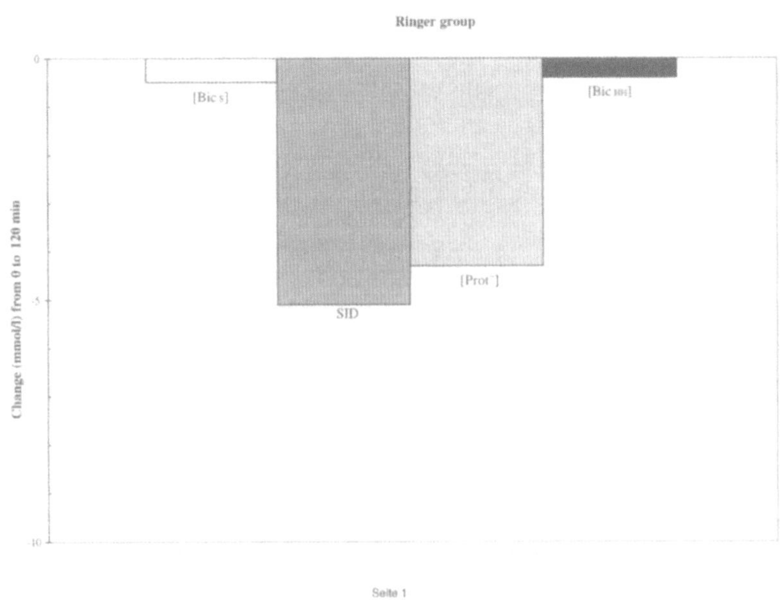

volume,i.e., the distribution space of colloids, have to be considered separately.

In study 2 we studied 20 female patients without apparent cardiac, pulmonary, or renal diseases (ASA class II) scheduled for radical hysterectomy due to cancer of the cervix. The patients were randomly assigned to receive either 6% HES (HES group, N=10) or 5% albumin solution (HA group, N=10). The HES solution contained 154 mmol/l of Na^+ and 154 mmol/l of Cl^- (pH 5.44, Fresenius, Bad Homburg, Germany) and the HA solution contained 158 mmol/l of Na^+ and 150 mmol/l of Cl^-, 4 mmol/l of octanoate, and 4 mmol/l of n_l-acetyltryptophanate (pH 6.86, Centeon Pharma, Marburg, Germany). Neither solution contained bicarbonate or citrate. After the induction of general anesthesia, mechanical ventilation was performed to maintain paO_2 at 250 - 300 mmHg and $paCO_2$ as close as possible to 40 mmHg. All measurements were taken before starting surgery during periods of stable anesthesia and hemodynamics. Before ANH, no intravenous infusions, and during ANH no crystalloids, were administered. Arterial blood samples were analyzed for the same variables using the same Radiometer analyzer as in study 1. Additionally, serum phosphate ($[PO_4]$, ultraviolet photometry of a phosphomolybdate complex), serum total protein concentration (Biuret method), and albumin concentration (colorimetry of bromocresol complex) were measured from the same blood samples. In contrast to study 1, the amount of weak plasma acid $[Prot^-]$ was calculated with the aid of a computer program developed by Figge et al. [19]. Standard serum bicarbonate concentration $[Bic_{HH}]$ and standard base excess $[BE_{HH}]$ were taken from the blood gas analyzer.

After baseline measurements, blood was removed at a rate of about 60 ml/min and was simultaneously replaced with 5% albumin solution (HA) or 6% HES at nearly the same rate as the blood was removed. After the completion of ANH and a steady-state interval of 20 min without any further infusions and before starting surgery, measurements of all variables were performed in the same way as before ANH. The predicted change in $[Bic_S]$ during ANH according to the Stewart approach [4] was calculated as: predicted change in $[Bic_S]$ = change in SID – change in $[Prot^-]$.

As all measured and calculated data described above were normally distributed (tested by Kolmogorov-Smirnov tests), they are presented as mean values with standard deviations. For demographic data, t-tests for unpaired data were performed. t-tests for paired or unpaired samples were performed as appropriate to compare intragroup and intergroup differences before and after ANH. A p value of 0.05 for intergroup differences before ANH and a value of 0.002 for intergroup differences after ANH and intragroup differences (with adjustment according to Bonferroni 0.05/25) for acid-base variables were considered to be statistically significant.

Table 2. Study 2 Patients' characteristics, amount of blood and plasma removed, and colloid supply during acute preoperative normovolemic hemodilution (ANH). Mean and standard deviation. Intergroup differences are indicated. (HES = hydroxyethyl starch, HA = human albumin)

	HES group (N=10)	HA group (N=10)
Age	39±8	46±8
Height (cm)	166±7	165±3
Weight (kg)	62±13	72±17
Body surface area (m²)	1.70±0.18	1.82.±0.21
Blood removed (ml)	1,269±217	1,579±228*
Plasma removed (ml)	863±158	1,050.±173*
Colloid infused (ml)	1,469±246	1,831±271*

* P< 0.05 difference between groups

There were no significant differences in weight, height, and body surface area (BSA) (Table 2). Due to slightly higher preoperative BSA and hematocrit values in the HA group, the amount of blood removed and colloid infused was significantly higher than in the HES group.

Table 3. Study 2 Measured and calculated values of acid-base balance, electrolyte, and protein (mean ±SD) (SID = strong ion difference)

	Before ANH	After ANH
	HES group	
pH	7.384±0.027	7.335±0.028*
Carbon dioxide (mmHg)	40.1 ±2.8	41.7±2.2
Actual bicarbonate (mmol/l)	23.6 ±1.0	21.6±1.2*
Standard base excess (mmol/l)	-0.9±1.3	-3,4±1.4*
Lactate (mmol/l)	0.6±0.1	0.5±0.1*
Sodium (mmol/l)	140 ±1.5	140±1.5.
Chloride (mmol/l)	105±1.7	111±2.3*
Potassium (mmol/l)	3.4±0.2.	3.4±0.2
SID (mmol/l)	37.0±1.2	31.7±1.8*
Prot⁻ (mmol/l)	11.5±1.2	6.5±0.7*
Phosphate (mmol/l)	1.2±0.2	1.2±0.2
Calcium (mmol/l)	1.1±0.1	1.0±0.1
Anion gap (mmol/l)	13.9±1.0	10.4±1.3*
	HA group	
pH	7.394±0.028	7.336*±0.032*
Carbon dioxide (mmHg)	38.6 ±3.0	40.2±3.2
Actual bicarbonate (mmol/l)	23.1 ±1.3	20.8±0.9*
Standard base excess (mmol/l)	-1,1 ±1.4	-4,0±1.0*
Lactate (mmol/l)	0.8±0.2	0.6±0.2*
Sodium (mmol/l)	141 ±1.5	142±1.5*,**
Chloride (mmol/l)	106±2.9	109±2.9*,**
Potassium (mmol/l)	3.4±0.3	3.3±0.2
SID (mmol/l)	37.3±2.2	35.7±1.7*,**
Prot⁻ (mmol/l)	11.5 ±1.1	12.8±0.9*,**
Phosphate (mmol/l)	1.1±0.1	1.2±0.1
Calcium (mmol/l)	1.0±0.1	1.0±0.1
Anion gap (mmol/l)	15.0 ±1.6	15.6±1.9*,**

* P <0.05 intragroup difference with respect to value; before ANH; ** P < 0.05 difference beween groups

In Table 3, pH, $paCO_2$, [Bic], [BE], [Lac^-], [Na^+], [Cl^-], [K^+], SID, [$Prot^-$], [PO_4], [Ca^{2+}], and the anion gap before and after ANH are shown. At baseline measurements, there were no differences in all of these variables between groups. In both groups, there was a significant decrease in pH from about 7.39 to 7.34, and $paCO_2$ did not show major deviations from 40mmHg. In the HES group, starting from respective baseline values of 23.6 and –0.9mmol/l, [Bic] and [BE] significantly decreased to 21.6 and –3.4 mmol/l, after ANH. A [Bic] value of 23.6 and a [BE] value of –1.1mmol/l before ANH significantly decreased to 21.0 and –4.0mmol/l, respectively, after ANH in the HA group. [Lac^-] did not change in either group. There were no relevant changes in [Na^+] and [K^+], whereas [Cl^-] significantly increased in both groups during ANH. This increase was larger after the administration of HES (+6 mmol/l) than after HA (+3 mmol/l). SID decreased by a mean of 5.3 mmol/l in the HES group, and did not change significantly in the HA group (-1.6 mmol/l). Due to the dilution with an albumin-free solution, [$Prot^-$] decreased by about 5 mmol/l in the HES group, in contrast to the HA group where it increased slightly but significantly during ANH. [Ca^{2+}] and [PO_4] remained fairly constant and did not show any relevant differences within or between groups. The anion gap significantly decreased in the HES group, whereas it did not significantly change in the HA group. After ANH, significant intergroup differences were found for SID, [$Prot^-$], and the anion gap.

The main finding of study 2 was a slight but significant metabolic acidosis after ANH, both with the albumin solution and the HES solution. Advocates of the classical Henderson-Hasselbalch approach could argue again that the measured changes in [Bic] and pH in both groups were simply caused by the dilution of ECV with bicarbonate-free solutions. This "dilution hypothesis" takes electrolyte concentrations in plasma volume and ECV (which should be similar), such as bicarbonate or chloride, and the amount of water in ECV into account. However, the effect of changes in plasma albumin concentration on acid-base equilibrium is not represented in this theory. The comparison between measured changes in [Bic_{HH}] and predicted changes in [Bic_S] according to the Stewart approach which were derived from the changes in SID and [$Prot^-$] during ANH are illustrated separately for both groups in Fig. 3. In the HA group, [$Prot^-$] increased and SID decreased slightly by about 1.5 mmol/l each, so that the measured decrease in [Bic_{HH}] by a mean of 2.5 mmol/l was in good agreement with the predicted decrease in [Bic_S], according to the Stewart equations. In contrast, both SID and [$Prot^-$] decreased by about 5 mmol/l in the HES group so that the measured decrease in [Bic_{HH}] by a mean of 2.5 mmol/l could not be explained adequately. This discrepancy between the predicted constancy in [Bic_S] during ANH in the HES group, according to the Stewart approach, and the measured decrease in [Bic_{HH}] (Fig. 3) could lead to the assumption that in this group the Stewart approach fails. The main link between the Stewart approach and the "dilution hypothesis" is found in the changes in SID. SID depends on the dilution of the respective cations and anions in ECV. However, if HES is used as a volume substitute, a second (smaller) compartment, namely plasma volume, has to be considered. The large decrease in [$Prot^-$] after the infusion of an artificial colloid free of albumin should be independent of and disproportional to the dilution of ECV. This is different from the infusion of crystalloid solutions (as in study 2), where the decrease in [$Prot^-$] should be proportional to the dilution of ECV. Another explanation for the discrepancy between [Bic_S] and [Bic_{HH}] during ANH in the HES group could be the occurrence of some unmeasured negative charges during the elimination or splitting of HES molecules. Consequently, the value of [$Prot^-$] after ANH with HES was possibly too small, as the respective calculation by the program of Figge et al. [19] is only based on the serum albumin concentration.

In conclusion, study 1 and 2 demonstrated that after the infusion of both crystalloid and colloid solutions a metabolic acidosis is the result of changes in SID and [$Prot^-$]. Mainly the changes in SID determine the changes in pH during the infusion of crystalloid solutions. The hypothesis that especially in case of crystalloid infusions Stewart's theory probably reflects the complete pathophysiological background of the described changes in acid-base chemistry suggests itself. With colloid infusions, especially if artificial colloids are used, the different distribution volumes of colloids (plasma volume) and of electrolytes (the entire ECV) and the possible occurrence of some unmeasured negative charges additional to those on the albumin molecule should be considered if Stewart's algorithms are used to explain the respective changes in acid-base equilibrium.

Fig. 3. Study 2. Changes of serum bicarbonate concentration using the Henderson-Hasselbalch equation [Bic_{HH}] or Stewart's formulae [Bic_S] and of SID and [$Prot^-$] after ANH with 6% hydroxyethylstarch (HES) and 5% albumin (HA) solution)

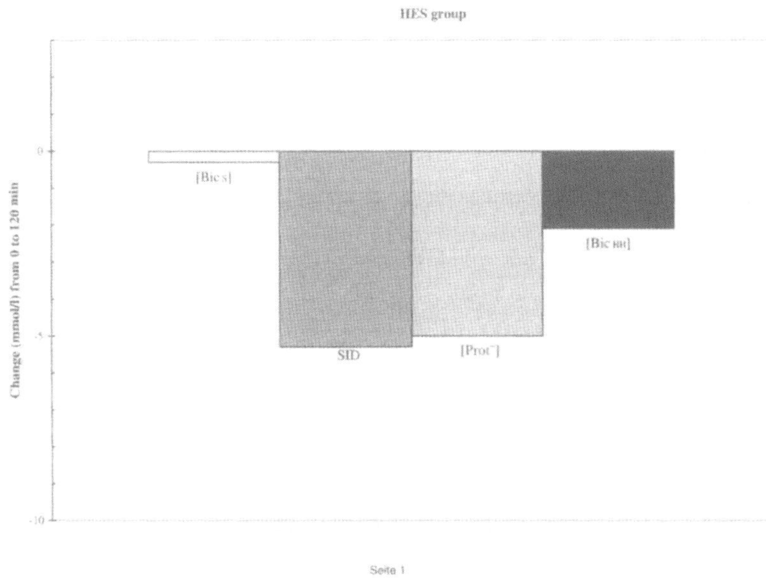

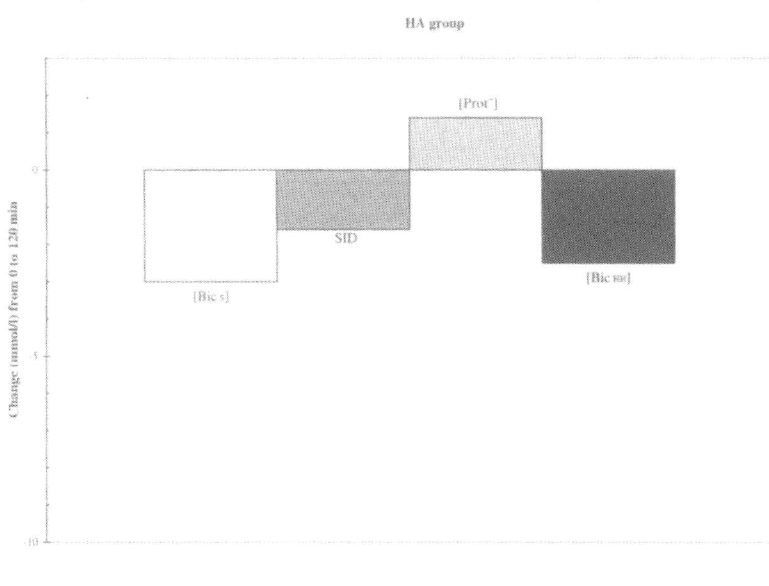

References

1. Shires GT, Holman J (1948) Dilution acidosis. Ann Intern Med 28:557-559
2. Peters J, van Slyke DD (1946) Quantitative clinical chemistry: Interpretations. Vol I, 1st edn. Williams and Wilkins, Baltimore
3. Sigaard-Andersen O (1976) The acid-base status of the blood, 4th edn. Williams and Wilkins, Baltimore
4. Stewart PA (1983) Modern quantitative acid-base chemistry. Can J Physiol Pharmacol 61:1444-1461
5. Fencl V, Leith DE (1993) Stewart's quantitative acid-base chemistry: applications in biology and medicine. Respir Physiol 91:1-16
6. Bellomo R, Ronco C (1999) New paradigms in acid-base physiology. Curr Opin Crit Care 5:427-428
7. Kellum JA (1999) Acid-base physiology in the post-Copernican era. Curr Opin Crit Care 5:429-435
8. Story DA, Bellomo R (1999) The acid-base physiology of crystalloid solutions. Curr Opin Crit Care 5:436-439
9. Liskaser, Story DA (1999) The acid-base physiology of colloid solutions. Curr Opin Crit Care 5:440-442
10. Tan HK, Bellomo R (1999) The effect of continuous hemofiltration on acid-base physiology. Curr Opin Crit Care 5:443-447
11. Feriani M, Dell'Aquila R, Ronco C, La Greca G (1999) The acid-base effects of peritoneal dialysis. Curr Opin Crit Care 5:448-451
12. Bellomo R, Ronco C (1999) The pathogenesis of lactic acidosis in sepsis. Curr Opin Crit Care 5:452-457
13. Kaplan LJ, Bailey H, Kellum J (1999) The etiology and significance of metabolic acidosis in trauma patients. Curr Opin Crit Care 5:458-463
14. Hayhoe M, Bellomo R (1999) The pathogenesis of acid-base changes during cardiopulmonary bypass. Curr Opin Crit Care 5:464-467
15. Leblanc M (1999) The acid-base effects of acute hemodialysis. Curr Opin Crit Care 5:468-478
16. Scheingraber S, Rehm M, Sehmisch C, Finsterer U (1999) Rapid saline infusion produces hyperchloremic acidosis in patients undergoing gynecologic surgery. Anesthesiology 90:1265--1270
17. Rehm M, Orth V, Scheingraber S, et al (2000) Acid-base changes caused by 5% albumin versus 6% hydroxyethylstarch solution in patients undergoing acute normovolemic hemodilution. Anesthesiology 93:1174-1183
18. Van Slyke DD, Hastings AB, Hiller A, Sendroy J (1928) Studies of gas and electrolyte equibrilia in blood. XIV. Amount of alkali bound by serum albumin and globulin. J Biol Chem 79:769-780

[illegible] J, Mydosh T, Fencl V (1992) Serum proteins and acid-base equilibria: a follow-up. J Lab Clin Med 120:713-719

Fluid Management in Gastrointestinal Surgery

M. G. Mythen, M. Hamilton, M. Grocott

Major gastrointestinal (GI) surgery is high risk, producing significant physiological disturbance in patients who are often frail prior to surgery. It is associated with considerable morbidity and mortality [1, 2]. Fluid therapy is a fundamental part of the management of the high-risk surgical patient [3]. Detailed knowledge of the pharmacology of the available intravenous solutions should guide their use. It is now clear that differentiation between the properties of the carrier solution and the dissolved colloid is of fundamental importance. Preoperative risk assessment should lead to institution of adequate perioperative monitoring to guide fluid therapy and allocation of an appropriate level of postoperative care, which in many cases will be in a dedicated critical care facility. Fluid therapy should be titrated to rational, physiological endpoints and not dictated by a recipe. Pro-active "optimization" of intravascular volume and organ blood flow has been shown to improve outcome. A "big picture" look at the available literature suggests that the "when" and "how much" of fluid therapy are far more important than the "what".

The challenge of perioperative fluid balance in GI surgery

Our basic understanding of fluid flux is that hydrostatic and osmotic forces dictate movement of fluid between the different compartments of the body across semi-permeable membranes. In health the balance of osmotic and hydrostatic forces results in a net pressure gradient from capillary lumen to interstitium, and this results in a constant fluid flow that is drained by the lymphatics. The osmotic pressure generated by a solute is proportional to the number of molecules or ions of solute and their charge characteristics. Solutes that can pass freely across a semi-permeable membrane do not generate any osmotic pressure. Capillary walls are made up of endothelial cells, which are freely permeable to small ions (Na^+ and Cl^-), but are relatively impermeable to larger molecules such as colloids (e.g., albumin and starches). The cell membrane is effectively impermeable to Na^+ and Cl^- ions due to the presence of the energy-dependent Na^+/K^+ pump. The composition of administered fluids should therefore dictate their distribution (Fig. 1). The vast majority of body water is intracellular (approximately 30 l) and the minority (about 5 l) is in the intravascular space [3].

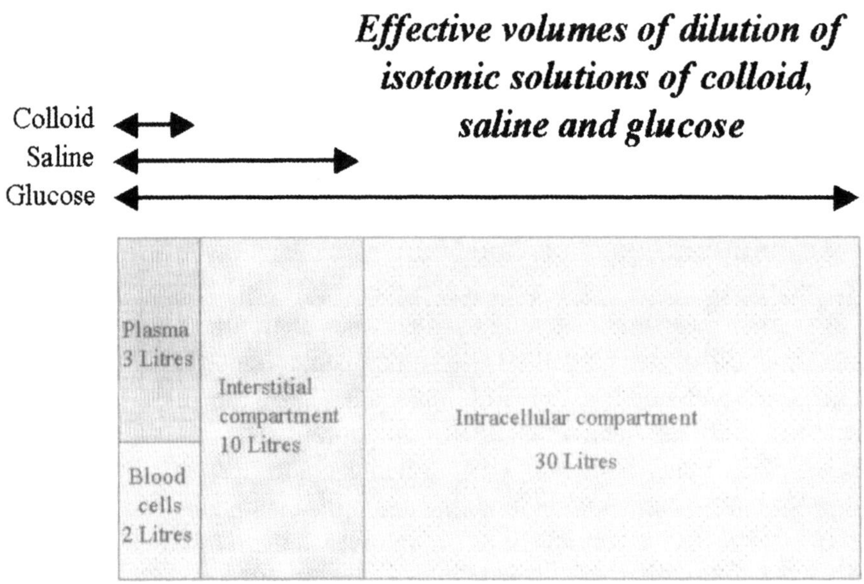

Fig.1. Simplified theoretical model of body water and volumes of distribution of infused isotonic solutions of an ideal colloid, balanced salt, and glucose

Major GI surgery perturbs the simplistic model of fluid distribution shown in Fig. 1. Preoperatively patients undergoing GI surgery may be grossly water and solute depleted due to decreased intake, e.g., preoperative fasting, and increased losses, e.g., bowel preparation. During the operation, fluid balance is disturbed by both anesthesia and the surgical procedure. Intravenous and inhalation anesthetic agents commonly produce relative hypovolemia as a result of vasodilation, and depress myocardial function, thus reducing cardiac output. Surgical losses include blood loss through hemorrhage, evaporative losses from exposed mucosal surfaces, and third-space losses from peritoneal exudation that may continue for many hours following intra-abdominal surgery [4]. In addition pro-inflammatory insults, including surgical trauma and the bacteremia, endotoxemia, and cytokinemia that often result from bowel injury, can lead to a systemic inflammatory response syndrome with increased endothelial permeability and loss of intravascular fluid into the interstitium [5,6].

Perioperative replacement of fluid losses and normo- and hypervolemic plasma expansion to maintain tissue perfusion should be a routine part of the perioperative care of the major GI surgical patient. The complex interplay of the various factors discussed produces a clinical situation in which maintaining a normal physiological milieu becomes a major fluid balance challenge. Invasive pressure monitoring and cardiac output/blood flow/perfusion monitoring may helpful in achieving this goal.

Choice of intravenous fluid

This section aims to briefly review the types of intravenous fluids available for use in clinical practice. Transfusion of red cells and other blood products, and the use of hyperosmolar and hyperoncotic solutions will not be considered here but are extensively reviewed elsewhere [3, 7, 8].

Crystalloid Solutions

Crystalloid is the term commonly used to refer to solutions in water of inorganic ions and small organic molecules used for intravenous therapy. They are either glucose or sodium chloride (saline) based, and may be isotonic, hypotonic, or hypertonic. In addition potassium, calcium, and lactate are common constituents added to make the composition of the intravenous fluid closer to that of plasma (Table 1). A 1- litre infusion of so-called normal (0.9%) saline will result in less than 250 ml expansion of the circulating volume and a significant expansion of the extracellular volume [3]. Large-volume crystalloid resuscitation is associated with significant tissue, and in particular, bowel edema. There is also a growing body of evidence suggesting that large-volume crystalloid replacement of blood loss during major surgery may result in a delay in the recovery of postoperative GI tract function (T.J. Gan, Duke University, N.C., USA and E. Bennett-Guerrero, Columbia University, N.Y., USA; personal communications).

Colloid solutions

A colloid is a homogeneous non-crystalline substance consisting of large molecules or ultramicroscopic particles of one substance dispersed through a second substance – the particles do not settle and cannot be separated out by ordinary filtering or centrifuging like those of a suspension such as blood.

Table 1. Comparison of contents, osmolarity, and pH of crystalloid solutions for intravenous administration

Solution	**Osmolarity** mosmol L-1	**PH**	**Na^+** mmol L^{-1}	**Cl^-** mmol L^{-1}	**K^+** mmol L^{-1}	**Ca^{2+}** mmol L^{-1}	**Glucose** mg L^{-1}	**HCO_3^-** mmol L^{-1}	**Lactate** mmol L^{-1}	**Energy** Kcal L^{-1}
Glucose 5%	252		-	-	-	-	50	-	-	400
Glucose 25%	1260		-	-	-	-	250	-	-	2000
Glucose 50%	2520		-	-	-	-	500	-	-	4000
Sodium Chloride 0.9%	300	5.0	154.0	154.0	-	-	-	-	-	-
Sodium Chloride and Glucose	262		30.0	30.0	-	-	40	-	-	320
Ringer's solution	309		147.0	156.0	4.0	2.2	-	-	-	-
Compound Sodium Lactate*	278		131.0	111.0	5.0	2.0	-	-	29.0	-
Plasmlyte B	298.5	5.5	140	98	5	-	-	50	-	-

* Compound sodium lactate = Hartmann's solution or Ringer's Lactate solution

Human albumin solutions, plasma protein fraction, and fresh-frozen plasma are all human plasma derivatives that are colloid solutions. There are three principle types of semisynthetic colloid molecule commonly used in intravenous solutions – gelatins, dextrans, and starches. All colloids are presented dissolved in a crystalloid solution. Isotonic saline is the most commonly used carrier solution, but isotonic or hypertonic glucose, hypertonic saline and isotonic balanced electrolyte solutions are also used [3]. Colloid osmotic pressure is the osmotic pressure exerted by the macromolecules (the colloid molecules). This can be measured using a membrane transducer system in which the membrane is freely permeable to small ions and water, but largely impermeable to the colloid molecules. The pharmacology of the various colloids is exhaustively covered elsewhere [3, 7, 8]. The following paragraphs provide a summary review.

Human albumin solution is the predominant free intravascular macromolecule in humans and contributes about 75% of the plasma colloid osmotic pressure. It is a monodisperse protein colloid of around 68,000 daltons. Albumin passes across from the intravascular space into the interstitium relatively easily and is continuously circulated via the tissues and the lymphatics back into the systemic circulation [3, 7, 8].

Gelatins are prepared from hydrolyzed bovine collagen. Succinylated gelatin (Gelofusine) is prepared by enzymatic modification of the source gelatin peptide, which causes a conformational change resulting in increased molecular size with no increase in molecular weight [3, 7, 8].

Dextrans are produced commercially by the action of bacteria using the enzyme dextran sucrase on a sucrose-containing medium. Dextrans are commonly described by their number averaged molecular weight (MWn, arithmetic mean of molecular weights): dextran 40 and dextran 70 having MWns of 40,000 and 70,000 daltons, respectively. Dextran solutions are available presented in hypertonic saline, isotonic saline, and hypertonic or isotonic glucose solution [3, 7, 8].

Hydroxyethyl starches (HES) are produced by hydroxyethyl substitution of amylopectin, a D-glucose polymer, obtained from sorghum or maize. The pattern of hydroxyethyl substitution on glucose moieties influences the susceptibility to hydrolysis by non-specific amylases in the blood. A high C2 to C6 substitution ratio and a high overall degree of substitution (the proportion of glucose moieties that have been substituted) protect against enzymatic breakdown and so prolong the effective activity of HES as a plasma volume expander. The different HES products are commonly described by their weight -averaged molecular weight (MWw, number of molecules at each weight times the particle weight divided by the total weight of all the molecules) . They are also described by their degree of substitution: hetastarches (C2/C6 ratio 0.6-0.7), pentastarches (C2/C6 ratio approximately 0.5), and tetrastarches (C2/C6 ratio approximately 0.4). Starch usage varies between countries. In the United States the only starches available for clinical use are high molecular weight [>450 kilodaltons (kDa)] hetastarches presented in either normal saline (Hespan) or a lactate-buffered, glucose containing balanced electrolyte solution (Hextend). In the United Kingdom medium molecular weight (220kDa) pentastarches presented in 0.9% saline are more common, whilst in continental Europe the trend is towards the use of lower molecular weight (130kDa) tetrastarches presented in saline [3, 7, 8].

Differing properties of colloid solutions

Colloid solutions produce a variety of physiological effects and the products differ in a number of characteristics. They have a spectrum of activity in terms of the duration and magnitude of plasma volume expansion. In addition they have varying effects on hemostasis and hemorheology, and some products may have additional "drug effects". Adverse event profiles are also clearly differentiated.

Effective circulating volume expansion

Although it is commonly believed that immediate plasma volume expansion is similar for the commonly used colloid solutions, there is considerable variation in the magnitude and duration of intravascular volume expansion achieved. Intravascular retention is dependent on molecular size and charge characteristics. For example, gelatin molecules are relatively rapidly lost from the circulation, and at 90 min post infusion plasma expansion is similar to that achieved with crystalloid solutions (200 ml/l 1 infused for Haemaccel). The larger dextran and HES solutions (dextran 70, Hespan) produce an expansion of around 0.75 l/litre infused after 90 min. It is important to note that these results are from studies undertaken in healthy volunteers. Increased vascular permeability in major GI surgery will probably result in more-rapid loss of smaller molecules from the intravascular compartment [9, 10].

Hemostasis

Changes in coagulation variables can be detected after infusion of all intravenous solutions. The predominant effect is simple hemodilution of coagulation factors. It is increasingly recognized that crystalloid hemodilution can induce a hypercoagable state, but the clinical significance is uncertain. The synthetic colloids have varying effects on coagulation. Gelatin solutions probably have the least effect, but thromboelatograph studies suggest a decrease in total clot strength associated with these molecules. Dextrans are known to decrease factor VIII activity, increase plasminogen activation and fibrinolysis, and impair clot strength and platelet function. HES effects are thought to vary with molecular size, the larger molecules being particularly implicated. Both impairment of platelet function and a von Willebrand-like syndrome are recognized [3, 7, 8].

Hemorheology

Fluid therapy has a significant effect on the physics of blood flow. All intravenous isotonic fluids reduce whole-blood viscosity, and thereby increase flow, by hemodilution. The reduction in viscosity is proportional to the magnitude of plasma volume expansion, is therefore greater for colloids than crystalloids, and is proportional to the reduction in hematocrit. The prolonged intravascular persistence of the larger molecules will result in a more-prolonged overall improvement in hemorheology, not withstanding their effect on plasma viscosity [3, 7, 8].

Inflammatory activation

There is some evidence that the semi-synthetic colloids may modulate inflammatory activation. Endothelial cell activation can be reduced in vitro by treatment with HES, and animal studies have shown a reduction of trauma -induced macrophage suppression with HES infusion. In septic patients, HES therapy was associated with a reduction in circulating adhesion molecules when compared with fluid therapy with albumin. Dextran molecules (in hypertonic saline) may reduce postischemic leukocyte-endothelial interactions [3, 11]. However, the clinical relevance of such findings remains uncertain.

Cost of fluids

There is a significant cost differential between the different colloids. The gelatins commonly cost around £ 4.00 (U.S.$ 6.00) per 500 ml. Starch solutions are between 3 and 4 times as expensive (£12-16, U.S.$18-24), with albumin costing about 10 times as much as the gelatins [3]. Crystalloids are by far the least expensive.

Adverse event profile

Anaphylaxis and anaphylactoid events can occur with any of the intravenous colloids however the risk varies between individual preparations. The individual colloid types also have specific adverse effect profiles, and it is important to be familiar with the product information sheets of products being used in clinical practice.

Choosing the right fluid for major GI surgery

Crystalloid versus colloid and colloid versus colloid

Despite numerous prospective randomized control trials and meta-analyses, there is no easy answer to this age-old question [12-14]. In truth there are no adequately designed studies to answer these questions, and more specifically not in the context of major GI surgery. There are numerous studies with intermediate outcome variables that suggest superiority of almost every solution (colloid or crystalloid) when compared with almost every other, in any combination. A quick on-line visit to the Cochrane database leads one to conclude that there is inadequate evidence upon which one can make an evidence-based judgement [16]. At the end of the day, common sense based on first principals and personal experience in the context of resource availability leads most clinicians to conclude that a combination of both crystalloids and semisynthetic colloids is the ideal for major surgery. The electrolyte composition of the fluid administered and the dosage and timing of administration are probably far more important issues than the distinction between colloid and crystalloid [17, 18].

Balanced versus saline-based intravenous fluids

Maintaining electrolyte and acid-base balance is especially difficult during major GI surgery for all the reasons cited above. Most intravenous fluids are based on 0.9% sodium chloride [3]. There is now accumulating evidence that the administration of intravenous saline and saline-based fluids is the commonest avoidable cause of clinically relevant hyperchloremic acidosis [18, 19]. Moreover, the lack of additional essential electrolytes such as potassium and calcium, in pure saline-based fluids makes transient severe electrolyte disturbance unavoidable. Hyperchloremic metabolic acidosis (HCMA) is the clinical combination of a non-respiratory acidosis, i.e., metabolic acidosis, with an increase in the plasma concentration of chloride to supraphysiological levels (the elevation of chloride level being responsible for the metabolic acidosis). "Normal" saline (sodium chloride solution) has 154 mmol of sodium, which is compatible with that found in the extracellular space, and 154 mmol of chloride, which is supraphysiological (normal range 98 – 107 mmol/l). The explanation for the acidosis that ensues is explained elsewhere in this book, but is essentially due to a decrease in the strong ion difference of the plasma [20, 21]. More physiologically balanced solutions, such as lactated Ringer's or the colloid Hextend (6% HES in a balanced electrolyte and dextrose solution), have a lower chloride and physiological amounts of other electrolytes and buffer [17].

There is no doubt that HCMA occurs in humans. For example, Williams et al. [22] in a blinded cross-over study of the administration of 50 ml/kg of 0.9% saline compared with lactated Ringer's solution found that the saline-treated individuals developed a significant metabolic acidosis not seen with lactated Ringer's. Scheingraber et. al. [20] randomized two groups of patients undergoing intra-abdominal gynecological surgery to receive 0.9% saline or Ringer's lactate at an infusion rate of approximately 30 ml/kg per hour. In the saline group they observed a significant increase in their chloride level and a significant decrease in pH [20]. In an earlier study McFarlane and Lee [23] randomized 30 patients undergoing hepatobilary or pancreatic surgery to 15 ml/kg per hour of either 0.9% saline or Plasmalyte B. They found the saline group had a significant change in chloride, base excess, and standard bicarbonate [23]. More recently, we randomized 47 elderly patients mainly undergoing GI surgery into "unbalanced" and "balanced" fluid groups during major surgery. The "unbalanced" group received Hespan (6% HES in 0.9% saline) and 0.9% saline, whilst the "balanced" group received Hextend (6% HES in a balanced electrolyte and dextrose injection) and Ringer's lactate. We found a 67% incidence of hyperchloremic acidosis in the unbalanced group compared with a 0% incidence in the balanced group.

Is saline-induced acidosis clinically relevant?

There has been much discussion regarding the clinical relevance of HCMA seen in humans [18, 19]. Certainly in animal models of both hemorrhage and endotoxin shock, resuscitation with Ringer's lactate was associated with improved survival when compared with 0.9% saline [24, 25]. In humans it is generally accepted that the persistence of a metabolic acidosis is predictive of a poor outcome. However, the survival benefits of correcting or avoiding metabolic acidosis, or in this case HCMA, are not proven. If HCMA is clinically relevant, then one might reasonably expect the derangements in acid-base and electrolyte milieu to cause multi-system effects detectable as organ dysfunction and morbidity. There is now a reasonable body of human data to support this hypothesis, with studies demonstrating clinically significant central nervous system, renal, hemostatic, respiratory, and GI dysfunction. For example, in the study by Williams et al. [22] human volunteers experienced subjective mental changes, abdominal discomfort, and renal impairment when they received 0.9% saline, but not when infused with Ringer's lactate. Such findings should not be unexpected. Hyperchloremic acidosis occurs with ammonium chloride, and the symptoms and signs are described as nausea, vomiting, abdominal pain, headaches, thirst, and hyperventilation [27]. Wilcox found that chloride caused selective renal vasoconstriction and a decrease in glomerular filtration rate in greyhounds [28], and at least four prospective randomized human studies of saline versus balanced solutions in major surgery have reported an increased incidence of renal impairment in the saline-treated patients.

In our study of elderly surgical patients we found a significant increase in the CO_2 gap measured using gastric tonometry, suggesting gut hypoperfusion in the patients receiving saline base fluids. There was also significantly more postoperative nausea and vomiting and the use of rescue anti-emetics in the saline treated [26]. Chloride may have the same vasoconstrictive effect on the splanchnic circulation as it does on the renal circulation. This may lead to nausea and vomiting or general gut discomfort, either linked to a genuine gut hypoperfusion effect or to a chloride-specific effect [28, 29].

Strategies for perioperative fluid management

There are a number of different approaches to perioperative fluid management varying from the traditional recipe of x ml per kilogram per hour to more -complex techniques aimed at "optimizing" intravascular volume and organ blood flow. To have a usable strategy, it is important to define both trigger points for the institution of a therapy or technique, and rational endpoints.

An example of a technique that can trigger a particular therapeutic strategy is preoperative risk stratification – the identification of which patients are at increased risk of morbidity and mortality related to their surgery. This risk may be due to their underlying pathology, type of operation, comorbidity, or age. Traditionally this assessment has been a subjective process, but can be performed objectively using specific criteria. A more-sophisticated technique is the use of a validated scoring system such as the POSSUM score [30].

Although it is important to make an assessment of fluid losses and to replace them intravenously, we will argue that neither the assessment, nor the attempted replacement are usually adequate. The commonly used indices of adequacy of the circulation are largely pressure based–arterial, central venous, and pulmonary artery occlusion pressures. Unfortunately the pressure-volume relationship of the physical components of the circulation vary with their compliance.

This in turn is dependent on a number of factors including, critically, the action of the various vasoactive hormones produced and released in response to the relative hypovolemia produced by anesthesia, perioperative fluid losses, and the stress response to surgery.

Pressure directed fluid management

The traditional, and probably the commonest, approach to perioperative volume replacement is to maintain a standard background infusion (e.g., 15 ml /kg-per hour 0.9% saline) and to replace fluid losses with further crystalloid. Maintenance of an adequate blood pressure, and central venous pressure (CVP), if monitored, are accepted goals. The problem with this reactive approach based on pressure values is that the circulation is maintained at the lower limit, in terms of filling, of physiological compensation. In unanesthetised healthy volunteers, 20-25% of the intravascular volume can be removed without significant disturbance of arterial blood pressure or heart rate [31]. Similarly in patients undergoing major surgery it has been demonstrated repeatedly that maintenance of commonly measured cardio-respiratory variables (heart rate, arterial blood pressure) is commonly associated with reduced organ blood flow and a poor outcome [4-6, 32]. Static central venous pressure monitoring is all too commonly used as a brake to prevent "fluid overload" rather than a dynamic guide to fluid optimization.

The fluid challenge

An alternative approach to a pressure-based reactive strategy of fluid management is to "challenge" the circulation to establish whether further fluid can be accommodated within the intravascular space without precipitating cardiac failure due to hypervolemia – the concept of pre-load recruitable stroke volume or cardiac output. The fluid challenge is the main therapeutic maneuver used in strategies aimed at optimizing intravascular volume [33]. After observation of cardiovascular variables, a pre-determined volume of fluid is infused over a short period of time and the measured variables reassessed. The normal fluid bolus in adults is 200 ml, but in patients where there are concerns about ventricular function, or with a low body weight, a smaller volume can be used. A colloid solution is the logical choice of agent, as it will achieve the most -effective plasma volume expansion. Although this technique has some utility when only heart rate and blood pressure are monitored it is clearly difficult to identify an endpoint for repeated boluses in this situation. When CVP monitoring is available, a common approach is to continue bolusing fluid until a sustained rise in CVP occurs, e.g., >3mmHg after 15 min – rather than be limited by a predetermined CVP value.

Flow directed fluid therapy

The fluid challenge is particularly useful when information about stroke volume and cardiac output is available and the effects of a fluid bolus on these variables can be measured. A number of invasive and relatively non-invasive techniques are available that permit measurement of cardiac output and stroke volume. These include thermodilution using the pulmonary artery catheter, bioimpedence, descending aortic velocimetry (esophageal Doppler), and arterial pulse contour analysis. Measurement of some index of cardiac output opens up the possibility of strategies aimed at achieving optimal filling status by maximizing stroke volume or "optimizing" the patient to pre-defined oxygen delivery goals.

Increasing oxygen delivery to predefined goals

Cardiac function and reserve have been recognized as a predictor of postoperative outcome for many years. During the 1970s and 1980s Shoemaker et al. [34] observed that survivors of major operations had higher postoperative cardiac outputs and oxygen delivery [34]. They hypothesized that using the values for cardiac output and oxygen delivery from the survivors as goals for perioperative treatment in all major surgical patients would reduce mortality. This strategy was shown to be effective at reducing mortality in two large single-center trials, one from the United States and one from the United Kingdom [34, 35]. These trials used dobutamine and dopexamine respectively to attain the goals if fluid alone was not adequate. However, many argued that in fact this technique was selecting those patients with a greater physiological reserve who were able to reach the predetermined goals, and questioned the rationale of adding inotropes to achieve such specific goals in a heterogeneous group of patients. Several more-recent studies have shown that the philosophy of improving cardiac output and oxygen delivery perioperatively improves outcome and that in many patients this improvement is achieved with fluid therapy alone [36, 37]. There is probably a small extra gain from low-dose inotropic therapy in those that don't achieve the predefined targets with fluid alone, but overstressing patient physiology with high-dose inotropes is thought to be deleterious in this context.

Maximizing stroke volume

An alternative approach to optimizing to specific predetermined goals is to attempt to maximize stroke volume using fluid alone. Non-invasive techniques such as the esophageal Doppler monitor lend themselves to this. We prospectively studied 60 American Society of Anesthesiology grade III patients with preoperative left ventricular ejection fraction > 50% undergoing elective cardiac surgery [36]. Patients were allocated randomly to a control or protocol group. The control group were treated according to standard practices. After induction of general anesthesia, the protocol group received, in addition, 200 ml boluses of a 6% HES solution to obtain a maximum stroke volume as outlined above. This procedure was repeated every 15 min until the end of surgery, except when the patient was on cardiopulmonary by-pass. Patients were followed postoperatively until discharge from hospital or death. The incidence of gut mucosal hypoperfusion at the end of surgery was reduced in the protocol group (7% vs. 56%; $P < 0.01$), as was the number of patients developing major complications (0 vs. 6; $P < 0.01$), days spent in hospital [6.4 (range 5 – 9) vs. 10.1 (range 5 –48); $P < 0.05$] and days spent in the intensive care unit [1 (range 1 – 1) vs. 1.7 (range 1 – 11); $P < 0.05$] [36]. Similar results have subsequently been reported in patients undergoing operative repair of fractured neck of femur and non-cardiac major elective surgery, including major GI surgery [37].

Sinclair et al. [37] studied 40 patients undergoing repair of proximal femoral fracture under general anesthesia. Patients were randomly assigned to receive either conventional intraoperative fluid management, or additional repeated colloid fluid challenges guided by the esophageal Doppler monitor to maintain optimal stroke volume. Intraoperative intravascular fluid loading produced significantly greater changes in stroke volume than in the conventionally managed group. In the survivors, postoperative recovery was significantly faster in the protocol patients, with shorter times to being declared medically fit for discharge [median 10 (9 – 15) days vs. 15 (11 – 40) days, $P < 0.05$] and a 39% reduction in hospital stay [12 (8 – 13) days vs. 20 (10 – 61) days, $P < 0.05$].

More recently, in a prospective, randomized study, Gan et al., (T.J. Gan, Duke University Medical Center, N.C., USA; personal communication) assessed the effect of intraoperative fluid optimization guided by esophageal Doppler monitor on length of postoperative hospital stay following major non-cardiac surgery. They studied 100 patients who were to undergo major elective surgery with an anticipated blood loss > of 500 ml. Patients were randomly assigned to a control group (N=50) that received best standard intraoperative care or to a protocol group (N=50) that, in addition, received intraoperative plasma volume expansion guided by the esophageal Doppler monitor to maintain optimal stroke volume. Groups were similar with respect to demographics, surgical procedures, and baseline hemodynamic variables. The protocol group had a significantly higher stroke volume and cardiac output at the end of surgery compared with the control. Patients in the protocol group had a shorter duration of hospital stay compared with the control group, 5 ± 3 versus 7 ± 3 days (mean ± SD), with a median of 6 versus 7 days respectively (P=0.03). These patients also tolerated an oral intake of solid regimen earlier than the control group, 3 ± 0.5 versus 4.7 ± 0.5 days (mean ± SD), with a median of 3 versus 5 days, respectively (P=0.01).

Gut directed therapy?

Global indicators are often normal in the presence of significant regional hypoperfusion. GI blood flow is known to be reduced early in relative hypovolemia [4-6, 32] and perfusion of the GI mucosa is compromised early due to the presence of the microvillus countercurrent. In the context of major GI surgery a measure of the adequacy of GI perfusion would seem like a rational end point for fluid resuscitation if achievable. The GI tonometer is an established and validated method of assessing GI perfusion [32]. The presence of an elevated GI luminal PCO_2 relative to arterial PCO_2 has been shown in a number of studies to be a sensitive predictor of poor postoperative outcome. Additionally patients randomized to a fluid-loading algorithm have been demonstrated to have both a significant improvement in gut perfusion at the end of surgery and improved outcome [36]. However, there are currently no trials that demonstrate that intervening specifically to correct abnormal GI tonometry results in normalization of the perfusion defect and/or subsequent improved outcome.

Conclusion

Effective fluid therapy is at the core of the management of patients undergoing major GI surgery. The available crystalloid and colloid solutions have specific clearly defined pharmaco-kinetic and –dynamic properties. When considering the choice of intravenous solutions it is important to remember the considerable challenge of maintaining pH and electrolyte balance during major GI surgery. A combination of blood and blood products, crystalloids and colloids, ideally as physiologically normal as possible, is required to achieve optimal fluid balance. Accurate titration of fluid therapy in major GI surgery often requires invasive monitoring. The use of specific pro-active fluid management algorithms coupled with techniques to assess cardiac output leads to improved outcome.

References

1. Report of the National Confidential Enquiry into Perioperative Deaths (NCEPOD) 1997/1998 (1999) NCEPOD, London
2. Bennett-Guerrero E, Welsby I, Dunn TJ, et al (1999) The use of post operative morbidity to evaluate patients with prolonged hospitalization after routine. moderate-risk, elective surgery. Anesth Anal 89:514-519
3. Grocott MPW, Mythen MG (1999) Fluid therapy. In: Ballieres Clin Anaesthesiol; 13: 363-381
4. Mythen MG, Webb AR (1994) The role of gut mucosal hypoperfusion in the pathogenesis of post-operative organ dysfunction. Intensive Care Med 20: 203-209
5. Ackland G, Grocott MP, Mythen MG (2000) Understanding gastrointestinal perfusion in critical care: so near, and yet so far. Crit Care 4:269-281
6. Mythen MG, Fink M (1999) The role of gut derived endotoxin in the pathogenesis of multiple organ dysfunction. In: Brade, Morrison, Opal, Vogel (eds) Endotoxin in health and disease, Dekker, New York
7. Salmon JB, Mythen MG (1993) Pharmacology and physiology of colloids. Blood Rev 7:114-120
8. Haljamae H, Dahlqvist M, Walentin F (1997) Artificial colloids in clinical practise: pros and cons. Baillieres Clin Anaesthesiol 11:49-79
9. Lamke LO, Liljedahl SO (1976) Plasma volume changes after infusion of various plasma expanders. Resuscitation 5:93-102
10. Webb AR, Barclay SA, Bennett ED (1989) In vitro colloid osmotic pressure of commonly used plasma expanders and substitutes: a study of the diffusibility of colloid molecules. Intensive Care Med 15:116-120.
11. Webb AR, Moss RF, Tighe D, et al (1992) A narrow range, medium molecular weight pentastarch reduces structural organ damage in a hyperdynamic porcine model of sepsis. Intensive Care Med 18:348-355.
12. Velanovich V (1989) Crystalloid versus colloid fluid resuscitation: a meta-analysis of mortality. Surgery 105:65-71
13. Schierhout G, Roberts I (1998) Fluid resuscitation with colloid or crystalloid solutions in critically ill patients: a systematic review of randomised trials. BMJ 316:961-964.
14. Anonymous (1998) Human albumin administration in critically ill patients: systematic review of randomised controlled trials. Cochrane Injuries Group Albumin Reviewers . BMJ 317:235-240.
15. Bunn F, Alderson P, Hawkins V (2000) Colloid solutions for fluid resuscitation (Cochrane Review). In: The Cochrane Library, issue 4
16. www.cochrane.org
17. Gan TJ, Bennett-Guerrero E, Phillips-Bute B, et al (1999) Hextend, a physiological balanced plasma expander for large volume use in major surgery: a randomized phase III clinical trial. Anaesth Anal 88:992-998
18. Stephens RC, Mythen MG (2000) Saline-based fluids can cause a significant acidosis that may be clinically relevant. Crit Care Med 28:3375-3377.
19. Prough DS, Bidani A (1999) Hyperchloremic metabolic acidosis is a predictable consequence of intraoperative infusion of 0.9% saline. Anesthesiology 90:1247-1249.
20. Scheingraber S, Rehm M, Sehmisch C, Finsterer U (1999) Rapid saline infusion produces hyperchloremic acidosis in patients undergoing gynecologic surgery. Anesthesiology 90: 1265 -1270
21. Ref from TRICE (2001)
22. Williams EL, Hildebrand KL, McCormick SA, Bedel MJ (1999) The effect of intravenous lactated Ringer's solution versus 0.9% sodium chloride solution on serum osmolality in human volunteers. Anesth Analg 88: 999 - 1003
23. McFarlane C, Lee A (1994) A comparison of Plasmalyte 148 and 0.9% saline for intra-operative fluid replacement. Anaesthesia 49:779-781
24. Healey MA, Davis RE, Liu FC, et al (1998) Lactated Ringer's is superior to normal saline in a model of massive hemorrhage and resuscitation. J Trauma 45: 894 - 899

25 Kellum JA, Schenigel J, Venkataraman R (2000) Fluid resuscitation and hyperchloraemic acidosis in experimental sepsis: improved survival and acid-base balance with a synthetic colloid in a balanced electrolyte solution compared to saline. Crit Care Med 28: A199
26. Wilkes NJ, Woolf R, Stephens R, et al (2001) The effects of balanced versus saline based intravenous solutions on acid base status and gastric mucosal perfusion in elderly surgical patients. Anesth Analg (in press)
27. Megarbane B, Bruneel F, Bedos J-P, Regnier B (2000) Ammonium chloride poisoning: a misunderstood cause of metabolic acidosis with normal anion gap. Intensive Care Med Online publication 9 November 2000
28. Gan TJ, Mythen MG, Glass PSA (1997) Intraoperative gut hypoperfusion may be a risk factor for postoperative nausea and vomiting. Br J Anaesth 78: 476
28. Wilcox CS (1983) Regulation of renal blood flow by plasma chloride. J Clin Invest 71: 726-735
29. Tournadre JP, Allaouchiche B, Malbert CH, Chassard D (2000) Metabolic acidosis and respiratory acidosis impair gastro-pyloric motility in anesthetized pigs. Anesth Analg 90: 74 - 79
30. Copeland GP, Jones D, Walters M (1991) POSSUM: a scoring system for surgical audit. Br J Surg 78:355-360.
31. Hamilton-Davies C, Mythen MG, Salmon JB, et al (1997) Comparison of commonly used clinical indicators of hypovolaemia with gastrointestinal tonometry. Intensive Care Med 23:276-281
32. Chapman MV, Mythen MG Webb AR, Vincent JL (2000) Gastrointestinal tonometry: state of the art. Intensive Care Med 26:613-622
33. Webb AR (1997) Fluid management in intensive care – the avoidance of hypovolaemia. Br J Intensive Care 7
34. Shoemaker WC, Appel PL, Kram HB, et al (1988) Prospective trial of supranormal values of survivors as therapeutic goals in high-risk surgical patients. Chest 94:1176-1186.
35. Boyd O, Grounds RM, Bennett ED (1993) A randomized clinical trial of the effect of deliberate perioperative increase of oxygen delivery on mortality in high-risk surgical patients. JAMA 270:2699-2707
36. Mythen MG, Webb AR (1995) Perioperative plasma volume expansion reduces the incidence of gut mucosal hypoperfusion during cardiac surgery. Arch Surg 130:423-429
37. Sinclair S, James S, Singer M (1997) Intraoperative intravascular volume optimisation and length of hospital stay after repair of proximal femoral fracture: randomised controlled trial. BMJ 315:909-912

Postoperative Fluid Management

G. Berlot, A. Tomasini, U. Lucangelo

Major surgery is associated with a number of fluid, electrolyte, and acid-base disorders, which can be ascribed to a number of different causes, including blood loss, volume resuscitation, tissue trauma, cardiovascular instability, changes in body temperature and renal dysfunction. In both the immediate and late postoperative phases, the increased reabsorption of sodium and water, driven by the trauma-induced neurohormonal response to stress, further aggravate the ongoing disturbances of the internal milieu [1]. Thus, both the choice of fluids and the strategy of their administration are of paramount importance in order to prevent or reduce the occurrence of potentially harmful disturbances of fluid and electrolytes.

Principles of water distribution

Total body water (TBW) accounts for 60% of body weight, and is contained in two separate but communicating compartments: the intracellular and extracellular spaces [2]. The latter, which accounts for one-third of the TBW can be further subdivided into the interstitial space, the plasma, and the red blood cells. The passage of fluids from the microvascular network to the tissues and back is governed by difference in hydrostatic and osmotic pressures through the capillary wall and by the efficiency of the extravascular fluid removal by the lymph flow (Starling's law) [3]. Under steady-state conditions, water volumes and solute concentrations remain fairly constant due to a precise regulatory action exerted by the renal ability to handle sudden changes of water and electrolytes. At the tissue and cellular level, other energy consuming mechanisms contribute to maintain the local concentration of solutes within relatively narrow ranges. A number of conditions, including advanced age, the presence of cardiac and renal disease, and drug-induced disturbances of renal tubular function can reduce these fine-tuned regulatory mechanisms [4]. In the perioperative phase, all these regulatory mechanisms can be altered. The intravascular hydrostatic pressure can be raised or lowered, the serum colloid osmotic pressure (COP) is often reduced due to decreased albumin levels, and the permeability of the capillary wall is increased due to a more- or less-widespread inflammatory reaction triggered by the surgical trauma and/or by possible infectious complications [5]. The consequence of these disturbance is an escape of the intravascular water toward the interstitial space, thus creating or widening the "third space", an ill-defined functional compartment whose ultimate clinical and morphological expression is edema. It should be remembered that (1) edema is extremely frequent in critically ill patients [6] and that (2) it cannot be considered only a benign or cosmetic problem. In a group of surgical patients the weight gain in the postoperative phase, indicating a net fluid accumulation was associated with an increased rate of complications, as well as reduced survival [7]. The same findings have been recently demonstrated in a group of critically ill septic patients [8]. In our experience, in a group of patients undergoing elective surgery, the postoperative fluid accumulation was associated with a worsening of the clinical conditions, an increased rate of complications, and a reduced survival (unpublished data).

The effects of surgery and anesthesia on the water regulatory mechanisms

In the perioperative phase, the body handling of fluids and electrolytes is influenced by the dual effects of anesthesia and surgery itself [9], working in association with the actions exerted by the neurohormonal response to stress. The final effect is an increase and a redistribution of the TBW. In general terms, both intravenous and inhaled anesthetic agents exert more- or less-pronounced cardiodepressant and vasodilating effects, thus potentially leading to a reduction of the organ perfusion. At the renal level, the reduced cardiac output (CO) is associated with a decrease of the glomerular filtration rate, and this effect can be further exacerbated by the administration of drugs such as angiotensin converting enzyme inhibitors. Obviously, the overall effect is more marked in patients with preexisting reduced cardiac or renal reserve. Furthermore, general anesthesia influences the secretion of antiduretic hormone (ADH), although the results of several studies addressing the issue are not unequivocal, since other factors, including serum osmolality and preoperative volume status, are implicated in its production and release. The anesthesia-induced vasodilation augments the fluids needed to maintain the CO and the arterial pressure, and this effect can be further increased by the block of the sympathetic flow induced by conduction anesthesia, especially when the upper spinal segments are involved.

The immediate but long-lasting consequence is the reduced ability to eliminate a volume load, which accumulates in the tissues. The effects of surgery on volume status largely depend on its characteristics. Whereas minor procedures do not determine relevant volume changes, extensive interventions, such as those involving the thorax and the abdomen, determine a more-marked disturbance due to several concomitant factors, including the blood loss, the sequestration of fluid inside the traumatized tissue, and the evaporative losses from the open body cavities. Another often unrecognized source of fluid loss is the evaporation via the tracheobronchial tree during mechanical ventilation.

Surgical procedures can also affect the renal handling of fluids through the often unrecognized increase of the intraabdominal pressure (IAP). Actually, the uncontrolled rise of the IAP causes a reduction of the diuresis up to the occurrence of full-blown acute renal failure (ARF) through different mechanisms, including a concomitant increased pressure of excretory conduits and the reduced venous return with subsequent decreased CO [10].

The neurohormonal response to stress

The response to stress includes a wide array of hormonal changes involving the hypothalamus, the pituitary, and the adrenal glands, and a widespread network of mediator-producing cells teleologically aimed at maintaining the CO and substrate supply to the tissues in the post-injury phase [1] (Table 1). Although

Table 1. Neurohormonal response to stress

Sympathetic nervous system activation
Endocrine stress response
- Pituitary hormone secretion
- Insulin resistance
Immuno-hematological changes
- cytokine production
- acute phase reaction
- neutrophil leukocytosis
- lymphocyte proliferation and differentiation

many endocrine changes have been described (Table 2), the increased secretion of aldosterone and ADH are the most important as far as the volume status is concerned. Their secretion enhances the renal reabsorption of Na^+ and free water, thus contributing to the well-known phenomenon of postoperative fluid retention. The stress response can blunted but not completely abolished by

Table 2. Hormonal changes in response to surgery (ACTH = adrenocorticotropic hormone, GH = growth hormone, TSH = thyroid-stimulating hormone, LH-FSH = luteinizing hormone – follicle-stimulating hormone, ADH = antiduretic hormone)

Endocrine gland	Hormones	Change in secretion
Aterior hypophysis	ACTH	↓
	GH	¯
	TSH	¯ or ¯
	LH-FSH	↓ or ↓
Posterior hypophysis	ADH	↓
Adrenal cortex	Aldosteron	¯
	Cortisol	↓
Pancreas	Insulin	¯ or¯
	Glucagon	↓
Thyroid	T3, T4	↓

epidural anesthesia started before the onset of surgery. In a classic study, Bromage et al. [11] were able to demonstrate that the epidural block extending up to the C5 level inhibited the surgery related glycemic changes, but not the increased secretion of cortisol. Moreover, a number of blood-borne mediators involved in the stress response work via extranervous pathways, making their blocking unlikely [12].

Choice of fluids

In the perioperative phase, the main goal of fluid administration is the restoration and maintenance of an adequate volemia and CO [13]. As the latter is usually far easier to assess, most studies focused more on the effects of fluid resuscitation on the overall cardiovascular performances than on the effects of different fluid regimens [14, 15]. A time-honored but always valid classifications divides the different fluids used in the volume resuscitation and maintenance phase according to their distributive properties, which ultimately account for their final cardiovascular properties. According to these characteristics, these agents have been classified into crystalloids and colloids.

Basically, the crystalloids are glucose or saline solutions that can be further subdivided into hypotonic (e.g., dextrose in water), isotonic (e.g., normal, saline, acetate, and lactated Ringer's solutions), and hypertonic (e.g., 7.5% saline solution) according to their osmolar properties [13]. Currently, the use of hypotonic solutions is not recommended in the postoperative volume replacement. Overall, crystalloids freely cross the capillary membrane and are distributed into the intravascular and interstitial space. Under normal conditions, after an equilibration period, only 25% of the infused crystalloids remain in the intravascular space, the remainder flowing into the interstitial space, thus facilitating the formation of edema. The increased microvascular permeability associated with sepsis, burns, and trauma, and the reduction of the colloid osmotic pressure (COP) associated with the administration of large volumes of crystalloids further increases the escape of water into the tissues. A more-recent study of the regulatory mechanisms of the acid-base equilibrium underscored the role of crystalloids in determining postoperative metabolic acidosis. The infusion of large amounts of Cl^-, such as those contained in normal or hypertonic saline, has been associated with the reduction in the strong ion differences (SID), thus prompting the dissociation of H_2O in H^+ and OH^-; the resulting increase of hydrogen ions accounts for the resulting hyperchloremic acidosis [16].

The colloids are a heterogeneous family of substances whose space of distribution under normal conditions is limited to the intravascular space. Consequently, their effect on the volemia is more pronounced than that of crystalloids, and in case of hemorrhage the replacement of the blood lost can occur on a 1:1 basis, provided that the permeability of the capillary wall is not impaired. Despite their heterogeneity, colloids share some side effects. First, their use can be associated with anaphylactic reaction, whose incidence appears to be related to the molecular weight [17]. Second, several hemocoagulative disorders have been described, which have been mainly related to different mechanisms, including decrease of von Willebrand's factor and enhanced fibrinolysys [18]. Finally, the colloid-induced brisk rise of COP has been associated with the occurrence of renal dysfunction, especially in dehydrated patients [17].

The available colloids differ in their pharmacological and clinical effects [17]. Albumin is the main natural colloid [19]. With a molecular weight of 69 kDa, it is associated with a relevant COP. Although it is produced from pooled donor plasma, the heating and ultrafiltration procedures used during the manufacturing provide an increased safety from transmissible diseases. Albumin 5% solutions are isooncotic, whereas 20% and 25% solutions are strongly hyperoncotic, thus exerting a much more-marked effect on volemia. Although an extremely effective plasma expander, its use has been recently questioned, as a meta-analysis demonstrated an excess mortality in critically ill patients given albumin as fluid resuscitation [20]. However, a more recent meta-analysis failed to confirm that colloids in general and albumin in particular were associated with a reduced survival in critically ill patients [21]; hence this issue can be considered still open [19].

Synthetic colloids differ from albumin, mainly due to their extremely diverse molecular weight present in each solution. The molecules with higher molecular weight contribute relatively to the increased volume effect, but maintain the effect for prolonged periods, whereas the smaller ones, which are far more effective as volume expanders, are rapidly eliminated by the kidney. According to their nature, synthetic colloids can be subdivided into the following [13].

Gelatins are manufactured from beef collagen and were the first to be used, their clinical use dating from the 1st world war. Currently, they are available in three different types: (1) cross linked, (2) urea linked, and (3) succynilated, which basically differ in the amounts of electrolytes contained. The increase in blood volume is somewhat less than the one infused and, due to the relatively low average molecular weight (approx 35 kDa), their action is time limited, requiring repeated or prolonged infusions. The administration of gelatins has been associated with the occurrence of life-threatening anaphylactic reactions, which limited their use and prompted the development of other plasma expanders.

Hydroxyethyl starches (HES) are an extremely wide family of substances, with different molecular weight, half-lives, and pharmacological properties. Basically, the molecule of HES is a derived from amylopectine, a highly branched starch compound, which is rapidly metabolized by -amylase and eliminated by the kidney. The degradation is reduced by substituting hydroxyethyl residuals in different positions (but mainly at the C2 and C6 locations) of the native starch molecule. Different HES preparations can be characterized according to (1) the weight averaged mean molecular weight, (2) the number-averaged molecular weight, that is the median molecular weight of all HES molecules; (3) the molar substitution (MS) that is the molar ratio of the overall number of hydroxyethyl radicals to the total number of glucose molecule, and (4) the degree of substitution, that is of substituted glucose molecules to the total number of glucose molecules. Consequently, HES solutions are available in a number of formulations, with different concentrations (3, 6, 10%), molecular weight (low 70 kDa, medium 200-270 kDa, high 450 kDa), and MS (from 0.5 to 0.7). These pharmacological features are associated with different properties, in terms of volume expansion, possible side effects, and duration. The choice of a given HES preparation should be driven on the basis of the underlying patient's condition. A number of side effects have been associated with the administration of HES, including hyoperamilasemia, anaphylactic reactions, and disturbances of blood coagulation [22]. Recently, the administration of HES with elevated MW has been associated with the occurrence of ARF in a group of critically ill septic patients [23].

The transfusion of blood and derivates to postoperative patients has undergone a complete reappraisal in the last 15-20 years. Initially, the worldwide shortage of available blood and the risk of transmissible diseases made the time-honored rule of the 10 [g Hb/dl] – 30 [Ht] difficult to respect. Despite their widespread use, these figures were not supported by experimental or clinical investigations, but were largely used as they made physicians feel more comfortable in the presence of a mild anaemia. Later, concerns about the immunodepressant action of the transfused heterologous blood further discouraged its use and prompted the search for alternative treatments of perioperative anemia, including hemodilution, self-transfusion, and the administration of recombinant erythropoietin in subjects at risk of hemorrhage or refusing blood transfusions [24-26]. At the same time, the transfusional threshold, that is the value of Hb below which blood transfusion is warranted, decreased. Several clinical investigations account for this relevant change. First, the oxygen--carrying capabilities of erythrocytes appear to be influenced by their age. In a group of septic patients given packet red cells (PRC) stored for different periods Marik and Sibbald [27] demonstrated that the transfusion of "old" PRC could increase the calculated but not the directly measured oxygen consumption (VO_2), thus indicating a limited usefulness as far as a rapid restoration of aerobic metabolism is concerned; more disturbing, a significant decrease of the gastric intramuscosal pH (pHi), indicating a splanchnic ischemia, was observed in many patients who received old PRC. Second, in a recent randomized, multicenter study Hebert et al. [28] used two different transfusional thresholds in critically ill, normovolemic patients. In the high-threshold group, PRC were transfused with the aim of maintaining a Hb level between 10 and 12 g/dl, whereas in the other group the threshold was set to maintain Hb at 7-9 g/dl. Although the 30-day survival did not differ in the two groups, in-hospital mortality was lower in patients treated with the restrictive policy. Rather strikingly, mortality was comparable when patients perceived at increased risk, such as those with advanced age, underlying cardiac diseases, and higher APACHE II scores, were separately analyzed. Further analyses demonstrated that Hb levels of 7-9 g/dl were safe even in patients with cardiac diseases, with the possible exception of those with acute myocardial infarction or unstable angina [29]. Moreover, the duration of the mechanical ventilation did not reduce the length of the mechanical ventilation, nor the failure of the weaning in the two groups [30]. On the basis of these findings, it appears that the transfusion of PRC in stable postoperative patients without bleeding should be reserved for patients with underlying myocardial ischemia or failure. For reasons similar to those described for PRC, the transfusion of whole-blood derivates, including plasma, coagulation factors, and platelets, has undergone profound revision, and international guidelines have been issued and published [31].

Titration of the fluid administration

The current approach to fluid therapy is strongly influenced by two opposing concepts, one stating "keep them dry and watch them die", thus favoring a liberal fluid administration, whereas the other, sentencing that "the good lung is a dry lung", underscores the risk of fluid overload and of pulmonary edema. As in many other instances, the truth lies somewhere in between, and a guide to treatment is keenly warranted, possibly indicting when fluids alone are sufficient to restore a normal redox status or when vasoactive agents are needed. As the ultimate goal of volume resuscitation is to restore and maintain tissue oxygenation, its monitoring appears valuable in titrating postoperative fluid administration. Unfortunately, this remains a difficult task, since (1) systemic variables of oxygenation, including DO_2, VO_2, SvO_2, and lactate, do not reflect what is going on at a tissue level and (2) more-sophisticated techniques able to identify tissue hypoxia at the bedside are not widespread. In the vast majority of cases, the administration of volumes in the postoperative phase is based more on subjective perceptions and/or on unreliable clinical information than on precise markers of dysoxia or hypoxia. Some data deriving from investigations performed either in trauma and/or postoperative patients indicate that the volume resuscitation based on changes of cardiovascular variables is associated with better results compared with a blind fluid infusion. Miller et al. [32] prospectively studied a group of trauma patients treated with inotropes or volume expansion, the latter was titrated according to the right ventricular end-diastolic volume (RVEDV) and on the pHi. Despite comparable increases of the systemic oxygenation variables, complications, and length of the mechanical ventilation, in fluid-resuscitated patients the splanchnic perfusion improved without the feared pulmonary complications, possibly associated with the larger amounts of fluid infused. Similar findings have also been reported by other authors [33], who observed that a supranormal RVEDV was associated with a better outcome. Sinclair et al. [34] reported a better outcome and a shorter hospital stay in orthopedic patients whose fluid infusion was titrated according to the CO changes monitored with an esophageal echo-Doppler compared with the control group, in which volume administration was based on variations of the arterial pressure and of the heart rate. Hence, it appears that, independent of the choice of fluids, a protocol-guided volume infusion is superior to the blind administration of a fixed volume.

Conclusions

Although less fiercely debated than in the past, the long-lasting colloid-crystalloid controversy does not seem to have been resolved, as supporters of both sides still claim the superiority of one class over the other. There is no convincing proof that, in the absence of precise contraindications, one approach is superior to the other. Furthermore, due to the continuous improvement of technology and expanding knowledge of the basic pathophysiology of the microcirculation, a possible colloid-colloid controversy can be forecasted, as substances with characteristics suitable in different clinical settings are already available Too many confounding factors, including the number of patients enrolled, their ASA class, the type and length of surgery, and the heterogeneity of the study endpoints (which included in-hospital survival, length of hospital stay, complication rate, and many others) make it extremely difficult to draw definite conclusions. Despite these shortcomings, some points can be established. First, independent of its nature, volume should be titrated according to the changes of some easily monitored variables. Second, in volume-unresponsive patients or in the presence of clear restrictions to the liberal infusion of fluids, vasoactive drugs should be given early. Third, blood transfusion is no longer considered a mandatory therapeutic act in postoperative anemic patients, provided that bleeding has ceased and in the absence of active myocardial ischemia.

References

1. Desborough JP (2000) The stress response to trauma and surgery. Br J Anaesth 85: 109-117
2. Narins RG, Jones ER, Stom MC, et al (1982) Diagnostic strategies in disorders of fluid, electrolyte and acid base disorders. Am J Med 72: 496-520
3. Jones JG, Wardrop CAJ (2000) Measurement of blood volume in surgical and intensive care patients. Br J Anaesth 84: 226-235
4. Watters JM, McClaran JC (1990) The elderly surgical patient. In: Wilmore DW, Brennan MF, Herken AH (eds) Care of the surgical patient. Scientific American/Am Coll of Surgeons, New York
5. Kaminski MV, Haase TJ (1992) Albumin and colloid osmotic pressure implications for fluid resuscitation. Crit Care Clin 8: 311-321
6. Koomans HA, Boer WB (1997) Causes of edema in the intensive care unit. Kidney Int [Suppl] 59: 105-110.
7. Lowell JA, Schifferdecker C, Driscoll DF, et al (1990) Postoperative fluid overload: not a benign problem. Crit Care Med 18: 728-733
8. Alsous F, Khamiees M, DeGirolamo A, et al (2000) Negative fluid balance predicts survival in patients with septic shock – a retrospective pilot study. Chest 117: 1749-1754
9. Gold MS (1992) Perioperative fluid management. Crit Care Clin 8: 409-421
10. Cheatham ML (1999) Intra-abdominal hypertension and abdominal compartment syndrome. New Horiz 7: 96-115

11. Bromage PR, Shibata HR, Willoughby HW (1971) Influence of prolonged epidural blockade on blood sugar and cortisol responses to operations upon the upper part of the abdomen and thorax. Surg Gynecol Obstet 21: 330-335
12. Ader R, Cohen N, Felten D (1995) Psychoneuroimmunology, interactions between the nervous system and the immune system. Lancet 345: 99-103
13. Boldt J (2000) Volume replacement in the surgical patient – does the type of solution make a difference? Br J Anaesth 84: 783-793
14. Jones JG, Wardrop CAJ (2000) Measurement of blood volume in surgical and intensive care patients. Br J Anaesth 84: 226-235
15. Gomez CMH, Palazzo MGA (1998) Pulmonary artery catheterization in anaesthesia and intensive care. Br J Anaesth 81: 945-956
16. Kellum JA (1999) Curr Opin Crit Care 5: 429-435
17. Salmon JB, Mythen MG (1993) Pharmacology and physiology of colloids. Blood Transfus 7: 114-120
18. Jonge E de, Levi M (2001) Effects of different plasma substitutes on blood coagulation. A comparative review. Crit Care Med 29: 1261-1267
19. Ferguson ND, Stewart TE, Etchells EE (1999) Human albumin administration in critically ill patients. Intensive Care Med 25: 323-325
20. Cochrane Injuries Group Albumin Reviewer (1998) Albumin administration in critically ill patients: systematic review of randomised controlled trials. BMJ 317: 235-239
21. Choi PL, Yip G, Quinonez LG, Cook DJ (1999) Crystalloids vs colloids in fluid resucitation: a systematic review. Crit Care Med 27: 200-210
22. Warren BB, Durieux ME (1999) Hydroxyethyl starch: safe or not? Anesth Analg 84: 206-212
23. Schortgen F, Lacherade JC, Bruneel F, et al (2001) Effects of hydroxyethylstarch and gelatin on renal function in severe sepsis: a multicentre randomised study. Lancet 357: 911-918
24. Spahn DR, Casutt M (2000) Eliminating blood transfusion – new aspects and perspectives. Anesthesiology 93: 242-255
25. Nielsen HJ (1995) Detrimental effects of perioperative blood transfusion. Br J Surg 82: 582-587
26. Hebert PC, Szick S (2000) Transfusion in the intensive care unit: strategies under scrutiny. Curr Opin Anaesth 13: 119-123
27. Marik PE, Sibbald WJ (1993) Effect of stored blood transfusion on oxygen delivery in patients with sepsis. JAMA 269: 3024-3029
28. Hebert PC, Wells G, Blajchman MA, et al (1999) A multicentre, randomized controlled clinical trial of transfusion requirements in critical care. N Engl J Med 340: 409-417
29. Hebert PC, Yetisir E, Martin C, et al (2001) Is a low transfusion threshold safe in critically ill patients with cardiovascular diseases? Crit Care Med 29: 229-234
30. Hebert PC, Blajchman MA, Cook DJ (2001) Do blood transfusions improve outcomes related to mechanical ventilation? Chest 119: 1850-1857
31. American Society of Anesthesiologists Task Force on Blood Component Therapy (1996) Practice guidelines for blood component therapy. Anesthesiology 84: 732-747
32. Miller PR, Meredith JW, Chang MC (1998) Randomized, prospective comparison of increased preload versus inotropes in the resuscitation of trauma patients: effects on cardiopulmonary function and visceral perfusion. J Trauma 44: 107-113
33. Chang MC, Cheatham ML, Nelson LD, et al (1994) Gastric tonometry supplements information provided by systemic indicators of oxygen transport. J Trauma 37: 488-494
34. Sinclair S, James S, Singer M (1997) Intraoperative intravascular volume optimisation and length of hospital stay after repair of proxial femoral repair fracture: randmomised controlled trial. BMJ 31: 909-912

Treatment of Acidosis: Sodium Bicarbonate and Other Drugs

G. A. SCHMIDT

Lactic acidosis, defined as a *lactate* level > 5 mmol/l and a pH 7.35, is far and away the most-important acidosis during critical illness and most of this discussion of acidosis treatment will focus on treatment of lactic acidosis. Even in the face of maximal supportive therapy, lactic acidosis is associated with a mortality of 60-90%[1-4], so physicians have long relied on treatments to lower the [H+], such as sodium *bicarbonate*. Less common than lactic acidosis, and much more amenable to conventional treatments, are ketoacidoses and respiratory acidosis, but these too occasionally prompt consideration of alkalinizing therapies. Lowering the [H+] in blood depends on manipulating the strong ion difference ([*SID*]), total concentration of non-volatile weak acid buffer (A_{TOT}), or arterial CO_2 tension ($PaCO_2$), or raising the total concentration of weak bases, BTOT (normally sufficiently small that it can be ignored). Therefore, potential treatments include:

1. Raise [SID]: a) add strong cations: bicarbonate, *carbicarb*, dialysis
   b) remove strong anions: dichloroacetate (DCA), dialysis, thiamine, riboflavin, vasoactive drugs?
2. Lower the $paCO_2$: raise V_E or lower V_D/V_T or VCO_2
3. Reduce A_{TOT}: remove albumin, but very limited effect
4. Raise B_{TOT}: *tromethamine*

Sodium bicarbonate

The chain of reasoning supporting the use of bicarbonate is:

1. An elevated [H+], in and of itself, is harmful (mostly notably by impairing cardiovascular function)
2. Sodium bicarbonate can lower the [H+] when infused intravenously

3. Lowering the [H+] with sodium bicarbonate improves cardiovascular function or some other relevant outcome
4. Any adverse effects of sodium bicarbonate are outweighed by its benefits.

The first of these points has been addressed in a prior session so I will limit my discussion to points 2 through 4.

Can sodium bicarbonate lower the [H+] in vivo?

It seems straightforward that adding a base to acidic blood will lower the [H+] – the reality is more complex. Administration of exogenous sodium bicarbonate increases the [SID] (which tends to lower the [H+]) since sodium is a strong cation and bicarbonate is not a *strong ion* at all, but at the same time elevates the $paCO_2$ (which tends to raise [H+]). In animal models of lactic acidosis, sodium bicarbonate does not predictably lower the arterial [H+]. In some studies, [H+] remained constant or rose [5, 6]. Most whole-animal studies, however, have shown that [H+] can be lowered and even normalized [7-12]. Most relevant to clinical practice, in two studies of mechanically ventilated patients with lactic acidosis, intravenous infusion of sodium bicarbonate at doses of 2 mmol/kg over 15 min or 1 mmol/kg over 1-2 min raised the pH only 0.14 and 0.05 units, respectively [2, 13].

If the ability to increase alveolar ventilation is limited, as is commonly the case in mechanically ventilated patients, lowering the [H+] may be difficult or impossible. Rapid intravenous administration of 50 mEq sodium bicarbonate generates roughly 200 ml CO_2. In one series of mechanically ventilated patients with lactic acidosis, a modest infusion of sodium bicarbonate (2 mmol/kg over 15 min intravenously) boosted $paCO_2$ from 35 to 40 mmHg [2]. In six patients with severe *acute lung injury* and V_D/V_T of 0.7-0.8, administration of bicarbonate acutely worsened the acidosis [14].

Further complicating the effects of this potential therapy, bicarbonate administration may engender metabolic reactions that may secondarily alter [SID], A_{TOT}, or $paCO_2$. For example, in animals and humans, bicarbonate infusion can augment the production of lactic acid, a strong anion [5, 6, 8, 10, 15, 16]. Mechanisms to explain this remain speculative, but include a shift in the oxyhemoglobin saturation relationship [17], enhanced anaerobic glycolysis, perhaps mediated by the pH-sensitive, rate-limiting enzyme phosphofructokinase, and changes in hepatic blood flow or lactate uptake [18].

It is important to consider the body's multiple compartments, separated by membranes of differing permeabilities and systems of active transport. Even when sodium bicarbonate added to the central veins succeeds in lowering the arterial [H+], its effects on the cerebrospinal fluid (CSF) and intracellular spaces may not be concordant. This could happen because CO_2, produced when bicarbonate reacts with metabolic acids, diffuses readily across cell membranes and the blood-brain barrier, while bicarbonate cannot. Alternatively, as discussed above, bicarbonate may provoke reactions within cells, vessels, or organs that lower the local [SID] or raise the local pCO_2.

Sodium bicarbonate raised CSF [H+] in dogs with diabetic ketoacidosis (DKA) [19], dogs being resuscitated after a ventricular fibrillation arrest [20], and two patients with DKA, where it was associated with a decrease in mental status [21]. Intracellular [H+] has been measured in cells or animals using nuclear magnetic resonance spectroscopy, pH-sensitive fluorescent dyes, intramuscular electrodes, and the distribution of ^{14}C-labeled dimethadione. The results are inconsistent, with *intracellular [H+]* falling in 1 study [12], not changing in 6 studies [7, 10, 22-25], rising in 9 studies [5, 6, 26-32], and either rising or falling depending on the buffer used in 3 investigations [33-35]. In various studies, intracellular [H+] has been shown to rise with bicarbonate in red blood cells [5], muscle [32], liver [6], lymphocytes [30], and brain [27]. I am aware of only one human study involving determination by magnetic resonance spectroscopy of intracellular [H+] in brain [29]. When these normal volunteers were given sodium bicarbonate intravenously, brain [H+] rose significantly.

In summary, sodium bicarbonate can lower the blood [H+] when given intravenously in some patients, but it may be ineffective when alveolar ventilation is limited by severe, concomitant lung disease. Also, this therapy fails to reduce reliably the intracellular [H+]. Indeed, intracellular [H+] rises in most animal models and in most organs studied, but the effect is variable.

Does lowering the blood (H+) with sodium bicarbonate have any salutary effects?

In isolated hearts (rat, rabbit) perfused with acidic solutions, bicarbonate fails to augment ventricular contractility [22, 36]. In whole animals (including varied models of metabolic acidosis), the effects of bicarbonate on ventricular function are more difficult to tease out from its impact on systemic vessels. Further, one must take care not to interpret these studies too simplistically. For example, a fall in blood pressure is not necessarily detrimental (if cardiac output rises). Nevertheless, these studies uniformly fail to reveal any hemodynamic benefit for sodium bicarbonate when compared with iso-osmolar saline [5-10, 12, 15, 26, 28, 37-39]. When it has been measured, cardiac output either does not change [8, 10, 39] or falls [5, 6, 22]. Right ventricular contractility [37, 39] and hepatic blood flow [5, 6] fall. Perhaps the most-careful study of left ventricular function involved L-lactic acid infusion in anesthetized, ventilated, beta-blocked, and atrially paced dogs. Before and after bicarbonate infusion, the left ventricular pressure-volume relationship was determined with a ventricular Millar catheter and three orthogonal pairs of ultrasonic crystals imbedded in the ventricular walls [9]. Although sodium bicarbonate lowered the arterial [H+] and did not increase lactate levels, mean arterial pressure fell and cardiac output and ventricular contractility (slope of the end-systolic pressure-volume relationship) did not change. The hemodynamic effects were indistinguishable from those of saline.

There have been two studies of the hemodynamic impact of sodium bicarbonate in human lactic acidosis [2, 13]. In both studies, patients were mechanically ventilated, had a mean blood lactate between 7 and 8 mmol/l, and were receiving continuous infusions of vasoactive drugs (except 1 patient in 1 study). Although sodium bicarbonate lowered [H+] and raised serum bicarbonate levels, it did not improve hemodynamics or catecholamine responsiveness. Specifically, bicarbonate was indistinguishable from saline with regard to heart rate, central venous pressure, pulmonary artery pressure, mixed venous oxyhemoglobin saturation, systemic oxygen delivery, oxygen consumption, arterial blood pressure, pulmonary artery occlusion (wedge) pressure, and cardiac output [2, 13]. These findings suggest that the commonly observed hemodynamic response to bicarbonate administration in patients treated with vasoactive drug infusions may simply be one of preload augmentation (rather than enhanced catecholamine responsiveness). When the most severely acidemic (pH range 6.9-7.2) subset of patients was analyzed separately, these negative findings persisted [2]. This result does not support the practice of some physicians who withhold bicarbonate from patients with mild *acidemia* but feel compelled to give it to those with acidemia of greater magnitude.

During permissive hypercapnic ventilation, bicarbonate therapy has often been advocated [40, 41], but it has received little study. In mechanically ventilated ewes without lung injury, acute permissive hypercapnia ($paCO_2 = 8$ mmHg) raised cardiac output, organ blood flow, and intracranial pressure, all of which were attenuated by infusion of bicarbonate to maintain a normal pH [42]. In six patients with acute lung injury and concomitant acidosis, in whom hypercapnia (mean $paCO_2 = 53$, pH 7.21) was a consequence of impaired gas exchange and lung-protective ventilation, bicarbonate worsened the acidemia in all patients (mean pH fell to 7.1) [14].

In both prospective and retrospective studies of patients with DKA treated with or without sodium bicarbonate, there were no differences in the neurological status, incidence of hypokalemia or hypoglycemia, or rate of correction of acidemia [43, 44].

In summary, no controlled study has shown improved hemodynamics attributable to sodium bicarbonate infusion, regardless of the effect on [H+], and many show worsening of some hemodynamic variables.

Does sodium bicarbonate have negative side effects?

The most-obvious side effects of sodium bicarbonate are the fluid and sodium load. This can cause hypervolemia, hyperosmolarity and hypernatremia [45]. In one study of three patients treated with sodium bicarbonate (mean dose 90 mEq) during cardiac arrest, osmolality rose from 308 to 343 mosmol/kg [20]. Sodium bicarbonate given as a rapid intravenous bolus can cause a transient fall in mean arterial pressure and a transient rise in intracranial pressure [46] that is probably related to its hypertonicity, and is alleviated when given as a slow intravenous infusion. Sodium bicarbonate has been shown in three studies to lower paO_2 from 5 to 15 mmHg in both acidemic animals and non-acidemic patients with congestive heart failure [19, 47]. The mechanism for this is unclear, but the authors speculated that there might be worsening of intrapulmonary shunt.

When normal human volunteers were made acidemic with acetazolamide and then corrected with sodium bicarbonate, the acute correction of the [H+] caused increased hemoglobin affinity for oxygen that worsened oxygen delivery. This effect lasted about 8 h [17]. This was thought to be due to the immediate nature of the Bohr effect and the delayed nature of the 2,3- diphosphoglyceric acid effect on hemoglobin oxygen affinity.

Lactate levels increased with sodium bicarbonate infusion (over control) in animal studies of hypoxic lactic acidosis [6, 10, 15], phenformin-induced lactic acidosis [5, 32], hemorrhagic shock [8], and DKA [12, 19]. This finding has also been reported in cases of chronic lactic acidosis associated with malignancies [48]. It is possible that lactate rises in these settings because of impaired oxygen delivery to tissues. It is somewhat reassuring that in patients with lactic acidosis treated with sodium bicarbonate, no significant changes in venous lactate concentration, hemoglobin affinity for oxygen, total body oxygen consumption, oxygen extraction ratio, or transcutaneous oxygen pressure were seen, although the dose of bicarbonate was small (1 mmol/kg) [13]. Even if enhanced lactate production does not signal cellular hypoxia, bicarbonate-induced hyperlactatemia may be detrimental, since lactate itself, buffered to a pH of 7.4, can cause decreased cardiac contractility in animal models [49].

Serum ionized calcium concentration is reduced by sodium bicarbonate infusion. In a randomized, controlled study of intensive care units (ICU) patients with lactic acidosis, sodium bicarbonate lowered ionized calcium from

0.95 to 0.87 mmol/l [2]. In an animal study of cardiac arrest, sodium bicarbonate decreased ionized calcium, although this had no apparent detrimental effects [50]. Since left ventricular contractility has been shown to vary directly with ionized calcium concentration [51], any beneficial effects of [H+] correction may be masked by hypocalcemic ventricular depression.

Finally, in patients with DKA, bicarbonate delays clearance of ketones and lactate [52, 53] and is a risk factor for the development of cerebral edema [54].

In summary, many potentially detrimental effects of bicarbonate administration have been identified, but their clinical relevance has not been established. Sodium bicarbonate is often effective in lowering [H+] in critically ill patients, but may worsen acidosis in some with severe lung disease. Even when bicarbonate corrects arterial acidemia, no favorable cardiovascular effects have been demonstrated, even for patients with severe acidemia and receiving continuous infusions of catecholamines. Therefore, for lack of efficacy, bicarbonate should not be used routinely to treat acidosis, regardless of the degree of acidemia. Given the current evidence, any future role for bicarbonate in these patients depends on the formulation of new hypotheses of efficacy, followed by animal and clinical studies to seek any proposed benefit.

Carbicarb

Carbicarb is an equimolar mixture of sodium carbonate and sodium bicarbonate. Compared with sodium bicarbonate, Carbicarb raises the [SID] (thereby lowering the arterial [H+]) far more [8, 10, 11, 15, 26] and boosts the $paCO_2$ far less [8, 10, 28] when given intravenously to animals with metabolic acidosis. To the extent that the failure of sodium bicarbonate to effect hemodynamic improvement is due to the generation of carbon dioxide, Carbicarb might be superior. Carbicarb more consistently lowers intracellular [H+] [10, 22, 26-28, 55] and, while it improved hemodynamics in five studies [10, 15, 22, 26, 28], it did not in four others [7, 8, 12, 56]. This drug is not available clinically.

Dichloroacetate

Some component of the lactic acidosis of sepsis may be due to impaired pyruvate oxidation, rather than to tissue hypoxia [57, 58]. The *pyruvate dehydrogenase* complex (PDH) is a key controller of carbohydrate metabolism, representing the first irreversible step in pyruvate oxidation in the mitochondria (Fig. 1).

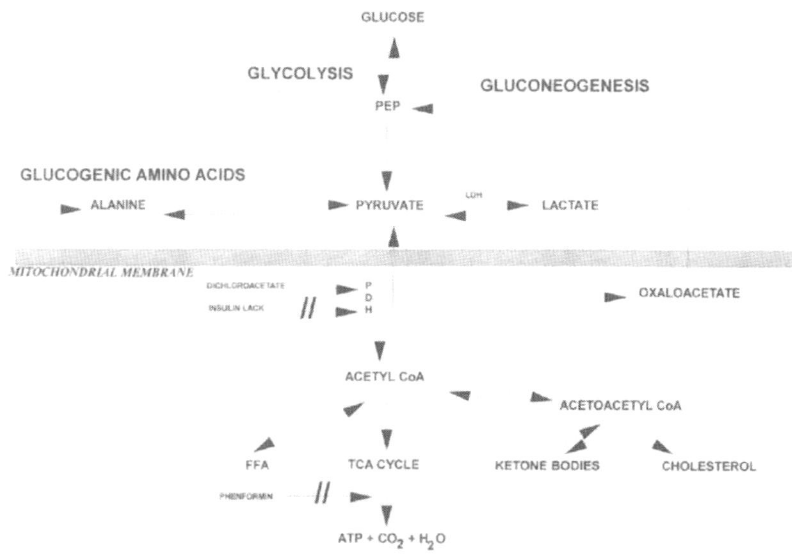

Fig. 1. Pyruvate connects glycolysis, gluconeogenesis, amino acid catabolism, and mitochondrial oxidation. It is also in equilibrium with lactate. Entry into the tricarboxylic acid cycle is governed by the activity of pyruvate dehydrogenase (PDH). PEP = phosphoenolpyruvate, LDH = lactate dehydrogenase, FFA = free fatty acids, TCA = tricarboxylic acid

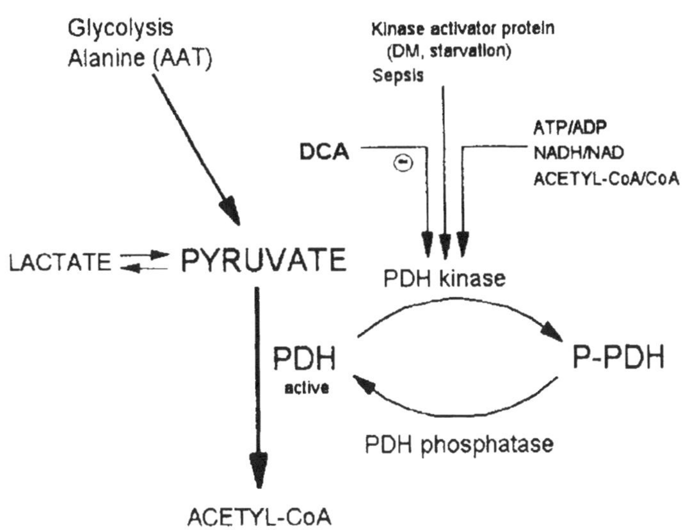

Fig. 2. The activity of PDH is down-regulated by a PDH-kinase, which itself can be activated during sepsis. Dichloroacetate (DCA) works in part through inhibition of this kinase, leading to accumulation of the active form of PDH. When PDH is largely in the inactive (phosphorylated) form, the pyruvate concentration rises, thereby increasing the lactate concentration. AAT = alanine aminotransferase; DM = diabetes mellitus

PDH activity is regulated, in part, by phosphorylation (inactivation), catalyzed by a PDH kinase (Fig. 2). This kinase may be activated in sepsis, down-regulating PDH and leading to accumulation of pyruvate (and, passively, lactate). Dichloroacetate (DCA) probably works by stimulating PDH, thus promoting the clearance of accumulated lactate. Other mechanisms of lactate clearance may also be operative, such as through enhanced gluconeogenesis [59]. In children with congenital lactic acidosis, a group of conditions characterized by defective pyruvate oxidation, DCA has sometimes been successful in ameliorating the acidosis and leading to overall clinical improvement [60].

Several animal trials showed that DCA could lower [H+] and raise bicarbonate concentration while lowering lactate levels [18, 61-63] in various models of lactic acidosis, including those of hypoxia, phenformin, and endotoxin. Further, in a rat model (*Plasmodium berghei* infection), DCA prolongs survival [64].

Studies in patients have also shown that DCA lowers lactate levels and ameliorates acidemia, with little apparent toxicity [65-67]. There has been one, large, randomized, placebo-controlled trial of DCA in patients with lactic acidosis due to sepsis, cardiogenic shock, or massive hemorrhage [3]. Patients had arterial blood lactate concentrations greater than 5 mmol/l (mean value 11.0) and pH 7.35 (mean 7.24). Treatment consisted of a 10% solution of DCA, 50 mg/kg body weight, infused over 30 min, then repeated at 2 h. DCA was much more likely to lower the arterial blood lactate concentration and [H+], but there was no effect on hemodynamics or survival.

The simplest interpretation of this study is that DCA is ineffective with respect to clinically important outcomes. Nevertheless, higher or more-prolonged doses of DCA might have more-dramatic effects than were demonstrated in this study, a supposition which is supported by the relatively short half-life of DCA during lactic acidosis (2.6 h)[68]. Since DCA not only improves acidosis but also may reverse impaired mitochondrial energy metabolism (unlike bicarbonate), it deserves further study in critically ill patients.

Tromethamine

Tris-hydroxymethyl aminomethane (tromethamine, THAM, tris, Tribonat) is a weak alkali (pK=7.8) that penetrates cells easily. Its potential to lower blood and intracellular [H+] without producing CO_2 has been confirmed in animal models of metabolic acidosis [69]. THAM also improved myocardial contraction and relaxation in an isolated rabbit heart preparation [36].

There has been extensive use of tromethamine outside of North America but, until recently, few systematic studies evaluating its effects. *Permissive hypercapnia* modestly reduces systemic vascular resistance, lowers myocardial contractility, raises pulmonary artery pressure, and raises cardiac output. In a study of 12 patients with acute respiratory distress syndrome (ARDS), when acidemia was corrected by tromethamine, the myocardial depression and pulmonary hypertension were significantly ameliorated [70]. In 10 ARDS patients with severe acidemia at the limits of mechanical ventilation, tromethamine at a mean dose of 1.07 mmol/kg par hour raised the pH from 7.14 to 7.26 and lowered $paCO_2$ from 63 to 50 [14].

Whether these effects are clinically relevant remains to be demonstrated, but tromethamine surely deserves additional study. Potentially detrimental effects of tromethamine include hypoglycemia, reduced arterial tone, respiratory depression, and hepatic necrosis (in neonates). It is excreted by the kidneys.

Thiamine

Occasionally, metabolic acidosis responds to *thiamine* administration. Patients with thiamine deficiency (beriberi due to alcoholism, malignancy, chronic illness, total parenteral nutrition) may improve dramatically following treatment with thiamine. HIV-infected patients receiving nucleoside analogues (e.g., stavudine, lamivudine, zidovudine) sometimes suffer mitochondrial dysfunction and lactic acidosis which can respond to thiamine [71] or to riboflavin [72]. These cases raise the possibility that thiamine, which is an essential cofactor for PDH, could reverse the mitochondrial dysfunction of sepsis, potentially improving mitochondrial energetics as well as treating acidosis.

Should acidemia be treated?

Although acidemia can be harmful, it is not self-evident that treatment of any kind is beneficial. Acidosis may have protective effects in critical illness. An elevated [H+] has been shown to delay the onset of cell death in isolated hepatocytes exposed to anoxia [73] and to chemical hypoxia [74]. Correcting the [H+] took away the protective effect and accelerated cell death. In addition, acidosis during reperfusion limits myocardial infarct size [75, 76]. Many other potentially beneficial effects of acidosis have been described [77]. Perhaps most relevant to critically ill patients is a study of acute lung injury induced by ischemia-reperfusion in ventilated rabbit lungs [78]. Hypercapnia prevented the usual increase in the pulmonary capillary filtration coefficient after reperfusion. Restoring the [H+] to normal worsened significantly the degree of vascular leakiness. Although it is a long leap from ex vivo rabbit lungs to human illness, these results should caution us that even the perfect alkalinizing agent (effective, safe, cheap) might not be good for patients.

References

1. Weil MH, Afifi AA (1970) Experimental and clinical studies on lactate and pyruvate as indicators of the severity of acute circulatory failure (shock). Circulation 41:989-1001
2. Cooper DJ, Walley KR, Wiggs BR, et al (1990) Bicarbonate does not improve hemodynamics in critically ill patients who have lactic acidosis: a prospective, controlled clinical study. Ann Intern Med 112:492-498
3. Stacpoole PW, Wright EC, Baumgartner TG, et al (1992) A controlled clinical trial of dichloroacetate for treatment of lactic acidosis in adults. N Engl J Med 327:1564-1569
4. Stacpoole PW, Wright EC, Baumgartner TG, et al (1994) Natural history and course of acquired lactic acidosis in adults. Am J Med 97:47-54
5. Arieff AI, Leach W, Park R, et al (1982) Systemic effects of NaHCO3 in experimental lactic acidosis in dogs. Am J Physiol 242:F586-F591
6. Graf H, Leach W, Arieff AI (1985) Metabolic effects of sodium bicarbonate in hypoxic lactic acidosis in dogs. Am J Physiol 249:F630-F635
7. Beech JS, Nolan KM, Iles RA, et al (1994) The effects of sodium bicarbonate and a mixture of sodium bicarbonate and carbonate (Carbicarb) on skeletal muscle pH and hemodynamic status in rats with hypovolemic shock. Metabolism 43:518-522
8. Benjamin E, Oropello JM, Abalos AM, et al (1994) Effects of acid base correction on hemodynamics, oxygen dynamics, and resuscitability in severe canine hemorrhagic shock. Crit Care Med 22:1616-1623
9. Cooper DJ, Herbertson MJ, Werner HA, et al (1993) Bicarbonate does not increase left ventricular contractility during L-lactic acidemia in pigs. Am Rev Respir Dis 148:317-322
10. Rhee KH, Toro LO, McDonald GG, et al (1993) Carbicarb, sodium bicarbonate, and sodium chloride in hypoxic lactic acidosis: effect on arterial blood gases, lactate concentrations, hemodynamic variables, and myocardial intracellular pH. Chest 104:913-918
11. Klepper ID, Kucera RF, Kindig NB, et al (1988) A comparative study of sodium bicarbonate and carbicarb in the treatment of metabolic acidosis induced by hemorrhagic shock. J Crit Care 3:256-261
12. Beech JS, Williams SCR, Iles RA, et al (1995) Haemodynamic and metabolic effects in diabetic ketoacidosis in rats of treatment with sodium bicarbonate or a mixture of sodium bicarbonate and sodium carbonate. Diabetologia 38:889-898
13. Mathieu D, Neviere R, Billard V, et al (1991) Effects of bicarbonate therapy on hemodynamics and tissue oxygenation in patients with lactic acidosis: a prospective, controlled clinical study. Crit Care Med 19:1352-1356
14. Kallet RH, Jasmer RM, Luce JM, et al (2000) The treatment of acidosis in acute lung injury with tris-hydroxymethyl aminomethane (THAM). Am J Respir Crit Care Med 161:1149-1153
15. Sun JH, Filley GF, Hord K, et al (1987) Carbicarb: an effective substitute for NaHCO3 for the treatment of acidosis. Surgery 5:835-839
16. Fraley DS, Adler S, Bruns FJ, et al (1980) Stimulation of lactate production by administration of bicarbonate in a patient with a solid neoplasm and lactic acidosis. N Engl J Med 303:1100-1102.
17. Bellingham AJ, Detter JC, Lenfant C (1971) Regulatory mechanisms of hemoglobin oxygen affinity in acidosis and alkalosis. J Clin Invest 50:700-706

18. Park R, Arieff AI (1982) Treatment of lactic acidosis with dichloroacetate in dogs. J Clin Invest 70:853-862
19. Bureau MA, Begin R, Berthiaume Y, et al (1980) Cerebral hypoxia from bicarbonate infusion in diabetic acidosis. J Pediatr 96:968-973
20. Bishop RL, Weisfeldt ML (1976) Sodium bicarbonate administration during cardiac arrest: effect on arterial pH, pCO2, and osmolality. JAMA 235:506-509
21. Posner JB, Plum F (1967) Spinal-fluid pH and neurologic symptoms in systemic acidosis. N Engl J Med 277:605-613
22. Shapiro JI. (1990) Functional and metabolic responses of isolated hearts to acidosis: effects of sodium bicarbonate and carbicarb. Am J Physiol 258:H1835-H1839
23. Bollaert PE, Robin-Lherbier B, Mallie JP, et al (1994) Effects of sodium bicarbonate on striated muscle metabolim and intracellular pH during endotoxic shock. Shock 1:196-200
24. Kette F, Weil MH, Planta M von, et al (1990) Buffer agents do not reverse intramyocardial acidosis during cardiac resuscitation. Circulation 81:1660-1666
25. Thompson CH, Syme PD, Williams EM, et al (1992) Effect of bicarbonate administration on skeletal muscle intracellular pH in the rat: implications for acute administration of bicarbonate in man. Clin Sci (Colch) 82:559-564
26. Bersin RM, Arieff AI (1988) Improved hemodynamic function during hypoxia with carbicarb, a new agent for the management of acidosis. Circulation 77:227-233
27. Li YC, Wiklund L, Tarkkila P, et al (1996) Influence of alkaline buffers on cytoplasmic pH in myocardial cells exposed to metabolic acidosis. Resuscitation 32:33-44
28. Shapiro JI, Whalen M, Chan L. (1990) Hemodynamic and hepatic pH responses to sodium bicarbonate and carbicarb during systemic acidosis. Magn Res on Med 16:403-410
29. Nakashima K, Yamashita T, Kashiwagi S, et al (1996) The effect of sodium bicarbonate on CBF and intracellular pH in man: stable Xe-CT and ^{31}P-MRS. Acta Neurol Scand [Suppl] 166:96-98
30. Bjerneroth G, Sammeli O, Li YC, et al (1994) Effects of alkaline buffers on cytoplasmic pH in lymphocytes. Crit Care Med 22:1550-1556
31. Ritter JM, Doktor HS, Benjamin N (1990) Paradoxical effect of bicarbonate on cytoplasmic pH. Lancet 335:1243-1246
32. Arieff AI, Leach WJ, Lazarowitz VC (1978) Effects of NaHCO3 in therapy of experimental lactic acidosis (abstract). Kidney Int 14: 645
33. Goldsmith DJA, Forni LG, Hilton PJ (1997) Bicarbonate therapy and intracellular acidosis. Clin Sci (Colch) 93:593-598
34. Levraut J, Labib Y, Chave S, et al (1996) Effect of sodium bicarbonate on intracellular pH under different buffering conditions. Kidney Int 49:1262-1267
35. Levraut J, Giunti C, Ciebiera JP, et al (2001) Initial effect of sodium bicarbonate on intracellular pH depends on the extracellular nonbicarbonate buffering capacity. Crit Care Med 29:1033-1039
36. Sirieix D, DeLayance S, Paris M, et al (1997) Tris-hydroxymethyl aminomethane and sodium bicarbonate to buffer metabolic acidosis in an isolated heart model. Am J Respir Crit Care Med 155:957-963
37. Tanaka M, Nishikawa T, Mizutani T. (1996) Normovolemic haemodilution attenuates cardiac depression induced by sodium bicarbonate in canine metabolic acidosis. Br J Anaesth 77:408-412
38. Basir MA, Bhatia J, Burdno DS, et al (1996) Effects of Carbicarb and sodium bicarbonate on hypoxic lactic acidosis in newborn pigs. J Invest Med 44:70-74
39. Tanaka M, Nishikawa T (1997) Acute haemodynamic effects of sodium bicarbonate administration in respiratory and metabolic acidosis in anaesthetized dogs. Anaesth Intensive Care 25:615-620
40. Menitove SM, Goldring RM (1983) Combined ventilator and bicarbonate strategy in the management of status asthmaticus. Am J Med 74:898-901
41. The Acute Respiratory Distress Syndrome Network (2000) Ventilation with lower tidal volumes as compared with traditional tidal volumes for acute lung injury and the acute respiratory distress syndrome. N Engl J Med 342:1301-1308

42. Cardenas VJ, Zwischenberger JB, Tao W, et al (1996) Correction of blood pH attenuates changes in hemodynamics and organ blood flow during permissive hypercapnia. Crit Care Med 24:827-834
43. Lever E, Jaspan JB (1983) Sodium bicarbonate therapy in severe diabetic ketoacidosis. Am J Med 75:263-268
44. Morris LR, Murphy MB, Kitabchi AE (1986) Bicarbonate therapy in severe diabetic ketoacidosis. Ann Intern Med 105:836-840
45. Máttar JA, Weil MH, Shubin H, et al (1974) Cardiac arrest in the critically ill. II. Hyperosmolal states following cardiac arrest. Am J Med 56:162-168
46. Huseby JS, Gumprecht DG (1981) Hemodynamic effects of rapid bolus hypertonic sodium bicarbonate. Chest 79:552-554
47. Bersin RM, Chatterjee K, Arieff AI (1989) Metabolic and hemodynamic consequences of sodium bicarbonate administration in patients with heart disease. Am J Med 87:7-14
48. Fields ALA, Wolman SL, Halperin ML (1981) Chronic lactic acidosis in a patient with cancer: therapy and metabolic consequences. Cancer 47:2026-2029
49. Yatani A, Fujino T, Kinoshita K, et al (1981) Excess lactate modulates ionic currents and tension components in frog atrial muscle. J Mol Cell Cardiol 13:147-161
50. Vukmir RB, Bircher NG, Radovsky A, et al (1995) Sodium bicarbonate may improve outcome in dogs with brief or prolonged cardiac arrest. Crit Care Med 23:515-522
51. Lang RM, Fellner SK, Neumann A, et al (1988) Left ventricular contractility varies directly with blood ionized calcium. Ann Intern Med 108:524-529
52. Hale PJ, Crase J, Nattrass M (1984) Metabolic effects of bicarbonate in the treatment of diabetic ketoacidosis. B M J 289:1035-1038
53. Okuda Y, Adrogué HJ, Field JB, et al (1996) Counterproductive effects of sodium bicarbonate in diabetic ketoacidosis. J Clin Endocrinol Metab 81:314-320
54. Glaser N, Barnett P, McCaslin I, et al (2001) Risk factors for cerebral edema in children with diabetic ketoacidosis. N Engl J Med 344:264-269
55. Shapiro JI, Whalen M, Kucera R, et al (1989) Brain pH responses to sodium bicarbonate and Carbicarb during systemic acidosis. Am J Physiol 256:H1316-H1321
56. Basir MA, Bhatia J, Burdno DS, et al (1996) Effects of Carbicarb and sodium bicarbonate on hypoxic lactic acidosis in newborn pigs. J Invest Med 44:70-74
57. Vary TC (1991) Increased pyruvate dehydrogenase kinase activity in response to sepsis. Am J Physiol 260:E669-E674
58. Lang CH, Bagby GJ, Blakesley HL, et al (1987) Glucose kinetics and pyruvate dehydrogenase activity in septic rats treated with dichloroacetate. Circ Shock 23:131-141
59. Kamel KS, Cheema-Dhadki S, Halperin ML (1992) Is accelerated oxidation of lactate required for dichloroacetate to lower the level of lactate in blood? Can J Physiol Pharmacol 70:1477-1482
60. Stacpoole PW, Barnes C, Hurbanis MD, et al (1997) Treatment of congenital lactic acidosis with dichloroacetate. Arch Dis Child 77:535-541
61. Curtis SE, Cain SM (1992) Regional and systemic oxygen/delivery uptake relations and lactate flux in hyperdynamic, endotoxin-treated dogs. Am Rev Respir Dis 145:348-354
62. Sheikh A, Fleisher G, Paredes CD, et al (1986) Effect of dichloroacetate in the treatment of anoxic lactic acidosis in dogs. Crit Care Med 14:970-973
63. Graf H, Leach W, Arieff AI (1985) Effects of dichloroacetate in the treatment of hypoxic lactic acidosis in dogs. J Clin Invest 76:919-923
64. Holloway PA, Knox K, Bajaj N, et al (1995) *Plasmodium berghei* infection: dichloroacetate improves survival in rats with lactic acidosis. Exp Parasitol 80:624-632
65. Stacpoole PW, Harman EM, Curry SH, et al (1983) Treatment of lactic acidosis with dichloroacetate. N Engl J Med 309:390-399
66. Stacpoole PW, Lorenz AC, Thomas RG, et al (1988) Dichloroacetate in the treatment of lactic acidosis. Ann Intern Med 108:58-63
67. Krishna S, Agbenyega T, Angus BJ, et al (1995) Pharmacokinetics and pharmacodynamics of dichloroacetate in children with lactic acidosis due to severe malaria. Q J Med 88:341-349

68. Stacpoole PW, Henderson GN, Yan Z, et al (1998) Pharmacokinetics, metabolism,and toxicology of dichloroacetate. Drug Metab Rev 30:499-539
69. Bjerneroth G. Tribonat (1999) A comprehensive summary of its properties. Crit Care Med 27:1009-1013
70. Weber T, Tschernich H, Sitzwohl C, et al (2000) Tromethamine buffer modifies the depressant effect of permissive hypercapnia on myocardial contractility in patients with acute respiratory distress syndrome. Am J Respir Crit Care Med 162:1361-1365
71. Schramm C, Wanitschke R, Galle PR (1999) Thiamine for the treatment of nucleoside analogue-induced severe lactic acidosis. Eur J Anaesthesiol 16:733-735
72. Fouty B, Frerman F, Reves R (1998) Riboflavin to treat nucleoside analogue-induced lactic acidosis. Lancet 352:291-292
73. Bonventre JV, Cheung JY (1985) Effects of metabolic acidosis on viability of cells exposed to anoxia. Am J Physiol 249:C149-C159
74. Gores GJ, Nieminen A-L, Wray BE, et al (1989) Intracellular pH during "chemical hypoxia" in cultured rat hepatocytes. J Clin Invest 83:386-396
75. Preckel B, Schlack W, Obal D, et al (1998) Effect of acidotic blood reperfusion on reperfusion injury after coronary artery occlusion in the dog heart. J Cardiovasc Pharmacal 31:179-186
76. Kitakaze M, Takashima S, Funaya H, et al (1997) Temporary acidosis during reperfusion limits myocardial infarct size in dogs. Am J Physiol 272:H2071-H2078
77. Laffey JG, Kavanagh BP (1999) Carbon dioxide and the critically ill-too little of a good thing? Lancet 354:1283-1286
78. Laffey JG, Engelberts D, Kavanagh BP (2000) Buffering hypercapnic acidosis worsens acute lung injury. Am J Respir Crit Care Med 161:141-146

Lactic Acidosis

G. A. SCHMIDT

Lactic acidosis

Definition and significance

Lactic acidosis is the most-common and most-important *metabolic acidosis* encountered in the intensive care unit (ICU). The acidemia has physiological significance and, more importantly, serves as a marker for a diverse group of serious underlying conditions. In addition, the presence, magnitude, and course of the acidosis have important prognostic implications.

Many patients in the ICU have small elevations in lactate level, usually in the range of 2-5 mmol/l, which are due to a variety of stimuli, including sympathetic activation. Mildly increased serum lactate levels in stable septic patients probably reflect impaired lactate clearance [1] or enhanced aerobic [2] or anaerobic [3] *glycolysis*, rather than *tissue hypoxia*. The definition of lactic acidosis is arbitrary; it is commonly defined as a lactate level greater than 5 mmol/ l with an arterial pH less than 7.35 [4]. Lactic acid is essentially fully dissociated in physiological solutions (pKa = 3.9), thereby acting as a strong anion, raising the strong ion difference ([SID]) and causing acidosis. Most cases of lactic acidosis encountered in the ICU occur secondarily to a handful of processes; shock is the most-common cause, with hypoxemia, seizures, regional ischemia (i.e., mesenteric or in an extremity), and toxin exposure accounting for a majority of the remaining cases.

The level of lactate is related to mortality. The in-hospital mortality for patients with a lactate level > 5 mmol/l was 83% and the median survival 2 days in the placebo arm of the dichloroacetate trial [5]. There is, however, considerable overlap in lactate levels between survivors and non-survivors. This inconsistent correlation is due, in part, to the influence on lactate levels of such factors as nutritional status and liver disease. However, the trend in lactate levels in a given patient can be helpful in gauging the effect of therapy and assessing prognosis. For example, in patients with septic shock, only those who ultimately survived showed a significant decrease in lactate level during the first 24 h of septic shock [6]. Survivors also had a shorter duration of *hyperlactatemia* and a smaller area under the curve for abnormal lactate levels.

Pathophysiology of lactic acidosis

Lactic acid is formed from pyruvate in a reaction catalyzed by lactate dehydrogenase (LDH), according to the following equation:

Pyruvate + $[H^+]$ + NADH = Lactate + NAD^+ (equation 1)

At equilibrium, the lactate concentration can be found as follows:
[Lact] = Keq x [Pyruvate] x [NADH]/$[NAD^+]$ x $[H^+]$ (equation 2)
where [Lact] is the lactic acid concentration at equilibrium; [NADH]/$[NAD^+]$ is the ratio of reduced to oxidized NAD^+, a measure of the adequacy of the oxygen supply; Keq is the equilibrium constant for the reaction; and $[H^+]$ is the hydrogen ion concentration.

Therefore, two fundamental derangements can underlie rising lactic acid production: (1) excessive accumulation of NADH when its oxidation to NAD in the mitochondrial respiratory chain is impaired, typically due to insufficient oxygen and (2) elevated pyruvate levels.

The first of these possibilities represents the mechanism of lactic acidosis when oxygen transport (QO_2) falls below a critical value (the critical QO_2; QcO_2). Since $QO_2 = CaO_2 \times Q_T$, where CaO_2 is arterial oxygen content and Q_T is cardiac output, either reduced arterial oxygen content (hypoxemia due to lung disease or intracardiac shunt, profound anemia, impaired binding of oxygen by hemoglobin) or reduced blood flow to the whole body or to a vascular bed (hypovolemia, pump dysfunction, splanchnic ischaemia) can leave the tissues with insufficient oxygen, prompting anaerobic metabolism. The QcO_2 in man has been determined to be roughly 4 ml O_2 per kg/min [7].

Whereas hypoxia is sufficient to cause lactic acidosis, it is not necessary. Since lactic acid is in equilibrium with *pyruvate*, an alternative origin for lactic acidosis is any condition that causes the pyruvate concentration to rise. In contrast to lactate, whose metabolic fate is simple (it can only be converted back to pyruvate), pyruvate lies at the nexus of no fewer than five relevant metabolic pathways (Fig. 1). A whole host of metabolic alterations can increase pyruvate levels, leading to non-hypoxic lactic acidosis, including enhanced glycolysis, impaired gluconeogenesis, excess catabolism of glucogenic amino acids, inactivation of pyruvate dehydrogenase activity, and any dysfunction in the *tricarboxylic acid cycle* or *oxidative phosphorylation* (see Table 1).

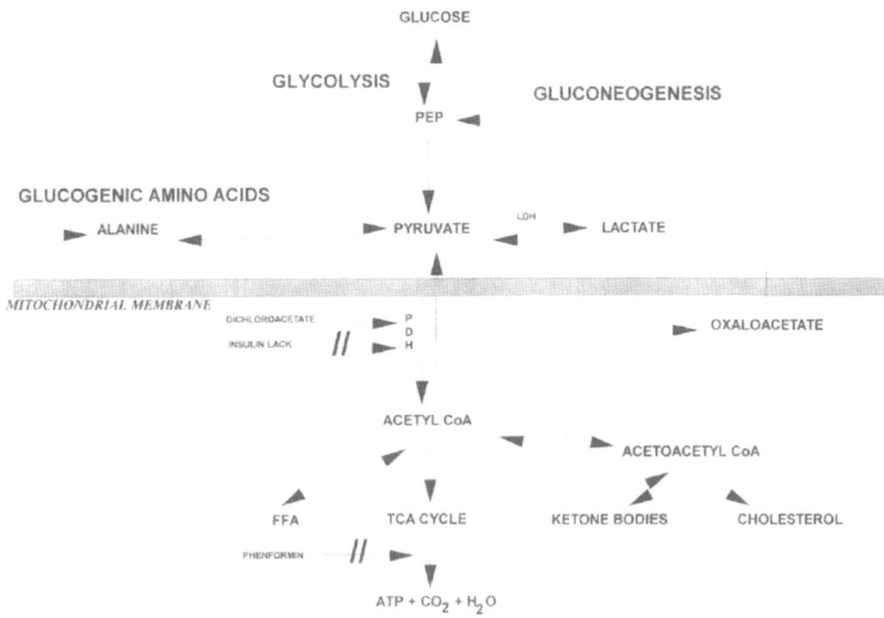

Fig. 1. Pyruvate is crucially involved in glycolysis, gluconeogenesis, amino acid catabolism, is in equilibrium with lactate, and serves as the entry point for the tricarboxylic acid (TCA) cycle. PEP = phophoenolpyruvate; LDH = lactate dehydrogenase; PDH = pyruvate dehydrogenase; FFA = free fatty acids

Table 1. Potential causes of lactic acidosis in sepsis (TCA = tricarboxylic acid; PDH = pyruvate dehydrogenase)

Insufficient O_2 to accept electrons at the terminal mitochondrial respiratory chain
Uncoupling of oxidative phosphorylation (e.g., dissipation of the strong ion gradient across the inner mitochondrial membrane) [8]
Inhibition of key enzymes in the mitochondrial respiratory chain (eg, NO inhibition of cytochrome aa3) [9]
Activation of poly-(ADP-ribosyl)-polymerase [PARP] which depletes NAD^+/NADH [10]
TCA cycle inhibition
PDH inhibition [11]
Lack of key cofactors for PDH or the TCA cycle (thiamine, riboflavin)
Catabolism of amino acids
Inhibition of gluconeogenesis
Enhanced aerobic glycolysis [2;12]

Until the last decade, the lactic acidosis of resuscitated septic shock was thought to represent an hypoxic phenomenon, but many studies have now challenged this view (Table 2) [13-24]. For example, if septic lactic acidosis were the consequence of hypoxia, the [NADH]:[NAD^+] ratio should be very high, forcing up the lactate: pyruvate ratio, yet the data fail to confirm this [13]. Further evidence that an oxygen deficit does not underlie septic lactic acidosis can be inferred from trials in which oxygen transport has been boosted by fluids, blood transfusion, or infusion of vasoactive drugs. First, raising QO_2 fails to enhance oxygen consumption (VO_2) [14, 16], even in patients with elevated lactate [15, 17] (i.e., there is no pathological supply dependence, at least at the whole-body level); and second, lactate levels do not fall when QO_2 is augmented [25]. More direct evidence that sepsis does not cause tissue hypoxia is available: measurements of tissue pO_2 by polarography [18], phosphorus-31 nuclear magnetic resonance spectroscopy [20], [^{18}F]fluoromisonidazole injection [21], and near infrared spectroscopy [22] fail to disclose hypoxia.

Table 2. Evidence that lactic acidosis of resuscitated sepsis is not hypoxic

QO_2 exceeds the critical QO_2
SvO_2 is normal or high
Lactate:pyruvate ratio not elevated [13]
Failure to demonstrate pathological supply dependence [14-16]
Failure of QO_2 augmentation to reduce lactate levels [15, 17]
Tissue PO_2 is not reduced
Polarography [18, 19]
Phosphorus-31 nuclear magnetic resonance spectroscopy [20]
[^{18}F]fluoromisonidazole injection [21]
Near-infrared spectroscopy [22]
Positive response to dichloroacetate [23]
Enhanced oxygen extraction in response to hypoxic hypoxia [24]

However, studies at the whole-body level may mask crucial regional truths. For example, were the gut to remain hypoxic despite resuscitation of the systemic circulation to supranormal levels of oxygen delivery, as has been shown in a canine model [26], studies of systemic QO_2, mixed venous oxyhemoglobin saturation, supply dependence, lactate:pyruvate ratio, and non-splanchnic tissue pO_2 might give falsely reassuring results about the adequacy of tissue oxygenation. Indeed, in septic patients (with or without lactic acidosis), tonometric measurements of gastric mucosal pCO_2 show that splanchnic and systemic perfusion may be poorly correlated [27], and support the hypothesis that the gut is hypoxic in human sepsis [28]. Further, in one series of patients with multiple organ failure, the hepatosplanchnic circulation was demonstrated to be a significant lactate producer [29]. Vasoactive drugs may worsen gastric mucosal perfusion and contribute to acidosis [30, 31].

In another vein, several possible causes of lactic acidosis rely not on lactate overproduction, but on decreased lactate clearance. Some tissues (most notably skin, erythrocytes, muscles, and, during sepsis, lung) metabolize glucose largely to pyruvate, convert the pyruvate to lactate, and transport lactate in the blood to the liver (and kidneys), where it is converted back to glucose through gluconeogenesis (or is metabolized further through the tricarboxylic acid cycle). Such regenerated glucose can travel to the tissues to be metabolized once again. This cycling of glucose to lactate and back to glucose again, called the Cori cycle, involves large quantities of lactate (Fig. 2). Interruption of the Cori cycle, owing to hepatic dysfunction, reduced hepatic blood flow, or impaired hepatic extraction of lactate, can produce clinically serious lactic acidosis in minutes to hours.

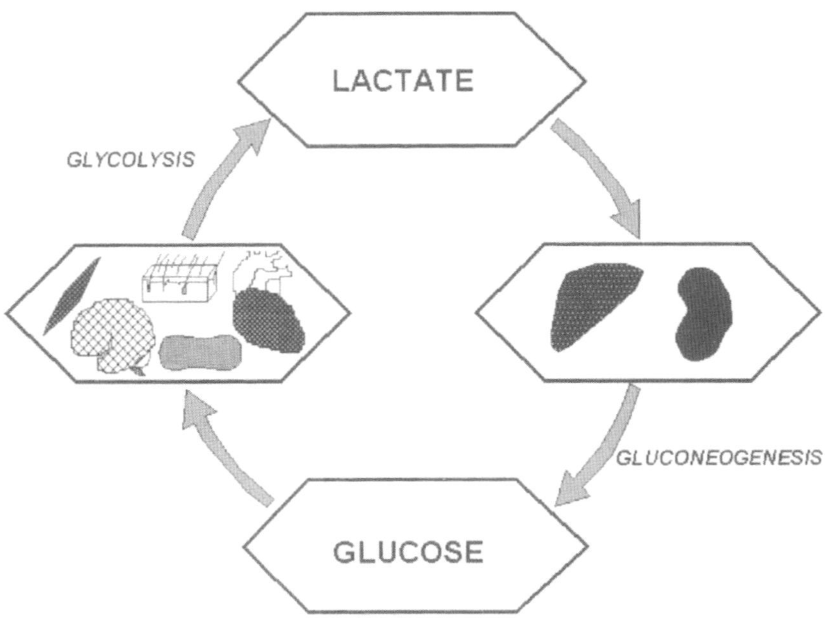

Fig. 2. Cori cycle. Some tissues, most notably the skin, red blood cells, and muscles metabolize glucose to lactate (glycolysis), which then is carried to the liver where it then is reconverted to glucose (gluconeogenesis) or metabolized to carbon dioxide and water. Glucose can return to the glycolytic tissues for additional energy production. This cycling of glucose and lactate represents a substantial flux of lactate, so that interruption of the gluconeogenic arm leads rapidly to lactic acidosis

The normal flux of lactate through the Cori cycle appears to be perturbed during sepsis and acute lung injury. For example, the lung normally is not a significant net lactate producer, but in both animals [32] and humans [33-35] with acute lung injury, the lung can become a major source of lactate. Also during sepsis, the liver, which normally consumes lactate, may switch to producing lactate [29, 36].

Effects of lactate

Lactate has physiological effects independent of changes in hydrogen ion concentration. Human neutrophils and fat cells in vitro show a decrease in β-adrenergic responsiveness with acidosis; this is exaggerated by increased lactate levels [37]. Animal experiments have shown direct lactate effects on the myocardium. These include inhibition of glyceraldehyde-3-phosphate dehydrogenase (and, thus, a decreased rate of glycolysis) and mitochondrial swelling (which decreases the ability to couple oxidative phosphorylation). Further, lactate decreases the slow inward calcium current, causing a negative inotropic effect even at a pH of 7.4 [38]. The clinical significance of these effects is uncertain.

Specific etiologies in the ICU

The etiologies of lactic acidosis are numerous and are listed in Table 3. A few examples will be discussed further, to give insight into the various mechanisms causing lactic acidosis.

Table 3. Etiologies of lactic acidosis

Increased oxygen consumption		
	Strenuous exercise	
	Grand mal seizure	
	Neuroleptic malignant syndrome	
	Severe asthma	
	Pheochromocytoma	
Decreased oxygen delivery		
	Decreased cardiac output	
		Hypovolemia
		Cardiogenic shock (including pericardial and pulmonary vascular disease)
	Decreased arterial oxygen content	
		Profound anemia
		Severe hypoxemia
	Regional ischemia (mesentery or extremity)	
Alterations in cellular metabolism		
	Sepsis	

Diabetes mellitus
Thiamine deficiency
Severe alkalemia
Hypoglycemia
Malignancy
Mitochondrial myopathies
AIDS?
Toxins and drugs
Carbon monoxide
Ethanol, methanol
Biguanides, e.g., metformin
Ethylene glycol, propylene glycol
Salicylates
Isoniazid
Streptozocin
Cyanide, nitroprusside
Papaverine
Acetaminophen
Nalidixic acid
Ritodrine
Terbutaline
Fructose, sorbitol, xylitol
Epinephrine, norepinephrine, cocaine
Zidovudine, other antiretroviral drugs
Kombucha tea
Propofol, lorazepam (via its vehicle, propylene glycol)
Congenital
Glucose-6-phosphatase deficiency
Fructose-1,6-diphosphatase deficiency
Pyruvate carboxylase deficiency
PDH deficiency
Oxidative phosphorylation defects
Decreased lactate clearance
Fulminant hepatic failure
D-Lactate
Short gut syndrome
Antibiotic-induced

Sepsis

Before patients with septic shock are resuscitated, hypovolemia and hypoxemia often contribute to hypoxic lactic acidosis, which improves with early shock management [39]. After resuscitation, when cardiac outputs and QO_2s of most septic patients are high, it is far more questionable whether tissue hypoxia exists. The answer to this question is important. If septic lactic acidosis represents hypoxia, therapies which serve to maximize QO_2 could be sensible. Alternatively, if oxygen lack does not underlie the acidosis, uncovering the true pathogenesis will be crucial to devising effective treatments or new drugs.

Seizures

Grand mal *seizures* cause tremendous muscle energy usage and glycogen breakdown, with much of the glucose converted to lactate. The lactic acidosis associated with seizures is illustrative of the handling of an acute lactate load. Immediately following a seizure, a lactic acidosis is present, with a lactate level often greater than 10 mmol/ l and a pH below 7.20. In 1 h, lactate levels fall to half their post-seizure levels and pH normalizes [40].

Malignancy

Lactic acidosis has been reported in a variety of malignancies, most commonly in leukemia and lymphoma. The excess lactate apparently is produced by the malignancy through enhanced glycolysis without the cellular control mechanisms that normally link glycolysis with oxidative phosphorylation. Extensive liver metastases are commonly found in lactic acidosis associated with solid tumours; diminished hepatic lactate extraction is contributory in many cases, although hepatic metastases are not required for lactic acidosis to occur. It is important to remember, however, that most cases of lactic acidosis in patients with malignancy are due to shock or sepsis.

Hepatic failure

The liver is the major lactate-metabolizing organ. With severe hepatic disease, lactate clearance is decreased. Because of the excess capacity for lactate metabolism that is normally available, stable patients with chronic liver disease do not manifest an elevation in serum lactate, even with severe hepatic dysfunction. However, the capacity to clear a lactate load is diminished, and any condition that increases lactate production will cause an exaggerated rise and delayed fall in blood lactate levels. In fulminant *hepatic failure*, patients may exhibit a lactic acidosis predominately on the basis of severely decreased lactate clearance.

Toxins

Toxin ingestion is an uncommon but important cause of increased anion gap acidosis. It should also be remembered that lactic acidosis can be caused by toxins, and that an increased lactate level does not rule out an acidosis from toxins. For example, in salicylate poisoning, the acidosis is predominantly a lactic acidosis, probably due to uncoupling of oxidative phosphorylation, perhaps because salicylate acts to dissipate the [SID] across the mitochondrial membrane created by oxidative phosphorylation [41].

Anti-retroviral therapy

Patients with AIDS are occasionally admitted to the ICU with significant lactic acidosis. Often this is due to sepsis or other causes of shock, but many patients have now been reported in whom lactic acidosis was due to anti-retroviral therapy, most often *zidovudine* [42-45]. Some patients will survive with discontinuation of the anti-retroviral agent, and there may be a role for thiamine [46] or riboflavin [47].

Treatment

The most-important treatment of lactic acidosis is treatment of the disease causing the metabolic derangements. Without successful treatment of the process precipitating lactic acidosis, survival is unlikely. Therapies aimed at ameliorating the lactic acidosis itself are attempts to prevent physiological deterioration until the primary process can be controlled, but it is not clear that any such therapy is effective, as detailed elsewhere.

References

1. Levraut J, Ciebiera JP, Chave S, et al (1998) Mild hyperlactatemia in stable septic patients is due to impaired lactate clearance rather than overproduction. Am J Respir Crit Care Med 157:1021-1026
2. James JH, Fang CH, Schrantz SJ, et al (1996) Linkage of aerobic glycolysis to sodium-potassium transport in rat skeletal muscle: implications for increased muscle lactate production in sepsis. J Clin Invest 98:2388-2397
3. Agbenyega T, Angus BJ, Bedu-Addo (2000) Glucose and lactate kinetics in children with severe malaria. J Clin Endocrinol Metab 85:1569-1576
4. Luft D, Deichsel G, Schmulling RM, et al (1983) Definition of clinically relevant lactic acidosis in patients with internal diseases. Am J Clin Pathol 80:484-489
5. Stacpoole PW, Wright EC, Baumgartner TG, et al (1994) Natural history and course of acquired lactic acidosis in adults. Am J Med 97:47-54
6. Bakker J, Gris P, Coffernils M, et al (1996) Serial blood lactate levels can predict the developement of multiple organ failure following septic shock. Am J Surg 171:221-226
7. Ronco JJ, Fenwick Jc, Tweeddale MG, et al (1993) Identification of the critical oxygen delivery for anaerobic metabolism in critically ill septic and nonseptic humans. JAMA 270:1724-1730
8. Mela L, Bacalzo LV Jr, Miller JD (1971) Defective oxidative metabolism of rat liver mitochondria in hemorrhagic and endotoxin shock. Am J Physiol 220:571-577

9. Takehara Y, Kanno T, Yoshioka T, et al (1995) Oxygen-dependent regulation of mitochondrial energy metabolism by nitric oxide. Arch Biochem Biophys 323:27-32
10. Szabo C, Cuzzocrea S, Zingarelli B, et al (1997) Endothelial dysfunction in a rat model of endotoxic shock: importance of the activation of poly (ADP-ribose) synthetase by peroxynitrite. J Clin Invest 100:723-735
11. Vary TC (1991) Increased pyruvate dehydrogenase kinase activity in response to sepsis. Am J Physiol 260:E669-E674
12. Widnell CC, Baldwin SA, Davies A, et al (1990) Cellular stress induces a redistribution of the glucose transporter. FASEB J 4:1634-1637
13. Cerra FB, Caprioli J, Siegel JH, et al (1979) Proline metabolism in sepsis, cirrhosis and general surgery: the peripheral energy deficit. Ann Surg 190:577-586
14. Russell JA, Phang PT (1994) The oxygen delivery/consumption controversy: approaches to management of the critically ill. Am J Respir Crit Care Med 149:533-537
15. Ronco JJ, Phang PT, Walley KR, et al (1991) Oxygen consumption is independent of changes in oxygen delivery in severe adult respiratory distress syndrome. Am Rev Respir Dis 143:1267-1273
16. Mira JP, Fabre JE, Baigorri F, et al (1994) Lack of oxygen supply dependency in patients with severe sepsis: a study of oxygen delivery increased by military antishock trouser and dobutamine. Chest 106:1524-1531
17. Hayes MA, Yau EH, Timmins AC, et al (1993) Response of critically ill patients to treatment aimed at achieving supranormal oxygen delivery and consumption: relationship to outcome. Chest 103:886-895
18. Boekstegers P, Weidenhöfer S, Kapsner T, et al (1994) Skeletal muscle partial pressure of oxygen in patients with sepsis. Crit Care Med 22:640-650
19. Hurtado FJ, Gutierrez AM, Silva N, et al (1992) Role of tissue hypoxia as the mechanism of lactic acidosis during *E coli* endotoxemia. J Appl Physiol 72:1895-1901
20. Hotchkiss RS, Long RC, Shires GT, et al (1989) An in vivo examination of rat brain during sepsis with 31P-NMR spectroscopy. Am J Physiol 257:C1055-C1061
21. Hotchkiss RS, Rust RS, Dence CS, et al (1991) Evaluation of the role of cellular hypoxia in sepsis by the hypoxic marker [18F] fluoromisonidazole. Am J Physiol 261:R965-R972
22. Taylor DE, Piantadosi CA (1995) Oxidative metabolism in sepsis and sepsis syndrome. J Crit Care 10:122-135
23. Stacpoole PW, Wright EC, Baumgartner TG, et al (1992) A controlled clinical trial of dichloroacetate for treatment of lactic acidosis in adults. N Engl J Med 327:1564-1569
24. Curtis SE, Cain SM (1992) Regional and systemic oxygen/delivery uptake relations and lactate flux in hyperdynamic, endotoxin-treated dogs. Am Rev Respir Dis 145:348-354
25. Silverman HJ (1991) Lack of a relationship between induced changes in oxygen consumption and changes in lactate levels. Chest 100:1012-1015
26. Vallet B, Lund N, Curtis SE, et al (1994) Gut and muscle tissue PO2 in endotoxemic dogs during shock and resuscitation. J Appl Physiol 76:793-800
27. Gutierrez G, Bismar H, Dantzker DR, et al (1992) Comparison of gastric intramucosal pH with measures of oxygen transport and consumption in critically ill patients. Crit Care Med 20:451-457
28. Gutierrez G, Clark C, Brown SD, et al (1994) Effect of dobutamine on oxygen consumption and gastric mucosal pH in septic patients. Am J Respir Crit Care Med 150:324-329
29. Douzinas EE, Tsidemiadou PD, Pitaridis MT, et al (1997) The regional production of cytokines and lactate in sepsis-related multiple organ failure. Am J Respir Crit Care Med 155:53-59
30. Marik PE, Mohedin M (1994) The contrasting effects of dopamine and norepinephrine on systemic and splanchnic oxygen utilization in hyperdynamic sepsis. JAMA 272:1354-1357
31. Neviere R, Mathieu D, Chagnon JL, et al (1996) The contrasting effects of dobutamine and dopamine on gastric mucosal perfusion in septic patients. Am J Respir Crit Care Med 154:1684 -1688
32. Bellomo R, Kellum JA, Pinsky MR (1996) Transvisceral lactate fluxes during early endotoxemia. Chest 110:198-204

33. Brown SD, Clark C, Gutierrez G (1996) Pulmonary lactate release in patients with sepsis and the adult respiratory distress syndrome. J Crit Care 11:2-8
34. Kellum JA, Kramer DJ, Lee K, et al (1997) Release of lactate by the lung in acute lung injury. Chest 111:1301-1305
35. De Backer D, Creteur J, Zhang H, et al (1997) Lactate production by the lungs in acute lung injury. Am J Respir Crit Care Med 156:1099-1104
36. Kellum JA, Bellomo R, Kramer DJ, et al (1995) Hepatic anion flux during acute endotoxemia. J Appl Physiol 78:2212-2217
37. Davies AO (1984) Rapid desensitization and uncoupling of human beta-adrenergic receptors in an in vitro model of lactic acidosis. J Clin Endocrinol Metab 59:398-405
38. Mochizuki S, Kobayashi K, Neely JR (1976) Effects of L-lactate on glyceraldehyde-3-P dehydrogenase in heart muscle. Recent Adv Stud Cardiac Struct Metab 12:175-182
39. Vincent JL, Dufaye P, Berre J, et al (1983) Serial lactate determinations during circulatory shock. Crit Care Med 11:449-451
40. Orringer CE, Eustace JC, Wunsch CD, et al (1977) Natural history of lactic acidosis after grand-mal seizures: a model for the study of an anion-gap acidosis not associated with hyperkalemia. N Engl J Med 297:796-799
41. Gutknecht J (1990) Salicylates and proton transport through lipid bilayer membranes: a model for salicylate-induced uncoupling and swelling in mitochondria. J Membr Biol 115:253-260
42. Chattha G, Arieff AI, Cummings C, et al (1993) Lactic acidosis complicating the acquired immunodeficiency syndrome. Ann Intern Med 118:37-39
43. Chariot P, Drogou I, Lacroix-Szmania I de, et al (1999) Zidovudine-induced mitochondrial disorder with massive liver steatosis, myopathy, lactic acidosis, and mitochondrial DNA depletion. J Hepatol 30:156-160
44. Shaer AJ, Rastegar A (2000) Lactic acidosis in the setting of antiretroviral therapy for the acquired immunodeficiency syndrome: a case report and review of the literature. Am J Nephrol 20:332-338
45. Bartley PB, Westacott L, Boots RJ, et al (2001) Large hepatic mitochondrial DNA deletions associated with L-lactic acidosis and highly active antiretroviral therapy. AIDS 15:419-420
46. Schramm C, Wanitschke R, Galle PR (1999) Thiamine for the treatment of nucleoside analogue-induced severe lactic acidosis. Eur J Anaesthesiol 16:733-735
47. Fouty B, Frerman F, Reves R (1998) Riboflavin to treat nucleoside analogue-induced lactic acidosis. Lancet 352:291-292

Acid-Base Balance during Renal Replacement Therapies

Z. Ricci, C. Ronco

According to established evidence, correction of metabolic acidosis is mandatory in acutely uremic patients. Bicarbonate, the physiological buffer, has almost totally replaced acetate in dialysis and has partially replaced lactate as a reinfusion solution in convective therapies. Bicarbonate does not require metabolic conversion and does not cause any known side effects, except for metabolic alkalosis deriving from excessive administration; it is also very well tolerated in the clinical setting, not interfering with cardiovascular and respiratory functions.

Bicarbonate has become the buffer of choice in continuous treatments in intensive care patients because of the frequent combination of acute renal failure with cardiovascular instability, hepatorenal failure, and metabolic acidosis derived from systemic inflammatory states or sepsis.

Buffer balance

The correction of metabolic acidosis in uremic patients is a primary indication for dialysis. Base gain during dialysis simulates the bicarbonate regeneration process by the normal kidneys. Fixed acids are produced by metabolic processes and taken up by gastrointestinal adsorption. Sulfuric acid is produced from oxidation of sulfur-containing amino acids, phosphoric acid is generated from proteins and phospholipids, and finally organic acids remain in the system when they are produced in excess of metabolic elimination capacity [1]. In patients without renal function, the maintenance of acid-base balance is only achieved when the dialytic base gain equals the patient's metabolic acid production. If hydrogen ion production exceeds the buffer gain from dialysis, the acidity would be continuously partially buffered by intracellular buffers, leading to undesired clinical consequences. While if the buffer gain prevails, an extracellular metabolic alkalosis would result.

An equation has been utilized in some mathematical models to predict post-dialysis blood bicarbonate values and dialytic base gain based on the concept of "space of distribution for bicarbonate":

$$ABS = (0.4 + 2.6/\text{blood } HCO_3^-) \times \text{body weight}$$

where ABS is apparent bicarbonate space, defined as the ratio of administered bicarbonate to the observed change in the plasma bicarbonate concentration, normally ranging between 40 and 50% the total body weight [2]. The extracellular bicarbonate system not only modulates the hydrogen concentration in the extracellular space but also exerts a buffering effect on the intracellular buffer systems that regulate the intracellular pH.

Acid production

Endogenous fixed acid production in normal subjects ranges between 0.7 and 1.2 mmol/kg per 24 h, mostly depending on diet and metabolism. In critically ill patients, this requires complex studies for a precise evaluation. Gotch et al. [3] reported that in normal subjects the ratio between net acid excretion in the urine and the protein catabolic rate (PCR) is constantly equal to 0.77. Daily acid production (H^+G_{24h}) is therefore calculated as

$$H^+G_{24h} = PCR \times 0.77$$

This relationship could not apply to critically ill patients, who are highly catabolic, and are fed by enteral or parenteral nutrition that does not contain the same ratio of amino acids as in normal food, thus generating a different amount of fixed acids per gram of nitrogen.

Dialytic buffer gain

Dialytic techniques cannot remove large amounts of free hydrogen ions because of their low concentration in the blood. Therefore H^+ removal is mainly achieved by the flux of the alkaline equivalents into the blood with replacement of the depleted buffers. Hence, during dialysis, fixed acids are converted to volatile acids. To achieve adequate correction of metabolic acidosis, the amount of buffers administered with dialysis should at least equal the overall production in the patient. In dialysis fluids bicarbonate has largely replaced acetate, because of the latter's deleterious effects on ventilation and hemodynamics; there is also a tendency to use bicarbonate in the replacement fluids during the convective treatment instead of the standard lactate solutions.

Factors affecting buffer balance in diffusive therapies

The amount of bicarbonate that diffuses across the membranes is a function of the concentration gradient between dialysate and blood; a role is also played by temperature and diffusivity, which is a constant and depends on membrane characteristics and on solute/solvent interaction. These parameters are fairly stable in clinical dialysis. Once the surface area of the dialyzer is defined, bicarbonate mass transfer rate (MTR) can be expressed as a function of dialysance (D) and bicarbonate average concentration gradient between dialysate and plasma (Cdi-Cpi).

$$MTR = D(Cdi - Cpi)$$

The exact amount of buffer to administer to balance the overall acid production in 24 h (net base gain = 0) can be achieved by varying the dialysate concentration of bicarbonate, the blood flow, the dialyzer surface area, or the duration of treatment session [4]. The individual requirement of buffer administration varies among patients, and the individualization of the dialysis bath is necessary to fulfil single needs, especially if intermittent dialysis sessions are carried out. When buffer depletion is occurring (because of renal failure itself, systemic inflammatory states, severe infections, congestive heart failure), higher bicarbonate concentration may be needed to achieve a positive balance. Furthermore, other substances move through the membrane according to a concentration gradient and affect the final "net base gain". Small amounts of acetate, in fact, are in the dialysate in order to prevent calcium and carbonate precipitation. This generates a flux of acetate into the blood ranging from 0.2 to 0.8 mmol/min. Converting to bicarbonate, acetate can produce a further base gain during bicarbonate dialysis (from 50 to 200 mmol per session of 4 h). Finally the mass transfer rate of organic anions (β-hydroxybutirate and acetoacetate) generally ranges between 0.2 and 0.5 mmol/min. This is an additional source of acid generation, since, if these anions are removed by dialysis, a consequent net accumulation of hydrogen ions occurs. However, only few free hydrogen ions cross the membrane, due to very low concentration gradients.

Factors affecting buffer balance in convective therapies

The kinetics of buffers in exclusively convective therapies (hemofiltration or ultrafiltration) is dependent on the characteristics of reinfusion solutions. Large quantities of bicarbonate are lost with convection, and the precise evaluation can be made only by measuring bicarbonate concentration in the ultrafiltrate. Nonetheless, bicarbonate loss can be estimated using the following formula:

$$HCO3^{-}(f) = UF \times HCO3^{-}(p) \times 1.124$$

where HCO3-(f) is bicarbonate in the ultrafiltrate and $HCO3^-$(p) is bicarbonate in plasma and 1.124 is average bicarbonate sieving coefficient. The average buffer concentration in the replacement solutions varies from 35 to 60 mmol/l. Bicarbonate solutions range from 30 to 40 mmol/l.

In convective treatments, solute transport is mostly governed by the membrane permeability [5-7]. Since non-diffusable anions, such as proteins, are present on one side of the membrane, bicarbonate concentration in the ultrafiltrate will be determined by the Donnan equilibrium, which will provide electrochemical equilibrium on both sides of the membrane. Therefore the bicarbonate concentration in the ultrafiltrate is generally higher then in plasma water, and sieving values range between 1.10 and 1.15, depending on plasma protein concentration at the inlet of the filter and the filtration fraction. The buffers infused via replacement solution must equal these losses to achieve stable serum bicarbonate levels, and may also give the excess amount of alkaline equivalents necessary to balance the metabolic acid production.

When continuous therapies are applied without fluid replacement (as in slow continuous ultra filtration) in order to reduce patient's fluid overload, bicarbonate losses are generally compensated by the reduction of the volume of distribution for bicarbonate, and the serum concentration does not change significantly. If hemofiltration is applied, the final balance will depend on the amount of buffer lost in the ultrafiltrate and the amount reinfused in the venous line after the filter. A different condition applies when pre-dilution is used. In the case of infusion of substitution fluid in the arterial line before the filter, part of the reinfused buffer is lost in the filtrate and the final balance is more complex.

Acid base in intermittent and continuous hemodialysis

In intermittent bicarbonate dialysis, blood pH and plasma bicarbonate progressively increase, while PCO2 shows stable values or a moderate increase [8, 9], so that at the end of the session a moderate metabolic alkalosis is observed. In the interdialytic period, blood pH and plasma bicarbonate progressively decrease until the subsequent session. Some authors [10] pointed out that during dialysis, bicarbonate delivery varies inversely with blood bicarbonate concentration. Hence, more alkali is gained when the plasma bicarbonate concentration is low and vice versa, thus making patient levels oscillate before reaching equilibrium. This hypothesis suggests that only in long-lasting treatments will acid-base balance reach the desired equilibrium. This indeed leads to speculation about the physiology of intermittent treatments and about the beneficial effects of continuous renal replacement therapies in acute renal failure and in critically ill patients.

Possible occurrence of hypoxemia during bicarbonate rather then acetate hemodialysis is still controversial. Some authors [11] observed , with dialysate concentration higher then 37 mmol/l, a rapid alkalinization of the patient, and a consequent compensatory hypoventilation.

Many examples are reported of a better effect of bicarbonate dialysis then acetate on hemodynamics: absence of acetate vasodilatory effect, less influence on heart rate, favorable effect of alkalosis on vascular reactivity [12], less effect on arterial PO_2. Despite the beneficial effects of bicarbonate instead of acetate, the most-accurate buffer balance and the most-constant metabolic correction is still achieved with continuous hemodialysis. In this treatment, a progressive correction of metabolic acidosis is achieved, and once the patient is stabilized, the equilibrium is maintained by a slow continuous buffer transfer from dialysate to the blood. In long-lasting treatments, it is important to establish the level of buffer at steady state and eventually correct the buffer concentration in the dialysate. Furthermore, the fluid balance should be considered in order to compensate for possible changes of bicarbonate distribution space.

Acid base in intermittent and continuous hemofiltration

Few acid-base studies have been carried out in patients treated by hemofiltration. The net base balance (in post-dilutional intermittent hemofiltration) is obtained by the difference of the base losses in the ultrafiltrate and the amount of base administered via replacement fluid. Comparative studies of intermittent acetate dialysis and intermittent lactate hemofiltration [13] have demonstrated in the second group a moderate decrease in PO_2 with stability of pCO_2 levels, and a progressive increase of bicarbonate and pH levels, significantly higher in the hemofiltration group.

Lactate is no longer the main buffer utilized in the replacement solution. Bicarbonate, proposed some years ago, is now the first choice, especially in the intensive care unit, and especially if high-volume hemofiltration is utilized. Lactate-based solutions can cause hyperlactacidemia and in some cases lactic acidosis. Davenport et al. [14] showed how in chronic end-stage renal failure, in acute renal, and/or hepatorenal failure, changes in pH could be inversely correlated with the plasma lactate levels. This was especially evident in the hepatorenal failure group. Moreover, in cardiovascular failure and in all hemodynamically unstable patients, there is a risk that lactate-buffered solutions will exacerbate both metabolic acidosis and cardiovascular instability.

The problem of bicarbonate stability in a preformed solution has been solved, at least in Europe, by dividing the substitution fluid bag into two compartments: one acid solution containing calcium and magnesium, and one alkaline, containing bicarbonate. By breaking a valve in the partition wall, the solutions are mixed just before use without problems of calcium precipitation.

Continuous hemofiltration is much more physiological, as the correction of metabolic acidosis takes place progressively and slowly. Once the losses of bicarbonate are anticipated, steady-state, alkalinization or even acidification can be planned on the basis of the amount of buffer in the replacement solution and the liters of fluid exchanged in 24 h. Furthermore, the level of net ultrafiltration may cause a marked difference. Acid-base status may vary in conjunction with the variation of hydration of the patient.

While in most patients without lactate intolerance, lactate can still be advantageously used as a replacement solution, bicarbonate is absolutely mandatory when high-volume hemofiltration is utilized. The large amount of fluid exchange would lead to a lactate load that would be intolerable for the majority of patients, even in the absence of lactate intolerance.

Acid base in intermittent and continuous hemodiafiltration

In mixed diffusive-convective transport, base balance calculations are extremely complex. The net buffer fluxes depend on interaction between driving force (diffusive parameter) and ultrafiltration (convective parameter). If diffusive and convective transports are in the same direction, a higher negative net flux would result [4]. Furthermore, convective flux is always negative for any buffer, because ultrafiltration moves from patient to dialysate all the buffers contained in the patient's plasma. If diffusive and convective fluxes are in opposite directions, a decrease in expected positive net flux would occur. In addition some solvent/solution interactions occur, which limit diffusive entry of small molecules against a high convective current.

Based on these issues, the use of bicarbonate both in dialysate and in the replacement fluid has become common practice, in order to balance bicarbonate losses; a study carried out on intermittent hemodiafiltration showed that dialytic bicarbonate flux only becomes positive if the driving force is greater then 17.5 mmol/l at 50 ml/min of ultrafiltration, indicating that replacement buffer flux must be added to dialytic bicarbonate flux to predict balance in HDF [15]. In continuous therapies, since dialysate and ultrafiltration flows are relatively small, hemodiafilters operate almost inevitably at equilibrium, and a steady-state condition is commonly reached after a few hours of treatment.

Conclusions

Adequate correction of acid-base disturbances is one of the main targets of renal replacement therapies. In intermittent renal replacement therapies, a continuous shift from alkalemia to acidemia and vice versa occurs throughout the day. In contrast, in continuous renal replacement therapies a progressive correction is reached over a certain number of hours, and afterwards a steady equilibrium is maintained, reaching a higher level of treatment physiology. In patients with critical illness, this steady correction represents a definite advantage and makes continuous therapy the treatment of choice.

References

1. Lennon EJ, Lemann J Jr, Litzow JR (1996) The effects of diet and stool composition on the net external acid base of normal subjects. J Clin Invest 45:1601-1607
2. Fernandez PC, Cohem RM, Feldman GM (1989) The concept of bicarbonate distribution space: the cruial role of body buffers. Kidney Int 36: 747-752
3. Gotch FA, Sargent JA, Keen ML (1982) Hydrogen ion balance in dialysis therapy. Artif Organs 6: 388-395
4. Sargent JA, Gothc FA (1979) Bicarbonate and carbon dioxide transport during hemodialysis. ASAIO J 2:61-72
5. Sprenger KBG, Kratz W, Lewis AE, Stadtmûller U (1983) Kinetic modelling of hemodialysis, hemofiltration and hemodiafiltration. Kidney Int 24:143-149
6. Colton CK, Henderson LW, Ford CA, Lysaght MJ (1975) Kinetic of hemodiafiltration. *In vitro* transport characteristics of a hollow fiber blood ultrafilter. J Lab Clin Med 85:355-371
7. Henderson LW, Colton CK, Ford CA (1975) Kinetics of hemodiafiltration. Clinical characterization of a blood cleansing modality. J Lab Clin Med 85:372-394
8. Man NK, Fournier G, Thireau P, et al (1982) Effect of bicarbonate containing dialysate on chronic hemodialysis patient: a comparative study. Artif Organs 6:421-426
9. Nissenson AR (1980) Prevention of dialysis induced-hypoxemia by bicarbonate dialysis. Trans Am Soc Artif Intern Organs 26:339-343
10. Gennari FJ (1985) Acid-base balance in dialysis patient. Kidney Int 28:678-688
11. Eiser AR, Jayammane D, Kokseng C, et al (1982) Contrasting alteration in pulmonary gas exchange during acetate and bicarbonate hemodialysis. Am J Nephrol 2:123-128
12. Mitchell J, Wildenthal K, Johnson R (1972) The effects of acid base disturbances on cardiovascular and pulmonary function. Kidney Int 1:375-380
13. Bosch JP, Lauer A (1986) Acid-base balance in hemofiltration. In: Henderson LW, Quellhorst EA, Baldamus CA, Lysaght MJ (eds) Hemofiltratio. Springer, Berlin Heidelberg New York, pp 147-154
14. Davenport A, Will EJ, Davidson AM (1989) The effects of lactate buffered solutions on the acid-base status of patients with renal failure. Nephrol Dial Transplant 4:800-804
15. Feriani M, Ronco C, Biasioli S, et al (1990) Effects of dialysate and substitution fluid buffer on buffer flux in hemodiafiltration. Kidney Int 39:711-717

iPH and Splanchnic Dysfunction Management

S.M. Jakob

Definition and problems

There is evidence from experimental and clinical studies that the gastrointestinal tract is a key player in the development of endotoxemia, sepsis, and multiple organ failure [1-4]. Therefore, the assessment of perfusion and function of the splanchnic organs have become of major interest, both for investigators and clinicians. The currently available clinical tools are, among others, the assessment of gastrointestinal permeability, liver function tests, such as monoethylglycine xylidide (MEGX) production from lidocaine, and many others, regional and local blood flow measurements, such as estimation of splanchnic blood flow by hepatic uptake of substances that are metabolized by the liver and distributed in the plasma, such as indocyanine green, Laser Doppler flow, and tonometry. The estimation of gastric and intestinal mucosal pH by tonometry was introduced in the 1980, and further developed during the last 15 years to semi- and fully automated methods. An impressive number of both clinical and experimental studies has been conducted so far with tonometry, but the method has not yet gained clinical acceptance. There are many reasons for this. Some are listed in Table 1.

Table 1. Factors that make the interpretation of tonometry difficult

– Assumption that arterial and tissue bicarbonate are equal
– ipH is dependent on systemic metabolism
– Changes in oxygen saturation, hemoglobin, and pH alter the relationship between PCO_2 and CO_2 content
– Gastric acid is buffered by duodenal bicarbonate, resulting in increased CO_2 production
– Variability of the signal
– Gastric ipH may not reflect intestinal or colonic ipH

The mucosal pH can only be estimated by tonometry. It is calculated by the Henderson-Hasselbalch equation, and it is assumed that the mucosal bicarbonate equals the arterial bicarbonate. This may not be true [5]. Because the ipH partly reflects the systemic metabolic state, changes in this variable do not necessarily indicate alterations in splanchnic metabolism and/or perfusion. Therefore, it is recommended to use the mucosal PCO_2 or better the gradient between arterial and mucosal PCO_2 for the interpretation of changes in splanchnic perfusion and metabolism. The mucosal PCO_2 is used because it reflects the relationship between metabolism and blood flow: the lower the perfusion at a given metabolic rate (or CO_2 production), the higher the mucosal PCO_2. The quotient between CO_2 production [venous (mucosal) - arterial CO_2 content (ΔCO_2) blood flow] and blood flow is ΔCO_2. Because the venous (mucosal) – arterial PCO_2 gradient is linearly related to ΔCO_2, PCO_2 gradients instead of ΔCO_2 can be used for the assessment of changes in the relationship between metabolism and blood flow. However, changes in oxygen saturation, hemoglobin and pH alter the relationship between PCO_2 and CO_2 content ([6], Fig. 1). It is therefore difficult to indicate normal values for PCO_2 gradients because these depend on the local oxygenation, and, to a lesser extent, on hemoglobin and pH. Furthermore, if changes in these variables occur, they will

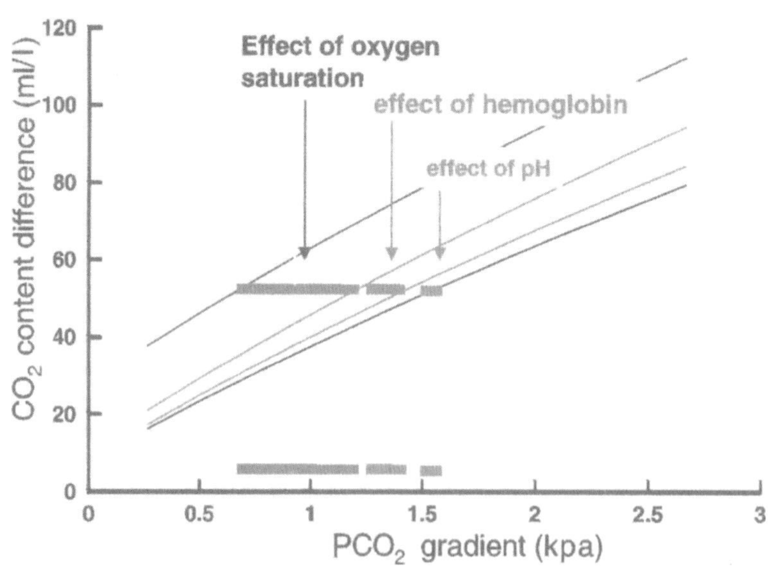

Fig. 1. Relationship between venous (mucosal) – arterial PCO_2 gradient and the respective CO_2 content difference: effects of oxygen saturation, hemoglobin, and pH

inevitably alter the relationship between CO_2 content and PCO_2 and make the interpretation of changes in PCO_2 gradients difficult.

Intraluminally produced CO_2, e.g., during enteral feeding or buffering of gastric acid ions by bicarbonate, can affect the tonometric measurements and cause misinterpretation. In addition, the mucosal PCO_2 is a physiological variable and therefore is subjected to variability. The coefficient of variation of tonometric measurements in critically ill patients is roughly 10% [7], but changes in this may occur by chance.

In the vast majority of experimental trials, jejunal or ileal tonometry has been studied. In the clinical setting, the placement of a tonometer in the small bowel is problematic, and in most of the clinical trials, gastric tonometry has been used. Since the colon is by far the most colonized part of the intestinal tract, it would be reasonable to assume that the phenomenon of increased permeability and translocation is most crucial in the colon. Stomach, small bowel and a large part of the colon are perfused by different vessels. Given the different effects of ischemia in these vascular beds [8], blood flow regulation may also be different Furthermore, anatomical variants are common. Hence, it is possible that changes occurring in one region do not reflect changes in another region. The significance of the resulting effects may also be different in different parts of the gut. Some or several of the above-mentioned issues may at least in part explain why the interpretation of tonometry in the gut is still difficult.

Relationship between ipH and splanchnic dysfunction

Since the splanchnic organs have so many different functions, there are many different methods to measure them (Table 2).

Table 2. Functions of splanchnic organs and methods to measure them

Functions:

- stomach and gut: transportation, dilution, secretion, absorption, digestion, barrier function, immunological-functions, etc.
- liver: degradation, synthesis, transformation of a great variety of physiological and non-physiological compounds

Methods for the assessment of splanchnic organ functions:

- gut and stomach: permeability measurements, regional and local measurements of perfusion, mucosal metabolism, measurements of cellular integrity
- liver: measurements of production, blood flow measurements, measurements of cellular integrity

As outlined above, the mucosal-arterial PCO_2 gradient is a measure of the relationship between local CO_2 production and blood flow that depends on local oxygenation. Because ipH is not measured directly but derived from the

Henderson-Hasselbalch equation (ipH = 6.1 + log abicarbonate/k*ipCO_2; k = solubility coefficient for carbon dioxide in blood), ipH is also a function of systemic (arterial) bicarbonate and hence arterial PCO_2 and pH. Changes in ipH may therefore reflect a variety of other disorders. This is illustrated in a simplified way in Table 3.

All metabolic and respiratory abnormalities result in a decreased ipH, even if they are compensated. It is therefore obvious that ipH is not a selective parameter for gastrointestinal dysfunction. Rather, the arterial-mucosal pH gradient should be used. However, even the pH gradient is affected by purely systemic changes (Table 3). While respiratory acidosis, regardless of the state of metabolic compensation, results in a decreased pH gradient, compensation of metabolic acidosis increases the pH gradient. Consequently, it seems best to use the mucosal-arterial PCO_2 gradient for the interpretation of gastrointestinal perfusion/metabolism abnormalities.

Management of splanchnic dysfunction

The functions of the splanchnic organs can only be partially replaced. Examples are substitution of factors normally synthesized by the liver (albumin, coagulation factors, etc.) and parenteral nutrition. In critically ill patients, blood flow and oxygen transport to the splanchnic organs is often inadequate [9-13]. Increasing splanchnic oxygen delivery should theoretically result in a better performance of the splanchnic organs. Gastrointestinal tonometry has been used to assess the effects of fluid, red blood cells, and vasoactive drugs on the splanchnic perfusion/metabolism relationship [9, 10, 12-14]. None of the currently available vasoactive drugs has selective beneficial effects on regional splanchnic blood flow. Because of the difficulties in the interpretation of tonometry (Table 1), effects on mucosal perfusion are much more difficult to assess. We suggest the following steps when using gastric tonometry to guide therapy in critically ill patients. First, the correct position of the tonometer should be confirmed and the stomach should be emptied (the new semi-continuous or continuous methods allow for a rapid sampling frequency; the PCO_2 in the fluid of a filled stomach may not equilibrate with the mucosal PCO_2 rapidly enough). Suppression of gastric acid secretion is not necessary in the critically ill [15]. Second, the mucosal-arterial PCO_2 gradient should be calculated. Because the mucosal PCO_2 is subjected to a certain variability [7], several $iPCO_2$ values should be averaged. Third, effects of the intervention on mucosal oxygenation should be either measured or at least taken into account. Changes in mucosal oxygenation have an effect on mucosal PCO_2 that is independent of

Table 3. Different clinical conditions affecting calculated ipH

	ipH	$iPCO_2$ (mm Hg)	$aPCO_2$ (mm Hg)	apH	abicarbonate (mmol/l)	ΔPCO_2 (mm Hg)	ΔpH
Normal state	7.35	45	40	7.40	24	5	0.05
Metabolic acidosis, no gastrointestinal dysfunction	7.17	45	40	7.23	16	5	0.05
Respiratory acidosis, no gastrointestinal dysfunction	7.23	60	55	7.26	24	5	0.03
Metabolic acidosis, respiratory compensation, no gastrointestinal dysfunction	7.28	35	30	7.35	16	5	0.07
Respiratory acidosis,metabolic compensation, no gastrointestinal dysfunction	7.31	60	55	7.35	29	5	0.04
Gastrointestinal dysfunction	7.23	60	40	7.40	24	20	0.17
Metabolic acidosis, gastrointestinal dysfunction	7.05	60	40	7.23	16	20	0.18
Respiratory acidosis, gastrointestinal dysfunction	7.13	75	55	7.26	24	20	0.13
Metabolic acidosis, respiratory compensation, gastrointestinal dysfunction	7.13	50	30	7.35	16	20	0.22
Respiratory acidosis, metabolic compensation, gastrointestinal dysfunction	7.21	75	55	7.35	29	20	0.14

IpH, apH, $iPCO_2$, $aPCO_2$: mucosal and arterial pH and PCO_2, respectively. ΔpH, ΔpCO_2 = arterial-mucosal pH and mucosal-arterial PCO_2 gradient, respectively changes in mucosal perfusion [6]. Even if this effect is small (a few mmHg), it may obscure major changes in the relationship between blood flow and metabolism (Fig. 1). Nevertheless, sustained changes in the mucosal-arterial PCO_2 gradient of at least 10 mmHg do reflect effects of the intervention on blood flow and/or metabolism. Finally, it is obvious that the mucosal PCO_2 reflects only changes in the organ where it is measured. Since stomach, small and large bowel are perfused by different vessels, and since there are many humans with variants in vascular anatomy [16], effects of a certain treatment may differ in different parts of the gastrointestinal tract. It is especially important to realize that there is an inverse relationship between blood flow changes in the portal vein (supplied by blood from the superior mesenteric artery and the celiac trunk) and in the hepatic artery (a branch form the celiac trunk): the so-called hepatic arterial buffer response [17]. The hepatic arterial buffer response describes the compensatory increase in hepatic arterial blood flow whenever protal venous blood flow decreases. It can be hypothesized that a decrease in mesenteric blood flow is also accompanied by an increase in perfusion of other branches of the celiac trunk, such as the splenic artery or gastric arteries. Nevertheless, if a drug with the potential to increase both systemic and global splanchnic blood flow (such as dobutamine or dopexamine) results in a sustained, significant decrease in mucosal-arterial PCO_2 gradient, it can be assumed that the local relationship between perfusion and metabolism has improved.

References

1. Kirton OC, Windsor J, Wedderburn R, et al (1998) Failure of splanchnic resuscitation in the acutely injured trauma patient correlates with multiple organ system failure and length of stay in the ICU. Chest 113:1064-1069
2. Swank GM, Deitch EA (1996) Role of the gut in multiple organ failure: bacterial translocation and permeability changes. World J Surg 20:411-417
3. Doglio GR, Pusajo JF, Egurrola MA, et al (1991) Gastric mucosal pH as a prognostic index of mortality in critically ill patients. Crit Care Med 19:1037-1040
4. Baker JW, Deitch EA, Li M, et al (1988) Hemorrhagic shock induces bacterial translocation from the gut. J Trauma 28:896-906
5. Benjamin E, Oropello JM (1996) Does gastric tonometry work? No. Crit Care Clin 12:587-601
6. Jakob SM, Kosonen P, Ruokonen E, et al (1999) The Haldane effect – an alternative explanation for increasing gastric mucosal pCO2 gradients? Br J Anaesth 83:740-746
7. Jakob SM, Parviainen I, Ruokonen E, et al (2000) Variability of continually measured gastric-mucosal Pco2 in critically ill patients and effect of ranitidine. Intensive Care Med 26:S429
8. Rendig SV, Premjit SC, Longhurst JC (1997) Cardiovascular reflex responses to ischemia during occlusion of celiac and/or superior mesenteric arteries. Am J Physiol 272:H791-H796
9. Fiddian-Green RG (1990) Gut mucosal ischemia during cardiac surgery. Semin Thorac Cardiovasc Surg 2:389-399
10. Landow L, Phillips DA, Heard SO, et al (1991) Gastric tonometry and venous oximetry in cardiac surgery patients. Crit Care Med 19:1226-1233

11. Ruokonen E, Takala J, Kari A (1993) Regional blood flow and oxygen transport in patients with the low cardiac output syndrome after cardiac surgery. Crit Care Med 21:1304-1311
12. Parviainen I, Ruokonen E, Takala J (1995) Dobutamine-induced dissociation between changes in splanchnic blood flow and gastric intramucosal pH after cardiac surgery. Br J Anaesth 74:277-282
13. Temmesfeld-Wollbruck B, Szalay A, Mayer K, et al (1998) Abnormalities of gastric mucosal oxygenation in septic shock: partial responsiveness to dopexamine. Am J Respir Crit Care Med 157:1586-1592
14. Uusaro A, Ruokonen E, Takala J (1995) Gastric mucosal pH does not reflect changes in splanchnic blood flow after cardiac surgery. Br J Anaesth 74:149-154
15. Vaisanen O, Ruokonen E, Parviainen I, et al (2000) Ranitidine or dobutamine alone or combined has no effect on gastric intramucosal-arterial PCO(2) difference after cardiac surgery. Intensive Care Med 26:45-51
16. Rosenblum JD, Boyle CM, Schwartz LB (1997) The mesenteric circulation. Anatomy and physiology. Surg Clin North Am 77:289-306
17. Lautt WW (1985) Mechanism and role of intrinsic regulation of hepatic arterial blood flow: the hepatic arterial buffer response. Am J Physiol 249:G549-G556

Crystalloids/Colloids: Controversies

C. SORBARA, D. PITTARELLO, M. PRIMADEI

Since 1918, intravenous fluid infusion in the treatment of shock has been fundamental to the resuscitation of critically ill patients [1]. Restoration of volume deficit is essential to survival of patients with hypovolemia; however, despite the importance of fluid therapy, controversy still exists over the choice of crystalloids or colloids as the ideal resuscitation fluid.

Maintenance of stable hemodynamics is crucial and an effective fluid therapy is a mainstay of managing hypovolemic patients. Yet, replacements of volume deficit require an understanding of the physiology of fluid compartments and the volume of distribution, as well as the pathophysiology of the underlying disease.

Use of crystalloid solutions for volume resuscitation is safe, well tolerated, and inexpensive, but most of the fluid, 80% and more, is rapidly lost to the interstitial space. Therefore, soft tissue edema is common when large volumes of crystalloids are administered to maintain intravascular volume. Colloids have a greater capacity to hold fluid within the intravascular space, but they have other limitations and side effects.

In spite of numerous studies on this topic, the question of the 'optimal' strategy for volume replacement is worldwide discussed very emotionally, and several guidelines, recommendations, and meta-analysis have been published.

There are a number of challenges in designing and interpreting the randomized trials in this area, yet, randomization is difficult in emergency life-threatening situations and heterogeneous populations may respond differently to different fluids. The treatment crossovers occur and cointerventions may not be recorded so that many studies are insufficiently powered to be conclusive on their own.

Moreover, the controversy concerning the 'ideal' kind of fluid for volume therapy does not only include the crystalloid/colloid debate but must be enlarged to a colloid/colloid debate.

Really, the choice of colloid, in particular the use of albumin, is a matter of considerable controversy [2, 3], and in spite of the absence of convincing supportive data, human albumin is still considered to be the fluid of first choice in many institutions. However, the rationale of using albumin is difficult to understand, and the indication for giving albumin should be revised in that modern low-priced nonprotein colloids [e.g., hydroxyethyl starch (HES), gelatins] do have economic advantages over albumin solution and should be preferred.

Therefore, even if the debate on the optimal fluid regimens for hypovolemic patients has been on going for decades and is still as intense as ever before, with new data and both new and old arguments, we will try to discuss this issue rememberig that the optimal approach will vary depending, not only on the underlying medical condition and its actual clinical stage, but also on the physical status and presence of complicating conditions of the patient.

Distribution characteristics of fluids

The total fluid flow between the intra- and extravascular compartments is influenced by hydrostatic as well as colloid osmotic gradients, as predicted by the Starling transcapillary fluid equilibrium equation. While the hydrostatic pressure depends on the capillary pressure, the osmotic pressure is due to the number of particles in solution. Each particle, regardless of its mass, exerts on average the same pressure because they have approximately the same kinetic energy. Larger particles move at slower velocities, while smaller particles move more quickly. Thus, on average, each particle has approximately equal kinetic energy.

The proteins are the only dissolved substances in the plasma that do not diffuse readily through capillary membranes. Because of this, the dissolved proteins in the interstitium and plasma exert the colloid osmotic pressure (COP) at the capillary membrane. COP is most commonly measured by a membrane transducer system, which detects volume of flow across a semipermeable membrane. The pore size of the membrane, the molecular weight of the protein and the surface area of the venous capillary bed affect the volume of flow across the capillary membrane [4].

Starling [5] noted that, under normal circumstances, the fluid filtered in the arterioles was nearly equal to the fluid reabsorbed in the venules. The fluid exchange across a capillary membrane is given by the Starling equation:

$$\mathbf{Q = Kf\,[\,(\,Pc - Pi\,) - \delta\,(\,\pi c - \pi i\,)\,]}$$

where Q is the flow of fluid, Kf is a coefficient of filtration, P is the hydrostatic pressure of the capillary (Pc) and interstitium (Pi), δ is the coefficient of reflection, π is the osmotic pressure of the capillary (πc), and interstitium (πi). The coefficient of reflection ranges from 0 to 1 and represents the transfer of colloid across the membrane. Zero indicates free passage, while 1 is totally impermeable to colloid transfer. The pulmonary capillaries have a value of 0.7, while most of the systemic circulation has a value of 0.95 [6].

The major contribution to the osmotic gradient is the difference in protein on each side of endothelium. The concentration of protein in the plasma is approximately 7.3 g/dl, while in the interstitial fluid it is 2 - 3 g/dl. When the capillary permeability is increased in same pathological states, the osmotic gradient between the capillary and interstitium is decreased and the net flux into the interstitium is increased. Normally measured COP of plasma ranges from 25 to 30 mmHg, while in the interstitium it is about 8 -10 mmHg.

Albumin, globulins and fibrinogen are the primary plasma proteins. Because albumin has a relatively small molecular weight (69,000 daltons) compared with the globulins, 1 g of albumin contains more molecules and thus exerts a greater COP (about 75% of the oncotic pressure of plasma).

The overall result is that the oncotic pressure gradient opposes the hydrostatic pressure gradient. As a result, there is a net flow of water into the interstitial space (the ionic composition of interstitial and intravascular fluids is the same) that supplies the lymphatic circulation. However, the capillary membrane is not totally impermeable to proteins, their movement depends on the membrane's characteristics, which in turn depends on the size, shape, and charge of the molecule.

Using these assumptions, to establish the plasma volume expansion (PVE) the following equation predicts that:

$$\mathbf{PVE = volume\ infused\ x\ (\ PV\ /\ Vd\ )}$$

where PVE is the plasma volume expansion, PV is the plasma volume, and Vd is the distribution volume of the fluid infused (Table 1).

Table 1. Fluid distribution volumes

Description	**% Total body weight**	**Volume (l/70Kg body weight)**
Total body water (TBW)	60	42
Intracellular volume (ICV)	40	28
Extracellular volume (ECV)	20	14
Plasma volume (PV)	4	3

From the equation we assume, for example, that PVE of 500 ml is to be achieved using 5% dextrose in water. Because the volume is sodium free and consequently the Vd is TBW (equal to 60% of total body weight), we would need a total volume of 7 l [500 ml = volume infused x (3/42)]. To replace 500 ml of blood loss with Ringer's solution or 0.9% saline, for which Vd = ECV, an infused volume of 3.3 l would be necessary. If membrane permeability is normal, colloids such as albumin, dextran, or HES preferentially expand PV rather than ECV or ICV. Knowing that each gram of intravascular albumin holds 15 ml of water in the PV [7], therefore, 500 ml of 5% albumin containing 25 g of albumin would expand PV by approximately 375 ml.

Fluid replacement in critically ill patients

Intravascular volume is a crucial factor in the maintenance of hemodynamic stability, tissue perfusion, and oxygenation, and organ function. A lack of intravascular volume may be the result of acute hemorrhage, trauma, burns, excessive vomiting, diarrhea, dehydration, fever, and therapy with diuretics or other compounds that reduce the intravascular volume or pathophysiological conditions involving increased microvascular permeability (e.g., systemic inflammatory response syndrome, sepsis) and anaphylaxis. Acute hypovolemia induces stimulation of the sympathoadrenergic and renin-angiotensin systems to maintain both cardiac output and arterial blood pressure. These compensatory mechanisms lead to redistribution of blood flow to the cerebral, coronary, and renal circulations. However, if extensive blood loss (> 30% of total blood volume) occurs and remains untreated, a number of pathophysiological abnormalities can be observed at the microcirculatory level (e.g., hypoxia, endothelial cell swelling, capillary leakage, and release of cytokines) that can promote multiple organ failure [8, 9]. An extensive loss of intravascular fluid that cannot be compensated for by physiological regulatory mechanisms in these critical situations leads to maldistribution of nutritional blood flow and generalized tissue hypoxia.

In severe sepsis or septic shock, hypovolemia is attributable to the effects of endotoxins or antigens released from microorganisms, with subsequent liberation of a variety of vasoactive mediators. Venous pooling and increased microvascular permeability induced by endothelial cell damage then occur, with extravasation of fluid and macromolecules such as albumin, followed by maldistribution of nutritional blood flow and disturbance of oxidative processes in the mitochondria [9-11].

It is therefore an essential task of critical care management to restore intravascular volume, to achieve adequate systemic circulation as well as sufficient microcirculation, especially in cases of generalized capillary leakage [12], because one of the most-important objectives of fluid therapy is to restore or guarantee tissue perfusion.

Concerning volemia, plasma volume responds differently to infusion of colloid and infusion of crystalloid in acute critical illness [13]. There are greater increases in plasma volume after infusion of equal volumes of colloid than there are for crystalloid in hypovolemic states (Fig. 1). The colloid moiety has a higher water-binding capacity than do the sodium cations (main constituent of crystalloid solutions) found in crystalloid and can retain a large fraction of infused water within the vascular space. After completion of infusion, the increase in plasma volume persists for longer periods with colloid than it does with crystalloid [13]. Many colloids have a long intravascular half-life, thereby prolonging retention of water within the vascular space.

Concerning hemodynamic status, fluids increase cardiac output (CO), stroke volume (SV), and stroke work (SW) in proportion to the increase in plasma volume and ventricular preload [13-15]. However, the CO response to similar increments in plasma volume is dependent on the type of fluid infused [14]. The relationship between CO and plasma volume for two types of fluids is

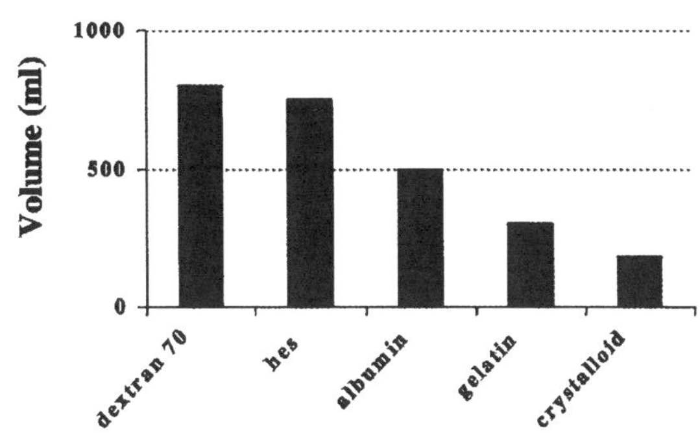

Fig. 1. Plasma volume responses to infusion of equal volumes (1,000 ml) of either colloid or crystalloid in acute hypovolemia

illustrated in Fig. 2. An interaction between the type of fluid given and left ventricular (LV) mechanical performance can explain the diverse CO response to similar plasma volume increments induced by either crystalloid or colloid fluid [16]. Hemodilution secondary to infusion of fluids reduces blood viscosity and lowers LV afterload. This effect may improve LV mechanical performance after resuscitation [17]. However, fluids may adversely affect myocardial performance in critically ill patients. Crystalloid can reduce LV compliance and contractility [18]. Myocardial edema, reperfusion injury secondary to free radical generation, and electrolyte shifts are some of the possible mechanisms by which crystalloid can depress LV mechanical performance [19]. Infusion of colloid is less prone to induce myocardial edema and may also scavenge free radicals and protect against reperfusion injury [19].

Infusion of fluid can increase O_2 delivery by improving CO in critically ill patients [14, 15, 20]. Although fluids also reduce arterial O_2 content by hemodilution, the net result on O_2 delivery represents the balance between the two opposing effects. Lactated Ringer's solutions and isotonic saline solution have been shown to cause significant hemodilution with moderate increases in CO and a relatively small increase in O_2 delivery [13, 14, 21]. In contrast, the colloids (e.g., albumin, dextran, HES) produce significant increases in CO

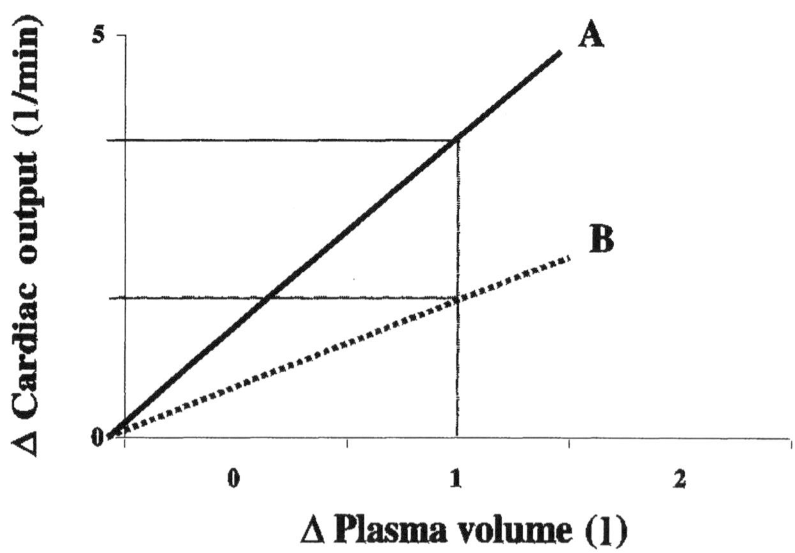

Fig, 2. The response of cardiac output to plasma increments produced by colloid (A) and crystalloid (B) at similar increments of plasma volume

with moderate hemodilution and larger increases in O_2 delivery [14, 15, 21, 22].

Concerning the demands of ischemic organ systems in hypovolemic critically ill patients, volume replacement with colloids (HES) preserved microcapillary integrity and resulted in less transvascular fluid filtration with better-preserved tissue oxygenation [23-26]. In particular, a clinical study conducted on septic patients [27] showed better splanchnic oxygenation, as measured by pHi, in patients treated with HES compared with those treated with albumin (Fig. 3). In this case the beneficial effects of HES seem to be more related to its action on inflammatory processes than to its action on COP.

Since isotonic crystalloid solutions are required in large infusion volumes to achieve an adequate hemodynamic response during initial resuscitation, their use may exacerbate interstitial fluid gain in critically ill patients [14, 28]. The gain in extravascular water content results in edema of many organ systems and can hinder the convection and diffusion of O_2 to these tissues.

Some investigators speculate that colloids also may leak into the interstitial space and exacerbate extravascular water gain in the presence of leaky capillaries in many organ systems [29]. However, this hypothesis is not always true, and depends on the characteristics of the molecules. Indeed, a large fraction of administered colloid remains in the intravascular space and can be efficiently cleared from extravascular fluid space [13, 14, 21, 30].

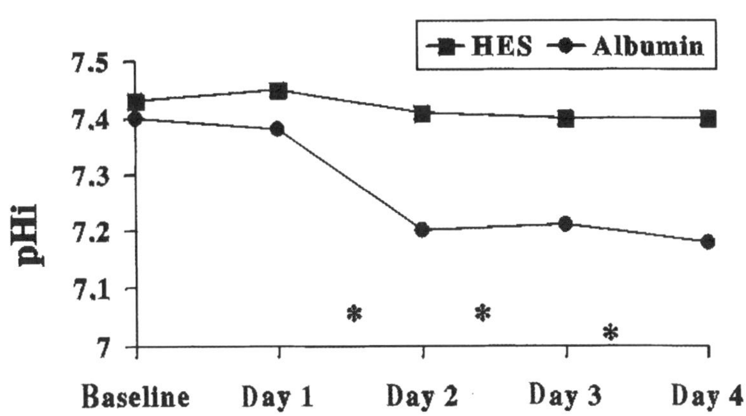

Fig. 3. Changes in gastric intramucosal pH (pHi) in septic patients treated with albumin or hydroxyethyl starch (HES) * P< 0.05 versus baseline

Crystalloid solutions

Isotonic crystalloid solutions (Ringer's lactate solution, 0.9% saline solution, balanced electrolyte solution) are usually the first choice for fluid replacement. They do not contain oncotically active macromolecules, so their effect on plasma volume expansion (approximately 200 ml for every 1,000 ml administered, with an intravascular half-time of 20 - 30 min) is very limited [10]. Moreover, it was demonstrated that crystalloids could not effectively restore microcirculatory blood flow in several organs in patients with shock [33]. In an animal study of normovolemic hemodilution, infusion of Ringer's lactate, equal to four times the blood withdrawn, maintained arterial pressure and filling pressures. However, tissue perfusion, as determined by counting the number of capillaries perfused, was significantly reduced by 62% and tissue oxygen partial pressure (pO_2) was reduced from 19 to 8 mmHg [34] (Fig. 4). Arguments in favor of the use of crystalloids include the observations that crystalloids expand the extracellular compartment more effectively with less increase in extravascular pulmonary water due to rapid equilibration [35,36], minimize the risk of anaphylactic reactions, and moreover cost less than colloids [37].

Recently, there has been growing interest in the use of small-volume hypertonic saline solutions for volume replacement. Hypertonic crystalloids (2,400 mosmol/l NaCl) increased osmolarity in extracellular fluid, which

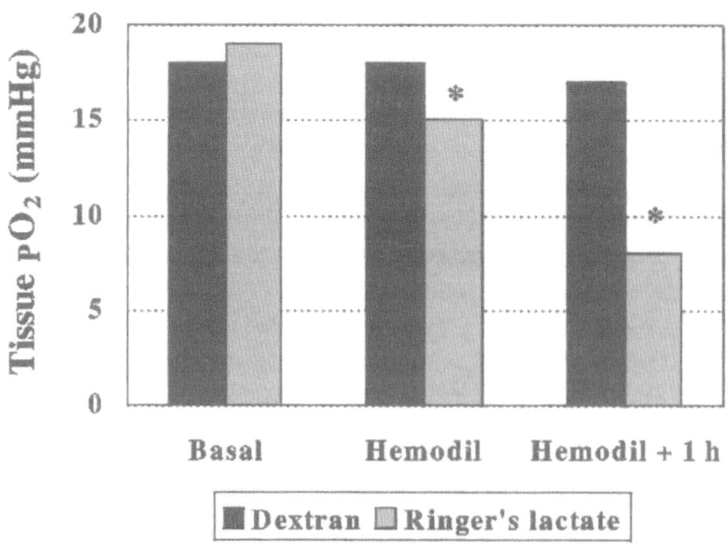

Fig. 4. Tissue PO_2 after hemodilution (hemodil) and exchange with Ringer's solution or dextran. * $P<0.05$ versus baseline

results in movement of water from the intracellular compartment to the interstitial and vascular compartments [38]. The addition of colloids prolongs the volume expansion, so that it is equal to 3 – 4 times the infused volume. Plasma volume expansion, however, does not suffice to explain the efficacy of hypertonic solutions, particularly as this effect is transitory. Their sustained duration of action is due to a reflex mechanism responsible for venous constriction and increased contractility [39]. Hyperosmolarity vasodilates the splanchnic and renal tissue beds [40]: an effect that is particularly useful in the setting of hemorrhagic and septic shock. Furthermore, this decreases intracranial pressure [41] and is responsible of intracellular dehydration and hypernatremia. For these reasons, hypertonic solutions should be considered to be not only volume expanders, but also real drugs with systemic and regional cardiovascular effects.

Colloid solutions

Colloids (Table 2) are described by both molecular weight and size. Solutions with small size or low molecular weight particles will be retained in the circulation for a shorter time than larger particles. For a given concentration (weight/volume), solutions with small particles will exert a greater oncotic effect than larger particles. Molecules are lost from the circulation by both renal clearance and losses into the interstitium.

Table 2. Comparison of colloid solutions

	Albumin 5%	Albumin 25%	Dextran 40 10%	Dextran 70 6%	HES 200/0.5 6%	Gelatin 3%
Average molecular weight (D)	70.000	70.000	40.000	70.000	200.000	30.000
Osmolarity (mosmol/l)	300	1500	308	308	326	NA
COP (mmHg)	20	100	170	26	26	24
Sodium level (mEq/l)	130-160	130-160	154	154	154	154
PV expansion (ml/500ml infused)	500	1700	500-1000	500-700	600-800	500
Duration of PV expansion	<24h	<24h	<6h	<24h	<12h	<4h
Dose limitation			≤2g/Kg/day	20 ml /Kg/day	33 ml /Kg/day	
Incidence of anaphylaxis (%)	0.129	0.129	0.273	0.273	0.058	0.345

HES = hydroxyethyl starch; COP = colloid osmotic pressure; PV = plasma volume; NA = not available

Colloid resuscitation requires less volume and time [42] than crystalloid. Their volume effect depends on the concentration, molecular weight, molecular structure, colloid osmotic pressure, metabolism, and elimination rate.

Albumin

The function of albumin in the blood is to maintain normal oncotic pressure and act as a carrier of various metabolites. Its use as the first natural colloid product dates back to World War I, and it has remained the standard colloidal agent for comparison. Albumin is a monodisperse solution, has an average molecular weight of 69,000 daltons and at physiological pH has a net charge of -17. Albumin is the predominant protein in human plasma, and comprises 70 - 80% of the normal colloid oncotic pressure and about 50 - 60% of plasma protein. The normal transcapillary leak rate is about 5%/h but increases up to 60-fold during sepsis [43]. Approximately 10% of the albumin in the body is broken down daily; however, the site of metabolism is uncertain but is probably the reticuloendothelial system [44]. Commercially available albumin is prepared from pooled human plasma, then heated for 10 h at 60°C for sterilization. It can be stored at normal room temperature (not to exceed 30°C). Given as a 5% solution, albumin has colloid oncotic pressure of 19 mmHg, providing an increase in intravascular volume equal to the volume infused; 25% albumin solution contains 12.5 g albumin in 50 ml of buffered normal saline, with an oncotic pressure of 100 mmHg, producing an increase of 300 - 500 ml in intravascular volume for 100 ml of infused solution [45]. The effect of infused albumin on plasma volume is variable, depending on volume deficits, initial oncotic pressure, vascular permeability, and the adequacy of the volume resuscitation. The expansion of the plasma volume primarily depends on the amount of albumin given, not on the concentration of the solution [46].

Although albumin has been used safely for decades as a volume expander, many studies have demonstrated possible complications with its use. Albumin, a derivative of blood, may cause adverse reactions similar to other transfusion reactions, such as chills, urticaria, fever, and vasodilatation, with a 0.129% incidence of anaphylaxis [47]. Another important complication is hypocalcemia. A study of trauma patients resuscitated with albumin demonstrated normal serum albumin and total calcium levels, but significantly reduced ionized calcium levels. Such a reduction, due to binding by albumin, may depress myocardial function [48]. A study in trauma patients receiving albumin for fluid resuscitation reported that intravascular volume requirements were higher, urine output lower, and renal function decreased compared with patients who received crystalloid resuscitation [49].

Dextrans

Dextrans are glucose polymers of various lengths, produced by bacteria grown on sucrose media. The solutions are polydisperse. Dextran 40 and dextran 70 are commercially available and differ according to the weighted average molecular weight (40,000 and 70,000 daltons, respectively). Dextran 40 is a 10% solution in normal saline, while dextran 70 is available as a 6% solution in normal saline. They can be stored at room temperature between 15 and 30°C. Both dextrans initially produce intravascular volume expansion due to increased osmotic load, but the effect is temporary. Smaller glucose polymers rapidly escape from the vascular compartment into the interstitial space or are excreted by the kidney. The plasma volume expansion is usually one-to twofold the volume of dextran 40 infused; however, 50% of the dextran is lost after 3 h, 60% within 6 h [45]. The remaining large glucose polymers are slowly eliminated by enzymatic degradation. Dextran 70, with a preponderance of larger polymers, is less rapidly lost from the intravascular space; within 12 h, 35% of the polymers are cleared. An additional characteristic of dextran solutions with clinical implications is their hematological effects. The dextrans alter blood viscosity. The changes in viscosity depend on the molecular weight of the dextran. Above 60,000 daltons the dextrans tend to aggregate red cells in vitro; however, below this weight, the tendency is to disaggregate them. The main advantages of the dextrans is their proven benefit of deep venous thrombosis prevention and of blood viscosity reduction [50]. Dextran administration is associated with a dilutional coagulopathy as well as decreased fibrin clot formation and reduced factor VIII activity [51]. Allergic reactions to dextrans include an anaphylactic reaction to high molecular weight dextrans with multiple branches and a true allergic reaction with pre-formed antibodies. Risk for anaphylactic reaction can be decreased by pre-treatment with monovalent hapten-dextran, which binds the antibodies [52].

Starches

HES is a very polydisperse solution of hydroxylated amylopectin. It is produced by partial hydrolysis of insoluble amylopectin, followed by substitution of hydroxyethyl groups at the C2, C3, and C6 positions on the glucose molecules.

A variety of different HES solutions exist worldwide, which differ greatly in their pharmacological properties. HES is classified according to its manufactured or *in vitro* molecular weight (MW) into high MW (450-480 kDa), medium MW (200 kDa), and low MW (70 kDa) starch preparations. However, this is not sufficient, because as HES is metabolized *in vivo*, its MW changes, and it is the *in vivo* MW that is responsible for the therapeutic and adverse effects of each HES. The role of metabolism depends mainly on the degree of hydroxyethyl substitution (ranging from 0.4 to 0.7), and the C2/C6 ratio of hydroxyethylation. A high degree of substitution and a high C2/C6 ratio lead to a slow metabolism of HES, resulting in a large *in vivo* MW. Slowly degradable high MW HES 450/0.7 (hetastarch) and medium MW HES 200/0.62 have a high *in vivo* MW and are eliminated slowly via the kidneys. As a result, these starches have a relatively long-lasting volume effect. When higher volumes (>1,500 ml) are administered, large molecules accumulate in the plasma. HES administration has been associated with a lower incidence of anaphylaxis (0.085%) [47] than other colloids.

With regard to the alteration of coagulation [53], this can result in bleeding complications due to reduction of factor VIII and von Willebrand factor activity, platelet function defects, incorporation into fibrin clots, and an unfavorable effect on rheological parameters with increased viscosity.

Rapidly degradable medium MW HES 200/0.5 or low MW HES 70/0.5 are quickly split *in vivo* into smaller, more-favorable molecular sizes, resulting in faster renal elimination, shorter volume effect, and fewer adverse effects on coagulation and rheological parameters. In Europe, a large variety of these HES solutions are available, dominated by medium MW, easily degradable HES (200/0.5) (pentastarch). This starch has a greater colloid osmotic pressure (40 mmHg) than hetastarch, and a greater expansion of the intravascular space, nearly twice that of the volume infused. However, the average half-life is only 2.5 h; 60% of an administered dose is excreted in the urine in 24 h and blood concentrations are undetectable within 96 h [54]. Thus, pentastarch may provide greater plasma volume expansion for the volume infused, with faster onset and more rapid elimination, than albumin or hetastarch [55]. Pentastarch administration is associated with hemodilution and decreased factor VIII von Willebrand complex [14]; moreover it increases the erythrocyte sedimentation rate and is used to enhance white cell separation by centrifugal means during leukapheresis.

A new HES, pentrafraction, which has been divested of most of the highest and lowest MW components present in other starch preparations, provides a medium MW range starch that has been used in animal studies [56]. Pentrafraction has a number averaged MW of 110,000 daltons, but the range of MW is less than in the case of hetastarch or pentastarch (100,000 - 500,000 daltons). Elimination of the very low MW molecules provides a more-sustained colloid osmotic effect, and should reduce fluid flux and edema formation compared with pentastarch.

Gelatins

Currently two types of gelatins are produced from bovine collagen. Both are initially treated with alkali, which causes the collagen to swell and hydrolyzes ester and peptide links, followed by suspension in aqueous solution. The urea-linked gelatins (Emagel) are prepared by cross-linking polypeptide chains with hexamethyl di-isocyanate, resulting in a weighted average MW of 35,000 daltons. The succinylated gelatins (Eufusin) use slightly higher weight polypeptide chains that are treated with succinic acid anhydrase. The weighted average MW of “Eufusin” is 30,000 daltons and the number averaged MW is 22,600 daltons. Both types of solutions are polydisperse. The small particles exert a large initial osmotic effect, but are rapidly lost from the circulation by glomerular filtration. The volume-expanding effect lasts approximately 3 h in a healthy circulation, but is shortened, during sepsis [50]. Urea-linked gelatin has much higher calcium (6.26 mmol/l) and potassium (5.1 mmol/l) levels than succinylated gelatin. This higher calcium level can lead to clotting if the urea-linked gelatin is infused with blood [57]. The modified gelatins have no effect on coagulation other than hemodilution [58], but are associated with allergic reactions, with an incidence of anaphylaxis of 0.345% [47].

Recent controversies on the use of crystalloids and colloids

The start of the recent phase of the crystalloid-colloid controversy was the publication in 1998 [32] on the mortality of critically ill patients resuscitated with either crystalloid or colloid. This report was based on a systemic review (meta-analysis) of 26 previously published randomized trials. The findings of the review indicated that the overall relative risk of death was higher for critically ill patients resuscitated with colloid compared with patients resuscitated with crystalloid. The relative risk of mortality was higher for trauma and burn patients than for those with increased capillary permeability due to other causes (e.g., sepsis). The meta-analysis suggested that resuscitation with colloid was associated with an absolute increase in the risk of mortality of 4%. In the light of such data, it was argued that, as colloids were not associated with improved survival and were considerably more expensive than crystalloid solutions, it was hard to see how their continued use, outside randomized controlled trials in subsets of patients of particular concern, could be justified. However the analysis by author [32] was not free of important limitations, because it included several studies that used experimental colloid solutions and hypertonic saline solutions. Furthermore, none of the studies analyzed used modern colloid solutions, which are the current standard of care. The colloids in the studies reviewed were albumin, dextrans, and gelatins, which in critically ill patients, with increased capillary permeability, allows molecules to pass into the interstitial space, thus compromising tissue oxygenation.

A similar difference in mortality in favor of crystalloid resuscitation of trauma victims was also reported by Choi et al. in 1999 [59], who presented a systemic review of 17 primary studies including 814 patients. His study, however, in addition to a subgroup of trauma patients, included all randomized trials of adult patients requiring fluid resuscitation. As part of this review, not only mortality but also the occurrence of pulmonary edema and length of hospital stay were documented. No overall differences in these two last variables between crystalloid-based compared with colloid-based resuscitation could be demonstrated.

Since the completion of our systematic review, two other meta-analyses of fluid resuscitation have been published by the Cochrane Injuries Group. The first [60] compared the effects of different colloid solutions in patients thought to need volume replacement. In this review 52 trials met the inclusion criteria, with a total of 3,311 patients, and the main outcomes were death, amount of whole blood transfused, and the incidence of adverse reactions. In this clinical trial there was no evidence that one colloid was more effective or safe than any other, although the confidence intervals were wide and did not exclude clinically significant differences between colloids. In this case, larger trials of fluid therapy are necessary if clinically significant differences in mortality are to be detected or excluded.

The second review [31] compared the effect of albumin or plasma protein fraction on all-cause mortality. Albumin is often used to treat hypoalbuminemia in intensive care patients [61]. On the basis of this systemic review of 30 randomized, controlled studies, including 1,419 critically ill patients suffering from hypovolemia, burns, or hypoalbuminemia, the Cochrane Injuries Group found increased mortality with albumin administration compared with crystalloids. The pooled results showed an excess risk of death of 6%. The authors found that there was no evidence of the efficacy of albumin over crystalloid; instead, albumin appeared to carry additional risk. As a result, the authors called for rigorously conducted randomized trials to determine the appropriate indications for human albumin. Pathophysiological mechanisms invoked by the authors and others in accompanying editorials to explain the increased risk included some anticoagulant properties, increased interstitial oncotic pressure in patients with increased capillary permeability, and the adverse hemodynamic consequences of rapid volume replacement [62,63].

In light of this, do the results from these meta-analyses suggest that colloid solutions should be banished from hospital formularies because of their higher costs and probable lack of benefit for survival?

The absence of a significant improvement in hospital or intensive care unit survival from the pooled results of studies is not altogether surprising, given the complexity of intensive care unit care and outcomes. What the results do suggest is that a 'magic bullet' intravenous solution does not exist for all clinical conditions. One solution may be preferred in some instances on the basis of pathophysiological principles and evidence from studies performed in restricted populations [61-65].

These findings do not suggest that fluid choice for resuscitation is unimportant. It is plausible that factors such as comorbidity, acute illness severity, and intensive care unit-acquired complications have a more-powerful influence on mortality than does resuscitative fluid. The variable choice of physiological end-points in these studies and different measurement strategies also preclude firm conclusions on outcomes other than mortality. Probably more-rigorous research in this field is necessary, given the emerging evidence that meta-analysis results may not be replicated in large, modern, randomized trials [66].

Recommendations for the use of fluids

The essential aims of volume replacement therapy are:

- Achieve and maintain normovolemia and hemodynamic stability
- Optimize oxygen delivery and oxygen consumption
- Restore fluid homeostasis in the different fluid compartments
- Ensure adequate plasma COP
- Improve microcirculatory perfusion
- Ensure appropriate inflammatory response and endothelial cell-leukocyte interactions.

In the past decades, the National Institutes of Health (NIH) of the United States has sponsored consensus conferences to develop guidelines for the use of several blood products, including fresh-frozen plasma, platelets, and packed red blood cells [67-69]. Not since the middle of the 1970s, however, has albumin been the subject of an NIH-sponsored guideline development effort, and subsequently clinical research and changes in medical practices have rendered the previous NIH recommendations obsolete.

Periodic reconsideration of clinical practice guidelines, incorporating the results of new research, is essential to ensure their currency and validity. The high cost and limited supply of albumin, the availability of nonprotein colloids, and the limited cost of crystalloid solutions underscore the importance of contemporary clinical practice guidelines to assure their appropriate use.

In 1995, new guidelines were published by Vermeulen et al. [70]. Because his study was performed systematically, after evaluation of a large volume of medical literature and consultation of a large group of experts. Furthermore, in recent years, other guidelines have appeared [71] and many clinical trials have defined indications somewhat more specifically [72, 73]. Although this information may sometimes be controversial, it might also have alerted physicians to the issue and made them more rational in prescribing fluid solutions.

In the past, plasma or its equivalent was the volume expander most commonly used. Considering the risk of transfer of infection and possible effects on immunocompetence associated with the infusion of blood products, it was obvious that plasma was not an optimal colloid for plasma volume support unless there was an indication to correct some hemostatic disorders.

Consensus statements on albumin, based on assessment of decision triggers in different clinical situations at different hospitals in various countries, have in recent years considerably influenced the discussions on its proper indications as a plasma volume expander [70, 74]. Although the scientific usefulness of such consensus conferences has been questioned [75], it is obvious that they have had a major impact on clinical routines and have resulted in a diminished 'abuse' of albumin which may in fact have improved medical practice. Therefore, it is obvious that:

- routine administration of albumin to critically ill patients on the basis of reduced plasma albumin levels cannot be recommended;
- albumin administration for intravascular volume expansion in critically ill patients seems questionable and crystalloid and/or nonprotein colloid should be preferred in most situations;
- at the present time the indications for albumin administration are restricted to general hypovolemic situations in which synthetic colloids are contraindicated or have been used to their maximal doses [70], and to specific hypovolemic situations, such as hemorrhagic shock if sodium restriction is required, hepatic resection in cases of dysfunction of the residual liver, significant diarrhea (> 2 l/day) associated with enteral feeding intolerance and with serum albumin less than 2.0 g/dl, and in the control of ascites and peripheral edema of postoperative liver transplant patients when serum albumin is less than 2.5 g/dl, pulmonary capillary wedge pressure is less than 12 mmHg, and hematocrit is more than 30%.

The optimal colloid for plasma volume support in different clinical situations is also a matter of considerable controversy [76]. While guidelines recommend the use of nonprotein colloids in hemorrhagic shock until blood products are available and in non-hemorrhagic shock after an initial infusion with crystalloid, artificial as well as natural colloids are commonly used in the clinical treatment of hypovolemia in critically ill patients. Specific indications for colloid products include a hypoproteinemic state, patients who require plasma volume expansion who cannot tolerate larger amount of fluid, and procedures requiring prevention of thrombus formation. Colloid therapy appears to be indicated in selected clinical situations where the patients require rapid plasma expansion and do not have significant endothelial injury. The decision to use one class of colloid over another should be subjected to the same critical thought process and reliance on evidence that ideally takes place with conventional drugs. All colloids are not created equal but a rationale approach to colloid administration is essential [77], and associated factors that have to be considered in their clinical choice are:

- plasma volume supporting capacity;
- intravascular persistence of the macromolecules;
- influence on microvascular blood flow;
- clinical safety of the preparation, including the potential risk of induction of adverse reactions [76, 78].

As far as crystalloids are concerned, they remain the volume replacement solutions of first choice, and their use provides essential benefit in the compensation of blood losses by correcting water and sodium deficits in the interstitial compartment. Crystalloids appear to be just as effective as colloids in the majority of clinical settings, suggesting that the more-expensive colloids may generally be overused. In the context of major hypovolemia, however, their use is not appropriate, since the amounts required do not allow for adequate treatment of shock and especially of microcirculatory disturbances, a key factor in limiting the effects of shock on tissues.

Although the fluid debate will continue, there are no definitive studies that demonstrate improved survival or reduced risk of acute injury with a specific therapy. Certainly the cost of solution makes the starches, dextrans, and gelatins compare favorably with albumin. However, crystalloid therapy remains the least-expensive method of plasma volume expansion, although it is rapidly lost to the interstitial space.

Conclusions

Resuscitation of intravascular volume and fluid replacement are essential in the treatment of hypovolemic patients. Restoration of macro- and microcirculatory perfusion is the primary goal of volume therapy, to prevent deleterious consequences such as organ dysfunction or multiple organ failure. Despite several studies and consensus conference recommendations, neither the 'ideal' resuscitation fluid for hypovolemic patients nor the 'best' resuscitation fluid for patients in the intensive care unit has been found. Most studies have compared a single colloid versus crystalloid therapy or compared two colloids, so definite recommendations on the 'best' fluid therapy remain elusive.

The only clear indications are related to the advantages for correction of fluid derangements. With reference to this, crystalloid solutions represent the basic treatment to correct water and electrolyte deficits after blood or fluid loss. Therefore, they are always the first choice for treatment of intravascular hypovolemia. However, for major hypovolemia, and particularly in cases with microcirculatory disturbances and increased capillary permeability, colloid solutions are necessary to guarantee sufficient tissue perfusion, and in cases of intravascular hypovolemia with reduced CO can restore intravascular volume and stabilize the hemodynamic conditions. There is growing evidence that albumin should not be routinely used for correction of hypovolemia or hypoalbuminemia in critically ill patients, but must be restricted to precisely defined indications, e.g., situations in which synthetic colloids are contraindicated or have been used to their maximal doses.

However, the debate on the optimal fluid regimens for critically ill patients is still as intense as ever before. Even though it is obvious that the ongoing discussions on the optimal fluid therapy of critically ill patients have had significant impact on present clinical routines, it must be remembered, however, that the fluid therapy of critically ill patients should be based on the specific needs of each individual patient. Really, the optimal approach will vary depending, not only on the underlying medical condition and its actual clinical stage, but also on the physical status, presence of complicating conditions, and age of the patient prior to the critical illness.

References

1. Cannon WB, Fraser J, Cowell EM (1918) The preventative treatment of wound shock. JAMA 70: 618-621
2. Haljamäe H (1998) Albumin: to use or not to use? Contemporary alternatives? In: Baron J-F, Treib J (eds) Volume replacement. Springer-Verlag, Berlin Heidelberg New York, pp 1-22
3. Margarson MP, Soni N (1998) Serum albumin: touchstone or totem? Anaesthesia 53: 789-803
4. Webb AR, Barclay SA, Bennett ED (1989) *In vitro* colloid osmotic pressure of commonly used plasma expanders and substitutes: a study of the diffusibility of colloid molecules. Intensive Care Med 15: 116-120
5. Starling EH (1986) On the absorption of fluids from the connective tissues spaces. J Physiol 19:312-326
6. Taylor AE (1981) Capillary fluid filtration: Starling forces and lymph flow. Circ Res 49: 557-575
7. Arfors KE, Buckley PB (1980) Role of artificial colloids in rational fluid therapy. In: Tuma RF, White JV, Messmer K (eds) The role of hemodilution in optimal patient care. Zuckschwerdt Verlag, Munich, pp 100-123

8. Parrillo JE (1993) Pathogenetic mechanisms of septic shock. N Engl J Med 328: 1471-1477
9. Baron JF (2000) Crystalloids versus colloids in the treatment of hypovolemic shock. In: Vincent J-L (ed) Yearbook of intensive care and emergency medicine. Springer, Berlin Heidelberg New York, pp 443-466
10. Kreimeier U, Peter K (1998) Strategies of volume therapy in sepsis and systemic inflammatory response syndrome. Kidney Int 53 [Suppl 64]: S75-S79
11. Hinshaw LB (1996) Sepsis/septic shock: participation of the microcirculation: an abbreviated review. Crit Care Med 24: 1072-1078
12. Boldt J (2000) Human albumin on the intensive care unit: can we live without it. In: Vincent J-L (ed) Yearbook of intensive care and emergency medicine. Springer, Berlin Heidelberg New York, pp 467-475
13. Hauser CJ, Shoemaker WC, et al (1980) Oxygen transport responses to colloid and crystalloid in critically ill surgical patients. Surg Gynecol Obstet 150: 811-816
14. Rackow EC, Mecher C, Astiz ME, et al (1989) Effects of pentastarch and albumin infusion on cardiorespiratory function and coagulation in patients with severe sepsis and systemic hypoperfusion. Crit Care Med 17: 394-398
15. Lazrove S, Waxman K, Shippy CR, et al (1980) Hemodynamic, blood volume and oxygen transport responses to albumin and hydroxyethyl starch infusions in critically ill postoperative patients. Crit Care Med 8: 302-306
16. Sibbald WJ (1985) Myocardial function in a critically ill: factors influencing left and right ventricular performance in patient with sepsis and trauma. Surg Clin North Am 65: 867-893
17. Voerman HJ, Groenveld AB (1989) Blood viscosity and circulatory shock. Intensive Care Med 15: 72-78
18. Foglia RP, Partington MT, Buckbeg GD et al (1986) Iatrogenic myocardial edema with crystalloid primes. Effect on left ventricular compliance, performance and perfusion. Curr Stud Hematol Blood Transfus 53: 53-63
19. Dart RC, Sanders AB (1998) Oxygen free radicals and myocardial reperfusion injury. Ann Emerg Med 17: 53-58
20. Edwards JD, Nightingale P, Wilkins RG, et al (1989) Hemodynamic and oxygen transport response to modified fluid gelatin in critically ill patients. Crit Care Med 17: 996-998
21. Shoemaker WC, Appel PL, Kram HB (1991) Oxygen transport measurements to evaluate tissue perfusion and titrate therapy: dobutamine and dopamine effects. Crit Care Med 19: 672-688
22. Matsuda H, Shoemaker WC (1975) Survivors' and nonsurvivors' responses to dextran 40. Hemodynamic and oxygen transport changes in critically ill patients. Arch Surg 110: 301-305
23. Wang P, Hauptman JG, Chaudry IH (1990) Hemorrhage produces depression in microvascular blood flow which persists despite fluid resuscitation. Circ Shock 32: 307-318
24. Antonsson JB, Boyle CC, Kruithoff KL, et al (1990) Validity of tonometric measures of gut intramural pH during endotoxemia and mesenteric occlusion in pigs. Am J Physiol 259: G519-G523
25. Mythen MG, Webb AR (1994) Intraoperative gut mucosal hypoperfusion is associated with increased post-operative complications and cost. Intensive Care Med 20: 99-104
26. Marik PE, Iglesias J, Maini B (1997) Gastric intramucosal pH changes after volume replacement with hydroxyethyl starch or crystalloid in patients undergoing elective abdominal aortic aneurysm repair. J Crit Care 12: 51-55
27. Boldt J, Muller M, Heesen M, et al (1996) Influence of different volume therapies and pentoxifylline infusion on circulating soluble adhesion molecules in critically ill patients. Crit Care Med 24: 385-391
28. Lowell JA, Schifferdecker C, Driscoll DF, et al (1990) Postoperative fluid overload: not a benign problem. Crit Care Med 18: 728-733
29. Holcroft JW, Trunkey DD (1975) Pulmonary extravasation of albumin during and after hemorrhagic shock in baboons. J Surg Res 18: 728-733
30. Kreimeier U, Bruckner UB, Niemczyck S, et al (1990) Hyperosmotic saline dextran for

resuscitation from hemorrhagic-traumatic hypotension: effect on regional blood flow. Circ Shock 32: 83-99
31. Cochrane Injuries Group Albumin Reviewers (1998) Human albumin administration in critically ill patients: systemic review of randomized controlled trials. BMJ 317: 235-239
32. Schierhout G, Roberts I (1998) Fluid resuscitation with colloids or crystalloids in critically ill patients: a systematic review of randomized trials. BMJ 316: 961-964
33. Kreimeier U, Ruiz- Morales M, Messmer K (1993) Comparison of the effects of volume resuscitation with dextran 60 vs. Ringer's lactate on central hemodynamics, regional blood flow, pulmonary function, and blood composition during hyperdynamic endotoxemia. Circ Shock 39: 89-99
34. Funk W, Baldinger V (1995) Microcirculatory perfusion during volume therapy. A comparative study using crystalloid or colloid in awake animals. Anesthesiology 82: 975-982
35. Gallagher JD, Moore RA, Kerns D, et al (1985) Effects of colloid or crystalloid administration on pulmonary extravascular lung water in the postoperative period after coronary artery bypass grafting. Anesth Analg 64: 753-758
36. Gallagher TJ, Banner MJ, Barnes P (1985) Large volume crystalloid resuscitation does not increase extravascular lung water. Anesth Analg 64: 323-326
37. Moss GS, Lowe RJ, Jilek J, et al (1981) Colloid or crystalloid in the resuscitation of hemorrhagic shock: A controlled clinical trial. Surgery 89: 434-438
38. Mazzoni MC, Borgstrom P, Arfors KE, et al (1988) Dynamic fluid redistribution in hyperosmotic resuscitation of hypovolemic hemorrhage. Am J Physiol 255: H629-H637
39. Lopes OU, Pontieri V, Rocha e Silva M Jr, et al (1981) Hyperosmotic NaCl and severe hemorrhagic shock: role of the innervated lung. Am J Physiol 241: H883-H890
40. Kien ND, Retain JA, White DA, et al (1991) Cardiac contractility and blood flow distribution following resuscitation with 7.5% hypertonic saline in anesthetized dogs. Circ Shock 35: 109-116
41. Prough DS, Whitley JM, Taylor CL, et al (1991) Regional cerebral blood flow following resuscitation from hemorrhagic shock with hypertonic saline. Influence of a subdural mass. Anesthesiology 75: 319-327
42. Rachow EC, Falk JL, Fein A, et al (1983) Fluid resuscitation in circulatory shock: a comparison of the cardiorespiratory effects of albumin, hetastarch, and saline solutions in patients with hypovolemic and septic shock. Crit Care Med 11: 839-850
43. Fleck A, Raines G, Hawker F, et al (1985) Increased intravascular permeability: a major cause of hypoalbuminemia in disease and injury. Lancet: 781-784
44. Mishler JM (1984) Synthetic plasma volume expanders their pharmacology, safety, and clinical efficacy. Clin Hematol 13: 75-92
45. Nearman HS, Herman ML (1981) Toxic effects of colloids in the intensive care units. Crit Care Clin 7: 713-723
46. Lamke LO, Liljedahl SO (1976) Plasma volume expansion after infusion of 5%, 20% and 25% albumin solutions in patients. Resuscitation 5: 85-92
47. Laxenaire MC, Charpentier C, Feldman L and the French Plasmasubstitutes Tolerance Study Group (1994) Anaphylactoid reactions to colloid plasma substitutes: incidence, risk factors, mechanisms. Ann Fr Anaesth Reanim 13: 301
48. Kovalik SG, Ledgerwood AM, Lucas CE, et al (1974) The cardiac effect of altered calcium homeostasis after albumin resuscitation. J Trauma 21: 275-279
49. Ledgerwood AM, Lucas CE (1974) Postresuscitation hypertension, etiology, morbidity and treatment. Arch Surg 108: 531-538
50. Salmon JB, Mythen MG (1993) Pharmacology and physiology of colloids. Blood Rev 7: 114-120
51. Bergqvist D (1982) Dextran and haemostasis: a review. Acta Chir Scand 148: 633-640
52. Laubenthal H, Messmer K (1992) Allergic reactions to dextrans. In: Baron JF (ed) Plasma volume expansion. Arnette Blackwell, Paris.
53. Strauss RG, Stump DC, Henriksen RA, et al (1985) Effects of hydroxyethyl starch on fibrinogen, fibrin clot formation, and fibrinolysis. Transfusion 25: 230-234

54. Mishler JM, Hester JP, Heustis DW, et al (1983) Dosage and scheduling regimens for erythrocyte-sedimenting macromolecules. J Clin Apheresis 1: 130-143
55. London MJ, HO JS, Triedman JK, et al (1989) A randomized clinical trial of 10% pentastarch (low molecular weight hydroxyethyl starch) versus 5% albumin for plasma volume expansion after cardiac operations. J Thorac Cardiovasc Surg 97: 785-797
56. Yeh T, Parmar JM, Rebeyka IM et al (1992) Limiting edema in neonatal cardiopulmonary bypass with narrow-range molecular weight hydroxyethyl starch. J Thorac Cardiovasc Surg 104: 659-665
57. Saddler JM, Horsey PJ (1987) The new generation gelatins. Anaesthesia 42: 998-1004
58. Lundsgaart-Hansen P, Tschirren B (1980) Clinical experience with 120,000 units of modified fluid gelatin. Dev Biol Stand 48: 251-256
59. Choi PT, Yip G, Quinonez LG, et al (1999) Crystalloids vs. colloids in fluid resuscitation: a systematic review. Crit Care Med 27: 200-210
60. Bunn F, Alderson P, Hawkins V (2001) Colloid solutions for fluid resuscitation (Cochrane Review). In: The Cochrane Library, Issue 2. Oxford: Update Software, pp 1-18
61. Boldt J, Lenz M, Kumle B, et al (1998) Volume replacement strategies on intensive care units: results from a postal survey. Intensive Care Med 24: 147-151
62. Berger A (1998) Why albumin may not work BMJ 317:240
63. Offringa M (1998) Excess mortality after human albumin administration in critically ill patients. BMJ 317: 223-224
64. Dung NM, Day NPJ, Tam DTH, et al (1999) Fluid replacement in dengue shock syndrome: a randomized, double-blind comparison of four intravenous-fluid regimens. Clin Infect Dis 29: 787-794
65. Van der Sande FM, Kooman JP, Barendregt JNM, et al (1999) Effect of intravenous saline, albumin, or hydroxyethyl starch on blood volume during combined ultrafiltration and hemodialysis. J Am Soc Nephrol 10: 1303-1308
66. Ioannidis PA, Cappeleri JC, Lau J (1998) Issues in comparisons between meta-analyses and large trials. JAMA 279: 1089-1093
67. Consensus Conference (1985) Fresh-frozen plasma: indications and risks. JAMA 253: 551-553
68. Consensus Conference (1987) Platelet transfusion therapy. JAMA 257: 1777-1780
69. Consensus Conference (1988) Perioperative red cell transfusion. JAMA 260: 2700-2703
70. Vermeulen L, Ratko TA, Erstad BL, et al (1995) A paradigm for consensus. The university hospital consortium guidelines for the use of albumin, nonprotein colloid and crystalloid solutions. Arch Intern Med 155: 373- 379
71. Mangues I, Lloberas N, Ferrer MI, et al (1995) Criterios de utilizacion de albumina. Farm Clin 12: 271-277
72. Gines P, Arroyo V, Quintero E, et al (1987) Comparison of paracentesis and diuretics in the treatment of cirrhotic with tense ascitis. Gastroenterology 93: 234-241
73. Planas R, Gines P, Arroyo V, et al (1990) Dextran 70 versus albumin as plasma expanders in cirrhotic patients with tense ascites treated with total paracentesis. Gastrenterology 99: 1736--1744
74. Subcommittee of the Victorian Drug Usage Advisory Committee (1992) Human albumin solutions: consensus statements for use in selected clinical situations. Med J Aust 157: 340-343
75. Durand-Zalesky I, Bonnet F, Rochant H, et al (1992) Usefulness of consensus conferences: the case of albumin. Lancet 340: 1388-1390
76. Haljamäe H, Dahlqvist M, Walentin F (1997) Artificial colloids in clinical practice: pros and cons. Baillieres Clin Anaesthesiol 11: 49-79
77. Mythen MG, Salmon JB, Webb AR (1993) The rational administration of colloids. Blood Rev 7: 223-228
78. Haljamäe H (1999) Use of fluids in trauma. Int J Intensive Care 6: 20-30

PERIOPERATIVE MEDICINE

Preoperative Assessment

A.F. HAMMERLE, C. TATSCHL, C. BAUMGARTNER

The goal of preoperative assessment

Information gathered during preoperative evaluation of patients should serve to identify risk factors that may contribute to perioperative complications related to anaesthesia.

Roizen [1] has subdivided the aims of preoperative assessments into the following categories:

- to obtain pertinent information about the patient's medical history and physical and mental conditions, in order to determine which tests and consultations are needed;
- to choose the care plans to be followed according to the patient preferences and the risk factors uncovered by medical history;
- to obtain informed consent;
- to inform the patient about anaesthesia, perioperative care, and pain treatments in the hope of reducing anxiety and facilitating recovery;
- to make perioperative care more efficient and less expensive.

It is the major task to screen for those physical conditions that can be improved by the choice of anaesthetic technique or by perioperative medical optimization. Therefore, diagnostic measures are only required, if the results obtained lead directly to interventions able to reduce the risk of an anaesthetic [2].

Assessing risk

Risk has been defined as the mathematical product of the *probability* of an event and *consequence* of this event [3]. This definition highlights the importance of being aware of the prevalence of a certain pathology in a given patient and the impact that its identification brings about. Especially in times of financial pressure and increased workload this simple formula may guide the anaesthesiologist's assessment strategy and may help to avoid unnecessary testing, that results in high costs and patient discomfort.

What are the factors influencing perioperative risk?

As demonstrated by Pedersen et al. [4] patient age, concomitant disease and type of surgery largely influence perioperative mortality. For example: a patient with chronic heart failure undergoing elective surgery who is less than fifty years old has a risk of in hospital mortality of 0.1%. By contrast, a patient with chronic heart failure and renal failure who is more than 70 years old and has to undergo emergency abdominal surgery will face a risk of in hospital mortality of 76%. Several indices to describe perioperative risk based on the condition of the patient have been developed:

General risk assessment

Mandated by the American Society of Anesthesiologists (ASA), Saklad published the original score for the description of the patient's preoperative physical condition in 1941 [5].

A modified version was adopted by the ASA in 1963 and is now known as the ASA-classification of physical status [6] (Table 1).

Table 1 ASA classification of physical status

ASA I	Normal healthy patient
ASA II	Patient with mild to moderate systemic disease with no functional limitation
ASA III	Patient with severe systemic disease with definite limitation of normal function
ASA IV	Patient with severe systemic disease that is a constant threat to life
ASA V	Moribund patient unlikely to survive 24 h with or without operation

Although initially developed to produce comparable patient collectives it has been recognized, that the ASA score correlates with perioperative complications [7-9].

Surgical risk assessment

A Consensus Group at the Johns Hopkins Medical Institutions has developed the classification system to describe the risk for the patient, that evolves from the type of surgery irrespective of the patient's physical condition or the type of anaesthesia. This score has been termed the Johns Hopkins Risk Classification System (JHRCS) and categorizes surgical procedures according to their invasiveness into 5 groups ranging from minimal to critical risk [10] (Table 2).

Table 2. The Johns Hopkins Risk Classification System (JHRCS) [10]

Category I	-	Minimal risk to the patient independent of anaesthesia
	-	Minimally invasive procedures with little or no blood loss
	-	Often done in an office setting with the operating room used principally for anaesthesia and monitoring
Category II	-	Minimally to moderately invasive procedure
	-	Blood loss < 500 cc
	-	Mild risk to patient independent of anaesthesia
Category III	-	Moderately to significantly invasive procedure
	-	Blood loss potential 500 – 1500 cc
	-	Moderate risk to patient independent of anaesthesia
Category IV	-	Highly invasive procedure
	-	Blood loss > 1 500 cc
	-	Major risk to patient independent of anaesthesia
Category V	-	Highly invasive procedure
	-	Blood loss > 1 500 cc
	-	Critical risk to patient independent of anaesthesia
	-	Usual postoperative ICU stay with invasive monitoring

Cardiac risk assessment

Goldman et al. (1977) developed a multifactorial index for the prediction of perioperative myocardial complications. According to this index patients are grouped into 4 categories. The risk for myocardial complications increases with the number of points attributed to the patient. In this index the major risk factors are Gallop rhythm or elevated jugular venous pressure, myocardial infarction in preceding 6 months and arrhythmias. No other concomitant cardiac diseases are considered as relevant risk factors, whereas age and urgency of surgery are thought to be relevant [11].

A modified version of the Goldman Cardiac Risk Index was published by Detsky et al. (1986). In this edition patients are categorized into three risk groups. The most severe risk factors are angina, suspected critical aortic stenosis, myocardial infarction within the last 6 months, pulmonary oedema within the last week and emergency surgery [12].

The ACC/AHA Task Force Report [13] subsumes medical comorbidities as major, intermediate or minor "clinical predictors of increased perioperative cardiovascular risk" for myocardial infarction, congestive heart failure and death. The major clinical predictors in this classification system are unstable coronary syndromes, decompensated congestive heart failure, significant arrhythmias and severe valvular disease. In addition these guidelines stratify surgical procedures according to their inherent cardiac risk into high, intermediate and low risk interventions. Both, clinical predictors and surgical procedures were integrated into a multistep algorithm that guides preoperative workup of cardiac risk patients awaiting non-cardiac surgery.

Pulmonary risk assessment

Attempts to identify patients with increased risk for pulmonary complications have been mostly inconclusive. Many patients with pulmonary risk factors display cardiac comorbidities. Several prediction systems have been tested.

Gerson et al. [14] demonstrated that the inability to perform two minutes of supine bicycle exercise with a heart rate above 99 beats per minute was the best predictor of cardiopulmonary complications in elderly patients when compared to assessment of clinical history, results of physical examination, electrocardiogram, chest radiograph, blood chemistry, pulmonary function test findings and Goldman cardiac risk factors.

In another study Epstein et al. [15] tested a cardiopulmonary risk index (CRPI) which is a combination of the Goldman cardiac risk index and pulmonary risk factors (obesity, productive cough, wheezing, tobacco use, ratio of the forced expiratory volume in 1 second over the forced vital capacity [FEV1/FVC] 70% and $PaCO_2$ 45 mmHg). Patients who had 4 or more of the cardiopulmonary risk factors were 22 times more likely to develop a cardiopulmonary complication compared to those who scored less than 4 points.

Shapiro et al. [16] have proposed a more detailed score including evaluation of the respiratory nervous and cardiovascular system, arterial blood gases and expected postoperative ambulation for the prediction of pulmonary complications.

The approach to the patient

The preoperative visit and the pre-anaesthetic assessment clinic

Commonly the preoperative visit takes place on the evening before surgery. However, increasing numbers of patients are met by the anaesthesiologist only on the day of surgery. It is not clear if this is disadvantageous for patients who are otherwise healthy. It has been demonstrated, that a pre-anaesthetic interview on the day of surgery may as well be safe and effective [17].

Another approach to preoperative patient evaluation is the institution of a preanesthetic assessment clinic. In such institutions the patients are interviewed by specially trained anaesthesiologists. Test results are discussed with experts of different specialities and the prescriptions are then transferred to the surgical ward. Such clinics are more efficient than bed side evaluation and are cost effective despite the increased requirements for trained staff [18].

Hierarchy in preoperative evaluation

The process of preoperative patient evaluation comprises several steps:
- medical history and physical examination;
- screening work-up (standard laboratory testing, chest x-ray, ECG);
- specific additional testing as indicated (echocardiography, lung function testing, specific coagulation abnormalities…).

Medical history and physical examination

A thorough study of the patient's medical history and careful physical examination are without doubt the mainstay of preoperative assessment. Based on the data from this initial step alone the anaesthesiological care plan had to be changed in up to 20% [19].

The physical examination contains:
- assessment of the patients general impression and nutritional status;
- brief assessment of the patient's mental status;
- measurement of blood pressure;
- evaluation of the anatomy of the oral region, mobility of the cervical spine, and dental status (screening for the difficult airway, see following paragraph);
- percussion and auscultation of the heart and lungs (e.g., valvular disease, asthma);
- palpation and auscultation of the abdomen (e.g., ileus, hepatic enlargement);
- inspection of the lower extremities (e.g., varicosis, oedema).

Oral anatomy and mobility of the cervical spine

The precise determination of the oral apertura, the relation of tongue size to the pharyngeal cavity as well as the proportion and flexibility of the neck region are essential to guarantee adequate oxygen delivery during induction. The respiratory catastrophe can only be prevented if, by timely recognition of the impending problem, adequate alternative measures (e.g., fiberoptic intubation, combitube) are instituted [20].

Several indices to predict difficult intubation have been published [21-23]. Noteworthy the predicted conditions for intubation should be documented in the patient record.

In most institutions standardized medical history forms are available to help both the patient and the anaesthesiologist to realize a comprehensive conception of the patient's condition. The following questions represent the questionnaire used in the Department of Anaesthesiology of the Vienna General Hospital:

- Age (years), Height (cm), Weight (kg)?
- What is your occupation at present?
- Do you smoke regularly? If yes, how many cigarettes (cigars, etc) per day?
- Do you drink alcohol regularly? If yes, what do you drink? How many glasses/bottles per day?
- Do you wear a hearing aid?
- Do you wear contact lenses?
- Do you wear removable dentures? Do you have any diseased teeth? Do you have any loose teeth?
- Have you consulted a physician recently? If yes, for what reason?
- Do you take medication regularly (e.g., analgesics, sleeping pills, cardiovascular drugs, anticoagulants such as warfarin, aspirin, etc.)? If yes, which medication do you take and in what doses per day?
- Have you ever been operated on before? If yes, when and for what reason? Were there any unusual occurrances during anaesthesia? If yes please describe.
- Have any of your blood relatives experienced unusual incidents during anaesthesia?
- Have you ever had a blood transfusion? If yes, were there any complications?
- Have you donated your own blood for the planned operation ? If yes, how much?
- Women of child-bearing age: Is there any possibility that you might be pregnant at the moment?
- Do you now suffer, or have suffered from any of the following diseases?

1. Heart disease (e.g., myocardial infarction, angina pectoris, heart defects, dyspnoea when climbing stairs, inflammation of the cardiac muscle (myocarditis), cardiac arrhythmias)?
2. Cardiovascular diseases (e.g., circulatory disturbances, abnormally high or low blood pressure, varicose veins, thromboses, embolism)?
3. Diseases of the lungs and respiratory tracts (e.g., tuberculosis, silicosis, pneumonia, pulmonary emphysema, asthma, chronic bronchitis) ?

4. Liver diseases (e.g., jaundice, hepatitis, fatty liver, cirrhosis) ?
5. Diseases of the kidneys or urinary tract (e.g., nephritis, pyelonephritis, kidney or bladder stones) ?
6. Diseases of the gastrointestinal tract (e.g., gastric disorders, chronic intestinal disorders) ?
7. Metabolic disorders (e.g., diabetes mellitus) ?
8. Thyroid disease (e.g., goiter, hyperthyroidism, hypothyroidism)
9. Diseases of the eye (e.g., glaucoma) ?
10. Disorders of the nervous system (e.g., epilepsy, paralysis) ?
11. Have you ever been treated for an emotional problem or disorder (e.g., depression)?
12. Diseases of the skeletal system (e.g., damage to the vertebral column, joint disease)?
13. Muscular disorders, muscular weakness (myasthenia), predisposition towards malignant hyperthermia?
14. Blood diseases or a tendency to bleed easily (Do you bruise for no apparent reason or have a tendency towards nose bleedings)?
15. Allergies/hypersensitivity reactions (e.g., hay fever, hypersensitivity to certain foods, medications, adhesive bandages or rubber gloves)?
16. Other diseases not listed above?
17. Miscellaneous points worth noting (e.g., accidents, serious injuries, special occupational circumstances)

Screening tests

Preoperative patient work up consisting of several laboratory tests, chest x-ray, and routine ECG theoretically serves to identify previously unknown physical alterations.

However, the findings, that routine testing leads to the detection of disturbances relevant to anaesthesiological practice only in a minority of cases, have lead to a change in testing philosophy. Several authors have proposed indications for different diagnostic procedures in advance of a surgical procedure. Over the years the age-related threshold for these tests have increased and the spectrum of patients in whom such testing should be undertaken has decreased [1].

One attractive example for the approach to the problem of decision making in context with preoperative testing has been proposed by Pasternak [10]. The indications for specific testing are grouped according to medical disease, patient age and the invasiveness of the surgical procedure. (Tables 2, 3].

Table 3. Laboratory testing required for the administration of anesthesia according to Pasternak (from reference [10])

Electrocardiogram	Age 50 or older Hypertension Current or past significant cardiac disease Current or past circulatory disease Diabetes mellitus (age 40 or older) Renal, thyroid or other metabolic disease Procedure category V
Chest x-ray	Asthma or COPD that is debilitating or with change of symptoms or acute episode within past 6 months Cardiothoracic procedure Procedure category V
Serum chemistries	Renal disease Adrenal or thyroid disorders Diuretic therapy Chemotherapy Procedure category V
Urine analysis	Diabetes mellitus Renal disease Genito-urologic procedure Recent genito-urinary infection Metabolic disorder involving renal function Procedure category V
Complete blood count	Haematological disorder Vascular procedure Chemotherapy Procedure level IV
Coagulation studies	Anticoagulation therapy Vascular procedure Procedure level V
Pregnancy testing	Patients for whom pregnancy might complicate the surgery Patients of uncertain status by history

Assessment of concomitant medication

Several medications directly interfere with anaesthesia, either by interacting with drugs applied during the anaesthetic or by altering the physiological status. It is one of the anaesthesiologist's tasks during preoperative evaluation to decide whether a given drug has to be discontinued or if it is beneficial to administer it on the day of surgery. In a series of articles the concept of perioperative drug administration recently has been reviewed [24-27]. Table 4 gives a survey of perioperative drug prescription.

Table 4. Continuation and discontinuation of concomitant medication

Drugs to be continued	Drugs to be discontinued
Antacid and gastrokinetic agents	Anticoagulant and antiplatelet drugs
Antiepileptics	MAOIs
Antihypertensives*, antanginal, and antiarrhythmic drugs	NSAIDs
	Diuretics
Antiparkinsonian drugs	Antidiabetic therapy
Immunosuppressants	Lithium
SSRIs	Oral contraceptives and hormone replacement therapy
Antipsychotics and anxiolytics	
Drugs for asthma	
Drugs of dependence	
Corticosteroids	

* Some authors [28] recommend to withhold angiotensin-converting enzyme inhibitors (ACEIs) on the morning of surgery. The rationale for this strategy is derived from the findings of Coriat and colleagues [29], who found that significantly more patients needed vasopressor support during induction of anaesthesia if ACEI-therapy was maintained until the morning of surgery than those patients, in whom ACEIs were withdrawn at least 12 hours (captopril) or 24 hours (enalapril) before anaesthesia.

Conclusions

Modern anaesthesia reflects the concept of perioperative medicine. To approach the goal of a constant quality of therapy, from the operating room through Postanaesthesia Care Unit (PACU) or intensive care unit (ICU) and vice versa the role of preoperative assessment may be extraordinary, as far as the reduction of morbidity and mortality can primarily be achieved by optimizing the patients risk profile in the preoperative period. Consequently, preoperative assessment is definitely reasonable when it is able to the augment patient safety.

References

1. Roizen MF, Foss JF, Fischer SP (2000) Preoperative evaluation. In: Miller RD (ed) Anesthesia. Churchill Livingstone, pp 824-884
2. Wilhelm W, Larsen R (1997) Preoperative evaluation for anesthesia. Anaesthesist 46:629-39
3. Arvidsson S (1996) Preparation of adult patients for anaesthesia and surgery. Acta Anaesthesiol Scand 40:962-970
4. Pedersen T, Eliasen K, Henriksen E (1990) A prospective study of mortality associated with anaesthesia and surgery: risk indicators of mortality in hospital. Acta Anaesthesiol Scand 34:176-182
5. Saklad M (1941) Grading of patients for surgical procedures. Anesthesiology 2:281

6. ASA (1963) New classification of physical status. Anesthesiology 234:111
7. Biondo S, Ramos E, Deiros M et al (2000) Prognostic factors for mortality in left colonic peritonitis: a new scoring system. J Am Coll Surg 191:635-642
8. Vacanti CJ, VanHouten RJ, Hill RC (1970) A statistical analysis of the relationship of physical status to postoperative mortality in 68 388 cases. Anesth Analg 49:564-566
9. Marx GF, Mateo CV, Orkin LR (1973) Computer analysis of postanesthetic deaths. Anesthesiology 39:54-58
10. Pasternak LR (1995) Perioperative evaluation - A systematic approach. In: Annual refresher course lectures, Inc. American Society of Anesthesiologists, Chapter 421, pp 1-7
11. Goldman L, Caldera DL, Nussbaum SR et al (1977) Multifactorial index of cardiac risk in noncardiac surgical procedures. N Engl J Med 297:845-850
12. Detsky AS, Abrams HB, McLaughlin JR et al (1986) Predicting cardiac complications in patients undergoing non-cardiac surgery. J Gen Intern Med 1:211-219
13. Eagle KA, Brundage BH, Chaitman BR et al (1996) Guidelines for perioperative cardiovascular evaluation for noncardiac surgery. Report of the American College of Cardiology/American Heart Association Task Force on Practice Guidelines. Committee on Perioperative Cardiovascular Evaluation for Noncardiac Surgery. Circulation 93:1278-1317
14. Gerson MC, Hurst JM, Hertzberg VS et al (1990) Prediction of cardiac and pulmonary complications related to elective abdominal and noncardiac thoracic surgery in geriatric patients. Am J Med 88:101-107
15. Epstein SK, Faling LJ, Daly BD et al (1993) Predicting complications after pulmonary resection. Preoperative exercise testing vs a multifactorial cardiopulmonary risk index. Chest 104:694-700
16. Shapiro BA, Harrison RA, Kacmarek RM (eds) (1985) Clinical applications of respiratory care, 3rd edition. Yearbook Publishers, Chicago
17. Twersky RS, Frank D, Lebovits A (1990) Timing of preoperative evaluation for surgical outpatients - Does it matter? Part II. Anesthesiology 73:A1
18. Prause G (1994) The preoperative outpatient clinic in Graz: The first 15 years. Anaesthesist 43: 223-228
19. Gibby GL, Gravenstein JS, Layon AF et al (1992) How often does the preoperative interview change anesthetic management? Anesthesiology 77:A1134
20. Krafft P, Frass M (2000) The difficult airway. Wien Klin Wochenschr 112:260-270
21. Mallampati SR, Gatt SP, Gugino LD et al (1985) A clinical sign to predict difficult intubation: a prospective study. Canadian Anaesthetists´ Society Journal 42:429-434
22. Samsoun GL, Young JR (1987) Difficult tracheal intubation: a retrospective study. Anesthesia 42:487-490
23. Wilson ME, Spiegelhalter JA, Robertson JA et al (1988) Predicting difficult intubation. Br J Anaesth 61:211-216
24. Anonymous (1999) Drugs in the peri-operative period 1 – Stopping or continuing drugs around surgery. Drug Ther Bull 37:62-64
25. Anonymous (1999) Drugs in the peri-operative period 2 – Corticosteroids and therapy for diabetes mellitus. Drug Ther Bull 37:68-70
26. Anonymous (1999) Drugs in the peri-operative period 3 – Hormonal contraceptives and hormone replacement therapy. Drug Ther Bull 37:78-80
27. Anonymous (1999) Drugs in the peri-operative period 4 – Cardiovascular drugs. Drug Ther Bull 37:89-91
28. Roizen MF (2000) Anesthetic implications of concurrent diseases. In: Miller RD (ed) Anesthesia. Churchill Livingstone, pp 903-1015
29. Coriat P, Richer C, Douraki T et al (1994) Influence of chronic angiotensin-converting enzyme inhibition on anesthetic induction. Anesthesiology 81:299-307

Patient Informed Consent

F. CARLI

One might believe that informed consent has been part of the Hippocratic oath, but until the twentieth century, physicians considered themselves extension of God and did not deign to confer with patients about medical care. With the industrial revolution and advances in medical care, codes of medical ethics started to be introduced, but no mention was made of patient-physician interaction or better informed consent [1]. With the advent of civil rights and consumer rights in the 1950s, individual liberties demanded a new interpretation of patient-physician conduct. Modern informed consent is beset by a tension between its spirit and legality. Overemphasis of the legal aspect leads to an adversarial framework for the relationship between patient and anesthesiologist. The balance between ethical responsibility and legal obligation provides a safeguard designed to help both physician and patient.

The elements of informed consent

Legal, philosophical, regulatory, medical, and psychological literature has often tried to define or analyze informed consent in terms of its elements. The following elements have been identified as fundamental to the concept: (1) disclosure, (2) comprehension, (3) voluntariness, (4) competence, and (5) consent. The postulate is that a person gives an informed consent to an intervention only if a person is competent to act, receives a thorough disclosure about the procedure, comprehends the disclosed information, acts voluntarily, and consents [2].

Patient-anesthesiologist relationship

Obtaining informed consent is an integral part of the special relationship existing between a patient and his anesthesiologist. Anesthesiologists do not have a long-term relationship necessary to build trust and rapport with their patients, and this might make anesthesia a unique specialty when it comes to informed consent. This relationship that started with the preoperative visit the night before surgery is now even more limited to meeting patients only minutes before surgery. The question therefore arises as to how can the anesthesiologist accomplish his responsibility to enhance patient comfort and confidence, to encourage patient's involvement in decision making, and to disclose material information.

Ethical and legal obligation

The patient and his anesthesiologist must develop a fiduciary relationship based on trust and confidence. Both terms fiduciary and trustee have ethical and legal implications. As the patient's trustee, the physician has the obligation to promote patient's interests. The fiduciary relationship implies the importance for the physician to treat each patient as an individual and to encourage his patient to participate in decisions about the care. Reciprocal truth telling is necessary for a patient-physician relationship to be valid [3].

Anesthesiologist's obligations

He or she must be clear in informing the patient about the relevant risks, benefits, and concerns of the anesthesia he wants to provide. Exception to this obligation may include patients who choose not to be informed, emergencies in which a valid informed consent cannot be obtained, and situations of therapeutic privilege. The latter, rarely used, when the physician chooses to withhold information because he/she believes disclosure would be significantly injurious to patient. Truth telling, however, is not forcing information on patients. Some specific events, such as instrumentation of the airway and complications of invasive monitoring, should be disclosed. Risks and benefits of each anesthetic technique should be discussed, as well as the possible use of a secondary plan. Anesthesiologists should be forthright about areas of uncertainty, whether it be in the anesthesiologists' or the anesthesia community knowledge. The patient should be informed if other health care providers (anesthesia specialist, residents in anesthesia, or nurse anesthetists) will be providing anesthesia care. Anesthesiologists should also discuss with the patient what will happen to them in sequence (clinical pathway from pre- to intra- to postoperative care) [4].

Patients have a right to confidentiality, implying that the fact communicated should not be shared with others without the patient's direct or implied consent. They should also be careful about casual conversation harming patient confidentiality.

Limitations to achieving a fiduciary relationship should be minimized. For example, variation in care as a result of skin color, socioeconomic status, sexual preference, disease process, type of health care coverage, and financial incentives, even in a well-meaning physician, could disrupt the relationship.

Anesthesiologists must recognize the importance and complexity of supporting a patient's religious belief, e.g., Jehovah's witness regarding blood product transfusion [5].

Disclosure and negligence

Each institution (hospital or clinic) defines what is the appropriate information standard and how it should be documented. Negligence in relation to the informed consent can be found if the anesthesiologist provides a disclosure that is insufficient to allow a patient to make an informed decision and an injury subsequently occurs, even if the injury was forseeable and in the absence of a treatment error. How does one determine whether sufficient and appropriate information was given? The courts assess whether the information provided meets standard of care (according to professional practice standards, e.g., national association guidelines). If the disclosure did not meet standards of care, then it may be considered breach of duty. Causation assesses whether sharing the omitted information would have caused the patient to choose a different option.

Courts may also consider how the information was given. For example, the informed consent discussion should occur in a setting conducive to decision making, giving the patient chance to ask questions. Talking to the patient as he enters the operating room is totally insufficient. Preprinted forms with all information cannot be relied on, and similarly a signed consent form may still expose the anesthesiologist legally if the document is signed in situations in which the patient is rushed.

Informing the patient about a risk does not eliminate liability for its occurrence. Anesthesiologists should not look at the disclosure process as a protection against medical malpractice liability if an adverse event happens. Liability is based on medical negligence and depends on whether the standard of care was met.

So, what and how an information should be disclosed? The depth of the discussion should vary in part with the level of risk. Of course it depends also on what the patient considers important information so that he control the extent of disclosure [6].

The need to obtain consent and the capacity to make a decision.

The majority of institutions have policies that specify the mechanisms and procedures for obtaining informed consent. However, a signed legal document does not necessarily achieve the goal of informed consent. When one obtains a consent this has to be fulfilled in both legal and ethical aspects.

It is important to establish that the patient has the ability to make decisions. Evidence that a person can make a decision includes the ability to understand the current situation, to assess the relevant information given by the physician, and to agree to what has been proposed to him/her.

It is clear that the capacity to decide depends upon the age, the mental status, the type of risk in the decision, and the disease process. There are some situations in which patients have limited decisions; for example a patient who is adjudged incompetent for health care decision or a child who has not reached the age of majority. Also there is the case of patients who cannot make any decision because their capacity is altered by sedation. Of course the clinician has to use his/her clinical judgement and establish whether he/she can make a specific decision. There are some situations where a patient has baseline difficulties to make a decision. In this case one should seek assistance from the hospital ethicist.

What about if the patient wants to follow a self-chosen plan voluntarily?

Respect for autonomy is sometimes misinterpreted as " do whatever the patient wants". This does not mean that the anesthesiologist cannot explain anesthetic options and offer an opinion as to which is best. Persuasion, the act of influencing through legitimate arguments, is a justifiable technique for educating patients. Coercion, the act of affecting behavior through the use of a credible threat, is not justifiable. One has to accept the possibility of informed refusal. If the patient refuses a procedure without all the relevant information, the physician can be legally liable for injury resulting from lack of information. When a patient refuses a recommended procedure, the anesthesiologist must provide additional information to the patient about the consequences of rejection [7].

The quality of consent

Problems about the quality and adequacy of consent probably cannot be resolved unless conventional disclosure rules are redirected toward the quality of understanding present in a consent. This approach focuses on the need for communication, dispensing with liability oriented discussions about proper legal standards of disclosure. The key to effective communication is to invite participation by patients or subjects in an exchange of information and dialogue. Asking questions, eliciting the concerns and interests of the patient or subject, and establishing a climate that encourages the patients or subjects to ask questions seem more important for medical ethics than do requirements of disclosure in law. If the proper climate is not introduced into the context of consent, a request from a professional that the patient or subject ask for information is as likely to result in silence as to elicit the desired result of a meaningful information exchange and consent. Patients find it difficult to approach physicians with questions and concerns, and even when they do not understand their physicians, many still do not ask questions. The extent to which a passive attitude characterizes research subjects is less clear. Although still understudied, it is a good guess that relatively little educating of this quality occurs at present in clinical practice or in research.

Can the physician refuse to provide care?

An anesthesiologist in ethical or moral disagreement with the patient will have difficulty providing the care requested and therefore should withdraw from or refuse patient care [8]. He/she may be obligated to make a reasonable effort to find a competent or willing replacement. However, there are situations where the clinician may not only refuse to participate in this procedure, but also opposes assisting the patient in finding another physician.

Refusing to provide care because a patient is infected with the human immunodeficiency virus is considered unethical. Withdrawing from the care of a patient when a relationship has already been established is unacceptable, unless the patients approves.

Emergency situations

In general, it is assumed that patients would give consent to treatment in emergency situations. The anesthesiologist needs to rely on his/her good judgement and should obtain as much informed consent as deemed possible.

When the anesthesiologists refuses to provide care and no alternative provider is available for an emergent situation, the reluctant anesthesiologist must be available.

References

1. Faden RR, Beauchamp TL (1986) A history of informed consent. Oxford University Press, New York
2. Gild WM (1989) Informed consent: a review. Anesth Analg 68: 649-653
3. Liang BA (1996) What needs to be said? Informed consent in the context of spinal anesthesia. J Clin Anesth 8: 525-527
4. Clark SK, Leighton BL, Seltzer JL (1991) A risk-specific anesthesia consent form may hinder the informed consent process. J Clin Anesth 3: 11-13
5. Hume MA, Kennedy B, Asbury AJ (1994) Patient knowledge of anaesthesia and perioperative care. Anaesthesia 49: 715-718
6. Lonsdale M, Hutchinson GL (1991) Patient's desire for information about anaesthesia. Anaesthesia 46: 410-412
7. Kerridge I, Lowe M, Mitchell K (1995) Competent patients, incompetent decisions. Ann Intern Med 123: 178-181
8. Dellinger A, Vickery AM (1995) When staff object to participating in care. J Health Hosp Law 28: 269-285

Coordination And Responsibilities In The Operating Theater

N. Weksler, G.M. Gurman

The operating theater is one of the most-complex places in a hospital, because many factors are involved during a normal working day. The most-costly place in a hospital is the operating theater. Since many health workers are involved in the care of any single patient (surgeons, anesthesiologists, nurses, and non-medical personnel), the salaries of an OR staff account for most of the OR costs.

The goal of the hospital administration is to optimize the utilization of the operating suites, in order to attain the largest amount of surgery per day, thus, increasing the income. The major determinant of OR costs is surgical time, and many models were proposed in order to optimize booking and scheduling of operating theaters, to assure maximal exploitation of ORs.

Another problem for the assessment of the operating theater schedule is the occurrence of non-scheduled urgent, emergenty or add-on surgery. Adding new cases to the operation list can cause cancellation or postponement of elective cases, affecting patients' satisfaction and hospital reputation.

Improving OR utilization

The scheduling process

Elective OR schedule is the basis of the daily work. An accurate calculation of the surgical time helps to predict staffing, availability of equipment, and results in a smooth-running OR. An inaccurate schedule, with multiple additions, cancellations, and substitutions on the day of surgery sends the entire system into disarray and with suboptimal utilization of manpower and equipment.

The open scheduling

The open scheduling is done on a first-come, first-serve basis. Generally the open schedule is accurate for a small operating suite. Such a system can work well when the workload is based on small procedures with an easily predicted surgical time. However, when large and different procedures are scheduled one after the other, such as neurosurgery following a laparoscopic cholecystectomy, an unacceptable turnaround time can occur, decreasing the OR time utilization.

The block scheduling-

With block scheduling, the OR is allocated to a specific surgeon, surgical speciality, or department for elective cases. Block scheduling allows predictability in OR utilization and control of the allotted time. However, when different surgeons use the block time it is difficult to adjust productivity. If block time is not used, it will negatively affect block utilization. On the other hand, a slow surgeon can slide from the day's lineup of cases, inducing postponement or cancelling of cases.

The creative block scheduling

With creative block scheduling, blocks are assigned to a surgeon based on the type of surgery performed and the surgeon's average time. Some advantages are that a realistic amount of time is provided for the procedure, turnover is minimized, and the schedule is more controllable.

Saving time in operating theater

The etiology of OR delays in an academic institution was assessed by Overdyk et al. in a prospective study. In this study, the causes of delay in the OR were divided into two phases. The first phase consisted of a daily observation of OR practice for 30 consecutive days, without notification of the surgeons, anesthesiologists, and OR staffing. The second phase consisted of an educational 2-week period, when the OR personnel were informed about the common causes of delay, and a change in the anesthesiologist practice, allowing him to bring the patient to the OR and prepare the patient simultaneously with OR nurses, rather then waiting until nursing tasks were completed.

Phase 1 data collection demonstrated that there was a disproportionate number of delays during the first case of the day, mostly due to personnel unavailability, congestion in staging areas, and delay in patient registration or transportation.

After the 2-week education program, a reduction of 22 min of waiting to start the first surgical case was noticed, as well as an average reduction of 16 min in the time of empty the OR.

The impact of a reduction in the anesthesiologist-controlled time (ACT) was very small, since the influence of the surgeon-controlled time is approximately 4-5 times greater than ACT. This small influence of the ACT on efficacy of OR utilization was previously reported by Dexter et al.

Based on these studies, production pressure should be transferred from the anesthesia team to optimization of cleaning time of the operating theater, shortening of the empty OR time, and in the operation time.

Saving money in the OR

Drugs

The costs of anesthesia are considerably influenced by the prices of the drugs. Newer anesthetic drugs have been launched, promising improved clinical outcomes, less side effects and complications, and better and faster anesthesia induction and recovery. However, these advantages should be weighed against their prices. It makes no sense to select an inexpensive drug if by so doing increased complications result. On the other hand, it is irrational to use more-expensive drugs if no advantage can be proved.

There is a universal tendency to use new anesthetic drugs, either in response to the pharmaceutical industry's propaganda, or as a consequence of the anesthesiologist's wish to be up to date.

Jackson and Myles compared the effectiveness of the new anesthetic drugs propofol and sevoflurane with thiopental and isoflurane in adults undergoing elective inpatient surgery. In this randomized controlled study they were unable to demonstrate any advantage of these new and expensive drugs over thiopental and isoflurane.

Implementing pharmaceutical practice guidelines may save a significant amount of money without affecting the quality of care. For outpatient or ambulatory surgery the impact of the new anesthetic drugs in decreasing the overall costs of surgery must be carefully evaluated. It is true that shortening the time of stay in the post-anesthesia care unit (PACU) may actually reduce the institution revenue, because patients are charged for time in PACU for offset fixed costs such as nurse salaries, maintenance fees, and building amortization. Shortening the PACU stay can actually decrease profits.

Creative manipulation of manpower

In many medical institutions patients who are submitted to surgery under MAC, peripheral blocks, sedation or light anesthesia, and were awake enough to be directly sent to the ward or to a step-down unit prior to discharge home, bypass PACU. This PACU bypass concept can be applied to patients anesthetized with the newer short-acting drugs who emerge from anesthesia rapidly.

Bypassing PACU increases the availability of nurses who can be cross-trained to become day surgery nurses, acute pain service staff, or preoperative assessment clinic nurses. In this form, newer short-acting anesthetic drugs can decrease costs by improving available manpower utilization without additional salaries.

Creative utilization of OR equipment

One of the major determinants of OR operational costs is related to equipment. Some of it is specific for anesthesia, but others can be shared by different specialities. Microscopes for instance can be shared by neurosurgeons, eye surgeons, ENT doctors, hands surgeons, etc. A rational scheduling of the use of this equipment can avoid unnecessary costs.

Scopes can be used for laparoscopic surgery, bronchoscopies, arthroscopies, fiberoptic intubation, etc. Plotting surgery against the availability of equipment can provide adequate care without any increase in these fixed expenses.

The physician and certified nurse anesthetist controversy

Reduction in costs without affecting the standard of care is one of the most-important issues in hospital administration. Anesthesia costs vary between 3% and 5% of the total health care expenditure. Salaries for service center personnel represent more than 50% of the expenses. The magnitude of the salary differential between certified nurse anesthetists (CRNAs) and anesthesiologists can be found by hospital administration as an opportunity for cost savings through an increase in hired CRNAs and a decrease in staff physicians. However, in a recent study Sibert showed a significant reduction in both 30-day mortality rate and mortality rate after complications, when anesthesia was delivered by a physician instead of a CRNA. Continuing with the policy of delivering unsupervised anesthesia by CRNAs may expose the health system to legal confrontation if complications occur.

Management organization

The Duke University Medical Center reorganized its OR management structure in 1995, when an anesthesiologist with full practice privileges was recruited to serve as a full-time director of the preoperative services, including medical direction and management responsibility for the OR as well as for preoperative preparation and recovery. This Director of Perioperative Services would report directly to the Chief Operating Officer of the hospital, with equal dotted-line relationships to the Chairman of Anesthesiology and the Chairman of Surgery.

A nurse would be recruited to serve as a Perioperative Nursing Coordinator, with responsibilities for all perioperative nursing functions, reporting jointly to the Director of Perioperative Services and to the Department of Nursing.

Previously the OR was directed by a committee constituted by an administrator and three physicians: one anesthesiologist and two surgeons. With this model, the decision-making process was very complicated and had difficulties in responding rapidly to new and unexpected situations, and in achieving consensus on important issues.

Why should the anesthesiologists be OR managers?

Anesthesiologists are present for and have the best understanding of the complete perioperative process, i.e., pre-anesthetic screening, preoperative medical consultations, patient preparation in holding area, anesthetic management, post-anesthesia recovery, pain control, treatment of post-operative nausea and vomiting, and effective discharge triage of patients to inpatients units or home. The anesthesiologist also understands the surgeon needs and is able to base decisions on medical judgement and a knowledge of surgery and individual surgeons.

What are we doing in the Soroka medical center?

Since 1995 a process for quality improvement has been developed. For this target, quality improvement teams were created, and the use of the hospital database became an important step for monitoring and early detection of problems.

One of the most-important obstacles in our hospital to database analysis is the existence of several different databanks, which are not necessarily linked, applying distinct languages (Magic, Clicks, RS/6000). Therefore, a program for data mining was required for centralization of data, allowing an effective analysis of data.

The methodology for collection of information consists of a nine-step process as proposed by Brachman et al. and shown below:

1. Definition of the goals, the information needed and the authorized users
2. Identification and localization of relevant information

3. Initial management and "cleaning" of the stored information
4. Condensation of information
5. Determination of tasks for data mining
6. Determination of algorithm for data mining
7. Data mining
8. Interpretation of data
9. Evaluation of the results

The quality improvement process consists of a seven-point methodology:
1. Definition of the problem
2. The actual situation
3. Research of factors
4. Proposition of solutions
5. Analysis of the results
6. Consolidation of the solutions
7. Diffusion of guidelines

The goal of the quality improvement team for the operating theater, is to optimize the utilization of the ORs, to improve the patients and families' satisfaction, and to localize and to resolve potential focus of complications, which can affect the hospital reputation and increase costs.

Suggested readings

1. Brachman R, Khabaza T, Kloesgen W, et al (1996) Industrial application of data mining and knowledge discovery. Communications of ACM. November
2. Dexter F (1998) Regional anesthesia does not significantly change surgical time versus general anesthesia – a meta-analysis of randomized studies. Reg Anesth Pain Med 23: 439-443
3. Dexter F, Coffin S, Tinker JH (1995) Decreases in anesthesia-controlled time cannot permit one additional surgical operation to be reliably scheduled during the workday. Anesth Analg 81: 1263- 1268
4. Dexter F, Macario A, Traub RD (1999) Which algorithm for scheduling add-on elective cases maximizes operating room utilization? Use of bin packing algorithms and fuzzy constraints in operating room management. Anesthesiology 91: 1491-1500
5. Gabel RA, Kulli JC, Lee BS, et al (1999) Operating room management. Butterworth-Heinemann
6. Glance LG (2000) The cost effectiveness of anesthesia workforce models: a simulation approach using decision-analysis modeling. Anesth Analg 90: 584-592
7. Jackson T, Myles PS (2000) Total episode costs in a randomized, controlled trial of the effectiveness of four anesthetics. Anesth Analg 91: 1170-1175
8. Macario A, Vitez TS, Dunn B, McDonald T (1995) Where are the costs in perioperative care? Analysis of hospital costs and charges for inpatient surgical care. Anesthesiology 83: 1138-1144
9. Malangoni MA (1997) Critical issues in operating room management. Lippincott-Raven
10. Overdyk FJ, Harvey SC, Fishman RL, Shippey F (1998) Successful strategies for improving operating room efficiency at academic institutions. Anesth Analg 86: 896-906

11. Roberts RR, Frutos PW, Ciavarella GG, et al (1999) Distribution of variable vs. fixed costs of hospital care. JAMA 17: 644-649
12. Sibert KS (1996) Operating room management for the 21st century. Annual Refresher Course Lectures, American Society of Anesthesiologists, Lecture 532
13. Silber JH, Kennedy SK, Even-Shoshan O, et al (2000) Anesthesiologist direction and patients outcome. Anesthesiology 93: 152-163
14. SWIPE Group (1997) The successful implementation of pharmaceutical practice guidelines. Analysis of associated outcomes and cost savings. Systematic Withdrawal of Perioperative Expenses. Anesthesiology 86: 1145-1160

How to Plan Anesthesia

N.G. VOLPE, R. ALEXANDER

Careful planning is one of the most important determinants for the success of any action. The degree of importance of planning varies depending on its objects; indeed it is of paramount importance in the anesthetic setting.

Many are the factors that play an important role in the choice of an anesthetic technique and the exclusion of another. Patient's health conditions and desire, environment, type of surgery, financial issues, anesthetist's skill, and equipment availability will influence the choice of safe and effective technique.

Improvement in life expectancy, social conditions, and patient's expectations have posed new challenges for the surgeon and the anesthetist. This has also occurred in an historical era where increase in healthcare needs have rarely been matched by availability of sufficient resources.

Many have been the end-points examined by a multitude of clinical and epidemiological studies in the last 20 years. The result has given us a better understanding of what we want to achieve with our clinical actions and what should be the ultimate outcome of our undertakings.

Outcome is a simple word whose real meaning is altered by the setting in which it is used. A successful outcome for a surgical operation is the survival of the patient who will gain all the benefits produced by the procedure with the minimization of expected or unexpected morbidity.

Surgical outcome, especially in patients with severely deranged physiology, is defined in terms of survival. Appropriate surgical and anesthetic intervention can sometimes make a difference.

With this in mind, especially as far as survival is concerned, it has not been shown that an anesthetic technique is better that another, indeed it has been shown with increasing evidence that good quality patient-oriented perioperative care may alter outcome.

The following review will very concisely examine the scientific rationale produced in the last 15 years that may influence, support, or exclude the utilization of a particular approach to perioperative care aimed at minimizing morbidity and improving outcome in critically ill surgical patients. The importance of maintaining physiological stability during the operative procedure will also be examined.

Risk evaluation

Postoperative cardiac complications

The most-frequent cause of morbidity and mortality in the perioperative period is represented by cardiovascular, respiratory adverse events [1, 2]. Various studies have has as their endpoint the evaluation and quantification of the risk of cardiovascular complications in patients undergoing non-cardiac surgery. Goldman et al. [3] identified nine variables that could predict the occurrence of perioperative cardiovascular events. The study of Detsky et al. [4] modified the Goldman Index by adding two other important predictors of increased risk, namely severe angina and remote myocardial infarction.

Recently, a report from a joint working party between the American College of Cardiology and the American Heart Association has published some guidelines for the evaluation of the risk of developing cardiovascular complications in the perioperative period [5]. This is quantified by examining some clinical markers of heart disease, the functional capacity of the patient, and the specific risk associated with the type of surgery . Furthermore, some clinical predictors have a varying degree of influence on the occurrence of myocardial infarction, congestive heart failure, and cardiovascular death (Table 1).

Table 1. Clinical predictors of increased risk of perioperative cardiovascular events

Major	Intermediate	Minor
Unstable angina	Mild angina	Advanced age
Decompensated CHF	Prior MI (>30 days)	Abnormal ECG
Significant arrhythmias	Compensated or prior CHF	Rhythm other than sinus
Severe valvular disease	Diabetes mellitus	Low functional capacity
		History of stroke
		Uncontrolled hypertension

MI = Myocardial infarction, CHF = congestive heart failure, ECG = electrocardiogram

It is also important to establish the patient's functional capacity because this variable is a reliable predictor of cardiac events. When major predictors are present, it is wise to delay or cancel surgery until the cardiac problem has been properly investigated and adequately treated.

In emergency cases, advanced organ support is mandatory and general anesthesia with adequate monitoring should be used. Some studies on surgical patients have shown that preoperative optimisation of cardiovascular function improves outcome in patients undergoing major surgery [6, 7]. In a study of 138 patients undergoing major elective surgery, Wilson et al. [8] have shown a significant decrease in mortality in the group of patients whose cardiovascular function was optimized preoperatively with the use of invasive cardiovascular monitoring and inotropes. In the protocol group, a 3% mortality was observed, whereas mortality reported for the control group was 17% (P=0.007). Economic analysis of the results of this trial also showed that the routine application of this method would be a significant and cost-effective improvement in perioperative care.

Although some controversies have arisen on the utilization of pulmonary artery catheters, our personal experience suggests that the benefits of their use in this particular setting outweigh the risks.

Studies on animals and humans have shown that the activation of the sympathetic system by surgical stimulation can increase cardiac morbidity and mortality [9]. Indeed, studies aimed at pharmacological intervention on the sympathetic system have shown a decrease in anesthetic requirements and in cardiovascular complications [10, 11-14]. We believe that any patient at risk of or with known coronary artery disease should receive perioperative sympathicolytic treatment if not contraindicated.

The choice of the anesthetic technique for patients with cardiovascular risk factors should also take into account the effects of epidural block on the stress response to surgery and to postoperative pain [15]. The results of many studies have supported the hypothesis that a reduction in the surgical stress responses (metabolic, endocrine, and inflammatory) will result in a reduced incidence of organ dysfunction in the postoperative period thereby improving outcome. The greatest reduction in surgical stress response has been observed only with regional anesthetic techniques and preferably continuous techniques with local anesthetics [16]. A recent meta-analysis has shown the utilization of intraoperative and early postoperative analgesia, provided either by single or multiple doses neuraxial techniques (spinal or epidural), reduces the incidence of deep vein thrombosis by 44%, pulmonary embolism by 55%, transfusion requirements by 50%, pneumonia by 39%, respiratory depression by 59%, myocardial infarction by 30%, and overall mortality by 30% [17]. These positive findings were found mainly after major orthopedic procedures; indeed no significant effects were found in urological, abdominal, and thoracic surgery.

The prognostic limitation of most of the studies examined in the above analysis is that single doses techniques were used; therefore no definitive conclusions can be drawn about the effects of continuous multidose techniques in the reduction of complications in the perioperative period.

While further data are required to establish with a high degree of certainty the role of neuraxial blockade in the reduction of cardiac complications, it is advisable to increase the use of these techniques because of the beneficial effects these produce.

Postoperative respiratory complications

From the data available in the international surgical and anesthetic literature, it is possible to establish that the incidence of pulmonary complications in the postoperative period ranges between 0.2 and 76% [18,19] depending on risk, factors. Complications affecting the respiratory system are the cause of significant morbidity and usage of healthcare resources. Patients who developed respiratory failure, pneumonia, or tracheobronchitis after abdominal surgery had a longer intensive care unit and hospital stay and a greater mortality rate [18].

Table 2 shows the variables that have been shown to be predictors of pulmonary complications after surgery [20-22].

Table 2: Risk factors for postoperative pulmonary complications

Factor	Odds ratio for increased risk
Age > 50 years	4.1
Age > 70 years	7.5
Smoking	4.2
Pre-existing pulmonary pathology	3.1
Duration of surgery 3 h	1.5
Major abdominal surgery	3.9
Emergency surgery	3.5

Pulmonary function tests can help to identify high-risk patients before major surgery, however their predictive value is inconsistent [22]. Preoperative preparation of patients with pre-existing pulmonary pathology is of great importance to prevent or diminish the risk of postoperative complications.

A decrease in the risk of pulmonary complications in patients with reversible obstructive diseases has been observed with the appropriate use of bronchodilators, as well as a reduction of the rate of postoperative infections when antibiotics are utilized [23].

The effect of smoking cessation on postoperative pulmonary complications remains uncertain. It is apparent from the data available that smokers have a much higher rate of respiratory complications than non-smokers [19]. The highest benefit from smoking cessation is obtained if it occurs 4 - 8 weeks before surgery [24].

Surgical and anesthetic technique can influence the development of pulmonary complications in high-risk patients. Laparoscopic techniques can reduce postoperative complications. One of these studies has shown a 15% decrease in the incidence of postoperative pulmonary complications (atelectasis, fever with positive cultures) in patients having their gallbladder removed laparoscopically compared with those who had an open upper abdominal procedure [25].

Spinal and epidural anaesthesia have little effect on respiratory function and may be used with a proved degree of success in lower abdominal and limb surgery [17].

As already stated above, excellent postoperative analgesia with a combination of local anesthetics and opioids can prevent atelectasis by promoting painless deep breathing [16]. Thoracic epidural analgesia has been shown to improve diaphragmatic function, which can be responsible, if altered, for V/Q mismatch and hence hypoxia [26].

Conclusions

In the last 20 years, significant progress has been made in our knowledge of the determinants of unfavorable outcome in the postoperative period. This knowledge has stimulated a series of studies that have improved the approach to better perioperative management of high-risk surgical patients with evident favorable prognostic effects. Further studies are needed to establish, the best way to produce a further reduction of perioperative morbidity and mortality.

References

1. Mangano DT (1990) Perioperative cardiac morbidity. Anesthesiology 72: 153-184
2. Bone RC. (1991) The pathogenesis of sepsis. Ann Intern Med 115: 457-469
3. Goldman L, Caldera DL, Nussbaum SR, et al (1977) Multifactorial index of cardiac risk in non cardiac surgical procedures. N Engl J Med 297: 845-850
4. Detsky AS, Abrams HB, McLaughlin JR, et al (1986) Predicting cardiac complications in patients undergoing non cardiac surgery. Gen Intern Med 1: 211-219
5. ACC/ AHA Task Force Report (1996) Guidelines for perioperative cardiovascular evaluation for non cardiac surgery. Circulation 93: 1278-1317
6. Berlauk JF, Abrams JH, Gilmour IJ, et al (1991) Preoperative optimisation of cardiovascular hemodynamics improves outcome in peripheral vascular surgery. A prospective, randomised clinical trial. Ann Surg 14: 289-297
7. Boyd O, Grounds RM, Bennett ED (1993) A randomised clinical trial of the effect of deliberate perioperative increase of oxygen delivery on mortality in high risk surgical patients. JAMA 270: 2699-2707
8. Wilson J, Woods I, Fawcett J, et al (1999) Reducing the risk of major elective surgery: randomised controlled trial of preoperative optimisation of oxygen delivery. BMJ 318: 1099-1103

9. Roizen MF (1988) Should we all have sympathectomy at birth? Or at least preoperatively. Anesthesiology 68: 482-484
10. Quintin L, Bonnet F, Maquin I, et al (1990) Aortic surgery: effects of clonidine on intraoperative catecholaminergic and circulatory stability. Acta Anaestesiol Scand 34: 132-137
11. Ellis JE, Drijvers G, Pedlow S, et al (1994) Premedication with oral and transdermal clonidine provides safe and efficacious postoperative sympatholysis. Anesth Analg 79: 1133-1140
12. Stone Jg, Foex P, Sear JW, et al (1988) Myocardial ischemia in untreated hypertensive patients: effect of a single oral dose of a beta adrenergic blocking agent. Anesthesiology 68: 495-500
13. Mangano DT, Layug EL, Wallace A, et al (1996) Effect of atenolol on mortality and cardiovascular morbidity after non cardiac surgery. Multicentre Study of Perioperative Ischemia Research Group. N Engl J Med 335: 1713-1720
14. Wallace A, Layug B, Tateo I, et al (1998) Prophylactic atenolol reduces postoperative myocardial ischemia. McSPI Research Group. Anesthesiology 88: 7-17
15. Kehlet H (1997) Multimodal approach to control postoperative pathophysiology and rehabilitation. Br J Anaesth 78: 606-617
16. Kehlet H (1998) Modification of responses to surgery by neural blockade: clinical implications. In: Cousins MJ, Brindebaughs (eds) Neural blockade in clinical anaesthesia and management of pain, 3rd edn. Lippincott-Raven, Philadelphia pp 129- 171
17. Rodgers A, Walker N, Shug S, et al (2000) Reduction of postoperative mortality and morbidity with epidural or spinal anaesthesia. Results from overview of randomised trials. Br Med J 321: 1493-1497
18. Lawrence VA, Hilsenbeck SG, Mulrow CD et al (1995) Incidence and hospital stay for cardiac and pulmonary complications after abdominal surgery. J Gen Intern Med 10: 671-678
19. Bluman LG, Mosca L, Newman N, et al (1998) Preoperative smoking habits and postoperative pulmonary complications. Chest 113: 883-889
20. Pedersen TV, Viby-Morgensen J, Ringsted C (1992) Anaesthetic practice and postoperative pulmonary complications. Acta Anaesth Scand 36: 812-818
21. Lawrence VA, Dhanda R, Hilsenbeck SG, et al (1996) Risk of pulmonary complications after elective abdominal surgery. Chest 110: 744-750
22. Keradmand F, Wiener-Kronish JP, Corry DB (1997) Assessment of operative risk for patients with advanced lung disease. Clin Chest Med 18: 483-494
23. O'Donohue WJ (1992) Postoperative pulmonary complications. When are preventive and therapeutic measures necessary? Postgrad Med 91: 167-170, 173-175
24. Brooks-Brunn JA (1997) Predictors of postoperative pulmonary complications following abdominal surgery. Chest 111: 564-571
25. Hall JC, Tarala RA, Hall JL (1996) A case-control study of postoperative pulmonary complications after laparoscopic and open cholecystectomy. J Laparoendosc Surg 6: 87-92
26. Pansard JL, Mankikian B, Bertrand M, et al (1993) Effects of thoracic extradural block on diaphragmatic electrical activity and contractility after upper abdominal surgery. Anesthesiology 78: 63-71

Monitoring and Assessment of Perioperative Vital Functions in Major Non-Cardiac Surgery

B. Allaria, M. Resta

In recent years, there has been a rise in the number of reports of perioperative and postoperative cardiovascular complications that once went unobserved. The study by Badner et al. [1] demonstrated that in-depth analysis can reveal the presence of acute myocardial infarction (AMI) in the perioperative phase of major non-cardiac surgery to a much greater extent than is usually noted. Using multiple-lead electrocardiography (ECG) in the operating theater, repeated postoperative ECG, regular enzymatic checks (troponin T twice a day for the entire postoperative period), and myocardial scintigraphy with technetium-99m pyrophosphate in case of doubt, the authors found 18 cases of AMI (5.6%) in 323 patients over the age of 50 years at risk for myocardial ischemia. Of these, most of these events (14) took place on the day surgery was performed or the next day. It is important to note that only 3 patients experienced precordial pain and that most (10) had a non-Q AMI. Consequently, it is clear that AMI is a complication that is anything but rare among risk patients undergoing major non-cardiac surgery. Given its characteristics, however, it may go unobserved and thus untreated.

The study by Lopez-Jimenez et al. [2] monitored troponin T throughout the entire hospitalization period of 772 patients over the age of 50 years who underwent major non-cardiac surgery. A total of 92 (12%) revealed altered levels of troponin T. The authors conducted a 6-month follow-up of all patients enrolled in the study, and found that the group of patients with positive troponin T levels also showed a much higher rate of cardiac complications over the follow-up period than the patient group with normal troponin T levels. This leads us to believe that there was a substantial group of patients with an unrecognized coronaropathy who had ischemic episodes during the perioperative phase, and thus had a higher likelihood of cardiovascular events over the subsequent 6-month period. Consequently, avoiding these episodes of silent ischemia is important.

There are two possible paths to follow that are not necessarily alternative to each other, and both are based on a common premise: that patients at risk must be identified. The paths that can be followed to protect them are listed below.

1. Close monitoring of the filling of the coronary circulus and perfusion, paying special attention to prevention and/or therapeutic treatment of situations that can promote myocardial ischemia, such as tachycardia, hypotension, hypertension, and O_2 desaturation.

2. Treatment during the perioperative phase with drugs that can prevent ischemia. Along these lines, in 1996 an interesting study was published by Mangano et al.[3]. The study enrolled 200 patients over the age of 50 years undergoing major non-cardiac surgery, treating half of the cohort with atenolol for the entire hospitalization period. During this period, no substantial differences were observed between the two patient groups from a cardiovascular standpoint, but in the 2-year follow-up the authors noted an important difference: the patients treated during hospitalization with atenolol had a much lower rate of cardiac complications than patients who received no treatment, and mortality for cardiac causes was 65% lower in the treated group. The authors concluded that atenolol had probably prevented ischemic alterations (that may have been present but not diagnosed in the untreated patients) and thus prevented coronary alterations that could potentially cause subsequent complications. We could discuss whether or not perioperative treatment with beta-blocking agents is in fact advisable in all patients at risk for ischemia (I personally do not share this opinion), but the study of Mangano et al. [3] is nevertheless important because it was one of the first to focus on undiagnosed perioperative events that could cause important complications even after a significant amount of time.

Very recent observations demonstrate that moderate infarctions, particularly if they occur in areas dependent on the left circumflex artery, can also occur with a completely normal ECG [4]. If we consider the fact that perioperative AMIs are often not accompanied by precordial pain and that creatine kinase in this phase is not indicative, we can easily understand how a coronary event can be completely underestimated.

Thus, the first thing to be done is to identify coronary risk patients. The risk factors are linked to lifestyle, physiological or biochemical characteristics and, lastly, personal characteristics.

Risk factors connected with lifestyle include: a diet rich in cholesterol, saturated fats, and calories. Biochemical characteristics include: hypertension, high low-density lipoprotein-cholesterol levels, low high-density lipoprotein-cholesterol levels, hypertriglyceridemia, obesity, and thrombogenic factors. Lastly, personal characteristics that increase the risk of coronary heart disease are: age, sex, familial vasculopathies, a positive family history of any coronary or vascular disorders.

In order to identify patients at risk for coronaropathies in whom all the monitoring and preventive techniques evaluated below should be applied perioperatively, it is helpful to use the *Coronary Risk Chart* furnished by the Joint European Societies Task Force [5], which considers sex, age, smoking habits, cholesterol, and blood pressure in non-diabetic and diabetic subjects. The *Coronary Risk Chart* makes it possible to divide the patients into five risk categories: slight, medium, moderate, high, and very high.

We feel that this type of assessment should be performed in all patients undergoing major non-cardiac surgery, and that risk levels 4 and 5 should entail the use of all monitoring and prevention methods throughout the entire perioperative phase.

The *Coronary Risk Chart* is a useful tool in order to make note of patients who are at greatest risk. However, it does not evaluate a series of risk factors of which the anesthesiologist should nevertheless be aware. We will briefly describe the most important ones.

1. **Thrombogenic factors:** the most-important one seems to be high fibrinogen, indicated as an independent factor increasing coronary risk [6]. Other factors have also proven to be useful in preventing coronary risk, such as factor VII and increased platelet aggregation, but the poor differentiation of measurement methods has not permitted the large-scale evaluation of these factors.

2. **Homocysteine:** high plasma concentrations of this factor are associated with the risk of coronary heart disease [7], above all if associated with smoking, hypertension, and hyperlipidemia [8].

3. **Inflammation markers:** clinical and experimental studies in recent years have made it possible to take a more in-depth look at the relationship between inflammation and coronaropathy. It has been observed that apparently healthy subjects have a higher risk of coronaropathy if their plasma concentration of *C-reactive protein* is also high [9]. It has been suggested that, together with an increased leukocyte count and a lower blood level of albumin, *interleukin 6* and *tumor necrosis factor* α, which regulate the production of C-reactive protein, play a role in the inflammatory genesis of arteriosclerosis. Moreover, this type of interpretation is also supported by the fact that fibrinogen (which, as we have noted, affects coronary risk) also increases during the acute inflammation phase [10].

While the relationship between inflammation and coronaropathy is currently an intriguing theory that must still be confirmed, we think that the evaluation of examinations that are performed routinely, such as C-reactive protein, fibrinogen, plasma albumin levels, and leukocyte counts, should be viewed with renewed interest by the anesthesiologist.

4. **Family history:** subjects with first-degree relatives with coronaropathies

should be considered to be particularly at risk – particularly if the pathology occurred prematurely (<55 years for men and <65 years for women).

Relatives with familial hypercholesterolemia (characterized by very high levels of cholesterol that can often exceed 300 mg/dl) reveal particular risk levels.

Coronary endothelial dysfunction

Patients at risk for coronaropathies do not necessarily have organic alterations of the coronary endothelium. The importance of coronary endothelial dysfunction has been known for a number of years and can exist even when there are no organically documented alterations. It widely known that the coronary endothelium of smokers, dyslipidemic patients, or simply relatives with a positive family history of coronaropathy can lose its normal function as a regulator of motility.

As early as 1986, Ludmer [11] reported that in certain patients with apparently healthy coronary arteries, the intracoronary instillation of acetylcholine [which normally triggers the secretion of nitrous oxide (NO) by the endothelium with ensuing vasodilatation] provokes vasoconstriction. In these patients, treatment with nitroderivatives maintains its effect as a coronary dilator. Thus, certain patients had lost the endothelial regulation of motility. Subsequently, there were also reports of abnormal vasoconstriction reactions at very low doses of amines that are not normally observed in patients with a normal endothelium. This is of paramount importance for the anesthesiologist, since it is evident that patients with coronary endothelial dysfunction can respond in a dangerous and rarely predictable way to both vagal and adrenergic stimulation.

The inhibitory effect that hypoxia plays on the endothelial formation of NO, which as we have noted is the most-important coronary dilator, has been known for many years [12].

However, hypoxia also performs a vasoconstrictive action by stimulating the endothelium to secrete endothelin 1, which may well be the most-important vasoconstrictor expressed by the human body [13], as well as at least two other substances, PDGF (platelet-derived growth factor) and VEGF (vascular endothelial growth factor) [14].

It is thus easy to understand the importance of this information for the anesthesiologist, who must frequently deal with vagal or adrenergic stimulation and/or hypoxia and thus with those factors that can cause coronary vasoconstriction in predisposed patients, i.e., those with endothelial dysfunction.

At this point, it becomes clear that it would be equally helpful to know if the patient who is about to undergo surgery has endothelial dysfunction. It is evident that the response to intracoronary acetylcholine can only be tested through an angiogram and this cannot be proposed in a clinical setting.

It is helpful to know that new tests are being perfected to study the motility of the peripheral arteries and they can offer helpful indications on the presence of coronary endothelial dysfunction. The method proposed in 1992 by Celermajer et al. [15] continues to be used, and has also been reported very recently by Fathi and Marwick [16], who attempted to standardize the procedure. It involves the ultrasound evaluation of the diameter of the brachial artery measured prior to occlusion, performed by inflating a cuff placed on the arm, and then again after the cuff is released. The reactive hyperemia that occurs as the cuff is deflated increases the diameter of the artery by about 10%. Increases under this level are indicative of endothelial dysfunction. The tests is completed by giving the subject 400 mg of nitroglycerin under the tongue, which should increase the diameter of the artery even if it was not modified in the reactive hyperemia phase. Flow-mediated vasodilatation (FMD) is thus considered an index of good endothelial function, while an inadequate increase in FMD after the cuff is deflated indicates endothelial dysfunction.

A simpler examination that can nevertheless be helpful in discovering subjects at risk for endothelial dysfunction is ultrasound imaging of the carotid wall. IMT measurement (intima medial thickness) is proposed for this and is a very simple test to perform, following the indications of Pignoli et al. [17]. A recent study by Hashimoto et al. [18] reveals the close correlation between FMD and IMT. Thus, we feel that IMT is a test that should be considered in order to identify patients at risk for ischemia, given the fact that it is far easier to perform than FMD. We must also add that the best point for measuring IMT is the distal-most 2-cm segment of the common carotid artery, just before the bifurcation. A very interesting study in this field was conducted recently by O'Leary et al. [19], who for a period of 6 years followed 5858 patients over the age of 65 years with no history or signs or cardiovascular disease, analyzing the relationship between IMT and the rate of cardiovascular disease during the observation period.

The patients with lower IMT levels (< 0.87 mm) had an incidence of stroke or myocardial infarction that was nearly four times less than the rate among patients with higher IMT levels (>1.18 mm).

At this point, we feel it is helpful to discuss at least two types of patients who, in addition to dyslipidemic subjects, smokers, hypertensive subjects, and those with a family history of coronaropathies have endothelial dysfunctions more frequently than others: obese and diabetic patients.

A study conducted by Al Suwaidi et al. [20] on coronary endothelial function is of significant interest. The study analyzed the response of coronary flow during angiography with a 200-to 300 μg bolus of acetylcholine in obese patients, noting a progressively reduced response as BMI (body mass index) increases.

The fact that diabetes per se must be considered a disease that increases the risk of myocardial ischemia has been known for years, but recently the mechanisms behind this risk have been clarified even further. Specifically, in patients with type II diabetes – who are frequently subjects on whom we must perform anesthesia – endothelial dysfunctions have been demonstrated a number of times [21, 22]. The mechanisms behind this dysfunction are not entirely clear, but greater credence is being given to the theory that insulin resistance plays an important role in causing this dysfunction. This seems to be confirmed by a recent study published by Mather et al. [23], who observed an improvement in endothelial dysfunction in type II diabetes when patients are treated with metformin, which is known to lower insulin resistance. The authors used a metformin dosage of 500 mg twice a day. This observation is also useful for the anesthesiologist, who must consider patients with type II diabetes as ischemic risk subjects, even when there are no documented organic alterations of the coronary circulus or related symptoms. It is also helpful to know that pretreating these patients with a drug that lowers insulin resistance can improve endothelial function and thus reduce the risk of perioperative ischemia.

Before moving on from the subject of coronary endothelial dysfunction, we feel it is appropriate to focus the attention of anesthesiologists on the effects that mental stress can have in patients with this type of pathology. In the immediate perioperative period, patients are often quite alarmed and an agitated mental state is not uncommon upon reawakening and in the postoperative phase, particularly if sedation and analgesia are not optimum. It is easy to see that if a stress-related abnormal response of coronary motility can be demonstrated, this would be of vital importance for the anesthesiologist.

It has long been known that mental stress increases the myocardial consumption of O_2, but it has only recently been found that there is a concomitant possibility of coronary vasoconstriction [24], which, associated with the increased demand for O_2, can lead to myocardial ischemia. On the other hand, it has been demonstrated many times that in heart patients who undergo ST ECG examination on an outpatient basis, stress can cause ischemic events, even if they are often asymptomatic, and the phenomenon is anything but rare if it is indeed true that the rate of transitory myocardial ischemia revealed by Holter monitoring following stress in heart patients is quite high (30-60%) [25]. Further confirmation of this also comes from a very recent study by Kop et al. [26], demonstrating that when heart patients undergo mental stress they show an increase in both arterial pressure and heart rate (and thus in the myocardial consumption of O_2), while at the same time there is also reduced flow, thus creating the classic conditions for myocardial ischemia.

Diagnostic confirmation of coronaropathy in the preoperative phase

In recent years, numerous tests have been proposed in order to discover the presence of coronaropathies. ECG and echocardiography continue to be the basic tests. If there is any doubt, a number of examination's can be proposed, such as resting or stress myocardial scintigraphy with thallium, resting or stress SPECT (single photon emission computed tomography), thallium-dipyridamole testing and echo/dobutamine testing. More recently, the EBCT (electron beam CT) has also been proposed. The latter is essentially an ultrafast radiograph of the coronary arteries that can reveal their calcium content despite cardiac movement. This technique has a sensitivity of 71% and a specificity of 91% in patients between 40 and 50 years, a sensitivity of 74% and a specificity of 70% for those between the ages of 50 and 60 years, and a sensitivity of 74% and a specificity of 81% for those aged 60-70 years [27].

The wealth of diagnostic proposals ends up confusing those who are faced with making a practical choice. Some help comes from the recent meta-analysis performed by Froelicher et al. [28]. This analysis demonstrates that none of the more-sophisticated tests (including the EBCT) show any greater sensitivity or specificity than the exercise ST ECG. Thus, none of the proposed tests can predict perioperative ischemia. However, positive results from these tests will help identify those patients who need special attention from the anesthesiologist and surgeon, not only in the selection of the techniques to use but also in the monitoring systems to apply. In clinical practice, patients with a history of AMI, angina, or ascertained coronaropathies need no further tests other than the ones designed to define the validity of the heart pump and any arrhythmia, since knowledge of these details can affect anesthetic and infusional behavior.

Patients who have no history of coronaropathy but who present the risk factors described above thus undergo exercise ST ECG testing and, only if they are unable to perform this test are they then studied via thallium-dipyridamole, echo/dobutamine, Holter monitor, or other tests. Coronary angiography is reserved for patients in whom imminent thrombosis is suspected (as in the case of unstable angina). In any event, angiography in the preoperative phase is significant above all if revascularization is a possibility prior to the scheduled surgery.

Prevention of myocardial ischemia

This can essentially be done in two ways:

1. Choice of anesthetic and monitoring techniques that can promptly prevent or correct hemodynamic imbalances that can potentially cause ischemia, above all the hypotension-tachycardia combination

It is fundamental for the anesthesiologist to have complete knowledge of the hemodynamic effects of anesthetics and of anesthesiology techniques for the effective prevention or prompt treatment of myocardial ischaemia

The anesthesiologist now has many means available for monitoring hemodynamics. Without adding invasive procedures such as the Swan-Ganz catheter or Pulsion-Cold system, or mini-invasive techniques such as *PICCO*, we must remember that today there are also non-invasive techniques available and if used correctly, they offer useful information. For example, we must mention evaluation via a filling test using stroke volume (SV) and pre-ejection period (PEP) as variables, permitted by thoracic impedance cardiography; a filling test using SV and ejection time (ET) as variables, permitted by transesophageal Doppler ultrasound imaging; and the non-invasive monitoring of cardiac output using the CO_2 partial rebreathing technique ($NICO_2$). Lastly, during surgery there is also the simple test of systolic pressure variation (SPV), which is very helpful in revealing and correcting circulus filling defects. If none of these techniques are available, there is also capnography, not to mention the importance of monitoring sudden drops in $PetCO_2$ and its recovery with a filling test. A comprehensive review of non-invasive techniques can be found in a recent study published by Allaria et al. [29].

2. Implementing drug treatments against the onset of ischemic events

We have already discussed Mangano's report on the usefulness of beta-blocking agents administered throughout the perioperative period, and this line of thought has also been supported by other authors [30].

The reason this treatment is effective lies in the fact that it impedes excessively high heart rates, which are doubly dangerous: they shorten diastole (during which perfusion of the left ventricle occurs) and they increase the RPP (PA syst x HR), which is directly correlated with myocardial consumption of O_2. Nevertheless, since the use of beta-blockers reduces the compensatory heart rate response in hypovolemia and can theoretically accentuate the myocardial depression caused by anesthetics, often in patients with reduced EF, we do not fully agree with using this method indiscriminately in patients at risk for ischemia.

A slowdown of sympathetic output by stimulating the central α_2 adrenergic receptors may be more viable, also because drugs like *clonidine, dexmedetomidine,* and *mivazerol* not only reduce potentially dangerous adrenergic responses but they also boost the effect of analgesics both intraoperatively and postoperatively. Moreover, they fight shivering, thus avoiding sources of high O_2 consumption that are often accompanied by O_2 desaturation and provoked by shivering. It has also been documented that with these drugs, there is a reduced incidence of AMI, at least in patients with coronary heart disease undergoing vascular surgery [31].

One of the most recently tested molecules is acadesine, which modulates the endothelial secretion of adenosine in the event of ischemia. A great deal has been written on the usefulness of this molecule. Mangano [32] performed a good meta-analysis of the subject, analyzing five randomized double-blind placebo-controlled studies involving 4,043 patients. The outcome of the meta-analysis indicates that in patients with coronary heart disease who undergo myocardial revascularization surgery, acadesine lowers in-hospital mortality, AMI, and cardiovascular alterations connected with this. While *calcium antagonists* are used widely, they do not seem to protect against perioperative ischemia [33].

Conclusions

In order to achieve the goal of lowering the incidence of perioperative myocardial ischemia, the most-effective weapons are prevention and early diagnosis. In order to put them to use, it is essential to identify risk patients who are not only subjects in whom a coronaropathy has been diagnosed, but above all those who, due to the presence of one or more risk factors (family history, dyslipidemia, diabetes, smoking, etc.), may have an undiagnosed organic coronaropathy or coronary endothelial dysfunction. In all these cases, which are undoubtedly the most numerous, perioperative diagnostic procedures must be used, starting with stress ECG – which continues to play an important role in detecting silent coronary heart disease – and moving on to more-complex procedures only in doubtful cases. Nevertheless, the most-important approach with risk patients is the close monitoring of the circulus for the entire perioperative phase, in order to avoid hemodynamic imbalances, often the cause of ischemia. Thus, cardiovascular monitoring must be increased, making ample use above all of the non-invasive procedures that are now widely available.

For the early diagnosis of ischemia, ECG continues to play a fundamental role, as long as it is performed with 12 leads, and the use of troponin T continues to grow in importance, with the recommendation that it be administered twice a day, at least during the first 2 days postoperatively.

The application of all the measures we have described here will undoubtedly be useful in reducing cardiovascular complications in the perioperative phase and in reducing the same complications even up to 2 years following surgery.

References

1. Badner NH, Knill RL, Brown JE, et al (1998) Myocardial infarction after noncardiac surgery. Anesthesiology 88: 572-578
2. Lopez-Jimenez F, Goldman L, Sacks DB, et al (1997) Prognostic value of cardiac Troponin T after noncardiac surgery: 6-month follow-up data. J Am Coll Cardiol 29: 1241-1245
3. Mangano DT, Layug EL, Wallace A, et al (1996) Effect of atenolol on mortality and cardiovascular morbidity after noncardiac surgery. Multicenter Study of Perioperative Ischemia Research Group. N Engl J Med 335: 1713-1720
4. Kontos MC, Kurdziel KA, Ornato JP, et al (2001) A non ischemic electrocardiogram does not always predict a small myocardial infarction: results with acute myocardial perfusion imaging. Am Heart J 141: 360-366
5. Joint European Societies task force "Coronary Risk Chart" (1998) Eur Heart J 19: 1434-1503
6. Kannel WB, Wolf PA, Castelli WP, et al (1987) Fibrinogen and risk of cardiovascular disease. The Framingham Study. JAMA 258: 1183-1186
7. Cardiovascular disease risk factors: news area for research – Report of WHO Scientific Group, WHO Technical Report Series 841 Geneva (1994) World Health Organization
8. Graham IM, Daly LE, Refsum HM, et al (1997) Plasma homocysteine as a risk factor for vascular disease. The European Concerted Action Project. JAMA 277: 1775-1781
9. Ridker PM, Cushman M, Stampfer MJ, et al (1997) Inflammation, aspirin, and the risk of cardiovascular disease in apparently healthy men. N Engl J Med 336: 973-979
10. Danesh J, Collins R, Appleby P, et al (1998) Association of fibrinogen, C reactive protein, albumin and leukocyte count with coronary heart disease: meta-analyses of prospective studies. JAMA 279: 1477-1482
11. Ludmer PL, Selwyn AP, Shook TL, at al (1986) Paradoxical vasoconstriction induced by acetylcholine in atherosclerotic coronary arteries. N Engl J Med 315: 1046-1051
12. McQuillan LP, Leung GK, Marsden PA, et al (1994) Hypoxia inhibits expression of eNOS via transcriptional and post-transcriptional mechanism. Am J Phsiol 267: H1921-1927
13. Kourembanas S, Marsden PA, McQuillan LP, et al (1991) Hypoxia induces endothelin gene expression and secretion in cultured human endothelium. J Clin Invest 88: 1054-1057
14. Karimova A, Piusky DJ (2001) The endothelial response to oxygen deprivation: biology and clinical implications. Intensive Care Med 27: 19-31
15. Celermajer DS, Sorensen KE, Gooch VM, et al (1992) Non-invasive detection of endothelial dysfunction in children and adults at risk of atherosclerosis. Lancet: 340, 1111-5
16. Fathi R, Marwick TH (2001) Noninvasive tests of vascular function and structure: why and how to perform them. Am Heart J 141: 694-703
17. Pignoli P, Tremoli E, Poli A, et al (1986) Intimal plus medial thickness of the arterial wall: a direct measurement with ultrasound imaging. Circulation 74: 1399-1406
18. Hashimoto M, Eto M, Akishita M, et al (1999) Correlation between flow-mediated vasodilatation of the brachial artery and intima-media thickness in the carotid artery in men. Arterioscl Thromb Vasc Biol 19: 2795-2800
19. O' Leary DH, Polak JF, Kronmal RA, et al (1999) Carotid artery intima and media thickness as

a risk factor for myocardial infarction and strike in older adults. Cardiovascular Health Study Collaborative Research Group. N Engl J Med 340: 14-22
20. Al Suwaidi J, Higano ST, Holmes DR Jr, et al (2001) Obesity is independently associated with coronary endothelial dysfunction in patients with normal or mildly diseased coronary arteries. J Am Coll Cardiol 37: 1523-1528
21. Mc Veigh GE, Brennan GM, Johnston GD, et al (1992) Impaired endothelium-dependent and independent vasodilation in patients with type 2 (non-insulin-dependent) diabetes mellitus. Diabetologia 35: 771-776
22. Williams SB, Cusco JA, Roddy MA, et al (1996) Impaired nitric oxide-mediated vasodilation in patients with non insulin dependent diabetes mellitus. J Am Coll Cardiol 27: 567-574
23. Mather KJ, Verma S, Anderson TJ (2001) Improved endothelial function with metformin in type 2 diabetes mellitus. J Am Coll Cardiol 37: 1344-1350
24. Lacy CR, Contrada RJ, Robbins ML, et al (1995) Coronary vasoconstriction induced by mental stress (simulated public speaking). Am J Cardiol 75: 503-505
25. Krantz DS, Kop WJ, Santiago HT, et al (1996) Mental stress as a trigger of myocardial ischemia and infarction. Cardiol Clin 14: 271-287
26. Kop WJ, Krantz DS, Howell RH, et al (2001) Effects of mental stress on coronary epicardial vasomotion and flow velocity in coronary artery disease: relationship with hemodynamic stress responses. J Am Coll Cardiol 37: 1359-1366
27. Agatston AS, Janowitz WR, Hildner FJ (1990) Quantification of coronary artery calcium using ultrafast computed tomography. J Am Coll Cardiol 15: 827-832
28. Froelicher VF, Fearon WF, Ferguson CM, et al (1999) Lesson learned from studies of the standard exercise ECG test. Chest 116: 1442-1451
29. Allaria B, Dei Poli M, Culotta D (1999) Perioperative hemodynamic monitoring. Invasive vs non invasive Crit Care Med 14: 291-299
30. Palda VA, Detsky AS (1997) Perioperative assessment and management of risk from coronary artery disease. Ann Intern Med 127: 313-28
31. Oliver MF, Goldman L, Julian DG, et al (1999) Effect of mivazerol on perioperative cardiac complications during non-cardiac surgery in patients with coronary heart disease: The European Mivazerol Trial (EMIT). Anesthesiology 91: 951-961
32. Mangano DT (1997) Effects of acadesine on myocardial infarction, stroke, and death following surgery. A meta-analysis of the 5 international randomized trials. The Multicenter Study of Perioperative Ischemia (McSPI) Research Group JAMA 277: 325-332
33. Foëx P (2000) Post operative myocardial ischemia and infarction. Yearbook of intensive care and emergency medicine, Springer, Berlin Heidelberg New York, pp. 365-376

How to Balance General Anesthesia

G. Torri

In 1950 Rees and Gray [1] suggested a definition of general anesthesia that included narcosis, analgesia, and relaxation. Time has proved that the term analgesia is unsatisfactory. Analgesia means freedom from pain. In order for pain exist, a conscious patient must elaborate impulse from the periphery as pain. If the patient is unconscious, then he cannot be aware of pain, that is to say analgesia is present. Of course during surgery there are important reactions to reflex stimuli that during consciousness would be painful. Moving from these concepts, the same authors [1] proposed the most widely accepted triad of anesthesia, which includes narcosis, relaxation and reflex depression.

The work of Gray was revisited by Pinsker in 1986 [2] who submitted the concept that unconsciousness, relaxation, and attenuation of stress response are the necessary and sufficient components of general anesthesia. The term "attenuation of stress reflexes" has been recently substituted by "control of pain reflexes".

Any combination of drug that can reversibly provide unconsciousness, muscle relaxation, and control of pain reflexes may be used in anesthesia, and control of these three components allows the control of general anesthesia. However the drug combination must agree with the basic principles of general anesthesia, including flexibility and control of anesthesia components.

Many techniques proposed in the past years (as neuroleptoanesthesia) provided a complete control of anesthesia components. However many unwanted side effects of neuroleptoanesthesia have been reported. They include prolonged recovery time, respiratory depression, muscle rigidity, increase in airways resistance, increase in nausea, vomiting, urinary retention, partial cardiovascular depression, and delayed recovery.

Total intravenous anesthesia (TIVA) has been improved by the clinical introduction of propofol. However many questions arise from all techniques of TIVA:

1. Is there a correlation between infusion rate and plasma concentration of drug?

2. Is there a relationship between infusion rate and effect of drug?
3. How may changes in protein binding may effect anesthesia?
4. How can we control the recovery from anesthesia?

From a theoretical point of view by combining a hypnotic with an analgesic and a muscle relaxant we can control all anesthesia components. In clinical practice, to prevent awareness, nitrous oxide is also often used by the anesthesiologist in this technique. Therefore the newest molecule still requires the oldest inhalation agent.

Modern balanced anesthesia is based on the combination of different drugs, each being used in minimal amount. They include barbiturate or propofol for induction of anesthesia, muscle relaxant, new short-acting analgesic, and inhalation agents for the maintenance of anesthesia.

The components of general anesthesia may be controlled by an accurate titration of those drugs with the least possible disturbance of physiological functions (cardiovascular, respiratory, and different metabolic functions), and with the smallest burden upon each of the different mechanism of metabolism and excretion of the used drugs.

In the last few years, two halogenated agents have been introduced in clinical practice. The low blood and tissue solubility of these agents can provide for a rapid uptake and elimination. Toxicity is very low and cardiovascular stability is frequently observed [3]. Furthermore, the recovery time from these drugs is not effected by anesthesia time [4]. When inhalation agents are used in the maintenance of general anesthesia, their end-tidal concentrations may be used to control the three components of anesthesia:

MAC 5 represents the alveolar concentration to obtain unconsciousness in 95% of patients [5, 6];

MAC 95 represents the alveolar concentration to prevent motor response to surgical stimulation in 95% of patients [7];

MAC bar 50 and 95 represent the alveolar concentrations to control the sympathetic response in 50% or 95% of patient to surgical stimulation [8].

These concentrations of inhalation agents represent the anesthetic requirements for the control of all anesthesia components when halogenated anesthetics are used alone. The value of MAC bar represents an alveolar concentration, which usually determines a marked depression on cardiovascular and respiratory systems.

When the halogenated agent is administered in combination with nitrous oxide and analgesic, the end-tidal concentrations required to control anesthesia components are reduced, allowing a correct cardiovascular stability. This is the basic principle of the modern balanced anesthesia.

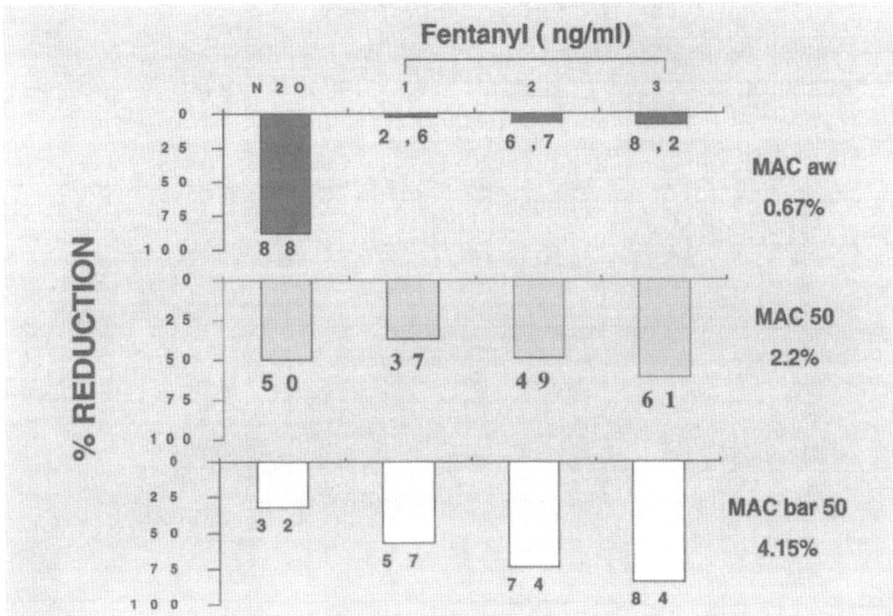

Fig. 1. Changes in minimal alveolar concentration (MAC) values of sevoflurane for the anesthesia components of nitrous oxide and fentanyl

In the interaction between halogenated agents and nitrous oxide or analgesic, the role of these two drugs on the MAC values is very different. As shown in Fig.1, nitrous oxide provides a large reduction of the value of MAC awake (-79%) of sevoflurane. In contrast, the effect of nitrous oxide is lower on MAC and very small on MAC bar (-39%).

In contrast, analgesics have a small effect in reducing MAC awake (from 10 to 24%), while they reduce MAC bar (from 57 to 83%).

These results indicate that nitrous oxide may be very useful to control unconsciousness in intravenous techniques and may reduce the required concentration of halogenated agent to control muscle relaxation and stress reflex control. However, this result underlines the fundamental role of analgesic in the control of reflex to surgical stimulation, as results from the large reduction of MAC bar.

The second result of this analysis is represented by the ceiling effect produced by analgesic when combined with halogenated agents. While small doses of analgesic can largely reduce MAC or MAC bar of anesthetic agents, increasing the dose of analgesic does not provide a similar effect. At a defined analgesic plasma concentration, an increase of this drug does not effect MAC or MAC bar.

At 2-3 ng/ml of fentanyl a further administration of analgesic does not reduce sevoflurane MAC (Fig. 1). A similar effect has been observed by Daniel et al [9] for isoflurane or desflurane: bolus of fentanyl of 1.5 mg/kg does not reduce the MAC bar values of these two inhalation agents (Fig. 2).

These data indicate that high doses of analgesic do not produce any advantage in the control of general anesthesia. However, these doses may produce some relevant problems during recovery.

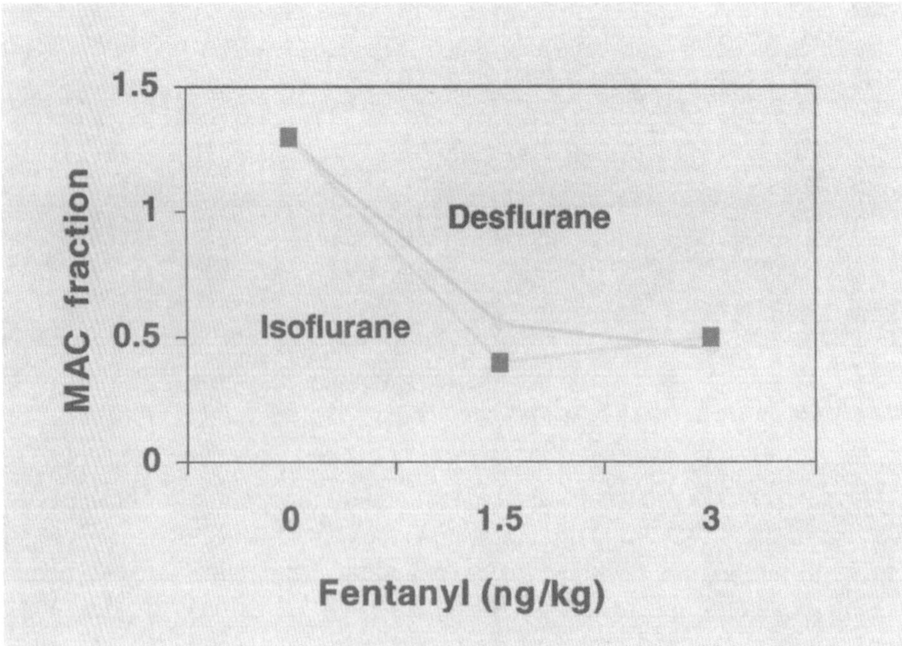

Fig. 2. Isoflurane and MAC reduction at different doses of fentanyl (modified from Daniel et al. [9])

How should we balance general anesthesia? Firstly we must consider that anesthesia must cover the different stress levels determined by surgical procedure or anesthesia maneuvers (tracheal intubation). Consequently the anesthetist must control the surgical stress using a halogenated concentration ranging from values of MAC bar 50 and MAC bar 95.

With particular reference to data of Katoh et al. [8] (Fig. 3), if the fentanyl plasma concentration is maintained at a value of 1 ng/ml and nitrous oxide is associated in the inspired mixture, the end-tidal concentration of sevoflurane required to control the sympathetic response to surgical stimulation ranges from 0.4 to 0.8. These values correspond respectively to MAC bar 50 and MAC bar 95 of sevoflurane.

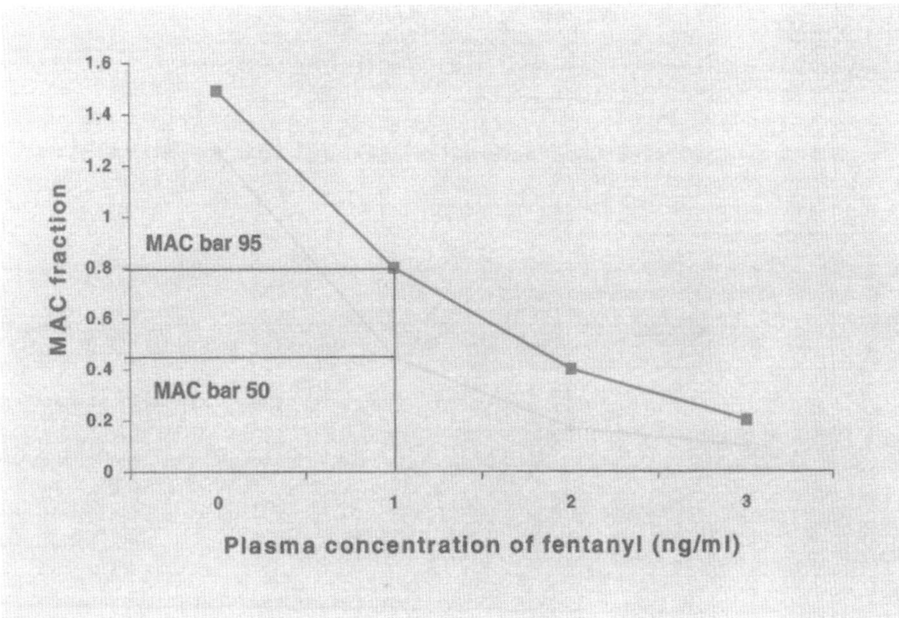

Fig. 3. Reduction of MAC bar 50 and MAC bar 95 of sevoflurane in 60% of nitrous oxide produced by different concentrations of fentanyl (modified from Katoh et al. [8])

Recently developed programs of pharmacokinetics allowing a constant target concentration in the blood [10] may easily control the plasma values of analgesic.

When anesthesia is not sufficiently adequate to control stress reflexes, the anesthesiologist can increase the halogenated end-tidal concentration instead of administering further doses of analgesic. Modern halogenated agents can provide a very short recovery time and are not dependent on the duration of anesthesia [11]. The rapid kinetics of these new drugs allows at every stage of surgery to rapidly increase the end-tidal concentration by changes in inspired concentration. Similarly the elimination kinetics allow a fast decrease in alveolar concentration of anesthetic and a fast recovery.

In conclusion, the combination of new halogenated agents with low plasma concentration of opioids and nitrous oxide allows a good control of anesthesia components, avoiding any respiratory depression [12] in the recovery phase. The incidence of other side effects (nausea, vomiting, and cough) may also be reduced.

Modern balanced anesthesia is a rational technique, and a scientific method to combine nitrous oxide, opioids, and halogenated agents to obtain maximal advantage together with few side effects.

References

1. Rees GJ, Gray TC (1950) Methyl-*n*-propyl-ether. Br J Anaesth 22:83
2. Pinsker MC (1986) Anesthesia: a pragmatic construct. Anesth Analg 65:819
3. Torri G, Casati A et al (2000) Cardiovascular homeostasis during inhalational general anesthesia: a clinical comparison between sevoflurane and isoflurane. J Clin Anaesth 12:117-122
4. Eger EI II, Johnson BH (1987) Rates of awakening from anesthesia with I-653, halothane, isoflurane, and sevoflurane: a test of the effect of anesthetic concentration and duration in rats. Anesth Analg 66:977-982
5. Katoh T, Ikeda K (1998) The effects of fentanyl on sevoflurane requirements for loss of consciousness and skin incision. Anesthesiology 88:18-24
6. Stoelting RK, Longnecker DE, Eger EI II (1970) Minimum alvolar concentration in man on awakening from methoxyflurane, halothane, ether and fluroxene anesthesia: MAC awake. Anesthesiology 33:5
7. De Jong RH, Eger EI I (1975). Mac expanded: AD and AD values 50 95 50 95 of common inhalation anesthetics in man. Anesthesiology 42:384
8. Katoh T, Kobayashi S et al (1999b) The effect of fentanyl on sevoflurane requirements for somatic and sympathetic responses to surgical incision. Anesthesiology 90:398-405
9. Daniel M, Weiskopf RB, Moorami M, Eger EI (1975) Fentanyl augments the blockade of the sympathetic response to incision (MAC-bar) produced by desflurane and isoflurane. Anesthesiology 42:384
10. Shafer SL, Varvel JR, Aziz N, Scott JC (1979) Pharmacokinetics of fentanyl administered by computer-controlled infusion pump. Anesthesiology 77:1091-1092
11. Glass PSA (1998) Anesthetic drug interactions: an insight into general anesthesia. Its mechanism and dosing strategies. Anesthesiology 88:5-6
12. Stoeckel RK, Hengstmann JH, Schuttler J (1979). Pharmacokinetics of fentanyl as a possible explanation for recurrence of respiratory depression. Br J Anaesth 51:771

Decision-Making during Anesthesia

G.M. GURMAN

"Hours of boredom, moments of terror", "85% boredom, 15% panic". These rather cynical definitions of the anesthesiologist's daily practice seem to confirm Beecher's classical saying : "anesthesia is usually terribly simple but sometimes simply terrible" [1].

Patients expect auxiliary procedures such as radiology or anesthesiology to be devoid of adverse effects while, ironically, the anesthesiologist's daily activities in actuality produce a temporary and reversible pharmacological intoxication of the patient. The practice of anesthesia involves a complex integration of mental and physical activities that require profound theoretical knowledge, highly developed manual skills, an absolute understanding of the needs of other professionals, particularly surgeons, and a permanent state of vigilance.

Anesthesiologists often deal with "healthy patients", e.g., women undergoing cesarean section or youngsters undergoing cosmetic surgery, so even though anesthesia entails an inherent danger, a tragic anesthesia-related outcome is completely unacceptable to the public, which has come to expect that anesthesiologists can reduce to a minimum the possibility of unfavorable outcomes.

One way to deal with this complex social, medical, economic, and legal situation is to maintain the decision-making capacity of the anesthesiologist at the highest possible level. This paper reviews different aspects of decision making in anesthesiology and presents some ideas for its improvement.

Decision-making in elective procedures and emergencies. What do they have in common?

Although circumstances are very different for routine decisions compared with crisis management, both situations require appropriate professional and ethical actions to prevent or minimize unfavorable outcomes. Whether handling a routine case or dealing with an emergency, anesthesiologists must take into consideration the three main factors that influence the decision-making process: the patient, the equipment, and the environment (the operating room team, production pressure, etc.). In both cases a plan must be devised. Even though creating a plan in a crisis situation necessitates rapid action, time is nonetheless required to identify the problems and come up with solutions to avoid further deterioration in the patient's condition. Skilled planning is as critical to patient safety as is skilled execution of the plan [2], and it is critical to accurately assess the patient's condition so as to ensure that the plan is appropriate to the specific situation.

In contrast to some authorities who consider pre-anesthetic assessment in ASA 1 and 2 patients to be unnecessary, Gibby et al. [3] reviewed 2,801 anesthesia records and found that a pre-anesthesia visit would have changed the anesthetic protocol in 564 cases. The majority of the study patients (63%) were classified as ASA 1 or 2.

A good plan sometimes renders the theoretical question of selecting the anesthesia technique immaterial. When a complete pre-operative plan was devised for all patients who had undergone vascular procedures, no difference was observed in the results obtained with different anesthetic regimens [4].

At this point, however, the similarity between routine and emergency situations with respect to the decision-making process comes to an end. For instance, it is obvious that a crisis in the operating room (OR) would not leave too much time for creating an alternate plan or gathering additional data on the patient. For this reason, we discuss alternative approaches in a variety of situations which might require entirely different decision-making processes.

Decision-making during routine procedures

Anesthesiologist are often confronted with a situation in which a decision is to be taken on the spot, and this could happen at any stage of their routine activity. Let's take the example of a 53-year-old patient scheduled for elective laparoscopic cholecystectomy. The evening before surgery, during a pre-anesthetic visit, the anesthesiologist is told by the patient about some undefined chest pain experienced during mild exertion, such as climbing a single flight of stairs. Neither the patient's family physician nor the surgeon paid particular attention to this vague complaint. The patient is known to suffer from chronic cervical spine arthritis and she has been receiving non-steroidal anti-inflammatory drug therapy for 3 years.

What should the anesthesiologist's approach be in this case? Should he/she go ahead with the scheduled surgery or postpone it for cardiological assessment? Insertion of an epidural catheter for intra- and postoperative analgesia is commonly practised today in patients undergoing aortic aneurysm surgery. However, the danger of a bloody tap necessitates revision of this initial decision, since this patient will receive heparin that could result in an epidural hematoma. Should the anesthesiologist remove the catheter? Since the catheter is already in the epidural space, its removal could be worse than leaving it in place. The dilemma is evident.

Finally, logistical considerations are sometimes more important than medical ones. Should a patient be discharged from the recovery room to the ward with an IV morphine patient-controlled analgesia (PCA) pump for postoperative analgesia, when the anesthesiologist is well aware of the poor nursing supervision on that floor? Is it justified to give this patient, who suffers from coronary disease, intramuscular opiates at regular intervals to relieve pain, thus exposing him/her to possible respiratory depression that an overworked nurse might not become aware of in time?

These and similar cases occur routinely. In all cases a decision-making process is started and the anesthesiologist is entitled to use any means to reach the proper decision.

1. *Evidence-based data from literature.* When published data or recommendations leave no room for doubt, as is the case with compulsory close respiratory supervision when intravenous opiates are administered [5], there is no justification for jeopardizing the patient by sending him to an unsupervised floor.
2. *Clinical judgement.* The main problem with using one's personal experience lies in the subjective nature of that judgement. Nevertheless, one cannot overemphasize the importance of the physician's clinical experience based on theoretical knowledge, logic, careful observation of the patient, and a deep understanding of the specific situation.
3. *Patient's preference.* Today many patients are knowledgeable concerning their medical condition. Ease of access to electronic medical data and the popularization of medical knowledge help patients to formulate a position on therapeutic decisions. When provided sufficient information by the anesthesiologist, some patients might decide to go on with further investigations and postpone surgery.
4. *Cost and benefit analysis.* In the case of the patient scheduled for a cholecystectomy described above, performing a stress test on the afternoon before surgery might avert a coronary complication. The patient would be reassured that his/her heart condition raises no anesthetic or surgical problems and a gap in the next morning's OR schedule would be avoided.

5. Finally, *the medico-legal aspects* of the profession are also to be taken into consideration. No one is to blame for performing a bloody epidural tap, but ignoring it might be hard to defend in court if an epidural hematoma with neurological complications developed. Although any patient could claim battery (unauthorized touching of a person), or abandonment (failure to provide proper clinical monitoring), by far the most-common allegation in malpractice lawsuits and the most difficult to defend is negligence [6].

Difficulties encountered in the decision-making process

1. *Organisational failure.* The nurses in the surgical ward may be well aware of the need to supervise a patient on IV morphine PCA, but if at the same time another patient develops hypovolemic shock as a consequence of postoperative bleeding the attention of the nurses will be diverted to that patient. Nobody will remember the patient on PCA for the next 2 h. Has the anesthesiologist erred in deciding to transfer the patient on PCA to the surgical ward? A lack of pertinent information could lead, for example, to the fatal aspiration of gastric content during general anesthesia for cystoscopy [7].
2. *Need for flexibility.* Anesthesiology is a team profession and co-operation is the key to efficiency in the OR. A surgeon's request should be considered positively, but that does mean that every surgical order should be followed blindly. For example, an inguinal herniography can easily be performed either under general anesthesia or single epidural injection. Since the latter can be time consuming, the anesthesiologist might accept the surgeon's suggestion and use general anesthesia to shorten the time between two procedures. But unilateral spinal anesthesia or even a continuous titrated spinal dose might be preferred for the same surgical procedure in a 74-year--old coronary patient with evidence of congestive heart failure.
3. *The uncertainty of data in the literature.* Controversies are part and parcel of the doctor's world. Conflicting conclusions relating to the appropriate anesthesia technique for a specific patient often appear in the literature. For instance, even today some experts still claim the validity of Reiz's data [8], which showed that isoflurane causes a "coronary steal", making it unsuitable for anesthesia in cardiac surgery. But more-recent reports [9] have not confirmed these previous data. In a well-known editorial [10], Mangano determined that isoflurane, when used as a primary or secondary anesthetic, does not have a deleterious effect on the coronary patient if hemodynamics are well controlled. Nevertheless, Mangano [10] emphasi-

zed the need for more-rigorous studies to solve this controversy. This is a real-life example of the clinician's dilemma when a decision has to be based on solid data, rather than on anecdotal figures.

Factors influencing the decision-making process during routine activities

1. *Boredom.* Passive behavior on the part of the anesthesiologist in a "prosaic" case, during which each step is well known, could impair his/her ability to identify adverse events and take early corrective action. This theoretical situation could develop at any time, even though "there is mental activity going on when the anesthesiologist appears idle" [11].
2. *Automation.* Indirectly, the automation of part of the anesthesiologist's work in the OR (e.g., mechanical ventilation) can increase boredom and lack of prompt response to the steady flow of information coming from the OR environment. But it should also increase available time for observation, for instance, of the surgical field and monitoring equipment. Hendon et al. [12] showed that the automatic recording of anesthesia was accompanied by a clear trend toward increased direct patient care during cardiac anesthesia.
3. *Production pressure (overt or covert pressures on personnel and incentives to place production, not safety, as their first priority).* Based on data collected from 354 Californian anesthesiologists, Gaba et al. [13] demonstrated the negative impact of production pressure on decision-making capacity: the fear of cancelling a case and the alteration of normal practice in order to hasten the start of surgery. During the 3 years prior to the survey, most of the respondents (54%) in the study had witnessed elective surgery that was conducted despite insufficient pre-operative patient evaluation.
4. *Noise and distraction.* Murthy et al. [14] studied the detrimental effect of noise on 20 anesthesia residents. The two cognitive functions studied – mental efficiency and short-term memory – were reduced when background OR noise reached 77 dB. Cooper et al. [15] analyzed the types and etiology of serious accidents during anesthesia. Distractions were responsible for 71 of 1,089 critical incidents. They found 70 incidents with substantive negative outcomes (mortality, cardiac arrest, etc.), 23 the result of judgmental errors such as wrong drugs, wrong decisions regarding airway management, etc.
5. *Hazardous attitudes.* Gaba [16], in a review of the human work environment and simulators, stated that invulnerability and macho attitudes are particularly hazardous for the anesthesiologist. He offered some examples

of hazardous attitudes, such as "it won't happen to me" or "I can intubate the trachea of anyone". It seems that the false feeling of security derived from ignorance or denying attitudes could influence "the anesthesiologist's ability to react instinctively and flawlessly every time a problem arises" [17].

Decision-making processes during anesthesia crisis

Webster's dictionary defines crisis as "a time of great danger or trouble whose outcome decides whether possible consequences will follow". Gaba et al. [17] describe anesthesiology as a field of complexity and dynamism, which makes crisis much more likely and more difficult to deal with. But another dimension should be added to these descriptions: that of a sudden and unexpected occurrence. The anesthesiologist is always prepared to encounter a significant drop in blood pressure in the case of a ruptured spleen caused, for example, by a motor vehicle accident. But a sudden decrease in systolic blood pressure during induction of general anesthesia for an abdominal hysterectomy in an ASA 2 patient (Fig. 1) is a much more-dramatic and unexpected complication that might catch the anesthesiologist less prepared.

Many aspects of a crisis during anesthesia are in fact beyond the physician's control: histamine release after suxamethonium, significant blood loss resulting from the lack of surgical hemostasis, or air emboli during craniotomy. An anesthesia error could even lead to a true catastrophe: death, permanent brain damage, peripheral nerve lesions.

Causes of anesthesia crisis

1. The inability to control underlying causes of pathological events is characteristic of an anesthesiologist's daily working conditions. The patient is not a robot and was not built according to a controlled design. Individual response to different pharmacological agents and invasive maneuvers may vary substantially from one patient to another. Mitral valve prolapse syndrome, coronary artery spasm (Prinzmetal's angina), or prolonged Q-T interval syndrome can all lead to sudden death, even without evidence of the cause at autopsy [18].
2. *Equipment malfunction.* Even when the physician has observed all steps in a routine check list, a unidirectional valve could get stuck or monitors could offer false-positive or false-negative data.
3. *Surgery* can complicate the anesthetized patient's condition. High intra-abdominal pressure produced by CO_2 insufflation for a laparoscopic proce-

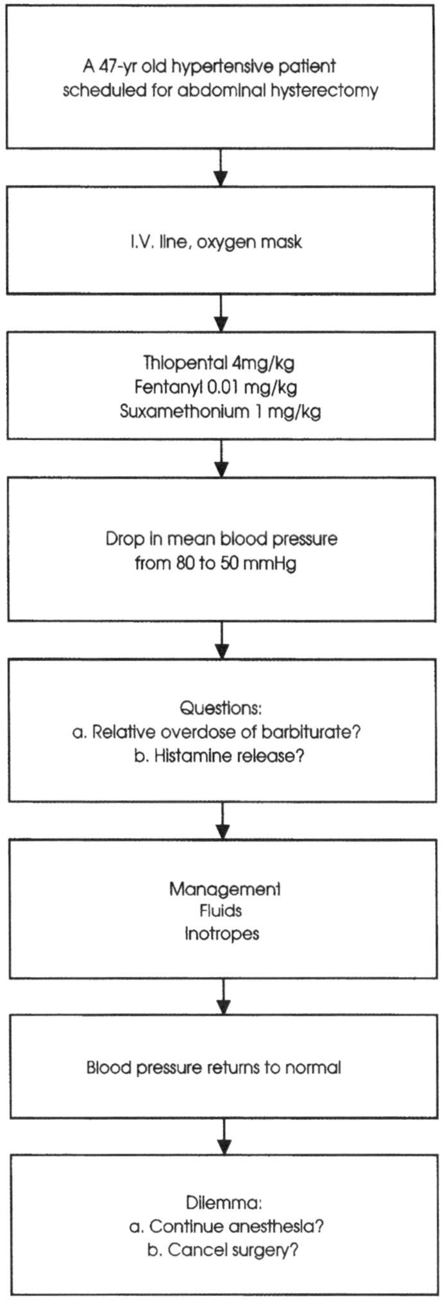

Fig. 1. A sudden drop in blood pressure (BP) during induction of general anesthesia, as an unexpected event

dure could lead to an exaggerated increase in systemic vascular resistance and a coronary ischemic event [19].

4. *Human error* can also be responsible for a crisis. In a follow-up study, Cooper et al. [15] found that more than 90% of substantive negative outcomes were the result of human error. In 24% of cases the error involved improper drug administration. The misuse of anesthesia machines was responsible in that study for 22% of the human errors. In most cases crises produced by human error have fatal outcomes. A Dutch study of accidents during anesthesia performed in 1990 showed that half of the patients with anesthesia-related cardiac arrests could not be resuscitated [20]. Many factors can explain human error during anesthesia, with lack of vigilance one of the most-common causes. Vigilance is the basic element of observation, the first step in recognition and management of an anesthesia crisis. Sleep deprivation, fatigue, boredom, and noise all result in reduced vigilance, which means a decrease in the anesthesiologist's alertness and readiness to deal with an unfavorable turn of events.

The response to crisis

As previously mentioned, crises during anesthesia are frequent. Gaba [16] quoted the results of a multicenter study on general anaesthesia published in 1988. Of 17,200 patients enrolled in the study, 86% had at least one undesirable outcome during anesthesia. More than 5% of the patients developed a condition requiring "significant therapy". These results indicate that in a majority of cases under their supervision, anesthesiologists need to change their original plan and initiate a new decision-making process.

Rasmussen [21] mentioned in his book on information processing the need to deal with command and control of all available resources in the decision-making process during an acute crisis. When analyzing an anesthesia crisis one can distinguish two kinds of activities. The first is recognition-primed decision making [22], in which case the event is well known and the required decision is self-evident. Anesthesia circuit disconnection is one of the examples. It is easily diagnosed and needs a simple maneuver to restore the situation to normal. Clinical observation and monitoring tools help the anesthesiologist to reach the correct diagnosis and decision. This kind of adverse event can also be easily simulated and rehearsed.

Figure 2 presents a much more-complex situation, an event that is cumbersome and difficult to explain. In this case the anesthesiologist is presented with a sudden and unexplained increase in peak inspiratory pressure during mechanical ventilation in the course of general anesthesia. The first step would be to reach a

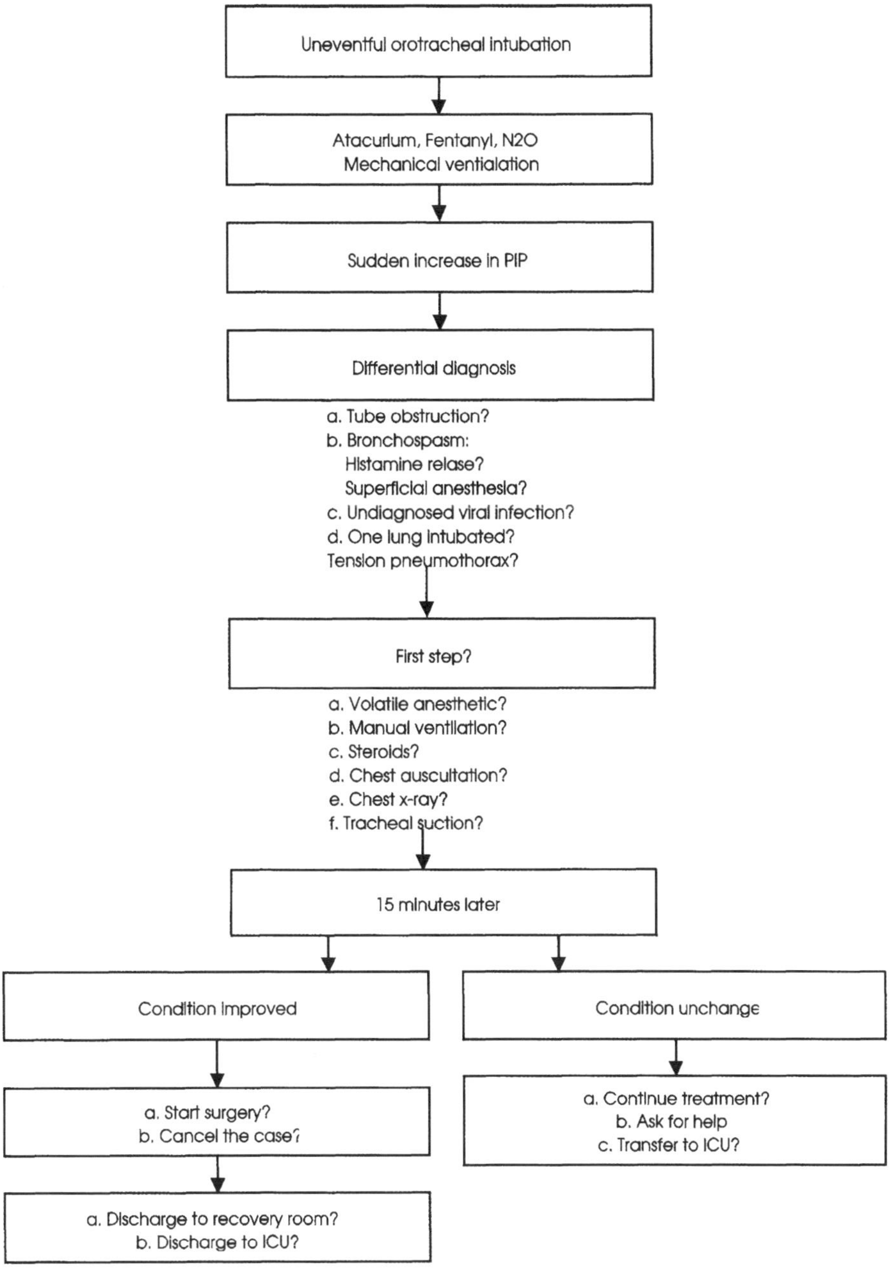

Fig. 2. Schematic representation of a sudden increase in peak inspiratory pressure (PIP) during general anesthesia, necessitating a complex chain of decisions

correct diagnosis, then to initiate specific treatment. But immediately after this another important decision has to be reached, i.e., whether to continue or not with the surgical procedure. This decision depends on the patient's condition, the possible damage already done, and the stage of surgery at that time. Finally, a new decision is to be reached, this time related to the location of post-operative patient management, i.e., regular ward, recovery room, or intensive care.

In these two examples, the similarity of the steps initiated by the practitioner – observation, verification, decision, action, and re-evaluation – are easily identified. Table 1 presents the decision-making process involved in responding to a significant reduction in systolic blood pressure during surgery. Each step is well defined and solutions are presented, but obstacles to implementation of the decisions are also presented. Clearly the main barrier to solving an OR crisis is reluctance to switch from "business as usual" mode to "emergency" mode, even when serious problems are detected. Erring too far in the direction of "wait and see" can be especially dangerous [17].

Table 1. Steps to be taken by the anesthesiologist to address a sudden decrease in blood pressure (BP). Each step could be aggravated by dangerous developments

Activity	Clinical situation/step	Danger
Observation	Decrease in BP	Boredom, "wait and see syndrome"
Verification	Invasive vs. noninvasive measurements, heart rate, surgical field, measure central venous pressure (CVP)	Work overload: giving fluids, preparing drugs (inotropes, etc.)
Decision	Consider hypovolemia, treat hypotension	Gambling on a single explanation
Action	Open an additional IV line, order blood, give colloids	Colloids or crystalloids?
Reevaluation	Measure BP, CVP, urinary output	Automation (not thinking of metabolic consequences such as lactic acidosis, which requires blood gases analysis)

The response to a crisis during anesthesia must include an efficient distribution of the workload among the members of the anesthesia team. It also implies mobilization of all available resources, including manpower, equipment, drugs. At the same time, however, even during an ongoing crisis the anesthesiologist is obliged to cope with psychological pressure from the surgeon, who is the person ultimately responsible for the patient, from the OR administration, who are eager to go on with the original schedule, and eventually from the patient and/or family members when explanations are required. Clearly, managing an OR crisis may become, in some circumstances, a difficult and hazardous task.

How to improve performance during crisis management

Simulators are one clear answer to the above problem. Although expensive, simulators can simulate real clinical situations, record the physician's reactions and decisions and react accordingly. When management of malignant hyperthermia was practised on simulators [23], it led to a significant improvement in performance at retest a few months later. Steadman et al. [24] randomly selected 39 anesthesiologists to receive either simulator-based or slide-based training on remifentanil. All the participants managed a new simulator scenario using remifentanil. Deviations in blood pressure from baseline were statistically more significant in the lecture group than in the simulator group.

New simulators can reproduce almost any clinical situation in the OR. In the near future they will become indispensable tools for improving human performance and increasing the chance that serious anesthesia-related crisis will be resolved successfully. Until that time, however, there are some practical issues to be taken into consideration for this purpose.

Table 2 presents a list of recommendations to be followed during training in the OR, as described in a comprehensive review of anesthesia training in Israel [25]. One of the most obvious is not to leave the resident alone with the patient during the initial period of his training. Training without a teacher is basically flawed and could lead to frustration and disappointment. It can also lead to a catastrophic development during anesthesia, just when the absent supervisor is most needed.

Table 2. Teaching principles in the operating room

1. Anesthesiologist's obligation to remain at all times at the side of the anesthetized patient, constantly observing and exercising clinical judgement
2. Assess all instruments, assuring their functionality before and during anesthesia
3. Call for help whenever the presence of a more-experienced physician or an additional pair of hands is required
4. Teach by being present in the operating room. Teaching is impossible in the absence of a teacher!
5. Gradually develop clinical skills in routine anesthesia techniques
6. Keep accurate data records and take notes whenever the situation requires

Increasing vigilance involves a complex of measures for coping with crisis in anesthesia, including continuous observation of the surgical field, the patient's vital signs, and the equipment. Inaccuracies in data gathering are to be noted immediately, especially when a given parameter is recorded by more than one device (invasive and non-invasive blood pressure, heart rate from ECG and pulse oximeter, FiO_2 from the monitor and ventilator, etc.). Incoming phone calls, inappropriate background music, and any other kind of noise should be avoided.

Finally, one must manage the workload properly by correctly scheduling the procedure list, leaving enough time between cases to prepare equipment and drugs reducing production pressure and, if necessary, cancelling non-emergency cases. Financial incentives must be ignored when the patient's condition is not fit for anesthesia or surgery. "All of us must be vigilant and not buckle under pressure to get the case going until we feel that the patient's interests have been best served" [26].

Conclusions

Although most crises during anesthesia can be prevented, or their adverse outcome minimized, anesthesiologists should be prepared to take care of acute unfavorable events in "straightforward" cases. Crisis management in anesthesia can be taught and practised, but it is vital that every opportunity be exploited to improve the practitioner's ability to act properly, accurately assess the new condition, and initiate a decision-making process for successful resolution of the crisis. This is the ongoing task of both teacher and trainee, but it is also the responsibility of the surgeons and OR administration to create and maintain a proper atmosphere that facilitates patient safety during anesthesia.

References

1. Beecher HK, Todd DP (1954) A study of the deaths associated with anesthesia and surgery. Am Surg 140:2-10
2. Cook RI, Woods DD, McDonald JS (1991) Human performance in anesthesia: a corpus of cases. Cognitive Systems Engineering Laboratory Report, prepared for Anesthesia Patient Safety Foundation, April: 18-25
3. Gibby GL, Gravenstein JS, Layon AJ (1992) How often does the preoperative interview change anesthetic management? Anesthesiology 77:A1134
4. Rode RH, Lewis KP, Zarich SW (1996) Cardiac outcome after peripheral vascular surgery: comparison of general and regional anesthesia. Anesthesiology 84:3-11.
5. Sevarino FB, Preble LM (1992) Appendices to Part I. In: Sevarino FB, Preble LM (eds) A manual for acute postoperative pain management. Raven, New York
6. Tinker JH, Hesson WW (1998) Legal issues in anesthesiology. In: Longenecker DE, Tinker JH, Morgan GE (eds) Principles and practice of anesthesiology. Mosby, St. Louis, pp 2461-2469
7. Eagle CJ, Davies JM (1992) Accident analysis of large-scaled technological disasters applied to an anesthetic complication. Can J Anaesthesiol 39:118-122
8. Reiz S, Balfors E, Sorensen MB (1983) Isoflurane-a powerful coronary vasodilator in patients with coronary artery disease. Anesthesiology 59:91-97
9. Tuman KJ, McCarthy RJ, Spiess BD (1989) Does choice of anesthetic agent significantly affect outcome after coronary artery surgery? Anesthesiology 70:189-198
10. Mangano DT (1989) Anesthetics, coronary artery disease and outcome. Anesthesiology 70:175--178

11. Drui AB, Behm RJ, Martin WE (1973) Predesign investigation of the anesthesia operational environment. Anesth Analg 52:584-589
12. Hendon OW, Weinger MB, Zornow MH, Gaba DM (1993) The use of automatic record keeping saves time in complicated anesthetic procedures. Anesth Analg 74:S79
13. Gaba DM, Howard SK, Jump B (1994) Production pressure in the work environment. California anesthesiologists' attitudes and experience. Anesthesiology 81:488-500
14. Murthy VS, Malhorta SK, Bala I (1995) Detrimental effects of noise on anesthetists. Can J Anaesthesiol 42:608-611
15. Cooper JB, Newbower RS, Kitz RJ (1984) An analysis of major errors and equipment failures in anesthesia management: considerations for prevention and detection. Anesthesiology 60:34--42
16. Gaba DM (1994) Human work environment and simulators. In: Miller RD (ed) Anesthesia, 4th edn. Churchill Livingstone, New York, pp 2635-2679
17. Gaba DM, Fish KJ, Howard SK (1994) Crisis management in anesthesiology. Churchill Livingstone, New York
18. Keats AS (1983) Role of anesthesia in surgical mortality. In: Orkin FK, Cooperman LH (eds) Complications in anesthesiology. Lippincott, Philadelphia pp 3-13
19. Desai S, Roaf E, Liu P (1982) Acute pulmonary edema during laparoscopy. Anesth Analg 61:699-703
20. Chopra V, Bocvill JG, Spierdijk J (1990) Accidents, near accidents and complications during anesthesia. Anaesthesia 45:3-10
21. Rasmussen J (1986) Information processing and human-machine interaction: an approach to cognitive engineering. Elsevier, New York
22. Klein GA (1989) Recognition-primed decisions. Adv Man-Machine Syst Res 5:47
23. Chopra V, Gesink BJ, Jong J de (1993) Does training on an anesthesia simulator lead to improvement in performance? Anesthesiology 79:A1117
24. Steadman RH, Oyesola B, Levin P, et al (1999) Does simulator training improve skill in administration of remifentanil? (Abstract) Anesthesiology 91:A1117
25. Gurman GM (1992) The education and teaching of anesthesiology in Israel. Breirot, Tel-Aviv, Israel
26. Blitt CD (2001) Patient safety and production pressure: private practice. APSF Newslett 16:6

Anesthesia for Abdominal Surgery

F. Carli

Morbidity and mortality associated with abdominal surgery have decreased over the years as a result of preoperative optimization of patient health status and improved anesthetic and surgical techniques. However, postoperative morbidity still occurs, even after elective surgical interventions. The key pathogenic factor in postoperative morbidity, excluding failure of surgical and anesthetic techniques, is the surgical stress response with subsequent increased demands on organ function.

These changes in organ function are thought to be mediated by trauma-induced endocrine and metabolic changes, and activation of several biological cascade systems (cytokines, free oxygen radicals, etc.). To understand postoperative morbidity it is therefore necessary to clarify the pathophysiological role of the various components of the surgical stress response and to determine if modification of such responses can improve surgical outcome.

Pathophysiology

Postoperative gastrointestinal tract (GIT) dysfunctions include disturbances of gastric emptying and disturbances of motility resulting in nausea, vomiting and ileus, and other functional deficiencies that reduce the barrier against translocation of endotoxin and bacteria from the intestinal lumen. Altered motility of GIT after anesthesia and surgery is manifested as the inability to tolerate food and fluids and a delay in the return of normal large bowel activity. Motility normally recovers within 4-5 days of major surgery, but more quickly after minor surgery. The causes for postoperative ileus are not entirely clear, but it is thought that a generalized increase in sympathetic tone is a major factor [1]. Postoperative ileus is defined as uncomplicated inhibition of gut motility lasting no more than 3 days. Paralytic ileus, in contrast, is defined as prolonged stasis greater than 3 days, and is usually caused by factors other than surgical trauma. Generally, bowel surgery is more likely to be followed by ileus than peripheral surgery. However, several studies have shown that postoperative inhibition of bowel function is not related to the degree of intraoperative handling of the bowel. Postoperative ileus delays normal recovery, increases the need for intravenous fluids and drugs, and delays postoperative mobilization, thereby increasing the overall cost of hospital stay [2]. Gastric emptying increases the risk of aspiration of gastric content in patients with obtunded protective reflexes in the early postoperative period, delays absorption of oral medicines, and increased the risk of postoperative nausea and vomiting.

The large bowel, especially the descending colon, takes the longest time to recover normal motility after surgery. Colonic ileus is recognized as abdominal distension and failure to pass flatus and stool. It results in third space loss of fluids and electrolytes and may impede respiration by diaphragmatic splinting. Increased intracolonic pressure may decrease colonic blood flow and adversely affect the integrity of bowel anastomosis by decreased perfusion and pressure effects. Impaired mucosal perfusion and ileus are associated with bacterial overgrowth, translocation of endotoxins, and development of organ failure [3].

Although the pathophysiological features of postoperative ileus remain ill defined, the most commonly accepted theory is that abdominal pain activates a spinal reflex arc that inhibits intestinal motility. In addition, surgical stress induces sympathetic hyperactivity, and an excessive sympathetic stimulation of the bowel inhibits organized propulsive activity. Thus, both nociceptive afferent and sympathetic efferent nerves are believed to be the key initiators of ileus. Although stimulation of sympathetic nerves inhibits contractile activity, therapeutic intervention with adrenergic blocking drugs does not speed resolution of the ileus. In contrast, the lack of efficacy of adrenergic blocking drugs on sympathetic innervation pathways to the GIT can block ileus after abdominal surgery. This observation provides a theoretical framework suggesting that blockade of abdominal nociceptive afferent or sympathetic efferent pathways might abolish inhibition of GIT motility induced by abdominal surgery.

Pharmacology and the GIT

Many drugs used for anesthesia affect postoperative gastric emptying, but opioids have the most-profound action [4]. Even the opioids given by the epidural route cause marked delay in gastric emptying [5]. The mechanism is unclear, although centrally mediated, and spinal sites of action have been suggested from animal studies. The effect of opioids on the large bowel is well known; there is a delay in passage of flatus or feces. The effect of volatile anesthetics is reversible and therefore clinically unimportant. Spinal and epidural local anesthetics have little effect on gastric emptying and improve colonic motility [6]. Epidural local anesthetics improve colonic motility through the blockade of nociceptive afferent pathways, therefore disrupting the afferent limb of the spinal reflex arc that has been postulated to mediate postoperative ileus. Furthermore, epidural local anesthetics can block the efferent limb of the reflex arc by blocking thoracolumbar sympathetic efferent nerves. Segmental neural blockade of thoracic dermatomes with local anesthetics will selectively block nociceptive afferent and sympathetic efferent nerves while leaving parasympathetic innervation (by the vagus and pelvic nerves) intact. The resulting modulation of autonomic balance toward a relative increase in parasympathetic tone during thoracic epidural should increase propulsive activity in the colon. Epidural local anesthetics may also increase GIT function through systemic absorption of local anesthetics and sympathetic pathways, and therefore may be less effective in reduction of ileus than local anesthetics. This is particularly true on the 3rd and 4th days after surgery. GIT motility can be increased with prokinetic agents such as cisapride and metoclopramide. Although the use of neostigmine has been associated with increased incidence of anastomotic leakage, there is no substantial evidence to support this effect.

Surgery and the GIT

The value of antibiotic prophylaxis is well established and the timing of administration, doses and duration of antibiotics have been clarified in recent years. This therapy has contributed to a great reduction in nosocomial infection [7]. The treatment of postoperative wound infections has also changed with the introduction of new suturing material and better understanding of suture techniques. Antithrombotic prophylaxis is well established during the postoperative period with a low-dose heparin regimen. The re-evaluation of postoperative nutritional traditions has shown that early restoration of oral intake is possible, and has beneficial effects in attenuating protein catabolism, controlling the ileus, and reducing postoperative septic complications [8]. One of the most-impressive changes has been the introduction of minimally invasive (endoscopic, laparoscopic) surgery. These developments have also contributed to increased use of ambulatory and semiambulatory settings for surgical procedures.

Perioperative program for upper GI surgery

The perioperative program for upper GIT surgery aims at reducing the incidence of postoperative complications. Two main complications occur after upper GIT surgery: pulmonary dysfunction and cardiovascular morbidity. The incidence of pulmonary dysfunction (atelectasis and pneumonia) between postoperative day (POD) 1 and 5 was reported to be around 26-35%. Diaphragmatic dysfunction induced by a neural reflex is the leading factor in respiratory changes after upper GI surgery. Myocardial infarction (MI) occurs during the first 3 days after surgery, as recently reported in a large study where serial enzymatic, ECG, and pathological indices of MI were conducted in a group of patients with history of ischemic heart disease undergoing major non-cardiac surgery [9].

Anesthetic care

Anesthesiologists can be actively involved in the perioperative program of upper GIT surgery by attempting to reduce postoperative complications. One way is to alleviate pain with epidural blockade. Epidural local anesthetics have been shown to attenuate postoperative pulmonary complications when compared with systemic opioids. However, it is not clear that epidural analgesia per se can provide cardiovascular protection. There is proven evidence whether epidural local anesthetics improve GIT motility when compared with systemic opioids. Maintenance of normothermia during surgery and attenuation of the inflammatory and adrenergic response to surgical stress need to be provided. A recent study compared the traditional regimen with a multimodal treatment of thoracic esophageal resection [10]. The multimodal protocol included: (1) intraoperative combination of general anesthesia and thoracic epidural block with bupivacaine plus sufentanil block to the fourth thoracic dermatome prior to surgery; (2) postoperative pain relief with patient-controlled epidural analgesia with low-dose bupivacaine and sufentanil treated to individual needs with VAS scores during rest and movement; (3) extubation at the end of surgery and mobilization as quickly as possible; (4) early oral nutrition. The results of this multimodal approach were (a) reduction of ICU stay, (b) significant difference in intermediate discharge, (c) tendency towards decreased in-hospital mortality.

Surgical care

With regards to the surgical approach, minimally invasive surgery can make upper GIT a fast-track surgery; for example laparoscopic approach without GIT resection compared with the open technique (laparotomy with resection). The program includes the following: (1) preoperative optimization of patient health status; (2) use of preoperative test to rule out dismotility; (3) aggressive antiemetics to avoid disruption of anastomosis; (4) effective analgesia - a precursor to early extubation and early weaning from respirator; (5) surgery to be performed as quickly as possible; judicious pre- and postoperative administration of i.v. fluids; (6) avoidance of supine position after surgery and oxygen therapy during the first 2 postoperative nights; (7) improved peripheral vascular circulation with early mobilization and ambulation.

Perioperative program for lower GII surgery

Major colonic surgery is performed for either benign or malignant tumors of the large intestine or for inflammatory bowel disease (IBD). Patients undergoing colonic surgery for tumors are generally over 60 years of age, while those with IBD tend to be in the younger age group. Associated diseases such as respiratory, cardiac, and metabolic diseases, are frequent in the elderly, as well as anemia and loss of muscle mass. Patients with IBD tend to have frequent pain and suffer psychological stress. Preoperative optimization of the patient's health status focuses on correction of anemia, stabilization of cardiopulmonary functions, psychological support and, if time allows, nutritional replenishment. In the preoperative clinic, patients can be informed of the measures taken during the hospital stay by using videotapes or leaflets prepared by the surgical team. The objectives of the preparation is to involve patients in the healing process.

Anesthetic care

The role of the anesthesiologist is to minimize the response to surgical stress and therefore choice has to be taken into account. Neural blockade with local anesthetics is strongly recommended, as this technique attenuates significantly the metabolic response. The block must be achieved before surgery is initiated, whether the latter is performed by either laparotomy or laparoscopy. Symmetrical sensory block must be extended from T3 to S5 dermatomes. The epidural catheter is introduced at thoracic dermatomes (T8-T10) and analgesia is maintained after surgery for 3-5 days. The requirements for general anesthesia are reduced, and large doses of opioids are discouraged. Nitrous oxide can be avoided when there is a risk of small and large bowel distension. The excellent quality of muscle relaxation provided by the epidural block can be maintained by a continuous infusion of local anesthetics to which a small amount of opioids can be added. As with an extensive sympathetic block, hypotension can occur, and this can be managed with careful administration of i.v. fluids (crystalloids) and use of vasopressors (phenylephrine and epinephrine). Great care must be taken to prevent heat loss from the exposed parts of the body by using active warming devices. At the end of surgery patients must be pain free and transferred to the recovery room in a semi-reclining position (20-30°).

Surgical care

Surgery can be performed by laparotomy or laparoscopy (full or assisted). The surgical incision can be limited to an area where the tumor is present or the bowel has to be resected in order to limit tissue damage. Laparoscopy is not favored in the presence of tumor for risk of dissemination. Nasogastric tube insertion is discouraged [11]. Heparin s.c. can be administered once the epidural catheter is in place and a successful block is achieved. It is advisable to administer antibiotics before surgery. Bladder catheterization is indicated to monitor fluid balance for a short period of time.

Postoperative care

Great care must be exercised during this period, and often patients are neglected with the risk of developing complications. Aspects of care to be considered in this group of patient are centred around recovery of gut function.

Optimal pain relief

Several retrospective, non-randomized and prospective controlled studies have been conducted on the merit of different methods of pain relief. Although all methods available (parenteral opioids, PCA opioids, and local anesthetics) can provide pain relief of a reasonable quality, it is clear that pain relief measures should also aim to continue the attenuation of surgical stress response and promote recovery. In this context, epidural combination of opioids and local anesthetics has been shown to provide optimal pain relief allowing patients to mobilize rather soon after surgery and achieve rapid recovery of GIT function [12].

Nutrition

There is no reason why patients undergoing elective procedures should fast after surgery for 3-4 days [13]. Incremental feeding can be achieved safely from the 1st postoperative day to minimize ileus. The use of metoclopromide or cisapride to accelerate gastric emptying is recommended.

Mobilization

Patients should be encouraged to stay out of bed, on a chair or walking. But to achieve this, pain relief must be optimal. Breathing exercises and adoption of semi-reclining posture are simple initiatives that have a beneficial effect on recovery. Patients should be discharged with a program of simple daily exercises.

Other measures

Oxygen therapy is advised for 48 h after surgery, particularly in patients with cardiopulmonary problems. A semi-sitting (45°) position should be maintained during the postoperative period. Bladder catheter should be removed 24-48 h after surgery and attention must be paid by staff to avoid unnecessary disruption of sleep pattern. Drains and tubes must be removed as soon as possible to facilitate patient's comfort.

Some examples of perioperative programs for surgical procedures

Cholecystectomy

There are no surgical barriers to a perioperative program for laparoscopic cholecystectomy. Anesthetic care includes small doses of opioids, adequate general anesthesia, preoperative infiltration of skin overlying the peritoneum with 0.5% bupivacaine, control of postoperative emesis with metoclopromide, and postoperative pain relief with a non-steroidal anti-inflammatory drug [14]. From the surgical point of view those patients selected for laparoscopic cholecystectomy should not present with common bile duct stones. In addition those patients in which there is a risk of conversion to open laparotomy should not be put in the fast-track program, as there is a 25% chance of conversion. For example, acute cholecystitis, older than 65 years of age, obesity, male gender, and thickened bladder wall on ultrasonography [15].

Hernia repair

Hernia repair is a procedure that is increasingly performed on an outpatient basis. Optimal anesthetic techniques associated with the shortest time to discharge include the use of local anesthesia with sedation or peripheral nerve blocks. A fast-track program includes a walk-in, walk-out protocol with same-day surgery and open, tension-free mesh repair and 1-2 day recommended convalescence [16]. The local-sedation technique includes: (1) low-dose midazolan premedication (mg); (2) propofol infusion 50Φ/kg per min initially and titrated to maintain patient comfort; (3) low-dose fentanyl (25-50)Φg given 3 - 4 min before local block; (4) an ileoinguinal-hypogastric block with a mixture of bupivacaine 0.5% and lidocaine 2% (30-40 ml). Subfascial administration of the local anesthetic has been shown to significantly reduce pain scores at rest, and with coughing and mobilization compared with subcutaneous infiltration. If supplemental analgesia is needed, IV ketoralac is suggested as this is effective and decreases time to ambulation.

Multimodal approach

A rational approach towards control of the postoperative period is therefore by multimodal intervention. Before surgery, detailed information about the accelerated stay program must be provided, possibly including a videotape program. Such detailed preoperative information has been demonstrated in itself to result in less pain and reduction of postoperative days. Stress reduction may be provided by currently available multimodal regimens. Most importantly, pain relief has to be used to facilitate ambulation and nutrition, in order to avoid postoperative functional impairment. Several studies, although not controlled and randomized, suggest that a multidisciplinary effort may result in pronounced improvements in surgical outcome and reduction in morbidity and hospital stay [17]. In this context, the combination of minimally invasive surgery, epidural local anesthetics, early nutrition and ambulation, and avoidance of opioids can reduce hospital stay and decrease postoperative fatigue and complications. In addition regionalization of major surgical procedures to one center may reduce costs and improve outcome. Finally, the organization of multidisciplinary intervention in rehabilitation units has to be the effort of anesthesiologists, surgeons, and surgical nurses.

References

1. Livingston EH, Passaro EP (1990) Postoperative ileus. Dig Dis Sci 35:121-132
2. Moss G, Regal ME, Lichtig LK (1986) Reducing postoperative pain, narcotics and length of hospitalization. Surgery 90:206-210
3. Deitch EA (1990) The role of intestinal barrier failure and bacterial translocation in the development of systemic infection and multiple organ failure. Arch Surg 125: 403-404
4. Nimmo WS, Heading RC, Wilson J, et al (1975) Inhibition of gastric emptying and drug absorption by narcotic analgesics. Br J Clin Pharmacol 2:121-125
5. Wattwil M (1988) Postoperative pain relief and GI motility. Acta Chir Scand 550[Suppl]:140-145
6. Liu S, Carpenter RL, Neal JM (1995) Epidural anesthesia and analgesia. Anesthesiology 82:1474-1506
7. Lau WY, Chu KW, Poon GP, et al (1988) Prophylactic antibiotics in elective colorectal surgery. Br J Surg 75: 782-785
8. Hessow I (1988) Oral feeding after uncomplicated surgery. Br J Clin Pract 42:275-280
9. Badner N, Knill RL, Brown JE, et al (1988) Myocardial infarction afternoon cardiac surgery. Anesthesiology 88:575-578
10. Brodner G, Pogatzki E, Van Aken H, et al (1998) A multimodal approach to control postoperative pathophysiology and rehabilitation in patients undergoing abdominothoracic esophagectomy. Anesth Analg 86:228-234
11. Cheatam ML, Chapman WC, Key SP, et al (1995) A meta-analysis of selective versus routine nasogastric decompression after elective laparotomy. Ann Surg 221:469-478
12. Liu S, Carpenter RL, Mackey DC, et al (1995) Effects of perioperative analgesic technique on the rate of recovery after colonic surgery. Anesthesiology 83:757-765
13. Stewart BT, Weeds RJ, Collopy BT, et al (1998) Early feeding after elective open colorectal resection: a prospective randomized trial. Aust N Z J Surg 68:125-128
14. Michaloliakou C, Chung F, Sharma S (1996) Preoperative multimodal analgesia facilitates recovery after ambulatory laparoscopic cholecystectomy. Anesth Analg 82:44-51
15. Fried GM, Barkun JS, Sigman HH, et al (1994) Factors determining conversion to laparotomy in patients undergoing laparoscopic cholecystectomy. Am J Surg 167:35-40
16. Callesen T, Beck K, Kehlet H (1998) The feasibility, safety and cost of infiltration anaesthesia for hernia repair. Anaesthesia 53:31-35
17. Bardram L, Funch-Jensen P, Jensen P et al (1995) Recovery after laparoscopic colonic surgery with epidural analgesia, early oral nutrition and enforced mobilization. Lancet 345:763-764

Suggested further reading

Carli F, Shricker T (2000) Combined epidural/general anesthesia for gastrointestinal surgery. Techn Reg Anesth Pain Management 4:77-84

Holte K, Kehlet H (2001) Epidural analgesia and risk of anastomotic leakage. Reg Anesth Pain Med 26: 111-117

Senagore AJ, Whalley D, Delaney CP (2000) Epidural anesthesia-analgesia shortens length of stay after laparoscopic segmental colectomy for benign pathology. Surgery 129: 672-676

Total Intravenous Anesthesia

R. ALEXANDER, N.G. VOLPE

The introduction of propofol in the 1980s led to resurgence in the development of total intravenous anesthesia (TIVA) since the loss of clinical interest due to the morbidity associated with the use of althesin and etomidate. Propofol has fewer side effects and a better pharmacokinetic profile for use in TIVA [1, 2]. Earlier recovery, compared with traditional anesthetic techniques, following its use has also been demonstrated, particularly in surgery of short to intermediate duration [3, 4].

Regimens based on a three-compartment model for propofol infusions were designed to achieve a blood propofol concentration of 3-4 μg/ml. This concentration is considered to be adequate for maintenance of surgical anesthesia when supplemented with nitrous oxide and/or an opioid. However, there were some drawbacks with infusions, which include the long time taken for the blood concentration to reach steady state when the infusion rate is altered. The administration of a bolus of propofol when attempting to increase the depth of anesthesia may lead to hemodynamic instability. The development of target controlled infusion in the latter half of the 1990s led to increased versatility and preference of use by anesthetists [5]. The software developed for infusion pumps can now control the pump to deliver either a calculated bolus dose or stop the infusion for an appropriate length of time. This reduces the risk of forgetting to switch the pump back when reducing the plasma concentration.

Pharmacokinetics

The pharmacokinetics of propofol has been studied extensively in humans [6, 7]. The decay of blood propofol concentration is best described using a tri-exponential equation, irrespective of the size of the bolus. The initial distribution half-life ranges from 2 to 3 min, the intermediate distribution half-life from 30 to 60 min, and the terminal phase 3-8 h. The central volume of distribution is approximately 228 ml/kg, but the steady-state volume of distribution ranges from 800 ml in healthy patients to 1,900 ml in elderly patients. A three-compartmental model shown below is required to describe the distribution, redistribution, and elimination of propofol.

It shows drug input into the central compartment (V_C), distribution to a shallow compartment (V_2) and to a remote compartment (V_3). The rate constants governing inter-compartmental drug distribution are K12, K21, K13, K31 and K10, which is the rate constant for elimination from the central compartment. The calculation of the maintenance infusion rate at any time after dosing initiation is: maintenance infusion rate (t) = $C_{ther}.V_C.(K_{10} + [K_{12}.e^{-K21.t}] + [K_{13}.e^{-K31.t}])$, where C_{ther} is a therapeutic concentration. More relevant, however, may be the concept of the context-sensitive half time, which is the time taken for the plasma concentration of a substance to decrease by 50% after administration by infusion [8]. Most of the hypnotic agents (excluding thiopentone and midazolam) have half times of less than 30 min after 4 h infusion. Propofol has a significantly shorter context-sensitive half time compared with other hypnotics for any duration of infusion, ensuring a more-rapid decline in blood concentration.

Advantages of intravenous compared with inhalation anesthesia

There have to be proven clinical benefits to patients and medical personnel before any new procedure or technique can be introduced into everyday practice. These include faster induction and rapid recovery and a reduction in postoperative nausea and vomiting when using TIVA compared with inhalation anesthesia using sevoflurane [9]. Intubation conditions without the use of muscle relaxant are better using propofol, with patients more likely to cough with sevoflurane [10]. Pollution of the operating environment can also be a significant problem, especially if using pediatric breathing circuits with no attachments for scavenging. Exposure to nitrous oxide at 11.8 ppm and isoflurane 0.5 ppm can cause genetic damage equivalent to 11-20 cigarettes per day [11]. Other complications of inhalation anesthetics include malignant hypothermia and potential hepatic and renal toxicity, which have been documented following the administration of sevoflurane and isoflurane [12-15]. Propofol has proved a safe alternative [16, 17].

Manual versus target-controlled infusion

The development of the software required to deliver target-controlled infusion

(TCI) in the 1990 s has led to the production of specialized TCI pumps, such as the Diprifusor from Graseby Simms Medical [18]. While there is a potential increase in capital costs when purchasing these specific syringe pumps, there are several clinical advantages to be gained. The dose of propofol required for loss of consciousness is less when using TCI compared with manual controlled infusions [19, 20]. This is because the calculated rate of infusion of the bolus is constantly changing with TCI so that while it takes slightly longer to reach desired effector site concentration, i.e., anesthesia, there is no overshoot in concentration. However, the total dose of propofol has been shown to be higher with TCI compared with administrating an induction bolus dose and using the 10 / 8 / 6 mg/kg per hour regimen for maintenance [21].

Remifentanil and total intravenous anesthesia

The administration of opioids reduces the minimum alveolar concentration (MAC) of volatile agents. There is also synergy in the pharmacodynamic interaction between propofol and alfentanil reducing the propofol infusion required [22, 23]. One of the problems however of infusing alfentanil is the increased duration of emergence from anesthesia at the end of surgery. If the infusion is discontinued too early, then the patient may emerge from anesthesia too soon. Remifentanil is a new, ultra-short-acting, selective mu-receptor agonist that is 20-30 times more potent than alfentanil [24]. Its ester linkage renders it susceptible to hydrolysis by blood and tissue non-specific esterases resulting in a short terminal half-time of less than 10 min at the site of action. Remifentanil has a context-sensitive half time of 3.65 min compared with 58.5 min with alfentanil after a 4-h infusion [24, 25]. These properties produce an extremely rapid termination of action. In addition, remifentanil has a rapid onset of action, with a time to peak effect of 60 s [26]. This pharmacokinetic profile makes remifentanil the ideal opioid for TIVA.

Early studies have shown greater patient satisfaction and less nausea with a remifentanil and propofol anesthetic compared with isoflurane and fentanyl [27]. Recovery of cognitive function is faster with a remifentanil-propofol technique compared with sevoflurane or desflurane [28]. There is also less nausea and analgesic consumption following laparoscopic cholecystectomy when using remifentanil-propofol compared with desflurane [29].

Costs

It is very difficult to compare costs of TCI with inhalation anesthesia due to the variety of anesthetic techniques in practice. The use of premedicants, opioids, and clonidine affect the required effector site concentration or MAC to attain and maintain surgical anesthesia. Low-flow anesthesia will also reduce the amount of inhalational agent used compared with coaxial circuits. This disparity is borne out by the differing conclusions of authors studying cost comparisons [10,30]. There are also cost differentials across various countries, due to the indigenous methods of purchasing pharmaceutical products.

References

1. Gepts E, Camu F, Cockshott ID, Douglas EJ (1987) Disposition of propofol administered as constant rate intravenous infusions in humans. Anesth Analg 66:1256-1263
2. Cockshott ID, Douglas EJ, Prys-Roberts C, et al (1990) The pharmacokinetics of propofol during and after intravenous infusion in man. Eur J Anaesthesiol 7:265-275
3. Doze VA, Shafer A, White PF (1988) Propofol-nitrous oxide versus thiopental-isoflurane-nitrous oxide for general anaesthesia. Anesthesiology 69:63-71
4. Millar JM, Jewkes CF (1988) Recovery and morbidity after day case anaesthesia. A comparison of propofol with thiopentone-enflurane with and without alfentanil. Anaesthesia 43:738-743
5. Russell D, Wilkes MP, Hunter SC, et al (1995) Manual compared with target controlled infusion of propofol. Br J Anaesth 75:562-566
6. White PF (1988) Propofol pharmacokinetics and pharmacodynamics. Semin Anesthesia 7:4-20
7. Kanto J, Gepts E (1989) Pharmacokinetic implications for the clinical use of propofol. Clin Pharmacokinet 17:308-326
8. Hughes MA, Glass PS, Jacobs JR (1992) Context-sensitive half-time in multicompartment pharmacokinetic models for intravenous anesthetic drugs. Anesthesiology 76:334-341
9. Smith I, Thwaites AJ (1998) Double-blind comparison of "single-agent" ambulatory anesthetics: TCI propofol versus sevoflurane (abstract). Anesthesiology 89 [Suppl]:A17
10. El Kettani C, Watremez C, Godet G, et al (2000) Anaesthesia with sevoflurane or TCI for propofol in vascular patients: comparison on quality of induction, quality of recovery and cost (abstract). Eur J Anaesthesiol 17: A310
11. Hoerauf KH, Wiesner G, Schroegendorfer KF, et al (1999) Waste anaesthetic gases induce sister chromatid exchanges in lymphocytes of operating room personnel.Br J Anaesth 82:764-766
12. Schmidt CC, Suttner SW, Piper SN, et al (1999) Comparison of the effects of desflurane and isoflurane anaesthesia on hepatocellular function assessed by alpha glutathione S-transferase. Anaesthesia 54:1207-1211
13. Shichinohe Y, Masuda Y, Takahashi H, et al (1992) A case of postoperative hepatic injury after sevoflurane anesthesia. Masui 41:1802-1805
14. Smith I, Ding Y, White PF (1992) Comparison of induction, maintenance, and recovery characteristics of sevoflurane-N2O and propofol-sevoflurane-N2O with propofol-isoflurane--N2O anesthesia. Anesth Analg 74:253-259
15. Murray JM, Trinick TR (1992) Plasma fluoride concentrations during and after prolonged anesthesia: a comparison of halothane and isoflurane. Anesth Analg 74:236-240
16. Murray JM, Trinick TR (1992) Hepatic function and indocyanine green clearance during and after prolonged anaesthesia with propofol. Br J Anaesth 69:643-644

17. Pollock AN, McKenzie AJ, Hodges M, Snoeck MM. (1997) Propofol and malignant hyperthermia susceptibility. Anaesth Intensive Care 25:583-585
18. Kenny GNC (1999) Target-controlled anaesthesia: concepts and first clinical experiences. Eur J Anaesthes 14[Suppl]:29-31
19. Servin FS (1998) TCI with compared manually controlled infusion of propofol: a multicentre study. Anaesthesia 53 [Suppl 1]: 82-86
20. Hunt-Smith J, Donaghy A, Leslie K, et al (1999) Safety and efficacy of target controlled infusion ("Diprifusor") vs manually controlled infusion of propofol for anaesthesia. Anaesth Intensive Care 27:260-264
21. Breslin D, Reid J, Kyle A, Mirakhur RK (2001) Manual versus target-controlled infusions of propofol; propofol dosage and BIS scores. Br J Anaesth 86: 305-306
22. Vuyk J (1997) Pharmacokinetic and pharmacodynamic interactions between opioids and propofol. J Clin Anesth 9:23S-26S
23. Vuyk J, Engbers FH, Burm AG, et al (1996) Pharmacodynamic interaction between propofol and alfentanil when given for induction of anesthesia. Anesthesiology 84:288-299
24. Glass PS, Hardman D, Kamiyama Y (1993) Preliminary pharmacokinetics and pharmacodynamics of an ultra-short-acting opioid: remifentanil (G187084B). Anesthes Analg 77:1031-1040
25. Egan TD, Lemmens JM, Fiset P, et al (1993) The pharmacokinetics of the new short-acting opiod remifentanil (GI87084B) in healthy adult male volunteers. Anesthesiology 79: 881-892
26. Minto CF, Schnider TW, Shafer SL (1997) Pharmacokinetics and pharmacodynamics of remifentanil. II. Model application. Anesthesiology 86:24-33
27. Epple J, Kubitz J, Schmidt H, et al (2001) Comparative analysis of costs of total intravenous anaesthesia with propofol and remifentanil vs. balanced anaesthesia with isoflurane and fentanyl. Eur J Anaesthesiol 18:20-28
28. Larsen B, Seitz A, Larsen R (2000) Recovery of cognitive function after remifentanil-propofol anesthesia: a comparison with desflurane and sevoflurane anesthesia. Anesthes Analg 90:168--174
29 Grundmann U, Silomon M, Bach F, et al (2001) Recovery profile and side effects of remifentanil–based anaesthesia with desflurane or propofol for laporoscopy cholecystectomy. Acta Anaesthesiol Scand 45: 320-326
30. Watson KR, Shah MV (2000) Clinical comparison of 'single agent' anaesthesia with sevoflurane versus target controlled infusion of propofol. Br J Anaesth 85:541-546

Dobutamine and Esmolol, Opposite Action or Sometimes Synergic Therapeutic Actions

R. Muchada

The utilization of exogenous cardiac vasoactive products to stabilize cardiovascular function, to optimize oxygen transportation, and to favor homogeneous cellular perfusion is common in anesthesia [1] and in intensive care medicine [2].

The action of the different drugs used can be predominantly on the cardiac or vascular sector, but unfortunately this does not imply a specific action. In general the stimulation or the inhibition of localized receptors acts at the cardiac level, at the vascular level, or on the two sectors.

After the description of [3] beta receptors by Ahlquist [4], their division into $beta_1$ and $beta_2$ and the identification of $alpha_1$ and $_2$ receptors, attention has been focused on effects of the different cardiovascular drugs at the receptor level.

At the cardiac level, the B stimulant products, acting on B1 receptors, are largely used, during left ventricular contractility failure. This positive inotropic effect is often accompanied by other effects (chronotropic, bathmotropic, and dromotropic) determined by B 1 stimulation [5].

These reactions can vary from patient to patient, and even in the same subject from one time to another.

This variability can be explained by several mechanisms, including: the number of receptors, the sensitivity of receptors, the availability of receptors, the bioavailability of the product used, the predominance of one of the actions of the products in relationship to the others, the level of the endogenous catecholamines, and the dose used.

However, some common actions have been attributed to the stimulation or inhibition of the $beta_1$ cardiac receptor, while acknowledging that the original mechanisms of the actions are different [6].

Two actions are exerted directly on cardiac muscular fibers. The positive or negative *inotropic* action involving stimulation or blocking of the beta-specific receptors operates via an increase of calcium inflow through the slow-stream of calcium channels, modifying pKA-dependent phosphorylsation, inducing an increase of fixed calcium on troponin C and a greater interaction of actin and myosin.

The *lusitropic* phenomenon is mediated by the stimulation of the calcium ATPase pump of the sarcoplasmic reticulum, which insures the re-pumping of calcium after contraction, due to phosphorylation, which is pkA dependent.

The *chronotropic* and the *bathmotropic* actions are essentially due to the activation of the AMP cycle, which effects the sinus automatism. The *dromotropic* effect is activated or inhibited by a regulation of entrance of calcium into the nodal sinus cells, modifying the potential action at the initial phase, with a modification of the propagation of the stimulus.

These different actions suggest the possibility of producing beta modulation by using apparently opposite properties of two therapeutic products, to achieve a functional myocardial balance.

This means, for instance, that use of the positive inotropic properties of dobutamine, but inhibition of the chronotropic positive effects with a beta--blocker. In this way it could be possible to preserve the contractility stimulation avoiding the ominous action of the increased heart rate (HR) on the overall myocardial oxygen consumption (MVO_2) in patients with coronary risk.

To test this hypothesis animal experiments have been undertaken in the pig.

Materials and methods

Animal preparation

The animal care committee of the University of Lyon approved the study; 5 white adult female pigs, weighing 25±5 kg were studied; 5 mg of ketamine i.m. was given 15 min before the induction of anesthesia, as premedication. The anesthesia was induced with propofol 4 mg/kg, fentanyl 20 µg/kg, and pancuronium 8 mg i.v. It was maintained with a perfusion of fentanyl at a rate of 0.8 µg/kg per min and isoflurane 1.2 %, inspiratory concentration, in O_2 (0.6) and air (0.4). After orotracheal intubation the animals were mechanically ventilated with a Modulus integrated device (Ohmeda, Madison, Wis., USA).

The left carotid artery and the internal jugular vein were exposed. A catheter was introduced into the jugular vein to perfuse the animals and to monitor the central venous pressure (CVP). Two other peripheral veins were catheterized to perfuse independently the cardio vasoactive drugs. A 16-gauge Teflon catheter (Vygon, Ecouen, France) was pushed into the carotid artery to record arterial pressure (AP). It was connected to a P 23 Db Gould Statham transducer zeroed to the mid chest position.

A special echo Doppler intra-esophageal probe [7] was used to measure the aortic blood flow (ABF). This was linked to a Dynemo 3000 module (Sometec, Suresnes, France), allowing integration of a hemodynamic profile. The association of Doppler and the ECG signals allowed measurement of the systolic time intervals [8].

The perfusion of dobutamine was performed with a specific electrical pump by an exclusively venous means. The dilution was of 250 mg of dobutamine in 50 ml of physiological solution the start dose was of 5 μg/kg per min with a progressive increase of 2 μg/kg/min for 3 min until the HR was 40 % higher than baseline.

Once the objective was reached a perfusion of Brevibloc (esmolol) was started by another specific venous route. The initial dose was 10 μg/kg/min. An increase by steps of 10 μg/kg per min over 5 min was carried out to obtain a diminution of the HR between - 5% and + 10 % of the starting HR.

The total i.v. perfusion of Ringer's lactate and drugs was 4± 0.25 ml/kg per hour.

On the continuous recording of the hemodynamic parameters (except for CVP) we selected the values corresponding to the steady state, before the introduction of the dobutamine (T0). This value corresponds to 100% of the relative values. A second point 10 min after reaching a stable increase of the HR under the dobutamine perfusion (T1) (10 min after T1), (T2) was also taken into account.

A third point under a stable esmolol perfusion and 10 min after that the HR had decreased to the pre-determined level (T3) and a fourth point 10 min after T3 with a stable dose of dopamine and esmolol (T4) were also considered.

A statistical study was performed to calculate the mean values and standard deviation. Student's t-test for matched series was used to compare the change of hemodynamic parameters. Wilcoxon rank test, applied to the small series, was used for the evaluation of the statistical significance of parametric variations. All p values < 0.05 were considered as statistically significant.

Results

The results are expressed in absolute values (Table 1) and as percentages (%) in relation to the starting values (Table 2).

Table 1. After the perfusion of dobutamine there is a significant increase of the heart rate (HR), the aortic blood flow (ABF), with a decrease of the pre-ejection period indexed to the heart rate (PEPi), the PEP/LVET rapport and the total systemic vascular resistance (TVSR). In contrast, there is no change in the stroke volume (SV). The esmolol reduces the HR, but increases ABF and SV. The TSVRS remained significant lower the in TI. The PEPi and the PEP/LVET rapport are always significant decreased, but values are not far away from the normal range (SAP= systolic arterial pressure, MAP = mean arterial pressure, DAP = diastolic arterial pressure, LVETi = left ventricular ejection time indexed to the HR, PEP/LVET= rapport, CVP= central venous pressure)

* P<0.05 ** P<0.01 *** P<0.001

	T0	T1	T2	T3	T4
HR (beats/min)	92±8	135±11***	133±13***	89±9	87±6
ABF (l/min)	1.5±0.25	1.98±0.38**	2.05±0.35**	2.12±0.21**	1.98±0.17**
SV (ml)	16±4	14±4.5	15±4	23±3**	22±3.5**
SAP (mmHg)	108±6	105±6	103±4	115±6	117±5
MAP (mmHg)	80±5	71±4	72±9	79±6	81±8
DAP (mmHg)	72 ±3	68±5	68±5	65±2	64±4
TSVR (Dyn.s.cm-5)	4,266±327	2,868±251**	2,809±176**	2,981±380**	3,170±272*
PEPi (ms)	162±11	118±9***	115±5***	136±8**	143±5**
LVETi (ms)	398±10	392±11	405±7	407±10	415±12
PEP/LVET	0.40±7	0.32±5**	0.28±3***	0.33±4**	0.34±3*
CVP (cm H_2O)	10±3	9±2	9±3	8±	8±2

Table 2. The values at T0 represent the absolute values. The variations of the hemodynamic parameters from T 1 to T4 are expressed as percentage variation from T0. It is interesting to note that although ABF is increased from T1 to T4, the HR is only increased under dobutamine but normalized under dobutamine + esmolol. In contrast, the SV, which is not changed under dobutamine, increases when the perfusion of Esmolol is attempted

	T0 (Absolute Value =100%)	T1 %	T2 %	T3 %	T4 %
HR (beats/min)	92	+46	+45	-3	-6
ABF (l/min)	1.5	+32	+36	+41	+32
SV(ml)	16	-12	-8	+43	+37
SAP (mmHg)	108	-3	-5	+ 9	+8
MAP (mmHg)	80	-12	-12	-1.5	+1
DAP (mmHg)	72	-1.5	-1.5	-9	-10
TSVR (Dyn.s.cm-5)	4,266	-33	-35	-31	-36
PEPi (ms)	162	-28	-30	-17	-15
LVETi (ms)	398	-2	-1.5	+2	+4
PEP/LVET	0.40	-20	-30	-18	-15
CVP (cm H_2O)	10	-10	-10	-20	-20

The average dose of dobutamine used to reach the HR at the plateau was 10.8 ±3.5 μg/ kg per min. The average dose of Brevibloc to reduce the HR was 32 ± 9.2 μg/ kg per min.

Under the action of the dobutamine the ABF increased in a significant manner, but this was HR dependent, since the stroke volume (SV) did not vary. The pre-ejection period (PEPi), the PEP/LVET, and total systemic vascular resistance (TSVR) showed a significant diminution.

The addition of the esmolol (T3) returned the HR to the level of departure, without significant change of the SV and of the ABF. However, the PEPi and the PEP/LVET remained below the initial level.

Comments

In this study, introduction of the cardiac drugs was begun after a period of anesthetic stabilization and without nociceptive stimulation. The non-invasive hemodynamic monitoring method used [9] guarded against any cardiovascular variation produced by the manipulation performed to obtain the measurements.

The continuous perfusion of the analgesic and the concentration of the halogen seem to be enough to avoid the manifestation of neuro-vegetative reactions. Nevertheless, the effects of this balanced anesthesia were seen on the cardiovascular sector, manifested as myocardial depression, translated into the diminution of the ABF and SV, by an increase of the PEPi and the PEP/LVET. The increase of the TSVR is probably determined by the fall of the ABF [10].

The positive inotropic action of the dobutamine is a known effect [11, 12]. Under this action there is an increase of the ABF, with an increase of the SV. However, when chronotropic effects exceed the inotropic effects, the ABF is certainly increased, but this is not entirely favorable for the hemodynamic equilibrium of the patients.

This experience shows that the dobutamine increases the ABF in a significant manner, but without increasing the SV. The ABF increase is herce HR dependent. The tachycardia is accompanied by a significant diminution of the PEPi and the PEP/LVET.

The reduction of these two parameters, measured with a method described and validated by our team [13], confirms the $beta_1$-chronotropic positive action of the dobutamine, under these experimental conditions.

The tachycardic action of dobutamine is known [14] and is dose dependent. A decreased pre-load worsens the effect. This last situation could be eliminated by a weak variation of the CVP, indicating at least a stability of the pre-load situation.

The tachycardia is a source of increase of the çonsumption of MVO_2. The shortening of the PEPi implies an acceleration of tension speed of the cardiac fiber, which according to Guyton [15] causes a consistent increase of the MVO_2, because it is during this period that 90% of the energy for the contraction is used. The increase of the HR reduces the diastolic period. This decreases the ventricular filling time and reduces the relaxation diastolic period.

These three elements act in a synergic and additive manner to compromise the coronary flow and the transport of oxygen to the myocardial structures.

The maintenance of the diastolic arterial pressure (PAD) during the perfusion of dobutamine would be, in this study, the only element allowing preservation of the coronary perfusion.

As in the study of Shakar et al. [16] the introduction of a beta-blocker, esmolol, produced a modulation of the $beta_1$-chronotropic effect of the dobutamine and a decrease of the time of the isovolumetric contraction. Nevertheless, the perfusion of the esmolol did not compromise the positive inotropic effect of the dobutamine, because the ABF did not change in a significant way, the SV increased, and the pre- and the after-load remained relatively stable.

This synergism of action could have been the result of the carefully adapted doses, due to adequate hemodynamic monitoring [17], without which it would be impossible to observe.

A sectorial functional specificity of the beta-receptors, at the myocardium level, has already been evoked [18,19]. This specificity could allow modulation of their actions with drugs, which have apparently opposite effects, but can, in a specific context, act in a synergic manner.

The synergism of the dobutamine and the esmolol in the present study, adding the positive inotropic effects of the first to the negative chronotropic effects of the second, could improve myocardial performance, but decrease the MVO_2 [20].

These effects would be due to an additive action on the diastolic relaxation, taking into account the synergic positive lusitropic effects of the dobutamine [21, 22] and the $beta_1$-blocker esmolol [23].

The association of two cardiovascular products whose actions could be considered as antagonistic is not new [24, 25]. The association of dobutamine and norepinephrine has been proposed for the treatment of septic shock with decreased vascular resistance, to take advantage of the inotropic cardiac beta 1 effects of the dobutamine, but opposing the beta 2 vascular effects by provoking a peripheral vasoconstriction, to preserve the tissue perfusion with a homogeneous distribution of the blood flow. At the same time, the increase of after-load determined by the norepinephrine can, by a reflex action, reduce the HR [26-29].

Our team has proposed the association of norepinephrine and esmolol for the treatment of some hyperkinetc septic shocks, when the diagnosis of a beta endogenous stimulation could be made [30].

The treatment of evolved cardiac failure with the association of intermittent perfusion of dopamine [31-34] and a bradycardic anti-arrhythmic, but also cardiodepressant, beta blocker [35] or amiodarone [36] has been eccective not only in improving the quality of life but also the duration of patient survival.

On the other hand, during brief periods of hypoxia, the resistance of the heart to the deficit of oxygenation can be increased by the mechanism of preconditioning. During the period of hypoxia, the cardiomyocytes demand an increased consumption of glucides by an increase of the intracellular transportation of glucides and activation of the intracellular glycolysis. This action is activated by the stimulation of the $alpha_1$-adrenoreceptors. During the period of hypoxia/ischemia, the number of $alpha_1$ receptors and the concentration of noradrenaline are locally increased [37, 38].

From a theoretical point of view if it is possible to preserve the stimulatory $alpha_1$ actions of the dobutamine [39-41] with, at least, a partial inhibition of its beta effects, with the esmolol, it would be possible to increase the activation of the alpha 1 receptors. The myocardial protection against hypoxia could be due not only to the diminution of the consumption of oxygen or effects on the diastolic period, but also to a better activation of the preconditioning.

Because our results are derived from animal experiments, extrapolation to man requires further testing. Secondly our study reports preliminary results on a small number of animals. Although the trends and the statistical study show apparently interesting results, it is necessary to widen the sample to increase the sensitivity of the study and to consolidate results. Thirdly, taking into account variations of beta-receptor sensitivities, endogenous catecholamines, and the individual metabolic level, the doses to be used should to be adapted precisely. Fourthly the therapeutic action has to be studied during clinic follow-up and hemodynamic monitoring comprising indirect or direct indices for the evaluation of left ventricle contractility.

Despite these limitations, this proposed association could be interesting for patients presenting with acute myocardial failure needing inotropic and lusitropic positive stimulation, while avoiding the therapeutic effects leading to an increase in MVO_2 or a loss of benefit of the preconditioning.

References

1. Muchada R, Haro D, Lamazou J, et al (1991) Efecto de la dobutamina sobre el transporte y el consumo de oxígeno durante la anestesia general con enflurano. Rev Esp Anestesiol Reanim 38 : 376-381
2. Martin C, Saux P, Eon B, et al (1990) Septic shock: a goal direct therapy using volume loading, dobutamine and/or epinephrine. Acta Anaesthesiol Scand 34:413-417
3. Dale HH (1906) On some physiological actions of Ergot. J Physiol 34 :163-167
4. Ahlquist RP (1948) A study of the adrenotropic receptors. Am J Physiol 135: 586-597
5. Lekfkowitz RJ (1974) Selectivity in beta – adrenergic responses. Clinical implication. Circulation 49:783-786
6. Lechat P (1998) Agonistes B-Adrenargiques (adénaline, dopamine, dobutamine, salbutamol); B-bloquants. Principes et regles d'utilisation. Rev Praticien 48:1115-1121
7. Lavandier B, Cathignol D, Muchada R (1985) Non invasive aortic blood flow measurement using an intraoesophageal probe. Ultrasound Med Biol 11:451-460
8. Muchada R. (1988) Continuous and non invasive hemodynamic profile monotoring including aortic blood flow, systolic time intervals and PetCO2 masurements. In: Kazuyuki I, Matsuyuki D, Tomiei K (eds) State of the art technology in anesthesia and intensive care. Elsevier, Amsterdam pp 75-85
9. Cariou A, Monchi M, Joly JL, et al (1998) Non invasive cardiac output monitoring by aortic blood flow determination: evaluation of the Sometec Dynemo – 3000 system. Crit Care Med 26: 2066-2072
10. Muchada R, Piriz H. Cathignol D, et al (1988) Monitorizacion no invasiva del gasto aórtico y otros parámetros hemodinámicos durante la anestesia con isoflurano y enflurano. Rev Esp Anestesiol Reanim 53:194-198
11. Leier CV, Unverferth DV (1985) Dobutamine. Ann Intern Med 99:490-496

12. Tuttle RR, Mills J (1975) Dobutamine: development of a new catecholamine to selectively increase cardiac contractility. Circ Res 36:185-196.
13. Tournadre J P, Muchada R, Lansiaux S, Chassard D (1999) Measurements of systolic time intervals using a transoeophageal pulsed echo Doppler. Br J Anaesth 83:630-636
14. Majerus TC, Dasta JF, Bauman JL, et al (1989) Dobutamine: ten years later. Pharamacotherapy 9:245-259
15. Guyton AC (1996) Heart muscle. The heart as a pump. In: Guyton AC, Hall JE (eds) Textbook of medical physiology. Saunders, Philadelphia, pp 113-114
16. Shakar SF, Abrham WT, Gilbert EM, et al (1998) Combined oral positive inotropic and B blockers therapy for treatment of refractory class IV heart failure. J Am Coll Cardiol 31: 1336-1340
17. Bernardin G, Tiger F, Fouché R, Mattei M (1998) Continuous noninvasive measurement of aortic blood flow in critical ill patients with a new esophageal echo – Doppler system. J. Crit Care 13: 177-183
18. Fowler MB, Lasser JA, Hopkins GL, et al (1986) Assessment of the B adrenergic receptor pathway on the intact failing human heart: progressive receptor down regulation and subsensitivity to agonist reponse. Circulation 74:191
19. Koch WJ, Lefkowitz RJ, Rockman HA (2000) Functional consequences of altering myocardial adrenergic receptors signaling. Annu Rev Physiol 62:237-260
20. Ahmed A B, Latimer D, Vuylesteke A (2000) Cardiovascular pharmacology: new drugs and new indications. Curr Opin Anaesthesiol 13:5-13
21. Harada K, Tamura M, Ito T et al (1996) Effects of low dose dobutamine on left ventricle diastolic filling in children. Pediatr Cardiol 17:220-225
22. Little WC, Rassi A, Freeman GL (1987) Comparison of effects of dobutamine and ouabain on left ventricular contraction and relaxation in closed chest dogs. J Clin Invest 80:613-620
23. Freemantle N, Cleland J, Young P, et al (1999) B blockers after myocardial infarction: systematic review and meta regression analysis. BMJ 1730-1737
24. Parker MP, Shelhamer JH, Bacharach SL, et al (1984) Profound but reversible myocardial depression in patients with septic shock. Ann Intern Med 100: 483-490
25. Lucas CE. (1994) A new look at dopamine and norepinephrine for hyperdynamicseptic shock. Chest 105:7-8
26. Martin C, Vialet R, Potié F, Thomachot L (1996) Interêt des associations de cathécholamines au cours du choc séptique et leur influence sur le pronostic. Reanim Urg 19: 507-516
27. Schaer GL. (1996) Norepinephrine plus low-dose dopamine: a beneficial combination. Crit Care Med 26 :205
28. Schaer GLF, Parrillo MP (1985) Norepinephrine alone versus norepinephrine plus low doses dopamine: enhanced renal blood flow with combination pressor therapy. Crit Care Med 13: 492-496
29. Groeneveld ABJ, Navita JJP, Thijs LG (1989) Peripheral resistance in septic shock: its relation with outcome. Intensive Care Med 14: 141-147
30. Muchada R (1999) Non invasive hemodynamic diagnositic of hyperkinetic septic shock treated with a B Blocker. Intensive Care Med 25 [Suppl 1]: 142
31. Collins J A, Skidmore M A, Melvin D B, et al (1990) Home intravenous dobutamine therapy in patients awaiting heart transplantation. J Heart Transplant 9:205-208
32. Miller L W (1991) Outpatient dobutamine for refractory congestive heart failure: advantages, techniques and results. J Heart Lung Transplant 10:482-487
33. Hodgson J McB, Aja M, Sorkin RP (1984) Intermittent ambulatory dobutamine infusion in patients awaiting for cardiac transplantation. Am J Cardiol 53:375-376
34. Liang C, Tuttle RR, Hood W B Jr, et al (1979) Conditioning effects of chronic infusion of dobutamine comparison with exercise training. J Clin Invest 64:613-619
35. Swedelberg K Hjmalrson A, Waagstein F, Wellentin (1979) Prolongation of survival in congestive cardiomyopathy by beta receptor blockade. Lancet I: 1374-1376

36. Nanas J N, Kontoyannis D A, Alexopoulos G P, et al (2001) Long term intermittent dobutamine infusion combined with oral amiodarone improves the survival of patients with severe congestive heart failure. Chest 119: 1173-1178
37. Salvi S (2001) Protecting the myocardium from ischemic injury. A critical role for Alpha 1 adrenoreceptors? Chest 119:142-149
38. Li K, He H, Li C, et al (1997) Myocardial alpha 1 adrenoreceptors: inotropic effects and physiologic implication. Life Sci 60: 1305-1318
39. Vernon DD, Garret JS, Banner W, Dean JM (1992) Hemodynamic effects of dobutamine in an intact animal model. Crit Care Med 20 :1322-1329
40. Lefkowitz RJ, Rockman HA, Koch WJ (2000) Catecholamines, cardiac beta adrenergic receptors and heart failure. Circulation 101:1634-1637
41. Feldman AM, McTiernan C (1998) New insight into the role of enhanced adrenergic receptor--effector coupling in the heart. Circulation 98:1783-1789

Intraoperative Spinal Cord Monitoring: Evoked Potentials and Cerebrospinal Fluid Oxygenation

J. LIPS, C.J. KALKMAN

Surgical procedures that involve occlusion of the spinal cord feeding arteries, application of corrective forces to the spine, invasion of the cord, or local osteotomy carry the risk of iatrogenic spinal cord injury. Current reports indicate that the incidence of paraplegia after aortic surgery ranges between less than 0.1% after repair of aortic coarctation and 15% after resection of thoracoabdominal aneurysms [1-3]. The incidence of neurological deficits after correction of kyphosis and congenital scoliosis varies between 1% and 2% [4]. Definite numbers of spinal cord injury after spinal neurosurgery are lacking, although an increasing use of spinal cord monitoring is reported in these procedures [5, 6].

The purpose of intraoperative monitoring of the spinal cord is the detection of spinal cord dysfunction before irreversible damage has occurred, allowing immediate corrective action. The worst-case scenario in surgical procedures that carry a risk for spinal cord ischemia is a patient who awakes paraplegic after an otherwise uneventful operation. Because the consequences of iatrogenic paraplegia are so devastating, spinal cord monitoring techniques should have a high sensitivity and minimal false-negative monitoring results. In general, the combination of fast and reliable detection of spinal cord dysfunction and the availability of successful surgical measures should reduce the number of unfavorable neurological outcomes. During spinal (neuro)surgery, such measures may include the reduction of traction on the spinal cord, guided decompressive surgery, or the increase of spinal cord perfusion pressure. During resection of thoracoabdominal aneurysms, retrograde perfusion of the spinal cord or reattachment of spinal cord feeding vessels in the graft can be applied to maintain spinal cord perfusion. In this review, currently used clinical methods of intraoperative spinal cord monitoring are described and their efficiency for the detection of spinal cord ischemia is discussed.

Spinal cord monitoring techniques

There are several techniques for intraoperative evaluation of spinal cord function. The classical wake-up test is very specific for spinal cord motor function, but has several practical drawbacks. The patient has to be awake and cooperative, surgical and anesthesiological proceedings might be disturbed, and monitoring is not continuous. Evoked potentials permit the noninvasive, functional assessment of spinal cord tracts transmitting sensory or motor information. Somatosensory evoked potentials to electrical stimulation of peripheral nerves (SSEP) are particulary widely used. A newer technique is myogenic motor evoked potentials to transcranial stimulation (tcMEP), which is very specific for ischemic dysfunction of the spinal cord motor pathways. Finally, intrathecal PO_2 measurements (CSF-PO_2) can be used to indirectly evaluate spinal cord oxygenation.

Somatosensory evoked potentials

SSEPs are electrophysiological responses of the central nervous system to stimulation of a peripheral nerve. Usually, stimulation is applied to the posterior tibial nerve at the ankle, because this site is readily accessible during the operation. Recordings are most commonly performed over the scalp (cortical SSEP), but can also be obtained from needle electrodes placed in the interspinous ligaments or the epidural space at different spinal cord levels. The SSEP displays the integrity of transmission through the ascending sensory tracts located in the dorsal columns of the spinal cord. The use of SSEP for the prevention of iatrogenic spinal cord injury is based on the hypothesis that severe ischemia of the ascending white matter tracts will result in significant changes in latency and amplitude of the cortical signal before irreversible neuronal damage occurs. The criterion for detection of spinal cord ischemia requiring intervention during vascular and spinal surgery was empirically defined as a decrease in signal amplitude of more than 50% or an increase of the signal latency of more than 10% [7]. Signal-averaging is necessary to separate the relatively small amplitude of SSEP [a factor 1,000 smaller than for example electrocardiographic (ECG) signals] from the background noise of biological and background signals in the operation room.

Motor evoked potentials

MEPs are the responses of the muscle, peripheral nerve, or spinal cord that result from electrical stimulation of the motor cortex or spinal cord. Although at least six combinations of stimulation and recording sites exist, the recording of muscle responses to a train of electrical or magnetic transcranial stimulations (tcMEP) appears to produce the most-efficient and stable signal. The tcMEP displays the integrity of transmission through the descending motor tracts and motoneuron synapses that are located in the ventral aspect of the spinal cord. The use of tcMEP for the prevention of iatrogenic spinal cord injury is based on the hypothesis that ischemia of the most-vulnerable segment in the cortico-spinal motor pathway, i.e., the motoneuronal synapses in the lumbar spinal cord, results in significant changes in amplitude of the myogenic response before irreversible neuronal damage occurs. The criterion for detection of spinal cord ischemia requiring intervention was defined on empirical grounds as a reduction of tcMEP amplitude to less than 25% of the baseline value [8]. The more--restrictive criterion for spinal cord dysfunction during tcMEP monitoring compared with SSEP recording was based on the relatively larger amplitude variability of tcMEP signals.

A possible reason for the delayed arrival of tcMEP monitoring in the operation room is that most anesthetic drugs, and especially volatile agents, decrease the excitability of the motor pathways [9, 10]. The myogenic tcMEP amplitude is of comparable size to ECG readings, and signal-acquisition is usually performed once a minute.

Spinal cord oxygenation

Indirect monitoring of spinal cord oxygenation is a relatively new technique that has been introduced recently during aortic surgery. Continuous measurement of parenchymal oxygenation via implanted microprobes has already been used clinically to detect cerebral ischemia after traumatic brain injury [11, 12], but direct measurement of spinal cord tissue oxygenation is not feasible with the current technology. However, the changes in cerebrospinal PO_2 (CSF-PO_2) values, which can be more readily determined, appear to parallel neuronal tissue oxygenation [13]. Recent observations in experimental models and in patients undergoing resection of thoracoabdominal aortic aneurysms indicate that intrathecal PO_2 decreases after aortic cross-clamping [14, 15]. CSF-PO_2 can be measured with fibreoptic devices and Clark-type electrodes that are inserted in the lumbar intrathecal space. Measurement of PO_2 values can be performed up to every 2 s. In a recent study (data not shown) a reduction of CSF-PO_2 by 50% correlated with clinical spinal cord ischemia as measured with tcMEP during experimental spinal cord ischemia. The technique seems to have a high temporal resolution for the detection of spinal cord ischemia and reperfusion.

Anesthesiological effects on evoked potentials

The recording of evoked potentials can be substantially influenced by many anesthetic agents that are commonly used in the operating room. Anesthetic drugs decrease the synaptic excitability in the central and peripheral nervous system. The cortical component of SSEP and the cortical and spinal motoneuronal component of tcMEP are especially vulnerable to reduction of neuronal excitability induced by volatile agents.

Recording of cortical and myogenic responses is possible with nitrous oxide 50%/opioid anesthesia, but evoked potentials are completely abolished when the mixture is combined with isoflurane 0.3% [9]. Intravenous agents that are known to possess muscle-relaxing properties, such as benzodiazepines, barbiturates, and propofol, severely depress myogenic tcMEP but do not substantially affect SSEP responses. However, application of multiple transcranial pulses within a short time interval can partly overcome the observed tcMEP amplitude reductions of these and most other anesthetic agents. Pharmacological agents that increase muscle tone, such as ketamine, fentanyl, sufentanil, and etomidate, do not affect tcMEP substantially. Etomidate is the only anesthetic drug known to increase SSEP amplitude. A widely accepted anesthetic technique during SSEP monitoring consists of the combination of the following agents: benzodiazepine premedication, barbiturate induction, bolus and continuous infusion of fentanyl, sufentanil, or alfentanil, and nitrous oxide 50%, with or without low concentrations (5 minimal alveolar concentration) of volatile agents. An anesthetic technique for the monitoring of myogenic tcMEP might consist of the following: benzodiazepine premedication, etomidate induction, sufentanil maintenance with a supplement bolus of ketamine. Alternatively, total intravenous anesthesia using continuous infusions of opioid and low-dose propofol may provide acceptable tcMEP recording conditions. During tcMEP recording, partial muscle relaxation can be maintained with a closed loop administration of vecuronium. In general, boluses of centrally active medication should be avoided during monitoring of evoked potentials. Temperature effects influence nerve conduction velocity, and this should be taken into account during interpretation of latency changes of the SSEP signal.

Comparison of monitoring techniques

Most studies indicating that the intraoperative use of SSEP can decrease the incidence of postoperative neurological deficits were carried out during orthopedic surgery. The correction of acute spinal injuries was associated with a smaller number of new neurological injuries in patients that were monitored with SSEP during the procedure compared with patients that were not monitored or underwent a wake-up test only [16]. In a retrospective multicenter study, SSEPs were used in the majority of scoliosis procedures, reducing the incidence of neurological deficits compared with procedures that were not monitored [17]. Although SSEP can increase the safety of certain orthopedic and neurosurgical procedures, the technique monitors mainly sensory spinal cord tracts, which are located in the dorsal aspect of the cord. This part of the spinal cord is perfused via another arterial system than the ventral spinal cord (which comprises the anterior horn motoneurons that innervate the leg musculature), and receives a more-robust input directly from the aorta. Furthermore, synaptic transmission in motoneurons is more sensitive to ischemia than white matter transmission. This might explain the long delay (more than 15 min) between onset and detection of ischemia with SSEP after aortic cross-clamping or hypoxia [18, 19]. Thus, there is a distinct though rare chance that a stable SSEP signal is measured throughout a surgical procedure in the presence of a motor pathway dysfunction. Indeed, several reports indicate false-negative monitoring results of SSEP that can reduce the application of the technique in procedures that carry a risk of spinal cord motor pathway ischemia [6, 20, 21]. Also, especially during resection of aortic aneurysms, in which immediate and continuous feedback is necessary to guide reattachment of spinal cord feeding arteries to the graft, the delayed detection time of SSEP might hinder the use of this technique for the detection of fast changes in spinal cord perfusion.

tcMEPs are highly specific for the integrity of motor pathway conduction and are lost almost immediately after cross-clamping of the thoracic aorta, probably as a result of ischemic synaptic failure in the anterior horn motoneurons. The loss of myogenic tcMEP correlates with a severe reduction of anterior spinal cord blood flow. Contributing to the variability of tcMEP amplitude is the use of partial muscle relaxation, which balances the surgical considerations of patient immobility and movements after transcranial stimulation and the minimal requirements for myogenic evoked potentials recording. The fast detection of spinal cord ischemia by tcMEP provided identification of segmental arteries that were critical to spinal cord perfusion in both the clinical and the experimental setting [22, 23]. Although the predictive value of intraoperative tcMEP for postoperative neurological outcome is presently unknown, there is evidence indicating that loss of tcMEP signals precedes irreversible damage during experimental spinal cord ischemia [24].

Functional assessment of the spinal cord seems more reliable than indirect measurements of spinal cord oxygenation. However, there are some advantages of CSF-PO_2 measurement compared with motor evoked potentials. Movement artefacts that are associated with partial neuromuscular blockade, the delivery of high-voltage stimuli to the brain, and the complexity of tcMEP monitoring may render CSF-PO_2 measurement more suitable for spinal neurosurgery than tcMEP. There seems to be considerable discussion as to the reliability of recording absolute PO_2 values, but the real-time relative CSF-PO_2 changes after occlusion of spinal cord feeding vessels appear valid. Several physiological parameters, such as end-tidal CO_2, mean arterial pressure, intracranial pressure, pH, and temperature, have to be controlled carefully to avoid artefacts in CSF-PO_2 measurement. More research is needed to determine if CSF-PO_2 detects spinal cord ischemia before irreversible neuronal damage has occurred. A first step might be a validation of the technique with functional measurements of the spinal cord during fast changes in experimentally induced spinal cord hypoperfusion.

Conclusions

The currently available techniques for intraoperative monitoring of the spinal cord aim to detect spinal cord ischemia before irreversible neuronal damage has occurred during spinal and vascular surgical procedures. Evoked potentials measure the conduction in motor, sensory, or a mixed motor/sensory spinal trajectory. Myogenic responses to transcranial stimulation are completely specific for motor pathway function and reduce rapidly during spinal cord ischemia, but can not be recorded when volatile agents or complete neuromuscular blockade are used. SSEP reliably detects global spinal cord ischemia after an initial delay, but lacks sensitivity for the detection of isolated motor pathway dysfunction. The continuous measurement of intrathecal oxygenation might be used intraoperatively in addition to motor evoked potentials, or in critical care environments.

References

1. Schepens MA, Vermeulen FE, Morshuis WJ, et al (1999) Impact of left heart bypass on the results of thoracoabdominal aortic aneurysm repair. Ann Thorac Surg 67: 1963-1967
2. Martin GH, O'Hara PJ, Hertzer NR, et al (2000) Surgical repair of aneurysms involving the suprarenal, visceral, and lower thoracic aortic segments: early results and late outcome. J Vasc Surg 31: 851-862
3. Svensson LG, Crawford ES, Hess KR, et al (1993) Experience with 1509 patients undergoing thoracoabdominal aortic operations. J Vasc Surg 17: 357-368
4. Dawson EG, Sherman JE, Kanim LE, Nuwer MR (1991) Spinal cord monitoring. Results of the Scoliosis Research Society and the European Spinal Deformity Society survey. Spine 16: S361-S364
5. Sala F, Niimi Y, Krzan MJ, et al (1999) Embolization of a spinal arteriovenous malformation: correlation between motor evoked potentials and angiographic findings: technical case report. Neurosurgery 45: 932-937

6. Deutsch H, Arginteanu M, Manhart K, et al (2000) Somatosensory evoked potential monitoring in anterior thoracic vertebrectomy. J Neurosurg 92: 155-161
7. York DH, Chabot RJ, Gaines RW (1987) Response variability of somatosensory evoked potentials during scoliosis surgery. Spine 12: 864-876
8. de Haan P, Kalkman CJ, de Mol BA, et al (1997) Efficacy of transcranial motor-evoked myogenic potentials to detect spinal cord ischemia during operations for thoracoabdominal aneurysms. J Thorac Cardiovasc Surg 113: 87-100
9. Kalkman CJ, Drummond JC, Ribberink AA (1991) Low concentrations of isoflurane abolish motor evoked responses to transcranial electrical stimulation during nitrous oxide/opioid anesthesia in humans. Anesth Analg 73: 410-415
10. King BS, Rampil IJ (1994) Anesthetic depression of spinal motor neurons may contribute to lack of movement in response to noxious stimuli. Anesthesiology 81: 1484-1492
11. Maas AI, Fleckenstein W, de Jong DA, van Santbrink H (1993) Monitoring cerebral oxygenation: experimental studies and preliminary clinical results of continuous monitoring of cerebrospinal fluid and brain tissue oxygen tension. Acta Neurochir (Wien) [Suppl] 59: 50-57
12. Valadka AB, Gopinath SP, Contant CF, et al (1998) Relationship of brain tissue PO2 to outcome after severe head injury. Crit Care Med 26: 1576-1581
13. Ishizaki M, Sugiyama S, Uchida H, et al (1997) Intrathecal oxygen concentration as a new indicator of spinal cord ischemia. Acta Med Okayama 51: 71-77
14. Hellberg A, Ulus AT, Christiansson L, et al (2001) Monitoring of intrathecal oxygen tension during experimental aortic occlusion predicts ultrastructural changes in the spinal cord. J Thorac Cardiovasc Surg 121: 316-323
15. Christiansson L, Karacagil S, Thelin S, Bergqvist D (1998) Continuous monitoring of intrathecal pO2, pCO2 and pH during surgical replacement of type II thoracoabdominal aortic aneurysm. Eur J Vasc Endovasc Surg 15: 78-81
16. Meyer PR Jr, Cotler HB, Gireesan GT (1988) Operative neurological complications resulting from thoracic and lumbar spine internal fixation. Clin Orthop : 125-131
17. Nuwer MR, Dawson EG, Carlson LG, et al (1995) Somatosensory evoked potential spinal cord monitoring reduces neurologic deficits after scoliosis surgery: results of a large multicenter survey. Electroencephalogr Clin Neurophysiol 96: 6-11
18. Cunningham JN Jr, Laschinger JC, Spencer FC (1987) Monitoring of somatosensory evoked potentials during surgical procedures on the thoracoabdominal aorta. IV. Clinical observations and results. J Thorac Cardiovasc Surg 94: 275-285
19. Kobrine AI, Evans DE, Rizzoli HV (1980) Effects of progressive hypoxia on long tract neural conduction in the spinal cord. Neurosurgery 7: 369-375
20. Lesser RP, Raudzens P, Luders H, et al (1986) Postoperative neurological deficits may occur despite unchanged intraoperative somatosensory evoked potentials. Ann Neurol 19: 22-25
21. Ben-David B, Haller G, Taylor P (1987) Anterior spinal fusion complicated by paraplegia. A case report of a false-negative somatosensory-evoked potential. Spine 12: 536-539
22. de Haan P, Kalkman CJ, Meylaerts SA et al (1999) Development of spinal cord ischemia after clamping of noncritical segmental arteries in the pig. Ann Thorac Surg 68: 1278-1284
23. Jacobs M, Meylaerts SA, de Haan P, et al (1999) Strategies to prevent neurologic deficit based on motor-evoked potentials in type I and II thoracoabdominal aortic aneurysm repair. J Vasc Surg 29: 48-57
24. Reuter DG, Tacker WA Jr, Badylak SF, et al (1992) Correlation of motor-evoked potential response to ischemic spinal cord damage. J Thorac Cardiovasc Surg 104: 262-272

Spinal Cord Injury in Thoracoabdominal Aneurysm Surgery: Methods of Intra-operative Protection of the Spinal Cord

E. P. VAN DONGEN, M.A. SCHEPENS, E.H. BOEZEMAN

Aneurysms extending from the descending thoracic aorta into the abdominal aorta are classified as thoracoabdominal aneurysms. The first thoracoabdominal aortic aneurysm was replaced by a homograft in 1954 [1]. With the current anaesthetic practice and advances in operative techniques, respiratory management, intensive care and graft materials the 30 days in-hospital- mortality and morbidity have been improved, but are still high. A mortality range of 8-35%, an incidence of paraplegia/paraparesis of 16-38%, an incidence of renal failure of 18-27% and re-exploration for bleeding in 7% of the cases have been reported [2-6].

Paraplegia, as a consequence of spinal cord ischaemia after aorta cross-clamping, is still one of the most serious complication of thoracoabdominal aortic aneurysm operations with prosthetic replacement. Many strategies for decreasing the risk of paraplegia have been proposed. Systemic or topical (epidural cooling) hypothermia can be used to protect the spinal cord [7-13]. Improving spinal cord blood supply can be achieved by cerebrospinal fluid (CSF) drainage, reducing the time of cross-clamping, reimplantation of intercostal arteries, left-heart bypass, and staged clamping to maximize the beneficial effect of the left-heart bypass [13-20]. The pharmacological strategy aims at increasing the ischaemic tolerance of the spinal cord [13, 15-26]. Neuroprotective treatment can be initiated before the ischaemic period to maximize neuroprotection.

In order to evaluate the benefits of the protection strategies mentioned, it is necessary to have a reliable spinal cord monitor. The measurement of biochemical markers of neuronal damage in the cerebrospinal fluid is another approach to monitor the metabolism in spinal cord neurons. Neurophysiological monitoring, recording of motor evoked potentials and somatosensory evoked potentials, of the spinal cord can detect ischaemia during the clamping period. Recording of myogenic motor evoked potentials evoked by transcranial electrical stimulation (tcMEP) is a method of monitoring the integrity of the vulnerable motor pathways. Somatosensory evoked potential (SEP) reflects the electrophysiologic status of the ascending tracts of the posterior columns. Recording both tcMEP and SEP during operations for thoracoabdominal aortic aneurysms may improve the accuracy in terms of sensitivity and specificity. However, most anaesthetic drugs and neuromuscular blocking agents decrease the tcMEP response. For reliable monitoring it is important to achieve maximal myogenic responses with the least possible within-patient variability.

There is a close relationship between the metabolic requirements of the spinal cord and its blood supply. Perfusion of the cord depends on one or two cervical, two or three thoracic and one or two lumbar vessels feeding the longitudinal anastomoses formed by the anterior and paired posterior spinal arteries. The artery of Adamkiewicz is one of these vessels, and is larger than the others. It arises between T8 and L1 in 85% of individuals, makes a hairpin bend and delivers most of its blood distal to its junction with the anterior spinal artery. The diameter of the anterior spinal artery just above this junction is extremely small compared to below this junction, facilitating cephalocaudal flow. So, the lower thoracic cord is the critical zone of the spinal cord blood supply [27]. The degree and duration of ischaemia to the spinal cord during aortic cross clamping and failure to reattach the vessels critical to the blood supply of the spinal cord appear to be the predominant causes of postoperative spinal injury. In this chapter we describe some aspects of the multimodality strategy.

Methods of intra-operative protection of the spinal cord

Moderate systemic hypothermia

The mechanism of hypothermic spinal cord protection is complex. The patient should be cooled prior to aortic cross-clamping to a temperature of 30-33 Celsius to increase ischaemic spinal cord tolerance. For each degree decrease in cord temperature the oxygen requirements in neural tissue will decrease by 6-7%. Furthermore, it has been hypothesized that there is a reduced release of excitatory neurotransmitters during hypothermia and better membrane stabilization.

Cerebrospinal drainage

The spinal canal consisting of bony vertebral, dura and spinal cord can act as a compartment syndrome. Increased CSF pressure, as a result of thoracic aortic cross-clamping, may increase the incidence of postoperative spinal cord injury. Furthermore, the CSF pressure is increased by administration of either glyceryl trinitrate or sodium nitroprusside to control arterial hypertension. At pressures of 10-15 cm H_2O or higher, freely CSF drainage during surgery and the continuation of CSF drainage for the first two days after surgery is recommended to enhance spinal cord perfusion.

Reimplantation of intercostal and lumbar arteries

It is our policy to reimplant all major intercostal arteries between T8 and L2 if technically feasible. Reattachment of intercostal arteries may reduce the impact of haemodynamic instability on the spinal cord during operation and thereafter, but may lead to a longer cross-clamp time. The use of motor evoked potential and somatosensory evoked potential can be used to identify segmental arteries that supply the spinal cord and to monitor the neurophysiological effects of reperfusion of those critical segmental arteries. Maintenance of distal aortic pressure during cross-clamping permits sequential aortic occlusion. When marked MEP changes occur after a few minutes of excluding a particular aortic segment, the intercostal arteries within this segment are considered critical to the spinal circulation and promptly reattached. Failure to reattach these critical vessels to the prosthesis together with postoperative hypoxia and hypotension can be responsible for the occurrence of paraplegia. Preoperative highly selective angiography and intraoperative identification of intercostals by hydrogen and pO_2 testing have been described [28, 29].

Distal aortic perfusion

Concerning intra-operative management two schools exist: a simple clamp-repair technique and the technique of distal perfusion [16, 17, 18, 30, 31]. Using "clamp and go", the aorta is cross-clamped and the aneurysm is replaced without spinal cord protective measures in less than 30 minutes (within this period there is a low risk of irreversible deficits). An open distal anastomosis is performed. Proximal hypertension can be treated with vasodilators or permissive partial backbleeding through the distal aorta and segmental vessels.

Perfusion of the distal aorta by partial left heart bypass (left atrium-femoral artery) with the use of a simple centrifugal pump facilitates both afterload reduction and increases distal aortic pressure. This device reduces the degree of ischaemia. Furthermore, the bypass avoids vasodilators, a heat exchanger can be applied and CSF pressures are maintained at baseline-levels during cross-clamping [32]. Minimal heparinisation is required.

Somatosensory evoked potential monitoring and transcranial motor evoked myogenic potential monitoring

The earliest reports of the employment of evoked potentials to monitor spinal cord function during TAA(A) surgery utilized the somatosensory response to stimulation of the posterior tibial nerve at the ankle or in the popliteal fossa. This electrical potential, obtained from the ongoing EEG, ranges from 0.2 - 5.0μV. Increasing the signal to noise ratio by signal averaging is the most common method to extract this signal from the EEG.

Two parameters are monitored: Latency of onset (in msec, measured as the time between stimulus and the onset of the potential) and amplitude (in μV, measured from baseline to peak, or peak to peak) of the response. For successful somatosensory pathway monitoring it is important to obtain baseline SEP recordings before the operation. Latency increase of more than 10% is considered as abnormal and signals the onset of spinal cord ischaemia. An amplitude reduction of more than 50% seems to correlate with persistent spinal cord ischaemia [33].

SEP changes may also occur as a consequence of anaesthetic agents, hypothermia, hypotension, intracranial pressure, hypoxemia, blood rheology (low haematocrit), ventilation ($pCO_2<2.5$ kPa), or positioning of the patient (due to compression of nerves or occlusion of blood vessels). These changes in the SEP are not associated with a surgical intervention related dysfunction anywhere along the somatosensory pathways. Therefore, all these factors may affect the specificity of SEP monitoring during TAA(A) surgery [33-35]. To allow differentiation between ischaemia of the spinal cord, central neurologic ischaemia or technical problems, SEPs from the median nerve at the wrist can be recorded simultaneously to cut the false positive rate down [36].

SEPs only reflect the electrophysiologic status of the ascending sensory tracts of the posterior columns, leaving the pyramidal tracts as well as the anterior horn cells undetected. Probably this is the reason why false negatives during monitoring of somatosensory evoked responses have been reported [37, 38].

There are two arguments supporting the addition of MEPs to an intraoperative spinal cord monitoring protocol. Firstly, the monitoring of MEPs can detect ischaemia of the anterior cord, that may leave the SEP recordings unaffected. Secondly, the area of the spinal cord supplied by the anterior spinal artery is more vulnerable to ischaemia [39].

Transcranial electrical stimulation activates directly the axons of pyramidal cells, causing the direct (D) waves, whereas indirect (I) waves, travelling down the same tract, arise from activation of cortical interneurons. The I waves show a phase delay of around 2 ms compared to D waves [40].

An advantage of transcranial stimulation during TAA(A) surgery is that the stimulation electrodes are placed outside the operative field.

The amplitude of the response in μV is usually measured as the voltage from the most negative component to the most positive component of the response. The onset latency in milliseconds is measured as the time from stimulation to the onset of the response. Injury to the motor pathways is perhaps seen as an increase in latency or a decrease in amplitude of the MEP. In case of ischaemia the amplitude of responses recorded from the spinal cord decreases more slowly than responses recorded from a peripheral nerve or muscle [41], because white matter is probably more resistant to ischaemia than grey matter of the anterior horn. Epidural recordings after transcranial stimulation do not show the integrity of the anterior horn grey matter, but monitor the corticospinal tracts only. Therefore, epidural recordings are possibly less important during resection of TAA(A), during which an ischaemic injury to the anterior horn might occur. Furthermore, recordings from the spinal cord and the peripheral nerve after spinal cord stimulation do not easily distinguish orthodromic signals in motor tracts from antidromic conduction in sensory pathways and so are not entirely specific for conduction alongside the motor pathways. In contrast to the NMEP, which is recorded from a mixed peripheral nerve with both motor and sensory fibres, the myogenic MEP is truly related to the functional integrity of motor pathways.

MEPs are similar to SEPs in being sensitive to nearly all types of anaesthetics, hypothermia, hypoxia and hypotension [33]. Anaesthetics depress the excitability of cortical motor neurons and probably spinal cord motor neurons [42, 43]. Nerve action potentials following spinal cord stimulation are less sensitive to volatile agents [44], but perhaps less sensitive to intraoperative injury due to the supposedly more suppressive effect of volatile agents to the motor component of the NMEP.

An additional disadvantage of the myogenic MEP is the need of neuromuscular blockade in aortic surgery [45, 46].

Multipulse stimulation may increase amplitude and the reproducibility of MEPs, probably as a result of temporal summation [56-58] To accomplish high sensitive as well as high specific spinal cord monitoring it is important to have a constant anaesthetic regimen, with a constant level of neuromuscular blockade.

De Haan et al. [48] described the use of transcranial motor evoked myogenic potentials during TAA(A) operations. They concluded that it was an effective method to detect spinal cord ischaemia within minutes.

Monitoring of evoked potentials requires a team approach of the surgeon, anaesthesiologist and clinical neurophysiologist. Every clinic has to define the anaesthetic strategy, the optimal stimulus parameter for perioperative MEP and

SEP monitoring to establish reliable criteria for spinal cord dysfunction. The most successful monitoring of intraoperative spinal cord integrity during TAA(A) surgery consists of a combination of SEP and MEP recording. Both, SEP and MEP, reflect an independent electrophysiological sign of spinal cord injury.

Spinal cord injury can also occur in the postoperative period. Hypotension and low flow states in the postoperative phase should be aggressively avoided and treated. MEP/SEP monitoring may be a method to evaluate the measures (haemodynamic, fluid and pharmacological interventions) to protect the spinal cord in the postoperative period as well.

Larger patient groups are needed to prove that MEP monitoring combined with SEP monitoring provide valuable information in predicting spinal cord ischaemia and in guiding the surgical strategy during TAA(A) surgery and in optimizing the postoperative management during intensive care.

Pharmacological neuroprotection

Many substances have been investigated in an effort to reduce the incidence of spinal cord injury after aortic cross-clamping. Indeed, additional damage to the spinal cord may result from reperfusion induced oxygen derived free radicals, lipid peroxydation, and oedema.

No agent has yet been shown to improve neurologic outcome in the clinical setting conclusively.

The list of neuroprotective substances include excitatory amino acid receptor blockers, calcium channel blockers, free radical scavengers, opiate receptor antagonists, corticosteroids, prostagladins, adenosine, GABA modulators, protein kinase C modulators, anaesthetics, inhibitors of leukocytes and monocytes, vasodilators, inhibitors of apoptosis, and modulators of coagulation and insulin [49].

Conclusion

In summary the goal of the above mentioned strategy is to optimize oxygen supply to the spinal cord, to reduce oxygen demand of the spinal cord and to reduce the development of the complex biochemical pathways of reperfusion injury. Much research will continue in the field of pharmaca and biochemical markers. The determination of the S-100 protein (e.g. in CSF) could be a marker of clinical value in evaluating the interventions taken and in detecting the patient at risk for spinal cord injury during the first postoperative hours or postoperative days [50]. The approach of combining the mentioned strategies and the information gained by the neurophysiological and biochemical monitor devices may contribute to an early detection and a reduction in spinal cord damage during and after thoracoabdominal surgery.

References

1. Etheredge SN, Yee J, Smith JV et al (1955) Successful resection of a large aneurysm of the upper abdominal aorta and replacement with homograft. Surgery 38: 1071-1081
2. Cox GS, O'Hara PJ, Hertzer NR et al (1992) Thoracoabdominal aneurysm repair: a representative experience. J Vasc Surg 15: 780-788
3. Golden MA, Donaldson MC, Whittemore MD et al (1993) Evolving experience with thoracoabdominal aortic aneurysm repair at a single institution. J Vasc Surg 13: 792-797
4. Schepens M, Dekker E, Hamerlijnck R et al (1996) Survival and aortic events after graft replacement for thoracoabdominal aortic aneurysms in 172 patients. Cardiovasc Surg 4: 713-719
5. Svensson LG, Crawford ES, Hess KR et al (1993) Experience with 1,509 patients undergoing thoraco-abdominal aortic operations. J Vasc Surg 17: 357-370
6. Hollier LH, Money SR, Naslund TC et al (1992) Risk of spinal cord dysfunction in patients undergoing thoracoabdominal aortic replacement. Am J Surg 164: 210-214
7. Allen BT, Davis CG, Osborne D et al (1994) Spinal cord ischemia and reperfusion metabolism: the effect of hypothermia. J Vasc Surg 19: 332-340
8. Kwun BD, Vacanti FX (1995) Mild hypothermia protects against irreversible damage during prolonged spinal cord ischemia. J Surg Res 59: 780-782
9. Marsala M, Vanick I, Yaksh TL (1994) Effect of graded hypothermia (27°C to 34°C) on behavorial function, histopathology, and spinal blood flow after spinal ischemia in rat. Stroke 25: 2038-2046
10. Salazano RP, Ellison LH, Altonji PF et al (1994) Regional deep hypothermia of the spinal cord protects against ischemic injury during thoracic aortic cross-clamping. Ann Thor Surg 57:65-70
11. Cambria RP, Davison JK, Zanetti S et al (1997) Clinical experience with epidural cooling for spinal cord protection during thoracic and thoracoabdominal aneurysm repair. J Vasc Surg 25: 234-243
12. Kouchoukos NT, Daily BB, Rokkas CK et al (1995) Hypothermic bypass and circulatory arrest for operations on the descending thoracic and thoracoabdominal aorta. Ann Thor Surg 60: 67-77
13. Acher CW, Wynn MM, Hoch JR et al (1994) Combined use of cerebrospinal fluid drainage and naloxone reduces the risk of paraplegia in thoracoabdominal aneurysm repair. J Vasc Surg 19: 236-248
14. Crawford ES, Svensson LG, Hess KR et al (1991) A prospective randomized study of cerebrospinal fluid drainage to prevent paraplegia after high-risk surgery on the thoracoabdominal aorta. J Vasc Surg 13: 36-46
15. Woloszyn TT, Marini CP, Coons MS et al (1990) Cerebrospinal fluid drainage and steroids provide better spinal cord protection during aortic cross-clamping than does either treatment alone. Ann Thor Surg 49: 78-82
16. Safi HJ, Bartoli S, Hess KR et al (1994) Neurologic deficit in patients at high risk with thoracoabdominal aortic aneurysms: the role of cerebrospinal fluid drainage and distal aortic perfusion. J Vasc Surg 20: 434-443
17. Schepens MA, Defauw JJ, Hamerlijnck RP et al (1995) The use of a left heart bypass in the surgical repair of thoracoabdominal aortic aneurysms. Ann Vasc Surg 9: 327-338
18. Svensson LG, Hess KR, Coselli JS et al (1994) Influence of segmental arteries, extent, and atriofemoral bypass on postoperative paraplegia after thoracoabdominal aortic operations. J Vasc Surg 20: 255-262

19. Safi HJ, Miller CC, Carr C et al (1998) Importance of intercostal artery reattachment during thoracoabdominal aortic aneurysm repair. J Vasc Surg 27: 58-68
20. Gharagozloo F, Larson J, Dausman MJ et al (1996) Spinal cord protection during surgical procedures on the descending thoracic and thoracoabdominal aorta. Chest 109: 799-809
21. Simpson JI, Eide TR, Schiff GA et al (1994) Intrathecal magnesium sulfaye protects the spinal cord from ischemic injury during thoracic aortic cross-clamping. Anesthesiology 81: 1493-1499
22. Wisselink W, Money SR, Crockett DE et al (1994) Ischemia-reperfusion injury of the spinal cord; protective effect of the hydroxyl radical scavenger dimethylthiourea. J Vasc Surg 20: 444-449
23. Elmore JR, Gloviczky P, Harper CM et al (1992) Spinal cord injury in experimental thoracic aortic occlusion: investigation of combined methods of protection. J Vasc Surg 15: 789-799
24. Svensson LG (1997) New and future approaches for spinal cord protection. Semin Thor Cardiovasc Surg 9: 206-221
25. Mauney MC, Blackbourne LH, Langenburg SE et al (1995) Prevention of spinal cord injury after repair of the thoracic or thoracoabdominal aorta. Thorac Surg 59: 245-252
26. Rokkas C, Helfrich LR, Lobner D et al (1994) Dextrorphan inhibits the release of excitatory amino acids during spinal cord ischemia. Ann Thorac Surg 58: 312-320
27. Domisse GF (1974) The blood supply of the spinal cord. J Bone and Joint Surg 56B(2): 225-235
28. Svensson LG (1996) Intraoperative identification of spinal cord blood supply during repairs of the descending aorta and thoracoabdominal aorta. J Thorac Cardiovasc Surg 112: 1455-1460
29. Williams GM, Perler BA, Burdick JF, et al (1991) Angiographic localization of spinal cord blood supply and its relationship to postoperative paraplegia. J Vasc Surg 13: 23-33
30. Cambria RP, Davison JK, Zanetti S, L'Italien G, Atamian S. (1997) Thoracoabdominal aortic aneurysm repair: Perspectives over a decade with the clamp-and-sew technique. Ann Surg 226(3): 294-303
31. Jacobs MJHM, Myhre HO, Norgern L. (1999) Thoracoabdominal aortic surgery with special reference to spinal cord protection and perfusion techniques. Eur J Vasc Endovasc Surg 17: 253-256
32. Kaplan DK, Atsumi N, D'Ambria MN, Vlahakes GJ (1995) Distal circulatory support for thoracic aortic operations: effects on intracranial pressure. Ann Thorac Surg 59(2): 448-452
33. Brown RH, Nash CL Jr, Berilla JA et al (1984) Cortical evoked potential monitoring. A system for intraoperative monitoring of spinal cord function Spine. 9 (3): 256-261
34. Drummond JC, Todd MM, U HS (1985) The effects of high dose sodium thiopental on brain stem auditory and median nerve somatosensory evoked responses in humans. Anesthesiology 63: 249-254
35. Sloan TB, Fugina ML, Toleikis JR (1990) Effects of midazolam on median nerve somatosensoryevoked potentials. Br J Anaesth 64: 590-593
36. Shahin GM, Hamerlijnck RP, Schepens MA et al (1996) Upper and lower extremity somatosensory evoked potential recording during surgery for aneurysms of the descending thoracic aorta. Eur J Cardio-thorac Surg 10: 299-304
37. Takaki O, Okumura F (1985) Application and limitation of somatosensory evoked potential monitoring during thoracic aortic aneurysm surgery: a case report. Anesthesiology 63: 700-703
38. Ginsburg HH, Shetter AG, Raudszens PA (1985) Postoperative paraplegia with preserved intraoperative somatosensory evoked potentials. J Neurosurg 63: 296-300
39. Brockstein B (1994) Bloodsupply to the spinal cord: anatomic and physiologic correlations. Ann Vasc Surg 8: 394-399
40. Rothwell J, Burke D, Hicks R et al (1994) Transcranial electrical stimulation of the motor cortex in man: further evidence for the site of activation. J Physiol 481: 243-250
41. de Haan, Kalkman CJ, Ubags LH et al (1996) A comparison of the sensitivity of epidural and myogenic transcranial motor-evoked responses in the detection of acute spinal cord ischemia in the rabbit. Anesth Analg 83: 1022-1027
42. van Dongen EP, ter Beek HT, Schepens MA et al (1999) Effect of nitrous oxide on myogenic

motor potentials evoked by a six pulse train of transcranial electrical stimuli: a possible monitor for aortic surgery. 82:323-328
43. Kalkman CJ, Drummond JC, Ribberink AA et al (1992) Effects of propofol, etomidate, midazolam and fentanyl on motor evoked responses to transcranial electrical or magnetic stimulation in humans. Anesthesiology 76:502-509
44. Bernard JM, Pereon Y, Fayet G et al (1996) Effects of isoflurane and desflurane on neurogenic motor- and somatosensory-evoked potential monitoring for scoliosis surgery. Anesthesiology 85: 1013-1019.
45. Kalkman CJ, Drummond JC, Kenelly NA et al(1992) Intraoperative monitoring of tibialis anterior muscle motor evoked responses to transcranial electrical stimulation during partial neuromuscular blockade. Anesth Analg 75: 584-89.
46. Dongen van EP, ter Beek HT, Schepens MA et al (1999) Within patiënt variability of myogenic motor evoked potentials to multi-pulse transcranial electrical stimulation during two levels of partial neuromuscular blockade in aortic surgery. 88:22-27
47. Kalkman CJ, Ubags LH, Been HD et al (1995) Improved amplitude of myogenic motor evoked responses after paired transcranial electrical stimulation during sufentani/nitrous oxide anesthesia. Anesthesiology 83: 270-276
48. de Haan P, Kalkman CJ, de Mol BA et al (1997) Efficacy of transcranial motor-evoked myogenic potentials to detect spinal cord ischemia during operations for thoracoabdominal aneurysms. J Thorac Cardiovasc Surg 113: 87-100
49. de Haan P, (1999) Spinal cord ischemia in thoracoabdominal aneurysm surgery: monitoring and conditioning the spinal cord. Tela Thesis: 43-71
50. van Dongen EP, ter Beek HT, Schepens MA et al (2000) The relationship between evoked potentials and measurements of S-100 protein in cerebrospinal fluid during and after thoracoabdominal aortic aneurysm surgery J Vasc Surg 30(2): 293-300

Ischaemic Spinal Cord Injury Following Thoracoabdominal Aneurysm Surgery

P. DE HAAN, J. KESECIOGLU

Thoracoabdominal or descending thoracic aneurysm surgery carries the risk of ischaemic spinal cord injury. Since the appearance of thoracoabdominal reconstructions in the early 1950's, the risk of paraplegia or paraparesis was soon recognized as a complication of these procedures. The paradigm for paraplegia causation, the interruption of the de-segmented blood supply to the anterior spinal artery, was established by Adams [1]. The extent of the aneurysm was found to be a significant predictor of spinal cord injury. Crawford classified thoracoabdominal aortic aneurysms (TAAA) as follows: type I involves the descending thoracic and upper abdominal aorta; type II includes the entire descending aorta and the abdominal aorta below the renal arteries, and is the most extensive; type III includes less then half of the descending thoracic aorta and most of the abdominal aorta; and type IV involves most or all of the abdominal aorta [2]. In 1 509 patients who had undergone repair for the treatment of thoracoabdominal aortic disease, Svensson found that type I, II, III, and IV aneurysms were associated with lower extremity neurological deficit rates of 15%, 31%, 7%, and 4% respectively [3]. The incidence of overall neurological deficits in that series was 16 %. In another large series of patients, which were equally distributed between types I to IV aneurysms, the long-term survivors (30 days) had a 4.4 % incidence of paraplegia and a 5% incidence of paraparesis[2]. In contrast, after elective abdominal aortic aneurysms surgery the incidence of lower extremity neurological deficits was 0.16 - 0.25 % [4, 5]. Repair of aneurysms confined to the descending thoracic aorta resulted in paraplegia in 6.5 % of the patients [6]. Despite recent advances in the treatment of thoracoabdominal aneurysms, postoperative paraparesis or paraplegia remains a distinct possibility after an otherwise successful operation. Variables predictive of neurologic deficits of the lower extremities include aortic clamp time, the presence of rupture or dissection, the extent of aneurysm, a history of smoking, postoperative hypotension, and age [2, 3, 7, 8].

The aetiology of neurological injury after aortic operations is thought to be a temporary or a permanent interruption of spinal cord blood supply, resulting in neuronal hypoxia. Irreversible injury to motor neurons and white matter axons will result in lower extremity neurological deficits. When the aorta is simply cross-clamped and replaced without adjuncts to protect the spinal cord, there is a sigmoidal relationship between the duration of thoracic aortic cross-clamping and the probability of spinal cord injury. If the time of aortic clamping does not exceed 30 minutes, the risk of postoperative neurological deficits appears. The probability of paraplegia increases linearly between 30 and 60 minutes of ischaemia, and to almost 90% after one hour of thoracic occlusion [9].

In the past four decades, numerous strategies have been described that protect the spinal cord during TAAA surgery. The prevention of irreversible ischaemic spinal cord injury is based on three principles. First, to minimize the degree and duration of ischaemia during the aortic crossclamping procedure, by means of techniques that maintain spinal cord blood flow. Second, to definitively restore spinal cord blood supply. This necessitates reattachment of the segmental arteries to the graft. Third, to apply neuroprotective strategies that improve neuronal survival following temporary spinal cord ischaemia, because prolonged transient spinal cord ischaemia will result in paraplegia despite adequate restoration of spinal cord blood supply.

Single clamp-repair

In TAAA surgery, the duration of aortic cross-clamping has consistently been a predictor of ischaemic spinal cord injury [2, 3,10-12]. Using a single clamp-repair technique ("clamp and sew", "clamp and go"), the aorta is simply cross-clamped and the aneurysm is rapidly replaced without spinal cord protective measures which might increase cross-clamp time, like distal aortic perfusion and segmental artery preservation. The rationale for this modality is to limit cross-clamp time to 30 minutes. This threshold is associated with a low risk of irreversible deficits [9]. Using a single clamp-repair technique, an open distal anastomosis is performed. Proximal hypertension is controlled with vasodilators and permissive partial exsanguination (back-bleeding through the distal aorta and through segmental vessels) [13, 14]. In patients with aneurysms confined to the descending thoracic aorta, Scheinin and Cooley described an average clamp time of 22 minutes [14]. In thoracic aneurysm repair with the single clamp-repair technique, Crawford reported a 0.9 % paraplegia rate [15]. However, in 260 patients with thoracoabdominal aneurysms, the single clamp-repair technique resulted in an incidence of paraplegia and paraparesis of 5% and 10%, respectively [11].

In conclusion, the single clamp-repair technique might be beneficial only for aneurysms confined to the descending thoracic aorta. In TAAA surgery, additional protective strategies that maintain and restore spinal cord blood supply should be applied.

Strategies to maintain adequate spinal cord blood flow

Distal aortic perfusion

When the aortic cross-clamp time exceeds 30 minutes, the risk of irreversible spinal cord damage rapidly increases. As a consequence additional protective measures are necessary to provide blood flow to the spinal cord during cross-clamping. Using retrograde or distal aortic perfusion, the aorta and corresponding segmental arteries can be perfused below the level of repair during graft inclusion. Distal aortic perfusion can be realized by a passive shunt or by various bypass techniques. In addition, these techniques reduce aortic pressure proximal to the clamp and decrease left ventricle afterload, often without the need of pharmacological interventions. An important division in currently used operation techniques for TAAA repair is based on the use of distal aortic perfusion; single clamp-repair vs. operations with distal perfusion, double aortic clamping, and sequential repairs.

Passive aortic shunts were first described by Gott [16]. A so-called Gott-shunt consists of a tube with a 5 - 6 mm internal diameter and a nonthrombogenic luminal coating, and is positioned (arterial-arterial) to bypass the cross-clamped aortic segment. As a result of the heparin coating, the shunt obviates the need for systemic heparinization. In 359 patients undergoing elective repair of aneurysms confined to the descending thoracic aorta, no lower extremity neurological deficits were encountered with the use of a Gott shunt [17]. There are several disadvantages of passive shunting. Maximum shunt flow is insufficient to unload the proximal circulation [18]. The static blood flow in the shunt can not be regulated to address specific problems encountered during cross-clamping. In addition, the Gott shunt only provided distal pressures less than 40 mmHg [19].

Among the various techniques to accomplish active distal aortic perfusion, partial cardiopulmonary bypass (femoral vein to femoral artery), has the distinct disadvantage of requiring full heparinization. Partial left heart bypass (left atrium-femoral artery) with the use of a simple centrifugal pump obviates the difficulties associated with active roller pumps as well as passive shunts. With this technique flow can be regulated, minimal heparinization is required, selective organ perfusion can be used, and a heat exchanger can be applied [20-22]. In a porcine experiment, active distal perfusion resulted in distal aortic pressures significantly higher than those achieved with passive shunting. Furthermore, the use of atrio-femoral bypass maintained cerebrospinal fluid (CSF) pressures at baseline levels during cross-clamping, while passive shunting increased CSF pressures significantly above baseline [19]. Distal aortic perfusion in combination with sequential and segmental repairs of the aorta maintained spinal cord electrophysiological activity while proximal anastomosis was performed [23]. Coselli and de Mol reported a reduced duration of intercostal ischaemic time with atrio-femoral bypass [24, 25].

Despite these obvious advantages, distal aortic perfusion with a centrifugal pump did not consistently improve neurologic outcome. In some clinical studies describing TAAA surgery , atrio-femoral bypass was associated with a decrease in the incidence of paraplegia and paraparesis [10, 12, 26, 27]. In a prospective non-randomized study of 99 patients, atrio-femoral bypass improved neurologic outcome, especially when distal bypass was combined with sequential aortic clamping and segmental repairs [10]. In a retrospective analysis of 370 patients, distal aortic perfusion and CSF drainage were beneficial if extended cross-clamp times were used, particularly in extensive aneurysms [27]. However, other studies reported both equal and increased rates of paraplegia in association with distal aortic perfusion techniques [3, 6, 24, 28-32].

There are several explanations for the fact that distal aortic perfusion did not consistently improve neurologic outcome. The use of a distal bypass technique increased the aortic clamp times in type I and II aneurysms by 50% [24]. The risk of paraplegia remained dependent on the duration of aortic clamping, even when distal aortic perfusion was employed [12]. The relation of aortic clamp time vs. the risk of paraplegia is merely shifted to the right. Consequently, if a shunt is protective, this protective effect might not outweigh the increased risk of neurological deficits that result from the increased clamping time. In addition, the spinal cord will remain ischaemic even in the presence of excellent distal aortic perfusion if the arteries supplying the anterior spinal artery arise from the excluded segment of the aorta [33]. In canine experiments and human observations it was reported that distal aortic pressure had to be maintained above a mean of 60-70 mmHg in order to have a protective effect on the spinal cord [34, 35]. Clinical data suggested that in some patients pressures higher than 80 mmHg were necessary to preserve electrophysiological function [23]. Therefore, merely applying distal aortic perfusion is insufficient to prevent spinal cord ischaemia; distal aortic pressures have to be maintained at least above 60 mmHg. Furthermore, if distal perfusion resulted in perfusion of the ARM, some authors demonstrated that only the lumbar cord flow was increased, whereas the thoracic spinal cord blood flow was not increased [36, 37]. This can be explained by human and animal anatomical observations, that the anterior spinal artery has a larger diameter below the junction of the ARM [36, 38, 39]. Because blood flow is inversely proportional to the fourth power of the radius (Poiseuille's equation), this caliber change has consequences for the distribution of blood flow to the thoraco-lumbar spinal cord. Calculations on post-mortem specimens in humans have revealed that the resistance to upward flow is at least 11 times greater, thus forcing blood in a caudal direction along the length of the spinal cord [36]. Accordingly, the ARM will preferentially perfuse the lumbar spinal cord, while the thoracic spinal cord remains at risk.

Shunts and bypass techniques are not without risk. Complications of distal perfusion techniques include the technical problems which may arise from cannulation of diseased femoral or iliac arteries or the left atrium, and emboli from the aneurysm sac thrombus during shunt perfusion (especially if sequential clamping is used). In addition, the use of a shunt or bypass with partial extracorporal circulation and heparinization resulted in a significant increase in bleeding and pulmonary complications [6, 30]. In an analysis of 596 patients undergoing surgery for traumatic rupture of the aorta, the mortality rate associated with bypass, passive shunts or a clamp and go technique was 16.7%, 11.4% and 5.8%, respectively [40]. In another study the mortality rate associated with atrio-femoral bypass was 4% compared to 11% with the use of cardiopulmonary bypass [41].

In conclusion, distal aortic perfusion, with left heart bypass and the use of a centrifugal pump, has the potential to decrease the incidence of paraplegia and paraparesis, especially when this technique is combined with sequential aortic clamping and segmental repairs. Distal aortic pressures should be maintained above 60 mmHg. The use of distal aortic perfusion does not automatically imply adequate spinal cord perfusion.

Cerebrospinal fluid drainage

A significant rise in CSF pressure after cross-clamping the aorta was described in animal studies [42, 43]. During TAAA resections, pressures up to 43 mmHg were observed after clamping the aorta [44, 45]. The spinal cord can be subjected to a compartment syndrome, because the bony vertebral channel and the dura can be regarded as non-distensible. The apparent compliance of the spinal canal is created by the volume of displaced blood by venous drainage. During thoracic aortic occlusion a volume distribution in the upper half of the body occurs, resulting in an increased central venous pressure (CVP) [46]. The resultant increase in volume of the venous capacitance beds within the dural space are thought to be the mechanism for the increased CSF pressure during aortic clamping [47]. Indeed, CSF pressure was observed to correlate with increases in CVP [43]. When CSF pressure exceeds the local venous pressure in the spinal cord, the drainage network is forced to contract and outflow resistance decreases the compliance of the spinal canal [47]. Spinal cord perfusion pressure (SCPP) is calculated by mean arterial pressure minus the CSF pressure or the CVP whichever of the two outflow pressures is greater. Consequently, a rise in CSF pressure will decrease SCPP. Spinal cord blood flow (SCBF) is autoregulated between perfusion pressures of 50 and 120 mmHg [48, 49]. Below pressures of 50 mmHg, flow decreases in proportion to SCPP. If a rise in CSF pressure decreases SCPP below 50 mmHg, SCBF will be affected. Therefore, CSF drainage (in order to maintain CSF pressure below 10 mmHg) was proposed as an adjunct to prevent paraplegia during TAAA surgery.

The importance of CSF drainage was asserted by observations that a SCPP of less than 20 mmHg was sufficient to preserve spinal cord integrity [42, 50-52]. Consequently, if atrio-femoral bypass is not used to maintain distal aortic pressure, CSF drainage is especially important in order to maintain a perfusion pressure above 20 mmHg.

The influence of CSF drainage on neurologic outcome in experimental studies was equivocal. In dogs, CSF drainage (cisterna magna) repeatedly reduced the incidence of paraplegia following periods of simple aortic cross-clamping [42, 44, 53-55]. In canine experiments, the improved neurological outcome with CSF drainage correlated with increased SCBF in the lower thoracic and lumbar spinal cord [56]. After double thoracic aortic cross-clamping CSF drainage was not effective in reducing the incidence of paraplegia in the dog [57]. In addition, CSF drainage was not able to reduce the degree of permanent spinal cord damage in the baboon or the pig [33, 43].

Most human studies describing CSF drainage had methodological limitations. They were uncontrolled (i.e., compared the results against a historical control group or were merely descriptive) [12, 27, 32, 44, 58-60]. Despite these limitations, it was consistently observed that CSF drainage, alone and combined with other spinal cord protective measures, provided significant protection using a single clamp-repair technique for aneurysm replacement [44, 58-60]. CSF drainage alone did not provide spinal cord protection during TAAA surgery with the use of distal aortic perfusion techniques [32], whereas CSF drainage combined with atrio-femoral bypass, was associated with a reduced incidence of lower limb neurological deficits [12, 27].

The only prospective randomized study of CSF drainage, in 98 patients undergoing TAAA surgery with the use of atrio-femoral bypass, did not demonstrate a reduction of neurological deficits [8]. Limitations of this study were a restriction of the volume of CSF drainage to 50 ml, and limiting CSF drainage in the intraoperative period. Therefore, spinal cord decompression was probably inadequate. In addition, the power analysis of this study assumed a fivefold decrease in neurological deficits, but considering the multifactorial aetiology of spinal cord ischaemia following TAAA surgery, a 50 % reduction would be more realistic. However, in the latter situation, the study group should have been three times larger [61]. Therefore, it is questionable if this investigation was able to detect a difference between the study groups.

In conclusion, there is circumstantial evidence that CSF drainage alone is protective if a "clamp and sew" technique for graft inclusion is performed. However, CSF drainage is simple and safe to perform and is probably a valuable adjunct in combination with a variety of other protective measures.

Control of proximal hypertension

Proximal hypertension following cross-clamping of the aorta is inherent to thoracic aortic surgery, if untreated, the proximal hypertension can cause left ventricular failure, myocardial infarction and/or haemorrhagic cerebral events. The measures used to control proximal hypertension have an effect on CSF pressure and SCPP. If these measures decrease the SCPP below 50 mmHg, they may play a role in the sequence of events resulting in ischaemic spinal cord injury.

Sodium nitroprusside is widely used to control proximal hypertension. However, nitroprusside has a deleterious effect on SCPP; it increases CSF pressure and decreases distal aortic pressure [51]. In addition, nitroprusside causes a loss of autoregulation of SCBF, and blood flow to the upper segments of the spinal cord is increased (nitroprusside steal) [51]. CSF drainage could not reverse the effect of nitroprusside infusion on CSF pressure, because the compliance of the spinal canal was reduced through nitroprusside induced oedema of the spinal cord itself [62]. The effect of nitroprusside on SCPP is especially detrimental if a single clamp-repair technique for graft inclusion is employed [63]. Aortic pressures below the clamp are reduced to values below 50 mmHg. In normal conditions (50 mmHg of SCPP) and in the presence of autoregulation of SCBF, an increase in CSF pressure does not influence SCBF. However, in the presence of an arterial pressure below 50 mmHg any nitroprusside induced increase in CSF pressure will compromise SCBF further.

Nitroglycerine has a different impact on CSF dynamics and autoregulation of blood flow. It also increased CSF pressure in a clinical and experimental setting [52, 64]. However, in contrast to nitroprusside, the nitroglycerine induced CSFP increase could be counteracted by CSF drainage [52].

It can be concluded that in order to control proximal pressures during aortic clamping, nitroprusside should be avoided, and nitroglycerine might be safer only if CSF drainage is performed. Active distal aortic perfusion also allows unloading of the proximal circulation. This technique obviates to a substantial extent the use of nitroglycerine and nitroprusside.

Management of intercostal arteries

The main questions in segmental artery management are whether intercostal or lumbar arteries should be preserved, and which arteries should be reattached. In order to prevent neurological deficits following TAAA surgery, blood supply to the spinal cord should be permanently restored. Accordingly, segmental arteries may need to be re-anastomosed. In the literature most attention was focused to reattach the ARM. However, considerable variation exists in the origin of this vessel. Additional anatomic diversity is created by the aneurysm, because atherosclerosis may occlude originally important segmental vessels, leaving the spinal cord dependent on unusual and diverse collaterals [65].

It was observed that most patients with a dissection had patent intercostal and lumbar arteries, with intense back-bleeding at all levels, while patients with non dissecting aneurysms had occlusion of many segmental arteries, some patients with complete occlusion at all levels [2]. These data are difficult to interpret, and are open for discussion. Occlusion of segmental arteries suggests the presence of substantial collateral circulation to the spinal cord. Or opposite, is the single intercostal artery with minimal back-bleeding of one of the few vessels that critically supply the cord, and thus should be reattached at all expense. In the case of dissection, the question is whether the frequently present, and profusely back-bleeding segmental arteries are the reflection of an extensive collateral supply of the spinal cord, and consequently no segmental arteries need to be reattached. In the opposite case, the question is whether back-bleeding is the result of the interconnected segmental arteries not reaching the cord, and should it be interpreted that alternate vessels to the cord have not developed. In the latter case all segmental vessels should be preserved in the hope that one gives rise to a radicular artery that reaches the spinal cord.

In the literature only some studies describe ligation of all segmental arteries [60], and in some studies the usefulness of segmental artery reattachment is questioned [7]. The majority of studies favour re-implantation of either some or all segmental arteries [10, 21, 24, 58, 66-68].

Despite the anatomical variation of the spinal cord blood supply, and the uncertainty regarding the necessity to re-anastomose segmental arteries, some general statements can be made on the management of intercostal and lumbar arteries.

When the aneurysm is opened, profusely back-bleeding intercostal arteries tend to drain blood away from the spinal cord. In porcine experiments, the prevention of this steal phenomenon significantly increased the pressure in the arterial vascular bed in the thoracic spinal cord [69, 70]. During TAAA surgery, the insertion of intravascular blockers, in order to stop back-bleeding could reverse electrophysiological evidence of spinal cord ischaemia [23].

Reattachment of the segmental arteries will decrease the rate of neurological deficits that are the result of a permanent interruption of blood supply. However, reattaching segmental arteries increases aortic cross-clamp time. Multiple studies have shown that the most important predictor of neurological deficit is the duration of aortic cross-clamping [2, 3, 26, 27, 32]. Therefore, preserving segmental arteries will increase the incidence of neurological lower limb deficits that are the result of temporary ischaemia. Consequently, the protection provided by segmental artery reattachment might not outweigh the risk associated with longer cross-clamp times. Indeed, using a single clamp-repair technique, reimplantation of segmental arteries had no beneficial effect on the incidence of postoperative neurological deficits, and even was a significant predictor of paraplegia and paresis [2]. In another series of patients, the paraplegia rate was increased almost threefold when segmental arteries were reattached using simple aortic cross-clamping [71]. Consequently, additional measures that maintain spinal cord perfusion should be applied if segmental arteries are preserved. When atrio-femoral bypass was used during TAAA surgery, reattachment of patent segmental arteries most likely to give rise to the ARM was associated with a significantly decreased risk of paraplegia or paresis [10, 66].

A problem of reattached segmental arteries is the possibility that they can occlude. Indeed, highly selective angiograms obtained postoperatively in patients with preserved segmental arteries revealed occlusion of these vessels in a significant percentage of patients [23, 72]. Occlusion of preserved vessels is probably the result of emboli or thrombosis.

It can be concluded that segmental artery reattachment without distal perfusion has no beneficial effect on neurologic outcome, because the reattached vessels probably do not compensate for the deleterious effect of longer cross-clamping. If distal perfusion techniques are employed in order to provide adequate time, preservation of segmental arteries decreased the rate of lower limb neurological deficits.

Identification of blood supply to the spinal cord

During TAAA repair, spinal cord blood supply should be restored. “Blindly” preserving a large cluster of back-bleeding intercostal arteries has gained widespread acceptance. A more logical approach would be to pre- or intra-operatively identify the vessels that supply the anterior spinal artery. This targeted reattachment might reduce cross-clamp time, which is the most important predictor of resultant paraplegia. This approach might also increase the rate of successful spinal cord revascularizations. The angiographic localization of spinal cord blood supply, however, has not become a routine because of the fear that manipulation with an atherosclerotic ostium or the direct injection of contrast material will result in lower limb neurological deficits. Indeed, the incidence of neurological deficits, including paraplegia, was 0 - 4.6%, after angiographic spinal cord blood supply localization [65, 73-76]. Other reported major complications associated with spinal arteriography are retroperitoneal haemorrhage, pancreatitis, cortical blindness, aneurysm rupture, fever, and atheromatous arterial emboli resulting in death [74, 75].

In the studies describing preoperative spinal cord angiography, the origin of the ARM could be found in 55% to 69% of the cases [65, 74-76]. Despite identification and reattachment of the ARM the incidence of neurological deficits remained as high as 14 % [65, 75]. No significant difference in occurrence of neurological injury was observed between patients in which the ARM could or could not be identified preoperatively [75]. If the thoracic radicular arteries supplying the spinal cord were also identified and preserved, a lower incidence of neurologic deficits was reported (5%) [74]. In the latter series distal aortic perfusion was not used. Postoperative neurological deficits are caused by a permanent interruption of spinal cord blood supply or by a temporary interruption of sufficient duration. Distal aortic perfusion might shorten spinal cord ischaemic time during TAAA repair, and reduce the risk of neurological deficits resulting from temporary ischaemia. Indeed, combined atrio-femoral bypass, preoperative spinal angiography and targeted intercostal preservation resulted in only 2.3 % of the lower limb neurological deficits [76].

An intra-operative technique for identifying the vessels supplying the spinal cord is the Hydrogen Induced Current. With this technique, a platinum electrode is placed intrathecally alongside the spinal cord. A saline solution saturated with hydrogen is injected into a clamped aortic segment or a segmental artery ostium. If hydrogen reaches the spinal cord, a Hydrogen Induced Current is generated from the electrode, indicating the segmental artery or the aortic section that had been injected supplied the spinal cord with blood [72, 77, 78]. In a porcine experiment, spinal cord blood supply could be accurately identified using this technique [72]. In a pilot study in humans undergoing TAAA repair, post operative angiography confirmed that this technique accurately identified spinal cord blood supply [72]. However, using the hydrogen technique postoperative paresis remained a distinct possibility (13 %) [72, 77].

It can be concluded that the identification of spinal cord blood supply provides additional value in a multimodality approach to reduce lower limb neurological deficits. However, the rate of serious complication associated with angiographic localization of spinal cord blood supply limits its clinical value.

Hypothermia

The rationale for the use of hypothermia during TAAA resections is to increase the tolerance of the spinal cord to ischaemia, so that blood flow can be re-established before the onset of irreversible damage. Hypothermia can be applied either regionally (confined to the spinal cord) or systemically.

Oxygen requirements in neural tissue are known to decrease 6 - 7 % for each degree decrement in the cord temperature [79]. The neuroprotective effect of hypothermia was presumed to be secondary to a decreased metabolic rate and to a generalized reduction of energy consuming processes in the cell. However, in 1944 it was demonstrated that the temperature coefficient of the processes ultimately resulting in destruction of nerve cells was consistently higher than that of the processes involved in the oxygen uptake of the spinal cord [80]. Thus, as the temperature was lowered, the destruction of nerve cells decreased to a greater extent than the oxygen uptake. Recently, it was shown that the mechanism of hypothermic spinal cord protection indeed is complex, involving the reduced release of excitatory neurotransmitters and membrane stabilization [81].

Profound hypothermia (15 -19 °C) and circulatory arrest is commonly used for surgery of the transverse aortic arch, and has also been described for TAAA surgery. It is an attractive technique because it provides cardiac, as well as visceral and spinal cord protection. Therefore, time to reattach all segmental arteries in extensive aneurysms is allowed [68, 82-84]. Lower extremity neurological deficits occurred up to 7.5 % in these series. However, this approach carries the risk of cerebral neurologic deficits, massive fluid shifts, and full heparinization and extracorporal circulation related problems like coagulopathy and haemorrhagic pulmonary complications. Therefore, Kouchoukos proposed to limit this technique to complex and therefore prolonged aortic surgery [68 82], while Safi recommended to leave this option as a last alternative in cases with massive intra-operative bleeding [85].

Moderate systemic hypothermia (30 - 33°C) can be accomplished either as permissive hypothermia (spontaneous cooling), or actively with an in-line heat exchanger combined with atrio-femoral bypass; the latter permits rapid cooling and rapid rewarming at the end of the procedure. The degree of hypothermia, achieved with this method, is limited by the potential for cardiac arrhythmia's. Moderate hypothermia was effective in experimental models of SCI and in clinical studies during TAAA surgery [58, 86, 87].

Mild systemic hypothermia (up to Δ - 4°C) exerted powerful neuroprotective properties in cerebral ischaemia [88]. Mild hypothermia in the setting of spinal cord ischaemia is discussed in chapter 6 of this thesis.

Regional cooling of the spinal cord has theoretical advantages, because lower cord temperatures can be achieved without the systemic complications. Subarachnoid perfusion (2 - 6 °C, 25 ml /min inflow, passive outflow), was demonstrated to be protective in several experimental models of spinal cord ischaemia. The spinal cord temperature could be decreased to temperatures of approximately 15 °C at the expense however, of increased CSF pressures [57, 89, 90]. Several authors showed that epidural infusion (5°C) protected against experimental spinal cord ischaemia [91-94]. In dogs, epidural perfusion (bolus 8 ml/kg and additional infusion of 20 ml/kg during aortic clamping) resulted in moderate levels of cord hypothermia (≈ 29°C) [92, 93]. Deep hypothermia was possibly not reached because the epidural space is less well insulated from the systemic circulation than the subarachnoid space. Spinal cord temperatures below 15 °C could only be reached with epidural cooling in a smaller animal model (rabbit), but lethal increases in CSF pressure occurred in some animals [91]. In clinical practice, iced saline (4 °C) was infused into the epidural space at the level of T11-12 in 70 patients [95]. The average infused volume was 1 400 ml, which resulted in a CSF temperature of 25 ± 1 °C. Using this technique, which included a "clamp and sew" protocol and segmental artery reattachment, 2.9 % lower extremity neurological deficits were reported. Remarkably, one patient in that series had a cervical cord infarction. The major disadvantage of this technique was the increased CSF pressure, which was more than doubled from baseline values [95, 96]. A rise in CSF pressure is thought to be a contributor to the development of postoperative paraplegia and paresis. Consequently, it can be postulated that the increased CSF pressure was distributed equal along the entire cord whereas the extent of protection provided by cooling was locally limited, which might account for the cervical infarction in this series of patients.

Another possibility to apply regional hypothermia is the direct infusion of cold perfusate into isolated aortic segments, with the intention that the spinal cord is cooled through the segmental arteries. In several experimental models, this technique provided protection against ischaemic spinal cord injury [79, 97-99]. Spinal cord temperatures as low as 18 - 20°C could be obtained [98].

An advantage of this technique was that additives like adenosine or lidocaine could be included in the perfusion solution [78, 100]. In 23 patients with extensive (type I and II) aneurysms, the aortic segment giving rise to the segmental arteries to be preserved (T8-L2) was perfused with 400 cc crystalloid solution containing heparin, methylprednisolone and mannitol at 8°C [101]. In this series, one patient (4.3%) awoke paraplegic after the operation.

Hypothermia can also be applied after the onset of ischaemia. It was demonstrated in 1968 that delayed localized cooling initiated 4 hours after spinal cord injury completely prevented neurological deficits. In a rat model of focal cerebral ischaemia mild hypothermia instituted within 30 minutes after the onset of ischaemia significantly reduced infarct size [102]. The delayed application of hypothermia after spinal cord ischaemia has not been described.

Some critical notes on hypothermia should be made. In experimental spinal cord ischaemia, hypothermia during the ischaemic period did not protect against late onset paraplegia [94]. Deep hypothermia may not be without risk, spinal cord temperatures of 10 °C have been described to result in irreversible neuronal injury [103].

In conclusion, induced hypothermia is a powerful strategy to increase ischaemic neuronal tolerance, and it appears that hypothermia always provides a marked degree of protection, irrespective of the method of cooling.

Delayed neurological deficits

One third of the neurological deficits after TAAA surgery developed in the postoperative period.[2] This phenomenon can not readily be explained. Several likely explications are provided.

Inadequate spinal cord blood supply. If segmental arteries feeding the spinal cord were severed during the operation, there might be areas of marginal perfusion. If spinal cord blood supply or spinal oxygenation is compromised further in the postoperative period, ischaemia can develop. Indeed, postoperative episodes of hypotension or increases in CSF pressure resulted in delayed neurological deficits [2, 58]. Decreased oxygen delivery as a result of postoperative respiratory insufficiency also resulted in delayed neurological deficits [104]. Another cause is the occlusion of reattached segmental arteries [23, 72]. A further deterioration of a compromised spinal cord blood supply, as explanation for delayed neurological deficits, is supported by the notion that acute CSF drainage reversed lower limb neurological deficits up to 14 days following TAAA repair in several studies (CSF drainage lowers CSF pressure and thus increases SCPP) [7, 58, 105, 106].

Reperfusion injury. During TAAA repair, a short period of SCI will probably not result in direct injury. However, following reperfusion, further neuronal damage may result from the burst of oxygen free radicals, cytotoxic actions of leukocytes and microglia, microcirculation defects by vasospastic prostaglandins, and vascular smooth muscle contractions [107-110]. These combined actions may ultimately lead to irreversible damage and delayed neurological deficits.

Apoptosis. Recent studies have suggested that delayed neuronal death after transient spinal cord ischaemia has apoptotic features [111-114]. In contrast to ischaemic cell death, apoptose is a form of programmed cell death, with the activation of a genetic program in which the apoptosis effector genes promote cell death. The advantage of apoptotic cell death is that the cell is smoothly removed by phagocytosis of neighbouring cells. In contrast, lysis that occurs with necrotic cell death is accompanied by excitatory amino acid release and macrophage activation, which might aggravate the insult [115].

Conclusion

Spinal cord ischaemic injury during TAAA surgery is the result of a permanent or temporary interruption of spinal cord blood supply. The permanent interruption is related both to the variable and unpredictable anatomy of the arterial vascularization of the spinal cord, as well as the extent of the aneurysm. The temporary interruption is dependent on the duration of aortic cross-clamping.

In order to restore cord blood supply, at least the intercostal arteries most likely to give rise to the ARM should be re-anastomosed to the graft. However, expending aortic clamp time for re-anastomosis of intercostal or lumbar vessels increases the risk of irreversible neurological deficits resulting from temporary ischaemia. Therefore, additional strategies need to be applied to maintain adequate spinal cord perfusion during aortic clamping. Distal aortic perfusion techniques, sequential aortic repairs, the maintenance of low CSF pressure using CSF drainage, and the avoidance of nitroprusside all have the potential to increase the tolerable duration of cross-clamping. In addition, if a period of ischaemia is likely to occur, the application of systemic or regional hypothermia will enhance neuronal survival.

References

1. Adams HD, Geertruyden H (1956) Neurologic complications of aortic surgery. Ann Surg 144:574-610
2. Crawford ES, Crawford JL, Safi HJ et al (1986) Thoracoabdominal aortic aneurysms: preoperative and intraoperative factors determining immediate and long-term results of operations in 605 patients. J Vasc Surg 3:389-404
3. Svensson LG, Crawford ES, Hess KR et al (1993) Experience with 1 509 patients undergoing thoracoabdominal aortic operations. J Vasc Surg 17:357-368
4. Joseph MG, Langsfeld MA, Lusby RJ (1989) Infrarenal aortic aneurysm: unusual cause of paraparesis. Aust N Z J Surg 59:743-744
5. Noirhomme P, Buche M, Louagie Y et al (1991) Ischemic complications of abdominal aortic surgery. J Cardiovasc Surg (Torino) 32:451-455
6. Livesay JJ, Cooley DA, Ventemiglia RA et al (1985) Surgical experience in descending thoracic aneurysmectomy with and without adjuncts to avoid ischemia. Ann Thorac Surg 39:37-46
7. Griepp RB, Ergin MA, Galla JD et al (1996) Looking for the artery of Adamkiewicz: a quest to minimize paraplegia after operations for aneurysms of the descending thoracic and thoracoabdominal aorta. J Thorac Cardiovasc Surg 112:1202-1213
8. Crawford ES, Svensson LG, Hess KR et al (1990) A prospective randomized study of cerebrospinal fluid drainage to prevent paraplegia after high-risk surgery on the thoracoabdominal aorta. J Vasc Surg 13:36-45
9. Katz NM, Blackstone EH, Kirklin JW et al (1981) Incremental risk factors for spinal cord injury following operation for acute traumatic aortic transection. J Thorac Cardiovasc Surg 81:669-674
10. Svensson LG, Hess KR, Coselli JS et al (1994) Influence of segmental arteries, extent, and atriofemoral bypass on postoperative paraplegia after thoracoabdominal aortic operations. J Vasc Surg 20:255-262
11. Grabitz K, Sandmann W, Stuhmeier K et al (1996) The risk of ischemic spinal cord injury in patients undergoing graft replacement for thoracoabdominal aortic aneurysms. J Vasc Surg 23:230-240
12. Safi HJ, Hess KR, Randel M et al (1996) Cerebrospinal fluid drainage and distal aortic perfusion - reducing neurologic complications in repair of thoracoabdominal aortic aneurysm types I and II. J Vasc Surg 23:223-228
13. Cooley DA, Baldwin RT (1992) Technique of open distal anastomosis fo repair of descending thoracic aortic aneurysms. Ann Thorac Surg 54:932-936
14. Scheinin SA, Cooley DA (1994) Graft replacement of the descending thoracic aorta: results of "open" distal anastomosis. Ann Thorac Surg 58:19-22
15. Crawford ES, Walker Hd, Saleh SA et al (1981) Graft replacement of aneurysm in descending thoracic aorta: results without bypass or shunting. Surgery 89:73-85
16. Gott VL (1972) Heparinized shunts for thoracic vascular operations. Ann Thorac Surg 14:219-222
17. Verdant A, Cossette R, Pagé A et al (1995) Aneurysms of the descending thoracic aorta: Three hundred sixty-six consecutive cases resected without paraplegia. J Vasc Surg 21:385-391
18. Molina JE, Cogordan J, Einzig S et al (1985) Adequacy of ascending aorta-descending aorta shunt during cross- clamping of the thoracic aorta for prevention of spinal cord injury. J Thorac Cardiovasc Surg 90:126-136
19. Kaplan DK, Atsumi N, D'Ambra MN et al (1995) Distal circulatory support for thoracic aortic operations: effects on intracranial pressure. Ann Thorac Surg 59:448-452
20. Connolly J, Wakabayashi A, German J et al (1971) Clinical experience with pulsatile left heart bypass without anticoagulation for thoracic aneurysms. J Thor Cardiovasc Surg 62:
21. Borst HG, Jurmann M, Buhner B et al (1994) Risk of replacement of descending aorta with a standardized left heart bypass technique. J Thorac Cardiovasc Surg 107:126-132
22. Jacobs MJ, de Mol BA, Legemate DA et al (1997) Retrograde aortic and selective organ perfusion during thoracoabdominal aortic aneurysm repair. Eur J Vasc Endovasc Surg 14:360-366

23. de Haan P, Kalkman CJ, de Mol BA et al (1997) Efficacy of transcranial motor-evoked myogenic potentials to detect spinal cord ischemia during operations for thoracoabdominal aneurysms. J Thorac Cardiovasc Surg 113:87-100
24. Coselli JS, LeMaire SA, de Figueiredo LP et al (1997) Paraplegia after thoracoabdominal aortic aneurysm repair: is dissection a risk factor? Ann Thorac Surg 63:28-35
25. de Mol B, Hamerlijnck R, Boezeman E et al (1990) Prevention of spinal cord ischemia in surgery of thoraco-abdominal aneurysms. The Bio Medicus pump, the recording of somatosensory evoked potentials and the impact on surgical strategy. Eur J Cardiothorac Surg 4:658-664
26. Coselli JS (1994) Thoracoabdominal aortic aneurysms: experience with 372 patients. J Card Surg 9:638-647
27. Safi HJ, Winnerkvist A, Miller CCr et al (1998) Effect of extended cross-clamp time during thoracoabdominal aortic aneurysm repair. Ann Thorac Surg 66:1204-1209
28. Crawford ES, Mizrahi EM, Hess KR et al (1988) The impact of distal aortic perfusion and somatosensory evoked potential monitoring on prevention of paraplegia after aortic aneurysm operation. J Thorac Cardiovasc Surg 95:357-367
29. Najafi H, Javid H, Hunter J et al (1980) Descending aortic aneurysmectomy without adjuncts to avoid ischemia. Ann Thorac Surg 30:326-335
30. Crawford ES, Rubio PA (1973) Reappraisal of adjuncts to avoid ischemia in the treatment of aneurysms of descending thoracic aorta. J Thorac Cardiovasc Surg 66:693-704
31. Schepens MA, Defauw JJ, Hamerlijnck RP et al (1995) Use of left heart bypass in the surgical repair of thoracoabdominal aortic aneurysms. Ann Vasc Surg 9:327-338
32. Murray MJ, Bower TC, Oliver WC et al (1993) Effects of CSF drainage in patients undergoing thoracic and thoracoabdominal aortic surgery. J Cardiothor Vasc Anesth 7:266-272
33. Svensson LG, Groeneveld HT, Rickards ES et al (1986) Cross-clamping of the thoracic aorta. Influence of aortic shunts, laminectomy, papaverine, calcium channel blocker, allopurinol, and superoxide dismutase on spinal cord blood flow and paraplegia in baboons. Ann Surg 204:38-47
34. Cunningham JJ, Laschinger JC, Spencer FC (1987) Monitoring of somatosensory evoked potentials during surgical procedures on the thoracoabdominal aorta. IV. Clinical observations and results. J Thor Cardiovasc Surg 94:275-285
35. Laschinger JC, Cunningham JJ, Baumann FG et al (1987) Monitoring of somatosensory evoked potentials during surgical procedures on the thoracoabdominal aorta. II. Use of somatosensory evoked potentials to assess adequacy of distal aortic bypass and perfusion after thoracic aortic cross-clamping. J Thor Cardiovasc Surg 94:266-270
36. Svensson LG, Rickards E, Coull A et al (1986) Relationship of spinal cord blood flow to vascular anatomy during thoracic aortic cross-clamping and shunting. J Thor Cardiovasc Surg 91:71-78
37. Maharajh G, Pascoe EA, Halliday WC et al (1996) Neurological outcome in a porcine model of descending thoracic aortic surgery. Stroke 27:2095-2101
38. Domisse GF (1974) The blood supply of the spinal cord. J Bone and Joint Surg 56B:225-235
39. Wissdorf H (1970) Die Gefässversorgung der Wirbelsäule und des Rückenmarkes vom Hausschwein, Tierärztliche Hochschule Hannover, Med Vet Habilschrift. Berlin, Parey-Verlag, 73-96
40. Svensson LG, Loop FD Prevention of spinal ischemia in aortic surgery. Bergan JJ, Yao JST (eds) (1988) Arterial surgery: new diagnostic and operative techniques. New York, Grune & Sratton, 273-285
41. Svensson LG, Crawford ES, Hess KR et al (1993) Variables predictive of outcome in 832 patients undergoing repairs of the descending thoracic aorta. Chest 104:1248-1253
42. Blaisdell FW, Cooley DA (1962) The mechanism of paraplegia after temporary thoracic aortic occlusion and its relationship to spinal fluid pressure. Surgery 51:351-355
43. Wadouh F, Lindeman EM, Arndt CF et al (1984) The arteria radicularis magna as a decisive factor influencing spinal cord damage during aortic occlusion. J Thor Cardiovasc Surg 88:1-10
44. McCullough JL, Hollier LH, Nugent M (1988) Paraplegia after thoracic aortic occlusion: influence of cerebrospinal fluid drainage. Experimental and early clinical results. J Vasc Surg 7:153-160

45. Berendes JN, Bredee JJ, Schipperheyn JJ et al (1982) Mechanisms of spinal cord injury after cross-clamping of the descending thoracic aorta. Circulation 66(suppl 1):112-116
46. Stokland O, Molaug M, Ilebekk A et al (1980) Mechanism of hemodynamic responses to occlusion of the descending thoracic aorta. Am J Physiol 238:H423-H429
47. Piano G, Gewertz BL (1990) Mechanism of increased cerebrospinal fluid pressure with thoracic aortic occlusion. J Vasc Surg 11:695-701
48. Griffiths IR, Pitts LH, Crawford RA et al (1978) Spinal cord compression and bloodflow. I. The effect of raised cerebrospinal fluid pressure on spinal cord blood flow. Neurology 28:1145-1151
49. Hickey R, Albin MS, Bunegin L et al (1986) Autoregulation of spinal cord blood flow: is the cord a microcosm of the brain? Stroke 17:1183-1189
50. Grubbs PE, Jr., Marini C, Toporoff B et al (1988) Somatosensory evoked potentials and spinal cord perfusion pressure are significant predictors of postoperative neurologic dysfunction. Surgery 104:216-223
51. Marini CP, Grubbs PE, Toporoff B et al (1989) Effect of sodium nitroprusside on spinal cord perfusion and paraplegia during aortic cross-clamping. Ann Thorac Surg 47:379-383
52. Marini CP, Nathan IM, Efron J et al (1997) Effect of nitroglycerin and cerebrospinal fluid drainage on spinal cord perfusion pressure and paraplegia during aortic cross-clamping. J Surg Res 70:61-65
53. Bower TC, Murray MJ, Gloviczki P et al (1988) Effects of thoracic aortic occlusion and cerebrospinal fluid drainage on regional spinal cord blood flow in dogs: correlation with neurologic outcome. J Vasc Surg 9:135-144
54. Woloszyn TT, Marini CP, Coons MS et al (1992) A multimodality approach lengthens warm ischemic time during aortic cross-clamping. J Surg Res 52:15-21
55. Woloszyn TT, Marini CP, Coons MS et al (1990) Cerebrospinal fluid drainage and steroids provide better spinal cord protection during aortic cross-clamping than does either treatment alone. Ann Thorac Surg 49:78-82
56. Elmore JR, Gloviczki P, Harper CM et al (1991) Failure of motor evoked potentials to predict neurologic outcome in experimental thoracic aortic occlusion. J Vasc Surg 14:131-139
57. Wisselink W, Becker MO, Nguyen JH et al (1994) Protecting the ischemic spinal cord during aortic clamping: the influence of selective hypothermia and spinal cord perfusion pressure. J Vasc Surg 19:788-795
58. Hollier LH, Money SR, Naslund TC et al(1992) Risk of spinal cord dysfunction in patients undergoing thoracoabdominal aortic replacement. Am J Surg 164:210-213
59. Acher CW, Wynn MM, Archibald J (1990) Naloxone and spinal fluid drainage as adjuncts in the surgical treatment of thoracoabdominal and thoracic aneurysms Surgery 108:755-761
60. Acher CW, Wynn MM, Hoch JR et al (1994) Combined use of cerebral spinal fluid drainage and naloxone reduces the risk of paraplegia in thoracoabdominal aneurysm repair. J Vasc Surg 19:236-246
61. Mutch WA (1995) Control of outflow pressure provides spinal cord protection during resection of descending thoracic aortic aneurysms. J Neurosurg Anesthesiol 7:133-138
62. Woloszyn TT, Marini CP, Coons MS et al (1989) Cerebrospinal fluid drainage does not counteract the negative effect of sodium nitroprusside on spinal cord perfusion pressure during aortic cross-clamping. Current Surgery 46:489-492
63. Marini CP, Levison J, Caliendo F et al (1998) Control of proximal hypertension during aortic cross-clamping: its effect on cerebrospinal fluid dynamics and spinal cord perfusion pressure. Semin Thorac Cardiovasc Surg 10:51-56
64. Dohi S, Matsumoto M, Takahashi T (1981) The effects of nitroglycerin on cerebrospinal fluid pressure in awake and anesthetized humans. Anesthesiology 54:511-514
65. Williams GM, Perler BA, Burdick JF et al (1991) Angiographic localization of spinal cord blood supply and its relationship to postoperative paraplegia. J Vasc Surg 13:23-33
66. Safi HJ, Miller CCr, Carr C et al (1998) Importance of intercostal artery reattachment during thoracoabdominal aortic aneurysm repair. J Vasc Surg 27:58-66

67. Svensson LG, Klepp P, Hinder RA (1986) Spinal cord anatomy of the baboon-comparison with man and implications for spinal cord blood flow during thoracic aortic cross-clamping. S Afr J Surg 24:32-34
68. Kouchoukos NT, Wareing TH, Izumoto H et al (1990) Elective hypothermic cardiopulmonary bypass and circulatory arrest for spinal cord protection during operations on the thoracoabdominal aorta. J Thorac Cardiovasc Surg 99:659-64
69. Wadouh F, Arndt CF, Oppermann E et al (1986) The mechanism of spinal cord injury after simple and double aortic cross-clamping. J Thorac Cardiovasc Surg 92:121-127
70. Dapunt OE, Midulla PS, Sadeghi AM et al (1994) Pathogenesis of spinal cord injury during simulated aneurysm repair in a chronic animal model. Ann Thorac Surg 58:689-696
71. Schepens MA, Defauw JJ, Hamerlijnck RP et al (1994) Surgical treatment of thoracoabdominal aortic aneurysms by simple cross-clamping. Risk factors and late results. J Thorac Cardiovasc Surg 107:134-142
72. Svensson LG, Patel V, Robinson MF et al (1991) Influence of preservation or perfusion of intraoperatively identified spinal cord blood supply on spinal motor evoked potentials and paraplegia after aortic surgery. J Vasc Surg 13:355-365
73. Szilagyi DE, Hageman JH, Smith RF et al (1978) Spinal cord damage in surgery of the abdominal aorta. Surgery 83:38-56
74. Kieffer E, Richard T, Chiras J et al (1989) Preoperative spinal cord arteriography in aneurysmal disease of the descending thoracic and thoracoabdominal aorta: Preliminary results in 45 patients. Ann Vasc Surg 3:34-46
75. Savader SJ, Williams GM, Trerotola SO et al (1993) Preoperative spinal artery localization and its relationship to postoperative neurologic complications. Radiology 189:165-171
76. Heinemann MK, Brassel F, Herzog T et al (1998) The role of spinal angiography in operations on the thoracic aorta: myth or reality? Ann Thorac Surg 65:346-351
77. Svensson LG (1996) Intraoperative identification of spinal cord blood supply during repairs of descending aorta and thoracoabdominal aorta. J Thorac Cardiovasc Surg 112:1455-1460
78. Svensson LG, Crawford ES, Patel V et al (1992) Spinal oxygenation, blood supply localization, cooling, and function with aortic clamping. Ann Thorac Surg 54:74-79
79. Allen BT, Davis CG, Osborne D et al (1994) Spinal cord ischemia and reperfusion metabolism: the effect of hypothermia. J Vasc Surg 19:332-339
80. Harreveld van A, Tyler DB (1944) Influence of temperature on spinal cord damage caused by asphyxiation. Am J Physiol 142:32
81. Rokkas CK, Cronin CS, Nitta T et al (1995) Profound systemic hypothermia inhibits the release of neurotransmitter amino acids in spinal cord ischemia. J Thorac Cardiovasc Surg 110:27-35
82. Kouchoukos NT, Daily BB, Rokkas CK et al (1995) Hypothermic bypass and circulatory arrest for operations on the descending thoracic and thoracoabdominal aorta. Ann Thorac Surg 60:67-76
83. Ergin MA, Galla JD, Lansman L et al (1994) Hypothermic circulatory arrest in operations on the thoracic aorta. Determinants of operative mortality and neurologic outcome. J Thorac Cardiovasc Surg 107:788-797
84. Kieffer E, Koskas F, Walden R et al (1994) Hypothermic circulatory arrest for thoracic aneurysmectomy through left-sided thoracotomy. J Vasc Surg 19:457-464
85. Safi HJ, Miller CCr, Subramaniam MH et al (1998) Thoracic and thoracoabdominal aortic aneurysm repair using cardiopulmonary bypass, profound hypothermia, and circulatory arrest via left side of the chest incision. J Vasc Surg 28:591-598
86. Frank SM, Parker SD, Rock P et al (1994) Moderate hypothermia, with partial bypass and segmental sequential repair for thoracoabdominal aortic aneurysm. J Vasc Surg 19:687-697
87. Marsala M, Vanicky I, Yaksh TL (1994) Effect of graded hypothermia (27 degrees to 34 degrees C) on behavioral function, histopathology, and spinal blood flow after spinal ischemia in rat. Stroke 25:2038-2046
88. Busto R, Dietrich W, Globus M et al (1987) Small differences in intraischemic brain temperature critically determine the extent of ischemic neuronal injury. J Cereb Blood Flow Metab 7:729-738

89. Salzano RJ, Ellison LH, Altonji PF et al (1994) Regional deep hypothermia of the spinal cord protects against ischemic injury during thoracic aortic cross-clamping. Ann Thorac Surg 57:65-70
90. Berguer R, Porto J, Fedoronko B et al (1992) Selective deep hypothermia of the spinal cord prevents paraplegia after aortic cross-clamping in the dog model. J Vasc Surg 15:62-71
91. Vanicky I, Marsala M, Galik J et al (1993) Epidural perfusion cooling protection against protracted spinal cord ischemia in rabbits. J Neurosurg 79:736-741
92. Marsala M, Vanicky I, Galik J et al (1993) Panmyelic epidural cooling protects against ischemic spinal cord damage. J Surg Res 55:21-31
93. Tabayashi K, Niibori K, Konno H et al (1993) Protection from postischemic spinal cord injury by perfusion cooling of the epidural space. Ann Thorac Surg 56:494-498
94. Gonzalez-Fajardo J, Beatriz A, Perez-Burkhardt JL et al (1996) Epidural regional hypothermia for prevention of paraplegia after aortic occlusion: experimental evaluation in a rabbit model. J Vasc Surg 23:446-452
95. Cambria RP, Davison JK, Zannetti S et al (1997) Clinical experience with epidural cooling for spinal cord protection during thoracic and thoracoabdominal aneurysm repair. J Vasc Surg 25:234-241
96. Davison JK, Cambria RP, Vierra DJ et al (1994) Epidural cooling for regional spinal cord hypothermia during thoracoabdominal aneurysm repair. J Vasc Surg 20:304-310
97. Colon R, Frazier OH, Cooley DA et al (1987) Hypothermic regional perfusion for protection of the spinal cord during periods of ischemia. Ann Thorac Surg 43:639-643
98. Coles JG, Wilson GJ, Sima AF et al (1983) Intraoperative management of thoracic aortic aneurysm, experimental evaluation of perfusion cooling of the spinal cord. J Thorac Cardiovasc Surg 85:292-299
99. Malatova Z, Vanicky I, Galik J et al (1995) Epidural perfusion cooling protects against spinal cord ischemia in rabbits. An evaluation of cholinergic function. Mol Chem Neuropathol 25:81-96
100. Herold JA, Kron IL, Langenburg SE et al (1994) Complete prevention of postischemic spinal cord injury by means of regional infusion with hypothermic saline and adenosine. J Thorac Cardiovasc Surg 107:536-541
101. Fehrenbacher JW, McCready RA, Hormuth DA et al (1993) One-stage segmental resection of extensive thoracoabdominal aneurysms with left-sided heart bypass. J Vasc Surg 18:366-370
102. Karibe H, Chen J, Zarow GJ et al (1994) Delayed induction of mild hypothermia to reduce infarct volume after temporary middle cerebral artery occlusion in rats. J Neurosurg 80:112-119
103. Craenen G, Jeftinija S, Grants I et al (1996) The role of excitatory amino acids in hypothermic injury to mammalian spinal cord neurons. J Neurotrauma 13:809-818
104. Svensson LG, Grum DF, Bednarski M et al (1990) Appraisal of cerebrospinal fluid alterations during aortic surgery with intrathecal papaverine administration and cerebrospinal fluid drainage. J Vasc Surg 11:423-429
105. Hill AB, Kalman PG, Johnston KW et al (1994) Reversal of delayed-onset paraplegia after thoracic aortic surgery with cerebrospinal fluid drainage. J Vasc Surg 20:315-317
106. Safi HJ, Miller CCr, Azizzadeh A et al (1997) Observations on delayed neurologic deficit after thoracoabdominal aortic aneurysm repair. J Vasc Surg 26:616-622
107. Wu YP, Ling EA (1998) Induction of microglial and astrocytic response in the adult rat lumbar spinal cord following middle cerebral artery occlusion. Exp Brain Res 118:235-242
108. Lindsberg PJ, Yue TL, Frerichs KU et al (1990) Evidence for platelet-activating factor as a novel mediator in experimental stroke in rabbits. Stroke 21:1452-1457
109. Lindsberg PJ, Siren AL, Feuerstein GZ et al (1995) Antagonism of neutrophil adherence in the deteriorating stroke model in rabbits. J Neurosurg 82:269-277
110. Barut S, Canbolat A, Bilge T et al (1993) Lipid peroxidation in experimental spinal cord injury: time-level relationship. Neurosurg Rev 16:53-59
111. Hayashi T, Sakurai M, Abe K et al (1998) Apoptosis of motor neurons with induction of caspases in the spinal cord after ischemia. Stroke 29:1007-1012

112. Kato H, Kanellopoulos GK, Matsuo S et al (1997) Neuronal apoptosis and necrosis following spinal cord ischemia in the rat. Exp Neurol 148:464-474
113. Sakurai M, Hayashi T, Abe K et al (1998) Delayed selective motor neuron death and Fas antigen induction after spinal cord ischemia in rabbits. Brain Res 797:23-28
114. Sakurai M, Hayashi T, Abe K et al (1998) Delayed and selective motor neuron death after transient spinal cord ischemia: a role of apoptosis? J Thorac Cardiovasc Surg 115:1310-1315
115. Bredesen DE (1995) Neural Apoptosis. Ann Neurol 38:839-851

The Elderly: from Physiopathology to Surveillance in the Perioperative Period

G. Galimberti, R. Muchada

Definition

Normally, a patient over 65 years is considered an elderly subject. More specifically, however, three age groups may be distinguished within the so-called elderly population, namely:
- the elderly subject, between 65 and 74 years of age,
- the old subject, between 75 and 84 years,
- the very old subject or geront, over 85 years of age.

In the absence of pathologies, the first age group still has a virtually normal social life that can be related to that of younger age groups. In contrast, over 75 years of age there is a more-significant decrease in strength, muscle elasticity, rapidity and motion co-ordination, leading to a parallel, gradual decrease of the normal physical and social activities.

Such a physical decay may be quicker or slower, more or less evident according to the genetic characteristics of the patient and to environmental and socioeconomic conditions [1]. Therefore, ageing is a natural, physiological, progressive process, which determines irreversible structural anatomical changes involving all tissues and organs. Further to these age-related physiopathological impairments, we can observe in the elderly patient pathological alterations that are independent of ageing, but which influence negatively the age-related impairment process [2].

Such a natural impairment of the organ system causes important changes in the composition of the organ system itself [3, 4]. For example, a man aged approximately 60 years generally has an average body weight 20-25% higher than he had at 20 years. Over this age, his weight usually tends to decrease again, reaching once again levels of youth. Even the lipid/water ratio inside tissues tends to change with age. In effect, in the elderly subject there is an increase in the global content of lipids and a parallel decrease in total body water; hence, the elderly patient tends to absorb more easily both anesthetic agents and all those drugs that are most liposoluble. This is more evident in women than in men, due to the physiological prevalence of adipose over muscular tissues. At the same time, in post-menopausal elderly women, a worsening of osteoporosis is observed, which determines a loss in bone tissue and evidences a global degeneration that involves all metabolically active support tissues. On the other hand, an important reduction of interstitial water prevails in men, probably due to a loss in muscle mass. The immediate consequence of this reduction of muscular function is a 30-50% decrease of the maximum oxygen intake during physical stress. In women, oxygen intake is significantly lower even at rest.

In either sex a progressive and significant decrease in metabolic activity occurs. This physiopathological alteration determines an important consequence for anesthetists, in that it is accompanied by a reduced thermogenesis, which makes the elderly subject unable to maintain a constant and adequate temperature in a cold environment, such as the air-conditioned operating theater, especially during general anesthesia or major surgery.

Furthermore, contrary to what was thought in the past, in the elderly there are no significant changes in plasma volume and, at the same time, the red and white blood cell content remains essentially constant, as well as the volume of platelets and of coagulation factors. In contrast, the replacement of all these elements is much slower and more difficult than in younger patients, due to a decreased marrow synthesis capacity. Similarly, especially after a loss or after an intense and sudden consumption, there is a slow replenishment of the number of platelets, coagulation factors, and white cells [5].

From an endocrine point of view, the basal secretion level of the elderly subject is virtually the same as that of the young adult, even though after intense stimulation, such as in the case of surgical or post-traumatic stress, the response is much slower and more limited than in young adults [6].

Cardiovascular function

Analysis of cardiovascular function in the elderly must take into consideration two independent but closely related factors, namely age-related physiopathological alterations of the cardiovascular system and the presence of associated cardiovascular pathologies [7-9].

With increasing age a decreased ventricular compliance is evidenced at the cardiac level, together with a moderate decrease in volemia and in venous capacity. Decreases in left ventricular compliance determine a parallel decrease in cardiac reserve in terms of output, due to a compromised telediastolic ventricular filling and a relative decrease of the left ventricular ejection volume. At the same time, an increased cardiac frequency may determine a severe decrease in cardiac output, due to the reduced telediastolic left ventricular filling caused by a reduction in ventricular release time and to a compromised coronary perfusion. In effect, coronary failure itself may be responsible for a worsening of the left ventricular function, either pre-existent or latent, thus contributing to a further decrease in cardiac output.

A slight change in plasma volume may lead to severe cardiovascular imbalance in the elderly. In fact, the elderly patient is at the same time dependent on the venous return to have an adequate cardiac output but also sensitive to an excessive preload that might compromise the unstable balance between adequate left ventricular filling and myocardial contractility.

Such changes in the preload may also be influenced by alterations in venous capacity. For example, if the latter is reduced, a hypervolemic status may result, with a sharp and sudden increase in the preload. In contrast, if a vasodilating stimulus is present (e.g., regional anesthesia, nitroderivate administration, etc.), an alteration in the container-content ratio may occur, so that there may be a situation of reduced preload even in normovolemic conditions.

Furthermore, the presence of supraventricular arrhythmia, either of atrial of junctional origin, may reduce the telediastolic left ventricular filling by almost 15% and, especially in recent tachyarrhythmias, it may cause acute cardiovascular failure [10].

It is worth remembering that a change in cardiovascular function (evidenced by invasive hemodynamic methods) is systemically present in almost 22% of patients over 65 years in the absence of clinical symptoms [11].

Another fundamental element of cardiac performance that is altered by the process of ageing is myocardial contractility. Furthermore, at the peripheral artery level, ageing determines a rise in the stiffness of the great artery walls, with a rise in aortic impendance and a consequent increase of the systolic arterial pressure that is not dependent on the left ventricular ejection volume.

Arterial hypertension provokes, in turn, a left ventricular hypertrophy that contributes to a decrease in left ventricular compliance, a decrease in the telediastolic ventricular volume and aggravates the volume-contractility ratio at the cardiac level.

The fall in peripheral artery elasticity also determines a decrease of the diastolic artery pressure of non-hypertensive patients. This decrease, associated with a rise in ventricular mass and a fall in ventricular compliance, compromises coronary perfusion and oxygen flow to the myocardium. All these factors, associated with alterations of the coronary system, increase the risk of ischemia in the elderly patient, mostly in the presence of tachycardia.

To sum up, all age-related cardiovascular changes lead to a fall in the cardiac load, with a reduced hematic intake from the center to the periphery. Such a fall may be seen as a physiological factor if we consider the parallel decrease in metabolic activity in the elderly. However, in the presence of an increase of peripheral oxygen demand as, for example, during an important stress or during surgical stress, it may determine a cardiovascular "defaillance", with serious parenchymal and tissue hypoperfusion [12, 13].

Respiratory function and cardiovascular system

The most-important change in respiratory function in the elderly patient is the loss of pulmonary and thoracic elasticity. Therefore, the elderly patient needs a greater oxygen intake to carry out the work of breathing equivalent to his younger counterparts [14].

This change in thoraco-pulmonary compliance is differently distributed in the various pulmonary zones, and it leads to a rise in the alveolar-artery oxygen gradient. The changes in pulmonary and thoracic structure associated with ageing determine a progressive fall in paO2. Under stress or in cases of increased requirements, such as during physical training, the elderly subject needs to increase cardiac output to compensate for his physiological fall in paO2 and to satisfy his respiratory muscle oxygen requirements.

Ageing alters the main function of the cardiac pump, which is that of maintaining an adequate systolic output; therefore, it may, in acute situations, favor the occurrence of respiratory failure due to a pulmonary perfusion pressure deficit and to a decreased oxygen flow.

Hepatic function and cardiovascular system

In elderly subjects over 80 years the hepatic parenchyma is decreased by almost 40% compared with young patients. Splanchnic flow decreases in proportion to the hepatic parenchyma; accordingly, with age splanchnic flow progressively decreases. Such a reduction in parenchymal volume and in hepatic flow may alter hepatic functions, thus modifying hematochemical functional tests and altering metabolic processes of biotransformation, mostly with regard to the molecules used during anesthesia [15].

Therefore, a further decrease in hepatic flow during general anesthesia may cause a worsening and failure of this basic physiopathological situation, thus determining a significant and evident reduction in the metabolic phase and in the phase of hepatic elimination of anesthetic drugs.

Renal function and cardiovascular system

As in other organs, in the kidneys ageing causes involutional anatomo-functional changes that lead to a progressive atrophy of the kidney parenchyma. Glomerular sclerosis causes a gradual suppression of the gradient between afferent and efferent arterioles to the glomerulus, with a consequent fall in glomerular filtration pressure and in glomerular function itself. The change in renal vascularization also causes a gradual decrease in renal blood flow, which falls by almost 10% every 10 years after the 65 years of age. This reduction is even more evident at the level of the renal cortex, while it remains basically the same in the marrow area. The logical consequence is a decrease in the glomerular filtration volume, which tends to decrease by almost 5 ml/min per m^2 of body surface area every 10 years over 65 years of age.

A systemic study of the renal function in surgical patients demonstrated that the prevalence of these renal alterations amounts to almost 30% in the elderly population [16]. Such degenerative renal alterations may further be worsened by a parallel fall in the cardiovascular function during surgery. The most important consequence of this physiopathological association is an increase in the half-life of elimination of anesthetic agents and of their metabolites, which have a mere or prevailing renal clearance.

Central nervous system and cardiovascular system

After 65 years of age there is a progressive reduction in the dimensions of the human brain. In men aged over 80 years there is a reduction of almost 20% compared with the dimensions of a 30-year-old subject [17, 18].

This loss in cerebral parenchymal mass amounts to almost 50,000 neurons a day. Furthermore, the number of neurons anatomically present inside the adult brain is of almost one billion, even though only a small percentage is functionally active. This causes neuronal cells to be progressively compensated by the activation of the remaining neurons. Such anatomical neuronal decrease is real, and the endocranial cavity is progressively filled by a greater quantity of cephalorachidian liquid, with a consequent occurrence of a physiological, normotensive hydrocephalus.

At the same time, with increasing age there is a progressive reduction in the resistance to endocranial compression, which makes the elderly much more sensitive to changes in endocranial pressure than a younger patient.

The cerebral flow of an 80-year-old patient is almost 20% lower than that of a young patient. This decrease in cerebral perfusion does not alter the electrical activity and the cerebral metabolism under physiological conditions, since self-regulation of vascular resistances and vasoconstriction caused by hyperventilation are preserved. However, in the elderly subject at risk of atherosclerosis, a reduced cerebral reactivity occurs, mostly in hypoxic conditions. The concomitant presence of hypoxia and of artery hypertension is particularly dangerous. In this case, the insufficient cerebral vascular self-regulation mechanism causes vasodilation, interstitial edema, an increase in the production of cephalorachidian liquid, and the worsening of the hydrocephalus, which, going from a normo- to a hypertensive state, may cause cerebral suffering.

Generally speaking, there are no important neurological alterations during general anesthesia; much more frequently minor functional alterations may be observed, such as memory loss, unrest, and postoperative confusion, which are proofs of cerebral perfusion alterations related to undiagnosed cardiovascular alterations [19-21].

Muscle function and cardiovascular system

The muscle mass in the elderly progressively decreases with increasing age, thus determining a progressive fall in muscular strength and in the ability to control and maintain the immobility of the upper extremities. This falls by 25-50% over the age of 80 years. At the same time, the neuromuscular junction becomes thicker at the level of the postjunctional membrane and there is a rise in extrajunctional cholinergic receptors. Such receptorial proliferation may be considered a symptom of the atrophy of the neuromuscular system, in that is constitutes a compensation mechanism to the decrease in density of motion units which occurs with the physical decay due to ageing [22].

The elderly patient's sensitivity to neuromuscular blockers is similar to that of the younger patient. However, it is generally agreed that there is an increase in the sensitivity to succinylcholine, due rather to a decrease in plasma pseudocholinesterase than to an alteration of the neuromuscular junction itself.

It must be remembered that the supply of neuromuscular blockers to the neuromuscular junction and their correct removal depends on an adequate local blood flow. Furthermore, it must also be emphasized that the main feature of ageing is the involvement of the cardiovascular system with a consequent decrease in cardiac load. Hence, if general anesthesia determines or emphasizes this basic hemodynamic alteration, a prolongation of the neuromuscular blockade action is to be expected due to reduced clearance by the local hypoperfusion.

Autonomic nervous system

The autonomic nervous system (ANS) allows maintenance of cardiovascular homeostasis in young subjects, but appears to be universally and progressively altered in elderly patients. Baroceptorial response, vasoconstriction at cold temperatures, and alterations in heart rate during position changes have a longer-range manifestation, while the range of adaptation is definitely lower. All the cardiovascular compensation mechanisms needed to maintain constant arterial blood pressure are thus less effective in the elderly patient.

Furthermore, the ANS in the elderly has an altered self-regulation characterized by a global reduction both in the number of adrenergic receptors and in the activation of down-regulation [23].

The most-important and fundamental consequence of all this is that anesthetic agents alter organ functions and reduce the plasma level of catecholamines more significantly in the elderly than in young patients, with a possible determination of a serious intraoperative hypotensive status [24].

Hypotension is even more evident when the patient presents a high adrenergic tone in the preoperative period, which is a sign of the activation of hemodynamic compensation mechanisms that may evidence a latent or subclinical cardiac failure not infrequent in elderly patients.

Perioperative risk and cardiovascular system

For the evaluation of perioperative complications after surgery the observation period is 30 days. The evolution of general anesthesia techniques has undoubtedly led to a progressive outcome improvement for elderly patients, thus allowing a reduction of the duration of hospitalization in both intensive care and surgical units. Furthermore, the possibility of monitoring elderly patients, greatly compromised from a functional point of view after surgery in resuscitation departments, has led to a drastic decrease in perioperative complications due to factors linked to anesthesia, which, up to a couple of years ago, amounted to almost 10% of all perioperative complications [25].

However, today it is much more difficult to distinguish among perioperative complications due to anesthesia itself and those determined by the operation or by pre-existing pathologies in the patient. For this reason, almost all the recent studies refer to perioperative survival, neither focussing on nor distinguishing among major and minor complications. The former, which are generally lethal and caused by surgical operations or by basic pathologies in patients, must be clearly distinguished from the latter, which are generally responsible for a prolongation of the period of hospitalization in the intensive care unit and are due to functional or organic alterations that have taken place mostly at the expense of the cardiovascular system during the perioperative period [26].

However, mortality in the elderly is undoubtedly higher than in young patients. At present such mortality in a population of subjects over 65 years of age amounts to almost 5-10% [27]. This incidence is equal to half of that evidenced in the same population 30 years ago and it corresponds to a 5 times higher value than in young patients.

Mortality 1 year after the operation rises approximately to 20% but, in the majority of cases, neither an anesthesiological nor a surgical cause may be evidenced.

There are three main factors acting on the mortality incidence, namely [28]: (1) emergency surgery, (2) site of operation, and (3) preoperative pathologies.

Emergency surgery does not allow a precise evaluation of the patient's conditions, or correction of the alterations present at the time of the intervention, such as absolute or relative hypovolemic status, hydroelectrolytic alterations, reduction in oxygen intake, anemia, heart, lung, or hepatic failure, etc.

The type of surgical lesion, determining hemorrhage or intraoperative ischemia, may cause or determine irreversible impairment in elderly patients, such as infections and sepsis, which are currently the two main causes of perioperative death in the elderly.

During the last few years, the progressive extension of the average life-span has led to a rise in the elderly population undergoing emergency surgical interventions.

Mortality due to the anatomical region where the intervention takes place has the same incidence in elective and emergency cases. However, the most-dangerous sites of operation in the elderly are the thorax, the abdomen, when there is colic resection or massive resection of the digestive tract, and major cardiovascular surgery. In effect, this type of surgery is associated with a 10-20 times greater risk than during inguinal hernia interventions or transuretral prostatic resection.

Age and preoperative pathologies involve an additional risk to that linked to ageing alone. Generally speaking, the higher the average age of the surgical population, the greater the number of associated pathologies; therefore, in this case the patient's physical conditions are more compromised. Almost 50% of elderly patients present cardiovascular alterations such as artery hypertension, silent coronaropathy, heart failure, arteritis, and an elevated pulmonary thromboembolic risk. Another part of the elderly population presents renal, hepatic or metabolic alterations that increase the perioperative risk even if the patient's conditions are stabilized by the therapy followed until the day of intervention. This visceral chronic pathology may be worsened in the perioperative period both due to an alteration in the cardiovascular system that provokes a perfusion decrease with a fall in oxygen intake, and to a recovery with consequent intake of catabolic agents.

Lastly, it must be remembered that over 40% of the elderly population has chronic respiratory distress, which increases significantly the risk of contracting infections in the perioperative period. Such infections, especially if localized at a pulmonary level, may overcome the elderly patient's weak compensation mechanisms, with a consequent occurrence of severe hypoxic conditions.

However, it is important to underline that the 80-year-old patient in good physical condition does not have a significantly higher risk of mortality and morbility than a younger patient in programmed surgery.

Therefore, the prognosis of the elderly patient undergoing surgery is highly influenced by the perioperative physical and pathological status, but it may also be strongly influenced, both negatively and positively, by the surgical technique, by the anesthesiological behavior, and by the choice and application of adequate monitoring, mostly cardiovascular monitoring. This must ensure continuous evaluation of cardiac performance and allow immediate and precise correction of all the alterations identified.

Surveillance of the elderly patient in the perioperative period

Even if we do not consider the patient's age, it is always necessary to make an accurate clinical evaluation in the preoperative period, if possible 7-10 days prior to the programmed intervention [29]. However, to date it has never been demonstrated conclusively that one anesthesia choice is safer than another in the elderly, in terms of morbility and mortality.

Several retrospective and prospective studies demonstrated that there are no significant differences in the postoperative evolution of the elderly patient when one anesthesia technique rather than another is used. In particular, the preference and greater safety for an elderly patient of general rather than regional or combined general-regional anesthesia has never been demonstrated. Only subarachnoid anesthesia, in the absence of intraoperative sedation, was found to interfere less than general anesthesia with the neurological functions of the elderly [30, 31].

The choice of the anesthesia technique must take into consideration the pathological situation and the organic alterations present in the elderly patient. In particular, the action of anesthetic drugs on the cardiovascular system must be closely monitored. In effect, the myocardiodepressant and vasodilating action is well known of drugs such as hypnotics, like sodium thiopentone and propofol, opioids, and some halogenated anesthetics, especially when used at high minimal alveolar concentrations or when rapidly injected at full dosage [32-35].

The organ functional reserve of the elderly patient can surely overcome a moderate work overload, but it can also lead to failure due to an anesthesiological action on the ANS, thus causing an increase of cardiovascular complications.

Cardiovascular monitoring must be very precise and accurate, and it must monitor the totality of the cardiovascular function, so as to allow a blood flow and a peripheral perfusion adequate to the metabolic and oxygen requirements of the tissues. The reaching of this objective is fundamental in order to preserve correct hepatic, renal, cerebral, splanchnic and cardiac functions. The correct functioning of the cardiovascular system may then ensure a correct and rapid metabolism of the opioids used. The logical consequence is a more-rapid neurological recovery due to a quicker plasma clearance of the drugs used.

Conclusions

Recent improvements in the physiopathological understanding of age-related alterations have prompted physicians to widen their assistance of the surgical patient, especially if of advanced age, from the intraoperative period to the overall perioperative period; this includes, besides correct and optimal preparation of the patient that has to undergo surgery, monitoring of vital parameters and of acute postoperative pain.

The loss of elasticity of almost all tissues, together with atrophy and organic fibrosis lead in the elderly patient to structural and functional alterations of the various parenchymas, which progress from maturity to old age.

In the absence of organic pathologies, even in elderly patients, the function of every organ remains balanced under basal conditions, but it may be inadequate under conditions of increased requirements. Therefore, there is an organ reserve that tends to progressively decrease with increasing age.

The elderly patient presents higher risks of perioperative morbidity and mortality than younger patients due to a greater incidence of associated pathologies.

The higher number of complications and their greater severity are signs of a reduced capacity to adapt to the increased requirements of the metabolism that may be observed during anesthesiological and surgical stress, and because of the co-existing pathology.

The optimal surveillance of the elderly patient needs a precise diagnostic capacity and adequate treatment so as to achieve a balance between the patient's pathology and the stimulus he is subject to.

Particular attention must be paid to the preparation of the patient in the preoperative and intraoperative periods in order to adequately survey the interaction between anesthetic drugs and the cardiovascular system. In order for this surveillance of the cardiovascular system to be accurate and effective, continuous and systemic monitoring is required, which must be able to provide all the data necessary to evaluate correctly the changes in the hemodynamic profile. Therefore, a correct interpretation of the cardiovascular pattern allows correct physiopathological diagnosis of the current alteration, a targeted choice of the therapy, verification of its therapeutic action, and to decide accordingly whether to proceed with it, change it, or modify it according to the different needs.

At this point, we should ask ourselves whether we consider the co-called standard hemodynamic surveillance systems (ECG, MAP, $PetCO_2$, SpO_2) to be enough to perform an adequate anesthesia in the elderly patient and to prevent perioperative complications, especially of cardiovascular origin.

References

1. Schneider EL, Reed J D Jr (1985) Life extension. N Engl J Med 312: 1159-1172
2. Williams ME (1984) Clinical implication of aging physiology. Am J Med 76: 1049-1054
3. Fülöp T Jr, Wórum I, Csongor J et al (1985) Body composition by multiscope method and the elimination kinetics of these isotopes in healthy elderly subjects. Gerontology 31: 6-19
4. Hussain S (1976) Disorder of homeostasis and thrombosis in the aged. Med Clin North Am 60: 1273-1285
5. Detraglia M, Cook FB, Stasiw DM, Cerny LC (1974) Erythrocytes fragility in aging. Biochim Biophys Acta 345:213-220
6. West CD, Brown H, Simons EL, et al (1961) Adrenocortical function and cortisol metabolism in old age. J Clin Endocrinol Metab 21: 1197-2009
7. Gerstenblith G, Renlud DG, Lakatta EG (1987) Cardiovascular response to excercise in younger and in old men. FASFB J 46:1834-1845
8. Rady MY, Ryan T, Starr NJ (1998) Perioperative determinant of morbility and mortality in elderly patients undergoing cardiac surgery. Crit Care Med 26:225-235
9. Kirsh M, Guesnier L, LeBesnerais P, et al (1998) Cardiac operations in octagenarians: perioperatives risk factors for death and impaired autonomy. Ann Thorac Surg 66: 60-67
10. Thomas DR, Ritchie CS (1995) Preoperative assessment of older adults. J Am Geriatr Soc 48: 811-821
11. Burns-Cox N, Campbell WB, van Nimmen BAJ, et al (1997) Surgical care and outcome for patients in their nineties. Br J Surg 84:496-498
12. Wesfeldt ML, Abben R (1981) Presbycardia. Johns Hopkins Med J 149: 203-212
13. Lakkata EG (1986) Diminished beta adrenergic modulation of cardiovascular function in advanced age. Cardiol Clin 4:185-196
14. Wahba WM (1983) Influence of aging on lung function – clinical significance of changes from age twenty. Anesth Analg 62: 764-781
15. Gepkas MC, Haverback BJ (1969) The aging gastrointestinal tract. Am J Surg 117: 881-892

16. MacLachlan MSF (1978) The aging kidney. Lancet II:143-156
17. Drummond GB (1975) The assessment of post operative mental function. Br J Anaesth 47: 130-142
18. Yamura H, Masatoshi I, Kubota K, Matsuzawa T (1980) Brain atrophy during aging: a quantitative study with computerized tomography. J Gerontol 32: 492-499
19. Beggren D, Gustafson Y, Eriksson B, et al (1987) Postoperative confusion aftre anaesthesia in elderly patients with femoral fractures. Anesth Analg 66: 497-504
20. Bigler D, Adelhoj B, Petring OU, et al (1985) Mental function and morbidity after acute hip surgery during spinal and general anesthesia. Anaesthesia 40: 672-676
21. Bedford PD (1955) Adverse cerebral effects of anaesthesia on old people. Lancet II: 259-263
22. Tomonaga M (1977) Histochemical and ultrastructural changes in senil human skeletal muscle. J Am Geriatr Soc 25: 125-134
23. Pan HYM, Hoffman BB, Pershe RA, Blashcke TF (1986) Decline in beta adrenergic receptor mediated vascular relaxation with aging in man. J Pharmacol Exp Ther 239: 802-811
24. Collins KJ, Exton – Smith AN, James MH, Olivier DJ (1980) Functional changes in autonomic nervous responses with aging. Age Ageing 9: 17-25
25. Vaz FG, Seymour DG (1989) A prospective study of elderly general surgical patients. I. Pre operative medical problems. Age Ageing 18: 309-315
26. Brander P, Kjellberg M, Tammisto T (1970) The effect of anaesthesia and general surgery on geriatric patients. Ann Chirug Gynaec Fenn 59: 138-145
27. Marx GF, Mateo CV, Orkin LR (1973) Computer analysis of post anesthesic deaths. Anesthesiology 39: 54-63
28. Forrester JB, Rheder K, Cahalan MK, Goldsmith CH (1992) Multicenter study of general anesthesia. III. Predictors of severe postoperative adverse outcomes. Anesthesiology 76: 3-12
29. Veering BT (1999) Management of anaesthesia in elderly patients. Curr Opin Anaesthesiol 12: 333-336
30. Chung F, Meier R, Lautenschlager E, et al (1987) General or spinal anesthesia: which is the best in the elderly. Anesthesiology 67: 422-427
31. Ghoneim MM, Hinrichs JV, O'Hara MW, et al (1988) Comparison of psychologic and cognitive functions after general or regional anesthesia. Anesthesiology 69: 507-515
32. Simpson BR, Williams M, Scott JF, Crampton Smith A (1961) The effect of anaesthesia and selective surgery in old people. Lancet II: 887-893
33. Gregory GA, Eger EI II, Munson ES (1969) The relationship between age and halothane requirement in man. Anesthesiology 30: 488-495
34. Scott JC, Stanski DR (1984) Decreased fentanyl and alfentanyl doses requirement with age : a simultaneous pharamacokinetic and pharmacodynamic evaluation. J Pharmacol Exp Ther 240: 159-164
35. Muravchik S (1984) Effect of age and premedication on thiopental sleep dose. Anesthesiology 61: 133-139

Priorities and Optimization of Care in the Elderly – Minimizing Disability

J. H. SILVERSTEIN

An elderly individual undergoing abdominal surgery is likely to spend a little more than 3 months recovering, if recovering is understood to mean returning to a preoperative level of independent function. Functional recovery goes beyond whether the patient's wound is healed or whether they awoke successfully from anesthesia to consider when, if ever, the patient resumes the life they were leading before they elected to have an operation [1]. With projections for increasing elderly populations in the next 2 decades in most countries, the degree of disability and services needed to provide for such disabilities becomes an important policy question.

From the perspective of mid-to-late life patients, symptoms and disability are the principle outcomes of most disease processes. Elective surgery is frequently the cause of disabilities that become the focus of protracted personal and medical care. The pathway to disability, originally described by Verbrugge and Jette [2], begins with a **disease or pathology**. Having a disease does not in itself imply and impairment (e.g. early hypertension). **Impairments** occur at the organ system level and are dysfunctional and structural abnormalities in specific body systems, such as cardiovascular or neurological systems. An example of impairment is congestive heart failure. **Functional limitations** subsequently occur at the organism, or entire being, level and comprise restrictions in basic physical and mental abilities, such as ambulation, reaching, bending, and communicating intelligibly. Relatively severe organ impairment can occur before functional limitations are evident. Early compensated congestive heart failure may not cause functional limitation, while advancing heart failure may severely limit physical functioning. **Disability** occurs when there is an insurmountable gap between an individual's capacities and environmental demands such that important activities are compromised. Disability, therefore, evolves in a patient's environment and socioeconomic conditions. Intra-individual (e.g., age, socioeconomic status) and extra-individual (e.g., acute medical events, preventive interventions) factors can influence the disablement process in either direction.

Valerie Lawrence, from the University of Texas Health Science Center has provided seminal information that delineates the difficulty elderly patients have in recovering from elective surgery. By examining activities of daily living (ADL) and independent activities of daily living (IADL), she found that recovery following elective abdominal surgery is frequently much more prolonged than would be estimated by many physicians. ADL activities include eating, toileting, dressing, grooming, ambulation, and bathing, and IADL include abilities to use the telephone, access transportation, purchase groceries, prepare meals, do housework, wash laundry, take medications, and manage money. Three-hundred and seventy-two patients were evaluated before and after elective abdominal surgery. For ADLs, mean change scores were significantly different from pre-operative assessment at 1, 3, and 6 weeks. For IADLs, mean scores were significantly decreased below baseline at 1, 3 and 6 weeks and 3 months. At 3 months after surgery, 14% of patients had disability in ADLs, while for IADLs, 20% had persistent disability at 6 months after surgery (personnel communication, V. Lawrence).

In designing perioperative care plans, we consider two types of pre-existing factors, or determinants: (1) *variable elements* of function that may be modifiable or amenable to interventions and (2) relatively *fixed elements* in the context of daily living, which shape function and the roles of the variable elements, but may not be feasible targets for improving recovery. Variable elements are a comprehensive array of psychosocial, behavioral, and preoperative biomedical factors that can influence the evolution of function directly or indirectly through their influences on, and/or interaction with, other determinants. Fixed elements are a separate constellation of contextual factors of daily living in which determinants and functional evolution interact and unfold.

We further consider the influence of an *acute event*, anesthesia and surgery, as a separate set of variable elements. Anesthesia incorporates pharmacological techniques to eliminate pain and the stress response attendant to surgical procedures. Improved surgical techniques have made the decision to undergo a surgical procedure more appealing to elderly patients.

What will be considered optimal care for the elderly will vary from country to country and area to area. Important variables include the overall socioeconomic status of the community, the local economics of health care, how health care is provided, the status of family units and the role of the elderly in family units. The following discussion is based on the following presumptions:

- There are no specific limits on the provision of health care to the elderly. Elective surgery may be appropriate for centenarians.
- The elderly value their independence and seek to preserve independent living.
- Hospitals actively attempt to decrease the length of stay.

Preoperative evaluation and management of the elderly surgical patient involves addressing the areas of variable co-morbidities and assessing fixed elements. The perioperative evaluation provides information for the immediate medical care of the patient, indicates what, if any rehabilitation program needs to be organized, provides the discharge planning team with sufficient information to plan for discharge, particularly if the patient will be going to somewhere other than their home, and finally permits the care team to prepare the patient and their family so that everyone is clear on what will happen surrounding the surgical procedure. Intensive care physicians, surgeons, and anesthesiologists are involved primarily in the medical management of these patients, while planning for proper rehabilitation and discharge planning are frequently the responsibility of other members of the care team and vary widely between centers. These last areas will not be addressed further in this article. Misconceptions about various aspects of medical care, particularly surgical care, are common among patients and their immediate relatives, and can be effectively addressed by physician members of the team.

Fixed variables include age, socioeconomic status, gender, and, in many cases, degree of assimilation into the society. Chronological age has been associated with perioperative morbidity and mortality. Ageing, however, is highly variable between individuals, and so chronological age may be a poor predictor. Tiret et al. [3] classically demonstrated that the disease burden of the individual is the greater predictor and that each additional disease has progressively more impact on the individual as they age. Socioeconomic status has been shown to have a profound impact on a variety of outcome variables [4, 5]. In some countries, socioeconomic status severely limits the accessible options for rehabilitation and nursing facilities. Although gender is a fixed variable, it has been associated with differing alterations in autonomic function [6], renal [7], and adrenocortical function [8]. With increasing mobility, elder patients are likely to find themselves requiring surgical care in a facility where they do not speak the principle language and/or have not assimilated into the prevailing culture.

The principle variable factors that should be addressed in the preoperative period are physical co-morbidities. Perioperative care, including intensive care, tends to follow what Muravchick [9] refers to as a vertical or systems approach. Cardiac disease tops the list of organ systems that have received attention among perioperative physicians. Pulmonary complications appear to be a more-common cause of morbidity and mortality in elderly patients [10]. In the following discussion, the cardiovascular system will be employed as our model organ system for demonstration purposes. The point is that there is a significant amount of knowledge relative to ageing that needs to be part of the armamentarium of practising physicians. This will be followed by a short discussion of central nervous system dysfunction following surgery.

Cardiovascular ageing

Ageing is associated with a decrease in connective tissue compliance and distensibility. This has been found due primarily to increasing cross bridging between elastin and collagen filaments. An elastic tube that undergoes regular stretching is the aorta. Given an average heart rate of 70, the aorta expands and contracts about 2.9×10^9 times by age 80 years. Elongation, stiffening and widening of the aorta, often noted in chest radiographs as "uncoiling" of the aorta, is a common result. Because the older aorta is stiffer, each ventricular systole is met with a higher peak pressure, i.e., there is a considerable increase in afterload. This same phenomenon exits throughout the entire vascular tree. So there is an increase in systemic vascular resistance. In addition, each pulse wave travels through the stiffer vascular tree and is reflected back towards the heart earlier and more strongly than in a young vascular tree. In young cardiovascular systems, the reflected pulse wave tends to arrive following systole, but in the elderly this component is appended to the end systolic afterload. Standard measurement of blood pressure by forearm sphygmomanometry fails to discern this aspect of pressure, as the reflected wave is not retransmitted significantly down the arterial tree. Thus, were you to measure blood pressure in the aortic root you would find that systolic hypertension, a common finding in elderly patients, is considerably more pronounced in the root of the aorta. The reflected pulse wave provides an important component to chronic increase in afterload experienced by the elderly heart [11].

Age-related alteration in aortic-arterial stiffness is probably the most-important and serious normal change that affects the ageing human cardiovascular system. The heart does not decrease in size with age, a unique feature compared with most other organs. There is a general hypertrophy of the cells and a marked increase in connective tissue, although there tends to be a decrease in total myocytes. Cardiac structural alterations in the human are not well represented by rat models. The two primary clinical alterations noted in elderly hearts, in the absence of disease states and severe deconditioning, are concentric left ventricular hypertrophy and a substantial decline in diastolic compliance. A prolonged action potential and isovolemic relaxation time in senescent hearts delays diastolic filling. The result is a 50% decline in early diastolic ventricular filling in the aged. The importance of atrial contraction to ventricular filling increases from 10% to 30% in elderly subjects [12]. By comparing highly fit individuals with a sedentary cohort, it was concluded that diastolic dysfunction is intrinsic to ageing rather than the result of a reduction in aerobic capacity [13].

Altered diastolic relaxation causes increased left ventricular end-diastolic pressure, both at rest and during exercise. Higher pressures are generated to achieve the same stroke volume. Stroke volume in the aged heart can be exquisitely sensitive to alterations in ventricular preload, particularly loss of the atrial systole. Frank-Starling relationships become increasingly important for aged patients. Despite multiple reports of progressive decline with age, cardiac output is essentially maintained in subjects who are carefully screened for occult disease [14].

While cardiac performance at rest may not be altered, major limitations become obvious during strenuous exercise. Maximum aerobic capacity decreases with age. There are essentially no direct observations of cardiac performance during surgery, so perioperative doctors seeking to discern a level of organ reserve have turned to the exercise response studies for insight. The presence of even occult coronary artery disease and individual conditioning, or deconditioning, play important limiting roles. While VO_2 max declines with age, Lakatta [11] has argued against concluding that this is entirely due to the alterations in the central circulation. It is possible that age-related alterations in oxidation capacity per unit muscle, ability to shunt blood to exercising muscles, and/or muscle mass could also contribute.

The physiology of the ageing cardiovascular system has to be kept in context. Disease load increases steadily with age and requires proper evaluation and treatment prior to elective surgery. Diastolic-based cardiac dysfunction has been distinguished from the more commonly recognized systolic dysfunction as a pathophysiology of heart failure. The reader is referred to a review by Wei [15] for the clinical distinctions of types of cardiac dysfunction. There is a significant and increasing prevalence of coronary artery disease in elderly patients in many countries. Thus, although pure age-related alterations in the cardiovascular system have been well delineated, it may be the rare patient in western civilizations with a cardiovascular system whose sole alteration is that associated with normal ageing.

A similar examination of other important vital systems associated with appropriate preoperative optimization should be conducted. Detailed descriptions of approaches to preoperative evaluation of geriatric patients have been published in recent years [9, 16].

Special mention is warranted for the cognitive and affective status of elderly patients. The elderly are subject to a variety of central neurological syndromes following operation, including postoperative delirium and postoperative cognitive dysfunction. Delirium, or acute confusional state, is characterized by acute onset, altered level of consciousness, fluctuating course and disturbances in orientation, memory, thought and behavior [17]. Delirium is fairly common during emergence from general anesthesia. Emergence delirium is particularly common in the pediatric age group but may be seen at any age. Emergence delirium is most commonly recognized by wild and dysfunctional behavior. Elderly patients do not frequently emerge from anesthesia delirious. Postoperative (in contrast to emergence delirium) delirium typically occurs 6-24 h following emergence from anesthesia, and is almost exclusively a disease of the elderly. Unlike emergence delirium, postoperative delirium is frequently not associated with wild or uncontrolled behavior. While there may be a complete lack of orientation to time, person, and place, the patient may suffer in quiet terror in their unfamiliar surroundings. This quiet form of delirium will be missed if the patient is not directly queried about their degree of orientation. There is at least one successful trial of a preventive orientation regimen that has been employed in medical patients [18]. There is a serious question as to whether postoperative delirium is the same disease as delirium in hospitalized medical patients [19]. There have been no trials to date of either a prophylactic or treatment regimen for elderly patients with postoperative delirium. The impact of delirium is severe, prolonging length of stay and increasing the potential for other life-threatening complications [20]. The likelihood of dying increases several fold once delirium appears. Risk factors for the development of postoperative delirium have been evaluated, however different studies have come to differing conclusions. Meperidine (pethedine) and benzodiazepines, but not other drugs, including choice of anesthetic agents, have been associated with the development of postoperative delirium [21]. It is believed that pre-existing cognitive difficulties are associated with a higher incidence of both postoperative delirium and postoperative cognitive dysfunction, but there is limited literature to date to support this contention.

Postoperative cognitive dysfunction (POCD) is a measurable deterioration of performance as defined by psychometric tests that probe specific cognitive tasks. This may not be clinically evident. There is commonly a dissociation between self-perception of cognitive decline and measured cognitive alterations. Cognitive decline is very common following open heart surgery with cardiopulmonary bypass [22]. Following non-cardiac surgery, POCD has been reported to occur in 25% of patients at 1 week after receiving general anesthesia, with 9.9% having measurable dysfunction at 3 months [23]. Although cerebral ischemia is a likely pathophysiological mechanism, the largest study of non-cardiac surgical patients failed to find a relationship between POCD and either hypotension or hypoxemia during either the pre, intra, or 3-day postoperative period [23]. To date there are no strategies that have been investigated to prevent or treat POCD.

There is little indication at the moment that any specific anesthetic regimen would be advantageous for elderly patients. An excellent review of particularly the difference between regional and general anesthetic techniques was recently presented by Roy [24].

Strategies for optimizing the care of elderly surgical patients clearly must be multi-factorial, seeking to minimize the impact of co-morbid conditions, providing sufficient education to the patient, and their families, so that they may participate in a useful manner during the recuperation period, and planning in advance for appropriate rehabilitation and placement.

References

1. Raja SN, Haythornthwaite JA (1999) Anesthetic management of the elderly: measuring function beyond the immediate perioperative horizon. Anesthesiology 91:909-911
2. Verbrugge LM, Jette AM (1994) The disablement process. Soc Sci Med 38:1-14
3. Tiret L, Hatton F, Desmonts JM, Vourch G (1988) Prediction of outcome of anesthesia in patients over 40 years: a multifactorial risk index. Stat Med 7:947-954
4. Pearlin LI (1994) The study of the oldest-old: some promises and puzzles. Int J Aging Hum Dev 38:91-98
5. Inouye SK, Albert MS, Mohs R, et al (1993) Cognitive performance in a high-functioning community-dwelling elderly population. J Gerontol 48:M146-M151
6. Barnett SR, Morin RJ, Kiely DK, et al (1999) Effects of age and gender on autonomic control of blood pressure dynamics. Hypertension 33:1195-1200
7. Malmrose LC, Gray SL, Pieper CF, et al (1993) Measured versus estimated creatinine clearance in a high-functioning elderly sample: MacArthur Foundation Study of Successful Aging. J Am Geriatr Soc 41:715-721
8. Born J, Ditschuneit I, Schreiber M, et al (1995) Effects of age and gender on pituitary-adreno-cortical responsiveness in humans. Eur J Endocrinol 132:705-711
9. Muravchick S (1997) Geroanesthesia. Principles for management of the elderly patient. Mosby, St. Louis
10. Polanczyk CA, Marcantonio E, Goldman L, et al (2001) Impact of age on perioperative complications and length of stay in patients undergoing noncardiac surgery. Ann Intern Med 134:637-643
11. Lakatta EG (1994) Cardiovascular reserve capacity in healthy older humans. Aging (Milano). 6:213-223
12. Alpert JS, Petersen P, Godtfredsen J (1988) Atrial fibrillation: natural history, complications, and management. Annu Rev Med 39:41-52
13. Folkow B, Svanborg A (1993) Physiology of cardiovascular aging. Physiol Rev 73:725-764
14. Lakatta EG (1990) Changes in cardiovascular function with aging. Eur Heart J 11 [Suppl C]:22-29
15. Wei JY (1992) Age and the cardiovascular system. N Engl J Med 327:1735-1739
16. Silverstein JH (2000) Geriatric anesthesia. Anesthesiol Clin North Am 18:1
17. Lipowski ZJ (1990) Delirium: acute confusional states. Oxford University Press, New York
18. Inouye SK, Bogardus ST Jr, Charpentier PA, et al (1999) A multicomponent intervention to prevent delirium in hospitalized older patients. N Engl J Med 340:669-676

19. Brauer C, Morrison RS, Silberzweig SB, et al (2000) The cause of delirium in patients with hip fracture. Arch Intern Med 160:1856-1860
20. Silverstein JH, Rasmussen LS, Moller JT, et al (1999) Risk factors and impact of postoperative delirium in elderly surgical patients (abstract). Anesthesiology
21. Marcantonio ER, Juarez G, Goldman L, et al (1994) The relationship of postoperative delirium with psychoactive medications. JAMA 272:1518-1522
22. Hlatky MA, Bacon C, Boothroyd D, et al (1997) Cognitive function 5 years after randomization to coronary angioplasty or coronary artery bypass graft surgery. Circulation 96:II-11-4
23. Moller JT, Cluitmans P, Rasmussen LS, et al (1998) Long-term postoperative cognitive dysfunction in the elderly ISPOCD1 study. Lancet 351:857-861
24. Roy RC (2000) Choosing general versus regional anesthesia for the elderly. Anesthes Clin North Am 18:91-104

Surgery in the Elderly – Outcome and Complication Pattern

L.S. Rasmussen

An increasing number of elderly patients is undergoing surgery. In addition, even elderly patients with significant concurrent disease are now frequently considered eligible for major surgical procedures. Generally, postoperative complications occur more frequently with increasing age. Age, however, is not in it self a very strong risk factor but the presence of chronic, age-related diseases increase with age and in addition, a predictable decrease in physiologic organ reserve is seen in the elderly. The elderly patient is therefore less able to compensate for any disturbance in organ function and clinical postoperative complications may result. Postoperative complications can be classified into cardiac, respiratory, infectious, and cerebral complications.

Cardiac complications

The primary cause of postoperative death is cardiac complications that include myocardial infarction (MI), unstable angina, serious dysrythmias, and congestive heart failure [1]. These complications may lead to postoperative cardiac death. In the postoperative phase, the complications may be difficult to detect. Many postoperative myocardial infarctions are associated with quite a few clinical symptoms and signs, chest pain may be attributed to other conditions and cardiac enzyme levels may to some extent be affected by surgery. Pulmonary oedema and other causes of respiratory insufficiency after surgery have similar features and dysrythmias may not be detected in the ward. Accordingly, many cardiac complications are probably not recognized. The incidence of perioperative MI is presumed to be approximately 1% after non-cardiac surgery but five times more common in patients with previous MI [1]. Recent MI (3-6 months) is probably more dangerous but the poor outcome in surgical patients with recent MI is related to cardiac function and the nature of the surgical procedures that such patients are undergoing [2].

The pathophysiology underlying these cardiac complications are thought to involve coronary artery thrombosis, spasm, and plaque rupture. A mismatch may easily occur between oxygen supply and perioperatively increased oxygen demand for instance in case of tachycardia and blood pressure changes where hypotension decreases coronary perfusion pressure and hypertension increases afterload. Many studies have focused on preoperative identification of patients at risk for cardiac complications. The most sensitive test are exercise stress testing, echocardiography, and ambulatory ECG monitoring. In selected cases, cardiac catherization and radionuclear imaging techniques may be used. Many abnormal findings will appear in the population of elderly patients and in daily practice, most patients will only have a history, a clinical examination, and a preoperative ECG. Actually, the aim is to identify the most well-established risk factors and which are recent MI and current congestive heart failure.

While no particular anaesthetic technique or anaesthetic drug seems to be documented as the most safe in patients at high-risk for cardiac complications, it is possible that beta-blockers may have a beneficial effect, especially in the elderly [3]. Atenolol was found to reduce mortality in patients with or at risk for coronary artery disease undergoing non-cardiac surgery [4]. Eight more cardiac deaths were observed in the placebo group ($p=0.03$). The findings in this study, however, are not easily interpreted. One problem is the inclusion criteria; for example all smokers aged 65 and older were considered risk patients. More important, diabetes mellitus turned out to be a more important predictor of death than atenolol and 7 more patients with diabetes mellitus were found in the placebo group. It would be interesting to know the effects of beta-blockade in the elderly surgical patient with diabetes mellitus.

Respiratory complications

While age is a commonly described risk factor for postoperative respiratory complications, other factors are usually more important. These risk factors consist of chronic pulmonary disease, smoking, obesity, and the type of surgery involving upper abdominal procedures with thoracic surgery being the most significant [5]. After upper abdominal surgery, the function of the diaphragm is inhibited probably due to inhibition by input of predominantly noxious stimuli [6]. This leads to pulmonary dysfunction with a decrease in functional residual capacity and small atelectasis that are visible on the chest CT-scan [7]. As closing capacity increases in the elderly, small airway closure already occurs in the supine position before surgery and clinical atelectasis are more likely. Residual curarization attenuates the airway protective mechanisms and increases the risk of pulmonary aspiration of gastric contents [8]. The response to hypoxaemia is also inhibited and residual curarization has been found to increase in the incidence of postoperative pulmonary dysfunction in the elderly [9, 10]. Postoperative arterial hypoxaemia is very common, especially on the second and third night after upper abdominal surgery, with approximately 10% having episodes or prolonged periods of desaturation [11, 12]. Nocturnal pulse oximetry may aid in the early detection of pulmonary dysfunction but, however, is not entirely reliable due to the common occurrence of artefacts caused by poor peripheral perfusion and patient movement [13]. It is still a matter of discussion whether postoperative pulmonary complications are influenced by the choice of anaesthetic technique, for instance by using epidural pain relief [14]. Application of positive end-expiratory pressure does not seem effective [15].

Infectious complications

As described, pulmonary infections are commonly seen in the elderly postoperative patient and other frequent infections after surgery include urinary tract infection and wound infection [16]. The immune response is altered in the elderly and the high incidence of diabetes mellitus and on-going medication with steroids and other immuno-modulating drugs probably explain the higher incidence of infections the elderly. Immunosuppresion is given not only for cancer and in transplant recipients, but also for numerous other conditions such as arthritis, connective tissue diseases and skin disorders. Postoperative septicaemia has a particular poor prognosis in old patients. Early and aggressive treatment with emphasis on the possibility for surgical debridement or drainage is essential [17]. Dosage of antibiotics must be guided by assessment of renal function and interaction with concurrent medication, especially when erythromycin or fluoroquinolones are given. Toxicity may otherwise result with subsequent additional complications. Perhaps it is possible to reduce the incidence of postoperative wound infections. Depletion buffy coat by filtration of blood decreases the white blood cell content and has been shown to decrease the incidence of wound infection after colorectal surgery presumably because lymphocytes and cytokines in allogenic blood inhibit the defence against bacteria [18]. In elderly patients, hypothermia is a common adverse event that increases postoperative morbidity. In a randomized study the incidence of wound infection was significantly less (6% versus 19%) when normothermia was assured in patients undergoing colorectal surgery [19].

Cerebral complications

Cerebral complications following anaesthesia and surgery cover a spectrum from uncommon and obvious occurrences such as stroke to the much more subtle and quite frequent cognitive disorders. Major cerebral complications may result in immediate death of the patient or major deficits. The major cerebral complications usually results from a stroke but generalized hypoxic brain damage has been reported. A perioperative stroke is defined as an episode of focal or global loss of cerebral function with symptoms lasting more than 24 hours or leading to death. The major cerebral complications are recognized through the typical symptoms and a brief neurological examination. The incidence of major cerebral complications following general surgery varies between 0.2 and 0.7% [20]. However, in selected patient groups the incidence is as high as 5%, presumably due to the associated risk factors of these patients (neck or cardiac surgery) [20, 21]. Outcome after a major perioperative cerebral complication is poor with a mortality of approximately 30% compared to approximately 15% in the general population. Several risk factors have been identified. Age seems to be an important factor. The perioperative stroke risk increases from 0.2% in patients below the age of 65 to 3.4% in those over 80 years of age [20]. Other important risk factors include type of surgery, cardiac disease, especially atrial fibrillation, peripheral vascular disease, previous cerebrovascular disease, and diabetes mellitus. Rarely, generalized hypoxic brain damage caused by profound perioperative hypoxaemia or haemodynamic instability result in insufficient cerebral blood flow. However, it is important to remember that the rare anaesthetic mishaps such as failed intubation and drug overdose are still reported as reasons for perioperative death or postoperative coma.

Perioperative cognitive disorders are characterized by clinically significant deficits in cognition and memory. They represent significant changes from a previous level of functioning.

Delirium is an acute disturbance of consciousness and a change in cognition that tends to fluctuate throughout the day. Postoperative delirium is a transient disorder dominated by disorientation, deficits in cognition and attention [22]. It is accompanied by lethargy or increased psychomotor activity. The onset is usually acute, the condition lasts for days or a few weeks and it fluctuates typically during the day, being most pronounced during the night with a disturbance in the sleep-wake cycle. The incidence of delirium after surgery is generally around 10% in elderly patients but it varies from 3-61% depending on the age, type of surgery, preoperative cognitive status, and preoperative medical status [22]. Elderly patients undergoing repair of hip fracture or cardiac surgery seem to be at very high-risk. Postoperative hospital stay is prolonged in those patients and rehabilitation is delayed. The pathophysiology of postoperative delirium is still poorly understood. Regarding aetiology or risk factors, delirium is usually the result of multiple causes rather than one specific factor. Important eliciting factors for postoperative delirium in the elderly include drugs (especially neuroleptics and anticholinergics), withdrawal states, infection, dehydration, and metabolic disturbances. Delirious patients may be unable to co-operate and are at high-risk for additional complications such as fractures and respiratory complications. While regional anaesthesia may be preferable due to a better maintenance of mental function for the first day after surgery, the difference fades away after a few days [22]. Adequate fluid and nutrition should be assured and a proper sensory environment including supportive nursing may be essential [23].

The more subtle postoperative cognitive dysfunction (POCD) is characterized by a deterioration in cognitive evidenced by neuropsychological testing. Typical findings are:

- memory impairment as identified by a reduced ability to learn or recall information;
- disturbance in executive functioning (i.e., planning, organising, sequencing, abstracting);
- disturbance in attention or speed of information processing;
- impairment in perceptual-motor abilities;
- impairment in language (i.e., comprehension, word finding).

POCD is detected in days or weeks after surgery and can last for weeks or months. In the worst degree, it may remain as a permanent disorder. Numerous neuropsychological tests exist and usually several are combined to be used in suitable test battery. Problems are associated with the application of the tests, with the statistical analysis, and the interpretation of the test results [24]. One problem is the pronounced variability between the individuals and the sessions of the individual patients. Another problem is the practice effect which, unfortunately, has been ignored to a large extent. Disregarding the practice effect may give a false impression of improvement or lead to the erroneous conclusion that no deterioration in cognitive function has occurred if the same result is obtained before and after surgery.

Most studies of postoperative cognitive dysfunction have focused on cardiac surgery patients who have a high incidence of POCD, 20-80% [25-28]. The aetiology behind POCD is thought to be related to the use of cardiopulmonary bypass (CPB) and the duration of CPB is an important risk factor and cerebral embolism is a common phenomenon during cardiac surgery. Some coronary artery bypass procedures can be performed without CPB. This would eliminate risk factors associated with CPB and perhaps improve outcome but the evidence is sparse [29].

After non-cardiac surgery, POCD is not well studied. In 1955 Bedford reported that 7% of 251 elderly patients undergoing surgery developed "gross dementia" [30]. The diagnosis was based on personal observation and questioning and no neuropsychological testing was attempted. In more recent studies, the application of neuropsychological tests on patients undergoing non-cardiac surgery has aimed at investigating potential differences in cognitive function between regional and general anaesthesia. This is a relevant issue often discussed with patients scheduled for an orthopaedic, urological or gynecological procedures. No significant difference has been found in neuropsychological test results between regional and general anaesthesia [31-33]. The primary purpose of these studies was not to estimate the incidence of POCD and in only one of them POCD was detected beyond the first postoperative week: in 262 patients undergoing knee replacement surgery, an incidence of 5% of POCD was found after 6 months [34]. In the multicentre study, the aim of the International Study of Postoperative Cognitive Dysfunction (ISPOCD was to specifically find the incidence of POCD after non-cardiac surgery in the elderly and to assess the importance of age, perioperative hypoxaemia and hypotension [11]. Oxygenation was measured by continuous pulse oximetry before surgery, throughout the operative day and during the first 3 postoperative nights. Blood pressure was recorded oscillometrically intraoperatively, throughout the day of surgery and the following night. A total of 1 218 patients were included and 7 days after surgery cognitive dysfunction was found in 25.8% of the patients. At the second postoperative test 3 months after the operation cognitive dysfunction was identified in 9.9% of the patients. In the control population, the criteria for cognitive dysfunction were fulfilled in 3.4% of the elderly volunteers at the one week time point and in 2.8% at 3 months. The difference in cognitive dysfunction between patients and controls were highly significant. A significant relationship was found between early POCD and increasing age, increasing duration of anaesthesia, low level of education, second operation, postoperative infection, and respiratory complication. POCD detected at the second postoperative test after 3 months was associated only with increasing age. No relationship could be demonstrated between different levels or duration of hypoxaemia or hypotension and POCD [11].

The ISPOCD study confirmed that POCD exists in after non-cardiac surgery and confirms the many anecdotal reports from clinicians who have observed patients who survived their operation and anaesthetic without any obvious injuries, but who complained of changes in cognition for weeks to months after surgery. The ISPOCD study raised a lot of new questions. For instance, the consequences on daily life are not well known although a significant relation was found between a deterioration in cognitive function and a decline in Activities of Daily Living. Occupational consequences are very relevant but difficult to assess in surgical patients, in particular in a population of elderly where many have retired or plan to retire in conjunction with major surgery. We do not know how much this POCD impairs quality of life or how often POCD leads to premature loss of independence. It must also be kept in mind that all of the included patients were above 60 years of age and that they underwent major surgical procedures with general anaesthesia. We do not know the incidence of POCD in younger patients, with regional anaesthesia, or after minor surgery. An increasing proportion of procedures is done on an out-patient basis and accordingly, the possible harmful effects of hospitalization on elderly patients could be reduced.

Conclusion

Although excellent surgical results may be obtained in elderly patients, increased attention to a co-existing disease is necessary to minimize postoperative complications. Functional organ reserve decreases with age and adverse events and minor complications are often poorly tolerated. The leading cause of postoperative death is cardiac complications but cerebral dysfunction with delirium or postoperative cognitive dysfunction seems to be the most common complication after major surgery in the elderly.

References

1. Mangano DT (1990) Perioperative cardiac morbidity. Anesthesiology. 72: 153-84.
2. Dirksen A, Kjoller E (1998) Cardiac predictors of death after non-cardiac surgery evaluated by intention to treat. BMJ 297: 1011-1013
3. Zaugg M, Tagliente T, Lucchinetti E et al (1999) Beneficial effects from beta-adrenergic blockade in elderly patients undergoing noncardiac surgery. Anesthesiology 91: 1674-1686
4. Mangano DT, Layug EL, Wallace A et al (1996). Effect of atenolol on mortality and cardiovascular morbidity after noncardiac surgery. Multicenter Study of Perioperative Ischemia Research Group. N Engl J Med 335: 1713-1720
5. Pedersen T, Eliasen K, Henriksen E (1990) A prospective study of risk factors and cardiopulmonary complications associated with anaesthesia and surgery: risk indicators of cardiopulmonary morbidity. Acta Anaesthesiol Scand 34: 144-155
6. Nimmo AF, Drummond GB (1996) Respiratory mechanics after abdominal surgery measured with continuous analysis of pressure, flow and volume signals. Br J Anaesth 1996 77: 317-326
7. Rothen HU, Sporre B, Engberg G et al(1993) Re-expansion of atelectasis during general anaesthesia: a computed tomography study. Br J Anaesth 71: 788-795
8. Viby-Mogensen J (2000) Postoperative residual curarization and evidence-based anaesthesia Br J Anaesth 84: 301-303

9. Eriksson LI, Sato M, Severinghaus JW (1993) Effect of a vecuronium-induced partial neuromuscular block on hypoxic ventilatory response. Anesthesiology 78: 693-699
10. Berg H, Roed J, Viby-Mogensen J et al (1997) Residual neuromuscular block is a risk factor for postoperative pulmonary complications. A prospective, randomized, and blinded study of postoperative pulmonary complications after atracurium, vecuronium and pancuronium Acta Anaesthesiol Scand 41: 1095-1103
11. Moller JT, Cluitmans P, Rasmussen LS et al (1998) Long-term postoperative cognitive dysfunction in the elderly: ISPOCD1 study. Lancet 351: 857-861
12. Rosenberg J, Ullstad T, Rasmussen J et al (1994) Time course of postoperative hypoxaemia. Eur J Surg 160: 137-143
13. Lewer BMF, Larsen PD, Torrance JM et al (1998) Artefactual episodic hypoxaemia during postoperative respiratory monitoring. Can J Anaesth 45: 182-185
14. Jayr C, Thomas H, Rey A et al (1993) Postoperative pulmonary complications. Epidural analgesia using bupivacaine and opioids versus parenteral opioids. Anesthesiology 78: 666-676
15. Wetterslev J, Hansen EG, Roikjaer O et al (2001) Optimizing perioperative compliance with PEEP during upper abdominal surgery: effects on perioperative oxygenation and complications in patients without preoperative cardiopulmonary dysfunction. Eur J Anaesthesiol 18: 358-365
16. Wallace WC, Cinat ME, Nastanski F et al (2000) New epidemiology for postoperative nosocomial infections. Am Surg 66: 874-878
17. Wacha H, Hau T, Dittmer R et al (1999) Risk factors associated with intraabdominal infections: a prospective multicenter study. Langenbecks Arch Surg 384: 24-32
18. Jensen LS, Kissmeyer-Nielsen P, Wolff B et al (1996) Randomized comparison of leucocyte-depleted versus buffy-coat-poor blood transfusion and complications after colorectal surgery. Lancet 348: 841-845
19. Kurz A, Sessler DI, Lenhardt R (1996) Perioperative normothermia to reduce the incidence of surgical-wound infection and shorten hospitalization. N Engl J Med 334: 1209-1215
20. Kam PCA, Calcroft RM.(1997) Peri-operative stroke in general surgical patients. Anaesthesia 52: 879-883
21. Nosan DK, Gomez CR, Maves MD (1993) Perioperative stroke in patients undergoing head and neck surgery Ann Otol Rhin Laryng 102: 717-723
22. O'Keefe ST, Chonchubhair AN (1994) Postoperative delirium in the elderly. Br J Anaesth 73: 673-687
23. Gustafson Y, Brännström B, Berggren D et al (1991) A geriatric-anesthesiologic program to reduce acute confusional states in elderly patients treated for femoral neck fractures. J Am Geriat Soc 39: 655-662
24. Rasmussen LS, Larsen K, Houx P et al (2001) The assessment of postoperative cognitive function. Acta Anaesthesiol Scand 45: 275-289
25. Savageau JA, Stanton B, Jenkins CD et al (1982) Neuropsychological dysfunction following elective cardiac operation. Early assessment. J Thorac Cardiovasc Surg 84: 585-594
26. Shaw PJ, Bates D, Cartlidge NEF et al (1987) Long-term intellectual dysfunction following coronary artery bypass graft surgery: a six month follow-up study. QJ Med 62: 259-268
27. Savageau JA, Stanton B, Jenkins CD et al (1982) Neuropsychological dysfunction following elective cardiac operation. II. A six-month reassessment. J Thorac Cardiovasc Surg 84: 595-600
28. Shaw PJ, Bates D, Cartlidge NEF et al (1986) Early intellectual dysfunction following coronary bypass surgery. QJ Med 58: 59-68
29. Malheiros SMF, Brucki SMD, Gabbai AA et al (1995) Neurological outcome in coronary artery surgery with and without cardiopulmonary bypass. Acta Neurol Scand 92: 256-260
30. Bedford PD (1955). Adverse cerebral effects of anaesthesia on old people. Lancet ii: 259-263
31. Ghoneim MM, Hinrichs JV, O'Hara MW et al (1988) Comparison of psychologic and cognitive functions after general or regional anesthesia. Anesthesiology 69: 507-515
32. Nielson WR, Gelb AW, Casey JE et al (1990) Long-term cognitive and social sequelae of general versus regional anesthesia during arthroplasty in the elderly. Anesthesiology 73: 1103-1109

33. Jones MJT, Piggot SE, Vaughan RS et al (1990) Cognitive and functional competence after anaesthesia in patients aged over 60: controlled trial of general and regional anaesthesia for elective hip or knee replacement. Br Med J 300: 1683-1687
34. Williams-Russo P, Sharrock NE, Mattis S et al (1995) Cognitive effects after epidural vs general anesthesia in older adults. JAMA 274: 44-50

Perioperative Challenges in Mentally Handicapped Patients

J. RUPREHT

Survival of mentally handicapped patients (MHP) from infancy into adulthood has significantly improved, and so have methods to assist them in their daily life. However, developments in perioperative care or in dentistry have generally not met many special challenges that surface when a mentally handicapped patient needs operative treatment. The revealing comparison with the pediatric patients shows that mentally handicapped patients do not receive special attention attuned to their needs, like children do. While normal children may be approached as a group of similar individuals this does not work for the handicapped for they are all different with a myriad of special needs. These needs are disadvantageous and complicating in the perioperative period. Vital needs are not always easy to identify, and may be difficult to meet when one follows a routine perioperative approach. Mental shortcomings and associated handicaps may be a credit for after life, but are no blessing on earth, neither for the sufferer nor for the care provider. MHP requiring anesthetic care present problems to the anesthetist that are challenging and may defeat the unprepared [1]. Psychiatric patients form a separate category of surgical population and are not considered in this perioperative context of MHP.

Mentally handicapped patients

Mental handicap may be inborn or acquired, it may be scientifically understood or not. Perinatal hypoxia or trauma are well known causes, so are some inflammatory infective diseases of the brain, but very often mental handicap is of unknown origin and labelled with *e causa ignota*. Severity of mental handicap knows no limits of diversity and may present itself as a barely perceptible deficit in an apparently normal person or as evident lack of any mental activity. The spectrum of mental handicaps may be combined with a broad range of disturbed physiological functions, with extremes in patients who have never heard, walked, seen, or eaten spontaneously. Some mentally handicapped survivors are worse off than a normal newborn baby. The degree of mental handicap is often denoted with the developmental stage of a normal child, and is expressed as retardation at the level of 1 year or more. Although apparently practical, such characterization of mental retardation does not account for the fact that mentally retarded patients also age and do not get better along the way.

Lack of understanding and reasoning is often combined with incapacity to learn. Many mentally retarded patients suffer from inability to cope with simple stresses of every day life, and certainly cannot cope with new surroundings and medical procedures when they are hospitalized. Fear and anxiety ensue, fear of dying often being there. If possible, the patient will try to escape from threatening events. All the traits of mental retardation can converge so that the patient does not co-operate [2]. Self-neglect is common in MHP and may be combined with any degree of self-mutilation. Lack of personal hygiene is tantalisingly measurable with the quality of dental health. Obesity is common among MHP and results from overfeeding, lack of movement, or from endocrinological abnormalities. Some MHP are chronically psychotic and this state may be combined with any degree of autism. Autistic patients are a particular challenge for medical professionals because they may not allow themselves to be touched or interacted with at all. Like an infant survives in symbiosis with the mother, many MHP depend in part or completely on symbiotical existence along with parents or care providers. Transfer of anxiety from the surrounding onto the patient is common in such symbiotical existence. Medical professionals must therefore rely on co-operation of symbiotic parents for a stress-free approach to the patient and to ensure a degree of co-operation. An example: a patient would not allow placement of a venous canula, but the mother instructed the anesthetist to loudly chant the slogan positive and by so doing the procedure was accomplished without further ado. Another Down syndrome patient would eventually take a seat in the dental chair but would insist on a small dance with the anesthetist before doing so. Symbiotical dependence on others must be exploited in management of MHP for smoother course of medical procedures. Problems of management of a MHP in the perioperative period can, of course, be twofold when parents or care-providers are not capable of coping with the demands of the medical treatment. For example, a rather asocial and not too intelligent mother gave breakfast to the MHP child despite the fasting instructions before anesthesia. Neglect of MHP by their parents is not uncommon, and this must be kept in mind when planning postoperative care following ambulatory anesthesia. The social context of providing anesthesia for MHP on a day-case basis is very important and one must be reasonably sure that instructions will be followed reliably and adequately in the perioperative period.

Challenge of gentle and protective restraint in MHP

It is not always medically responsible or practical for the anesthetist to prescribe an overdose of sedative medication to an uncooperative MHP, which may be required to ensure induction of anesthesia in a civilized manner. Medical contraindications may be weakened muscles or insufficient protective reflexes, in particular coughing and swallowing. In such cases reliable recovery of safe functioning following anesthesia cannot be guaranteed. Some MHP suffering from hypothyroidism or postencephalitic brain damage may appear overtly overactive but may take extremely long to recover vital functions after sedation and anesthesia. In such patients it appears better to plan short protective and gentle restraint for introduction of the venous cannula or for application of the anesthesia mask. Protective restraint should be additional to other methods of calming the MHP, must be short, agreed upon beforehand, and documented. No restraint is acceptable nowadays for the whole duration of dental, surgical, or diagnostic treatment, no matter how short.

Challenge of co-morbidity in MHP

In the realm of clinical syndromes [3, 4], many are characterized by mental retardation. Most MHP suffer from a myriad of concomitant diseases [5]. An instructive example is a Down syndrome patient who may harbor heart abnormalities [6], chronic respiratory infections, chronic hepatitis, abnormal anatomical features, oversensitivity to sedatives, and the feared prospect of sudden death. Worse, these patients age rapidly and are all different in regard to mental state and health. Atlanto-axial instability may be present in 20% of Down syndrome patients, and all should be screened for this disorder preoperatively [7]. Metabolic deficits in MHP are common and may be inborn or secondary to the way of life. Endocrinological disorders may escape diagnosis longer than in the normal population, examples being hypothyroidism, hyperthyroidism, or diabetes mellitus. Anemia is quite common. Obesity may accompany hypertension, and there is a statistically lower life-span expectancy in MHP in general.

Anatomical abnormalities are of great concern to the anesthetist, examples being contractures or kyphoscoliosis, which make positioning a challenge but may also be accompanied by respiratory deficiency. Accompanying neuro-muscular disorders should be feared because they may induce hyperthermic or hyperkalemic response during anesthesia. Simultaneous weakness of the myocardium may be present. Of strictly anesthesiological concern are abnormalities of the upper airways, like in Cornelia de Lange or in Cri du chat syndromes.

Epilepsy of any type and any degree is extremely common among the MHP, and so are the iatrogenic effects of medication. Phenylketonuria is a typical syndrome accompanied by epileptic fits. As in other groups of MHP, multi-medication can adversely affect perioperative course.

Spasticity is also very common in those who survive brain damage but not all spastic patients are mentally handicapped. Spasticity on its own is not a major anesthesiological difficulty.

Among the infamous syndromes for the anesthetist is Prader-Willi, characterized by Pickwickian-type hypoventilation, obesity, cor pulmonale, and hypoglycemia. In Rubenstein-Taybi, aspiration is a problem and cardiac dysrhythmias may occur. Cri du chat is also marred by congestive heart disease and physical retardation [8].

The very common presence of multiple co-morbidity in the MHP puts an extra strain on the anesthetist if the preoperative preparation is to be optimal and untoward problems during anesthesia prevented. It is prudent to communicate with other medical specialists before deciding on anesthesia, examples being geneticists, pediatricians, internists or neurologists. The interdisciplinary approach, including clinical psychologists where applicable, has proved very successful.

Choice of anesthetic technique and setting in MHP

It is a challenge to choose the optimal anesthetic technique for MHP given their co-morbidity and lack of coping. General anesthesia is by far preferable and assures a more-controllable operative course [2, 5]. Choice of anesthetic drugs is of lesser importance, but they should be followed by complete and swift recovery. An anesthetist is well advised to stick to one anesthetic method whenever possible, so as to be able better to deal with untoward reactions to anesthesia. Porphyria occurs in MHP, therefore barbiturates are better avoided.

Choice of setting is of paramount importance. The symbiotic person should be instructed how to help during induction, and the patient should return to the familiar surroundings as soon as possible. Whenever possible one should opt for day-care setting, provided that adequate and reliable aftercare is guaranteed.

Detailed documentation of the course of the perioperative period is mandatory in order to assure optimal approach to subsequent procedures. In particular, the effect of premedication and the quality of recovery are of interest for a safer and patient friendly individual approach. Overall the effect of anesthetic drugs should be registered in order to provide a smoother course next time.

Ethical and legal challenges of anesthesia in MHP

Dentists in many places complain of chronic shortage of anesthesia care for dental procedures in MHP. Public health systems often do not provide anesthetic assistance in dentistry, thereby causing much suffering in patients and inferior dental care for the MHP. Furthermore, most anesthesia residency programmes do not deal with specific challenges in the MHP, and anesthetists may not be particularly enthusiastic to help MHP. Bringing about change of the public and professional attitude to MHP is a novel challenge. It is not only to recognize the need for extra manpower for anesthesia in MHP but also to assure that adequate empathy towards these extra needy patients is taught, practised, and cultivated.

An ethical dilemma is never far from an anesthetist providing care in MHP. Abortions or sterilizations have been performed in MHP without foregoing procedural and ethical analysis. Each national society of anesthesiologists should ideally decide on the recommendations and guidelines of conduct in this field. Anesthesia professionals must be familiarized with the many specific demands of the MHP, and should be trained to respond to them no matter how challenging this may be.

Bordering on ethical challenges in MHP are the legal particularities of providing anesthesia for these patients. Very often one has to deal with two or three persons who need to be involved in consent for treatment, and it is not the patient who eventually sues the doctor but the parents or guardians. Therefore, learning to communicate with the symbiotic and social team which each MHP represents is indispensable. The medical preparation will be better and later complaints prevented. All instructions should be in writing and informed consent must be agreed on and signed before the treatment is planned [9]. Protective restraint, if applicable, should also be mentioned on the consent form.

Challenge to find anesthetic literature about MHP

It is not a new field of activity for operative medicine and for dentists to help MHP [1]. But it is a forgotten area of interest, deliberately or not, perhaps difficult to tackle and with little public appreciation. Whereas there are textbooks on pediatric or geriatric anesthesia or about cardiac anesthesia, only parts of one page may mention anesthetic management of mentally retarded patients even in major textbooks [5, 10, 11], interestingly, always as a minor part of the chapter dealing with anesthesia for dentistry. One would hope that specialized knowledge of how to provide optimal perioperative care for the MHP will soon appear in a monograph. First signs of improvement are there, now that major anesthesia congresses offer lectures dealing specifically with anesthetic care of MHP.

References

1. Diamond AW, Cochrane DF (1976) General anaesthesia for the mentally handicapped. Anaesthesia 31: 190-194
2. Rupreht J, Bouvy-Berends ECM (1998) Perioperative management of mentally handicapped patients. Anestezie (Prague) 9: 218-220
3. Wiedemann HR, Kume J, Dibbern H (1992) An atlas of clinical syndromes, 2nd edn. Wolfe, London.
4. Gorlin RJ, Cohen MM, Levin LS (1990) Syndromes of the head and neck, 3rd edn. Oxford University Press, New York
5. Padfield A (1996) Anaesthesia for dental and maxillofacial surgery. In: Prys-Roberts C, Brown Jr BR (eds) International practice of anaesthesia. Butterworth – Heinemann, Oxford, pp 2/109/1-11
6. Morray JP, MacGillivray R, Duker G (1986) Increased perioperative risk following repair of congenital heart disease in Down's syndrome. Anesthesiology 65: 221-224
7. Williams JP, Somerville GM, Miner ME, et al (1987) Atlanto-axial subluxation and trisomy-21: another perioperative complication. Anesthesiology 67: 253-254
8. Pollard BJ, Harrison MJ (1989) Anaesthesia for uncommon diseases. Blackwell, Oxford
9. Rupreht J, Erdmann W (1997) Voorwaarden voor het beoefenen van extramurale anesthesie. VBTGG, Index; May, pp 2-7 (in Dutch); Standards for practice of office-based anaesthesia
10. Gillies BS (1992) Anesthesia outside the operating room. In: Barash PG, et al (eds) Clinical anesthesia. Lippincott Company, Philadelphia, pp 1474-1475
11. Roizen MF (2000) Anesthetic implications of concurrent disease. In: Miller RD (ed) Anesthesia, 5th edn. Churchill Livingstone, Philadelphia pp 903-1032

Controversial Aspects in Perioperative Medicine

G. GALIMBERTI

Recently, current financial constraints across the medical sector, accompanied by increasing litigation by patients and/or relatives, has resulted in a renewed interest in the link between anesthesia and surgical outcome. Epidemiological studies have shown that cardiovascular disease continues as the leading cause for death in developed and in non-developed countries [1]. It is calculated that in year 2001 approximately 100 million patients will undergo surgery throughout the world, with one-third being more than 65 years of age or having two or more cardiovascular risk factors. Among these patients, 10% will suffer a perioperative myocardial ischemia causing a 50% reduction in their 2-year survival rate, and increasing world health care costs by an additional 50 billion dollars [2]. Although cardiovascular complications after surgery are well recognized, a great deal remains unknown and a number of controversies persist, not the least of which is the appropriate methodology for detection of perioperative morbidity and costly outcome. Furthermore, it is increasing the pressure on physicians of all specialties who have to account for their actions and supply supported reasoning for their actions. Evidence-based medicine, that is the approach to clinical practice based on knowledge of the evidence supported by literature appraisal and application, has been promoted as tool to provide physicians with the necessary means to evaluate the current basis for any proposed intervention.

Consequently, many controversial aspects involve the perioperative care of patient undergoing surgery, such as the perioperative evaluation, the type of intraoperative monitoring (invasive vs. non-invasive), the anesthetic technique (general vs. locoregional), and the postoperative pain management.

Routine preoperative evaluation

After the surgeon has been taken the decision to operate, the anesthetist plays a vital contributory role in the preparation of the patient and the timing of surgery. The anesthetist's duties during the perioperative period are to foresee difficulties, to enhance patient safety, to minimize the chance of errors, and to assess the global perioperative risk. Preoperative assessment must take into account several factors such as presenting conditions and concurrent medical history, anesthetic history, drug history with potential anesthetic interaction, and physical examination. More controversial is which laboratory tests or imaging techniques are relevant to anesthesia. In general, most investigators should not offer a battery of tests as a matter of routine but rather pursue investigations able to detect known or unknown abnormalities that are of significance, and that require changes to the patient's preoperative management or the conduct of anesthesia [3, 4]. In fact, preoperative tests are performed either to determine the progress of a known disease or to detect unsuspected abnormalities that could alter anesthetic and surgical management. Although the former is generally accepted, there is often dispute about the latter indication. The routine ordering of preoperative laboratory tests is common practice, because physicians generally believe that a clinical history and physical examination are insensitive and that preoperative investigations may protect against medicolegal complaints. In contrast, several studies have suggested that the clinical history and physical examination can adequately discriminate healthy patients (ASA I and II) who are suitable for surgery [5-11], most diagnostic tests ordered for other reasons during the year before surgery giving normal results could substitute for the preoperative tests [12], routine preoperative tests are not without risk and inconvenience to the patient, and increase the work of health care staff [7, 13, 14]. Moreover, the proportion of false-positive results is not negligible and one needs to consider the cost involved (financial and time), which is an important factor in the annual increase in hospital budgets [15-19].

Rather than employing a battery of investigations for every surgical admission, it is becoming more common to request preoperative tests taking into account (1) the incidence of abnormalities for that test in that age group, (2) the importance of that test result to perioperative outcome, (3) the cost of the test, (4) the ability to alter perioperative course favorably once an abnormal test result is obtained, (5) other benefits of the test to the patient, and (6) medicolegal issues. Preoperative assessment for minor procedures in relatively healthy patients and for complex surgical procedures in patients having conditions that adversely affect surgical outcome (i.e., hypertension, ischemic heart disease, cardiac dysrhythmias, chronic obstructive pulmonary disease, clotting disease, etc.) differ greatly. Generally, most patients with diseases are not totally asymptomatic and the screening history and physical examination will identify the majority of such patients.

Table 1. Definition of terms relating to laboratory test

Term	Definition
Sensitivity	Percentage of tests positive in disease: the percentage of patients who have the suspected disease and an abnormal (or positive) laboratory test result
Specificity	Percentage of tests negative in health: the percentage of healthy patients who have a normal (or negative) laboratory test result
False-positive rate	The percentage of healthy people who have an abnormal test result
Predictive false-positive rate	The percentage of abnormal test results belonging to healthy people determining this value requires knowledge of sensitivity, specificity, and prevalence of disease

It is well recognized that the normal range of laboratory tests is based on the statistical concept of the normal distribution of the Gaussian curve [20,21]. The quality of a test is based on its capacity to identify abnormalities (Table 1). Its clinical usefulness is strictly related to the positive predictive value and to the capacity to influence the anesthetic and surgical management (Table 2).

Table 2. Percentage of unexpected abnormalities and type of influences on the anesthetic and surgical management according to the result of the preoperative test (modified from [22]) (ECG = electrocardiogram, PCV = packed cell volume, PT = prothrombin time, PTT = partial thromboplastin time, WBC = white blood cell count, DC = differential cell count, BUN = blood urea nitrogen, SGOT-SGPT = serum glutamic-oxalacetic transaminase and serum glutamic-pyruvic transaminase, AP = alkaline phosphatase, ?GT = gamma-glutamyltranspeptidase, Na/K = sodium and potassium) [a] % Unexpected abnormalities = number of patients with unknown and unsuspected abnormalities/total number of patients tested x 100% [b] Influence = number of patients with unknown and unsuspected abnormalities with influence/total number of patients tested x 100

Preoperative test	% unsuspected abnormalities [a]	% influence [b]
Chest X-ray	8.6	0.56
ECG	5.6	0.46
Hematological		0.26
PCV	1.0	
Hemoglobin	0.8	
Platelet count	0.4	
PT	0.1	
PTT	0.2	
WBC	0.8	
DC	0.9	
Biochemical		0.32
Glucose	2.2	
BUN	1.9	
Creatinine	0.9	
SGOT-SGPT	1.9	
AP	1.2	
Proteingram	1.7	
Total protein	0.3	
?GT	3.2	
Na/K	0.4	
All tests (n= 3,106)	5.6	1.22

The percentages of patients whose management was changed by each test were: chest radiograph 0.56%, ECG 0.46%, hematological tests 0.26% and biochemical tests 0.32% (Table 2). Studies of the value of preoperative chest radiograph showed abnormality rates varied from 2.5% to 22.5% of patients, which were unexpected in 0.6%-10% and influenced subsequent management in only 0.56% [22-27]. The ACAPEM study [27], for example, showed, among patients with abnormal radiographs (6.2%) and free of risk factors who were undergoing general or gastrointestinal surgery, only 0.1% of anesthetic or surgical consequences. Furthermore, the Royal College of Radiologists found, in 3,154 patients undergoing non-acute, non-cardiopulmonary surgery, only small differences between the influence of abnormal and normal chest radiographs on the decision to operate (92% vs 96.2%) or on the decision to use inhalational anesthesia (96.1% vs. 96.7%) [28].

The preoperative ECG is a quick, safe test performed routinely in patients with the aim of detecting pre-existing cardiovascular disease, which, if abnormal (i.e., left ventricular hypertrophy, Q-waves, S-T segment abnormality, T wave abnormality, arrhythmia, conduction abnormality, etc.), is associated with increased postoperative risk [29, 30], particularly silent myocardial infarction and arrhythmias [31]. However the accumulated cost of the test is high (£ 15.00 per ECG) and, thus, the use of such tests needs to be reviewed frequently to ensure that they are being used in appropriate patients. Among the published results on the value of ECG abnormalities (known or unknown) in healthy patients, rates from 8.3% to 16% were found, but only 0.46% changed perioperative management [22, 26, 32]. Other studies of the utilization of preoperative ECG have shown that the incidence of ECG abnormalities increases with age and, therefore, an ECG should be performed routinely in all patients at risk of cardiac disease or over 50 years old [33-35]. Other authors raised the age limit for a routine ECG to 60 years, if there are no simple positive screening criteria (known cardiac disease or strong risk factors) [31, 34]. However, the preoperative ECG remains an important clinical investigation prior to anesthesia, as a baseline measurement and a helpful investigation in patients with other systemic diseases, such as significant respiratory disease. The presence of cardiac disease or risk factors for cardiac disease as an indication for a preoperative ECG uncovered a reasonably large number of abnormalities, missing very few, and was very simple to apply.

Table 3. Proposed guidelines for preoperative investigations (BUN = blood urea nitrogen)

Investigation	Indication
Chest X-ray	History suggestive of possible abnormality. A previously abnormal chest film. Any patient with thyroid enlargement. All patients over 30 years (smokers) or 40 years of age, and those without an available previous test 6 months before
	Patients with cardiovascular disease, male smokers >45 years old or all others >50 years old
ECG	All female adults. All males 50 years and all others with history of anemia or blood loss All patients over 65 years of age
Full blood count	
	Any history of liver disease History of coagulation disorder
BUN, creatinine, electrolytes	
Liver function tests	
Coagulation screen	

Hematological and biochemical tests are, generally, abnormal in 2.9% and 5.6% of patients and influence treatment in 0.26% and 0.32% respectively [22-24,26,36]. Abnormal laboratory tests are defined in probability terms based on the distribution of normal values. False-positive results would thus be expected even in healthy patients. In fact, 18% of patients with uncertain or unexpected abnormalities are usually normal on repeat testing. Retrospective review suggests that 75% of patients would not have required any preoperative test [22,36]. No significant differences were observed between the predictive value of screening tests and preoperative clinical history and physical examination [24]. Only 0.22% of preoperative abnormalities have some influence on anesthetic and surgical management [21,36]. Generally, the value of routine preoperative tests in detecting clinically inapparent abnormalities in ASA I and II patients is very small. Consequently, the preanesthetic visit is the best method of assessing the anesthetic and surgical risk of the patient and, thus the basis for the rational performance of preoperative investigations [37-40]. Most patients, after history and physical examination, have no preoperative indication for a laboratory test and can safely undergo anesthesia and surgery [41]. Nevertheless, a set of guidelines could be used in the majority of situations and could provided a guide to the minimum level of investigation (Table 3).

Anesthesia risk

Since 1960 the American Society of Anesthesiologists (ASA) five-point classification has been used to graduate the risks of perioperative complications [42,43], but unfortunately it is non-specific, poorly predictive of outcome when used alone, and does not identify factors that can be altered preoperatively to improve outcome.

Preoperative assessment of fitness score (PAFS), similar to the APACHE II system employed in critical care medicine, is used to obtain an objective assessment of the likelihood of perioperative survival. It has a low specificity, approximately 80%, but is very sensitive at predicting mortality and major complications after emergency and major elective abdominal surgery. The preoperative evaluation and management of the patient potentially at risk for cardiac complications of non-cardiac surgery require the identification of preoperative risk factors that are associated with an adverse cardiac event. This principle, which is quantified by Bayes theorem, explains why the same test result has different implications in patients with different prior probabilities of disease [44]. For example, if 10% of patients tested have the disease (prior probability = 10%), the probability of disease in a patient with a positive test result (positive predictive value) will be 67%, while the probability of no disease in a patient with a negative test result (negative predictive value) will be 99%. On the other hand, if 50% of patients tested have the disease (prior probability = 50%), the probability of disease in a patient with a positive test result (positive predictive value) will be 95%, while the probability of no disease in a patient with a negative test result (negative predictive value) will be 90%. The preoperative evaluation should be targeted at the following: establishing a reasonable estimate of the risk of complication; identifying factors that can be modified to reduce risk; planning a surgical approach and timing that will limit risk; and choosing an anesthetic most favorable for the specific patient and planned surgery. These goals should then lead to a preoperative plane that can provide those diagnostic and therapeutic interventations that will provide maximal risk reduction to the patient with minimal imposed risk at an acceptable cost. The most well-established multifactorial risk indexes for quantifying the potential risk of surgery in patients with underlying cardiac disease are summarized in Table 4.

Table 4. Cardiac risk stratification for non-cardiac surgery procedures (MI = myocardial infarction, PVCs = premature ventricular contraction, CCS = Canadian Cardiovascular Society)

Goldman's index [45]		Detsky's index [46]	
Factors	Points	Factors	Points
Age > 70 years	5	Age > 70 years	5
MI < 6 months	10	MI < 6 months	10
S3 gallop	11	CCS angina class III	10
Severe aortic stenosis	3	CCS angina class IV	20
Arrhythmias	7	Unstable angina < 6 months	10
> PVCs/min	7	Alveolar pulmonary edema:	
Other diseases	3	- < 1week	10
Thoracic or abdominal surgery	3	- ever	5
Emergency operation	4	Severe aortic stenosis	20
		Arrhythmias	5
		> PVCs/min	5
		Other diseases	5
		Emergency operation	10

Although risk prediction can be based on the references just mentioned, several points relating to risk are of major interest. For example, the traditional concern regarding recent myocardial infarction as a risk for reinfarction in the perioperative period must be tempered by more-recent observations [47,48]. Identification of factors that can be modified to reduce risk provides an opportunity for perioperative interventation that may improve outcome, but, unfortunately, most of the cardiac risk factors are not amenable. More controversial aspects are the surgical approach in patients at risk of cardiac complications [49], the anesthetic time [50], and the route and type of anesthetic drugs [51,52].

Cardiovascular monitoring

Another controversial aspect in anesthesia is the type of cardiovascular monitoring to use in the operating room. In particular, the debate continues between invasive and non-invasive monitoring. Standard cardiovascular monitoring in critically ill patients usually includes the ECG signal (3-5 leads), SpO2, PetCO2, and the measurement of the blood pressure (BP), central venous pressure (CVP), pulmonary capillary wedge pressure (PCWP), cardiac output (CO), oxygen delivery (DO_2), oxygen consumption (VO_2), left ventricular stroke work index (LVSWI), and right ventricular stroke work index (RVSWI) by a Swan-Ganz catheter inserted into the pulmonary artery (PAC). PAC, in hospitals around the world, is usually considered the "gold standard" in cardiovascular monitoring with respect to accuracy and reproducibility, although, recently, there have been indications of factors responsible for erroneous estimation of CO by thermodilution. Furthermore, PAC is associated with significant risks due to central venous catheterization and, at least in the traditional model, it allows measurement only of pressure indexes in an intermittent way. More recently some non-invasive devices have been introduced in the operating room, in particular the transesophageal echo-Doppler (TED) and transesophageal echocardiography (TEE).

TED is an aortic flowmeter able to measure continuously, contemporaneously, and at the same level of the esophagus the diameter of the descending thoracic aorta (d) and the average velocity of the blood (v) flowing through it. Thus, aortic blood flow (ABF) is calculated by the following formula:

ABF (t)= p *[d/2(t)2]* v(t)

An algorithm recognizes the Q and R wave on the ECG signal and the systolic beginning and end of the first derived from the blood velocity wave; so it can measure the systolic time intervals (STI), and in particular the PEP/LVET quotient that is strictly related to the ejection fraction determined by TEE.

TEE is the most-sensitive and probably most cost-effective method of detecting myocardial ischemia [53]. TEE is more sensitive for detection of myocardial ischemia than ECG or pulmonary capillary wedge pressure [54]. However, lack of a true reference standard for myocardial ischemia makes it uncertain that TEE regional wall motion abnormalities reflect true myocardial ischemia.

Anesthetic technique: general versus locoregional

Different authors agree about the issue of the stress response and its effects on the postoperative outcome. On the other hand, there is an important debate in hospitals worldwide about which anesthetic technique is best for the individual patient and is well tolerated, easy to administer, and produces a favorable risk/benefit ratio. Previous studies of different anesthetic techniques and surgical outcomes in extremely different groups of patients often obtained conflicting conclusions. For example, a recent meta-analysis of randomized and controlled trials showed only a significant reduction in deep venous thrombosis with regional versus general anesthesia [55]. The patient outcome for groups has been investigated in the past and is influenced by the following risk factors (Table 5).

Table 5. Identified risk factor affecting morbidity and mortality in anesthesia

Author	Study type	No. of patients	Identified risk
Marx et al. [56]	Retrospective	34,145	ASA, advanced age, emergent surgery
Farrow et al. [57]	Retrospective	108,878	Age, sex site of surgery, duration anesthesia
Holland [58]	Retrospective	5,262	Wrong choice of anesthesia, inadequate preparation and monitoring

It is more difficult to identify, for example, which ASA 1 patient will die as a result of anesthesia (1 in every 20,000) and to evaluate the impact of the anesthetic technique chosen on the patient outcome. Recently, several studies have tried to find a possible link between the choice of the anesthetic technique and patient outcome (Table 6). Nevertheless, there is disagreement among the results of the different studies, perhaps due to the study design and type of statistical analysis used. In fact, the link between outcome and anesthetic technique is a very difficult area that will obviously require many more cases to be studied, with an appropriate design, before any conclusion can be reached. Future outcome studies conducted to predict individual risk during surgery should be based on very large populations, knowing the prevalence of the researched variable and the interval of confidence chosen.

Table 6. Impact of the different anesthetic technique on the patient outcome. Some examples (GA = general anesthesia, CEGA = combined epidural and general anesthesia, epid = epidural; L = local anesthetic, F = fentanyl, A = aortic, P = peripheral)

References	Comparison	Surgery	Outcome
McQuay et al. [59]	GA vs GA+spinal (L)	Orthopedic	Preemptive analgesia
Salomaki et al. [60]	GA vs CEGA (F)	Thoracic	Modified hormonal resp.
Jayr et al. [61]	GA vs CEGA (L,M)	Abdominal	No differences
Galimberti et al. [62]	GA vs CEGA (L,F)	Abdominal	Lower hospitalization
Tuman et al. [63]	GA vs CEGA (L,F)	Vascular (A,P)	Fewer thrombotic events
Davies et al. [64]	GA vs CEGA (L)	Vascular (A)	No differences
Myles et al. [65]	GAvs spinal vs epid	Vascular (P)	No differences

Furthermore, these studies should be multicenter and consequently would be very expensive. The results should be correctly evaluated statistically; i.e., first, every variable is looked at separately by univariate analysis (i.e., chi squared test, odds ratios) then, by multivariate analysis using stepwise logistic regression [65]. Finally, results should be further validated by wide, prospective and controlled clinical trials.

These multicenter prospective structured studies are currently being performed in Europe and the United States, but it is expected to be some years before any definite conclusions can be reached due to the number of cases required (thousands). In any case, we know that several factors may influence the postoperative outcome, often having a synergistic action on the patient (Table 7).

Table 7. Factors involved in the postoperative outcome

Factors related to the:	
1) Patient	ASA, risk factors, monitoring, early mobilization
2) Anesthesia	anesthetic technique (GA, SA, EA, CSA, CSE, CEGA, n. blocks), analgesic technique (preemptive analgesia, wound infiltration, PCA, PACU, APS)
3) Surgery	site of surgery, surgical technique, surgeon skill, traditions (nursing quality system, routine monitoring)

Among the various factors that can interfere with patient outcome, the preoperative block of the afferent nociceptive pathways and the effective control of acute postoperative pain seem to be the most significant. In fact, only through a multi-modal approach to anesthesia and analgesia can these factors be eliminated from the stress response.

References

1. Murray CJL, Lopez AD (1997) From what will we die in 2020? Mortality by cause for eight regions of the world: global burden of disease study. Lancet 349: 1268-1276
2. Mangano DT (1994) Perioperative cardiac morbidity – Epidemiology, costs, problems, and solutions. West J Med 161: 87-89
3. Wyld R, Nimmo WAS (1988) Do patients fasting before and after operation receive their prescribed drug treatment? BMJ 296:744
4. Perez A, Planell J, Bacardaz C, et al (1995) Value of routine preoperative tests: a multicentre study in four general hospitals. Br J Anaesth 74: 250-256
5. Lurie P (1987) Toward optimal use of radiographs. Should admission and preoperative chest film be routine? Postgrad Med 62: 209-216
6. National Study by the Royal College of Radiologists (1979) Preoperative chest radiology. Lancet II: 83-86
7. Tape TG, Mushlin AI (1986) The utility of routine chest radiographs. Ann Intern Mede 104: 663-670
8. Turnbull JM, Buck C (1987) The value of preoperative screening investigations in otherwise healthy individuals. Arch Intern Med 147: 1101-1105

9. Jhonson H, Knee-Joli S, Butler TA, et al (1988) Are routine laboratory screening tests necessary to evaluate ambulatory surgical patients ? Surgery 104: 639-643
10. Wilson ME, Williams NB, Baskett PJF, et al (1980) Assessment of fitness for surgical procedures and the variability of anesthetics'judgement. Br Med J 1: 509-513
11. Macpherson DS (1993) Preoperative laboratory testing: should any test be "routine" before surgery? Med Clin North Am 77: 298-308
12. Macpherson DS, Snow S, Lofgren RP (1990) Preoperative screening: value of previous test. Ann Intern Med 113: 969-973
13. Roizen M (1989) Preoperative patient evaluation. Can J Anaesth 36: S13-S19
14. Goldberger AL, O'Konski M (1986) Utility of the routine electrocardiogram before surgery and on general hospital admission. Critical review and new guidelines. Ann Intern Med 105: 552-557
15. Kaplan EB, Sheiner LB, Boeckmann AJ, et al (1985) The usefulness of preoperative laboratory screening. J Am Med Assoc 253: 3576-3581
16. Adams JG Jr, Weigelt JA, Poulos E (1992) Usefulness of preoperative laboratory assessment of patients undergoing elective herniorrhaphy. Arch Surg 127: 801-805
17. Narr BJ, Hansen TR, Warner MA (1991) Preoperative laboratory screening in healthy Mayo patients: cost-effective elimination of test and unchanged outcomes. Mayo Clin Proc 66: 155-159
18. Robbins JA, Mushlin AI (1979) Preoperative evaluation of the healthy patient. Med Clin North Am 63: 1145-1156
19. Lawrence VA, Gafni A, Gross M (1989) The unproven utility of the preoperative urinalysis: economic evaluation. J Clin Epidemiol 42: 1185-1192
20. Krieg AF, Gambino R, Galen RS (1975) Why are clinical laboratory tests performed ? When are they valid? JAMA 233: 76
21. Gorry GA, Pauker SG, Schwartz WB (1978) The diagnostic importance of the normal finding. N Engl J Med 298: 486
22. Perez A, Planell J, Bacardaz A, et al (1995) Value of routine preoperative tests: a multicentre study in four general hospitals. Br J Anaesth 74: 250-256
23. Adams JG Jr, Weigelt JA, Poulos E (1992) Usefulness of preoperative laboratory assessment of patients undergoing elective herniorrhaphy. Arch Surg 127: 801-805
24. Narr BJ, Hansen TR, Warner MA (1991) Preoperative laboratory screening in healthy Mayo patients: cost-effective elimination of test and unchanged outcomes. Mayo Clin Proc 66: 155-159
25. Gagner M, Chiasson A (1990) Preoperative chest X-ray films in elective surgery. Can J Surg 33: 271-274
26. Turnboll JM, Buck C (1987) The value of preoperative screening investigations in otherwise healthy individuals. Arch Intern Med 147: 1101-1105
27. ACAPEM, Bouillot JL, Paquet JC, Hay JM, et al (1992) La radiographic thoracique preoperatoire systématique en chirurgie generale est-elle utile? Etude Prospective multicentrique sur 3959 malades. Ann Fr Anesth Reanim 11: 88-95
28. National Study by the Royal College of Radiologists (1979) Preoperative chest radiology. Lancet II: 83-86
29. Carliner NH, Fisher ML, Plotnick GD, et al (1985) Routine preoperative exercise testing in patients undergoing major noncardiac surgery. Am J Cardiol 56: 51-58
30. Von Knorring J (1981) Postoperative myocardial infarction: a prospective study in a risk group of surgical patients. Surg 90: 55-60
31. Goldman L, Caldera DL, Nussbaum SR, et al (1977) Multifactorial index of cardiac risk in noncardiac surgical procedures. N Engl J Med 297: 845-850
32. Goldberger AL, O'Konski M (1986) Utility of the routine electrocardiogram before surgery and on general hospital admission. Critical review and new guidelines. Ann Intern Med 105: 552-557
33. McKee RF, Scott EM (1987) The value of routine preoperative investigations. Ann R Coll Surg Engl 69: 160-162
34. Paterson KR, Caskie JP, Galloway DJ, et al (1983) The pre-operative electrocardiogram: an assessment. Scott Med J 28: 116-118

35. Elston RA, Taylor DJE (1984) The preoperative electrocardiogram. Lancet I: 349
36. Kaplan EB, Sheiner LB, Boeckmann AJ, et al (1985) The usefulness of preoperative laboratory screening. J Am Med Assoc 263: 3586-3581
37. Klazinga NS, Helsloot R (1989) Quality assurance of pre-operative assessment. A review of quality assurance activities related to pre-operative assessment in nine hospitals in The Netherlans. Qual Assur Health Care 1: 45-53
38. Roizen M (1989) Preoperative patient evaluation. Can J Anaesth 36: S13-S19
39. Robbins JA, Mushlin AI (1979) Preoperative evaluation of the healthy patients. Med Clin North Am 63: 1145-1156
40. Wong CA (1990) Preoperative patient preparation. J Post Anesth Nurs 5: 149-156
41. Narr BJ, Schroeder DR, Warner MA (1997) Outcomes of patients with no laboratory assessment before anesthesia and a surgical procedure. Mayo Clin Proc 72: 505-509
42. Vacanti CJ, Van Houten RJ, Hill RC (1969) A statistical analysis of the relationship of physical status to postoperative mortality in 68.388 cases. Anesth Analg 49: 564-566
43. Cohen MM, Duncan PG (1988) Physical status score and trends in anesthetic complications. J Clin Epidemiol 41: 83-90
44. Goldman L (1994) Quantitative aspects of clinical reasoning. In: Isselbacher KJ, Braunwald E, Wilson JD, et al (eds) Harrison's principles of internal medicine, 13 th edn McGraw-Hill, New York, pp 43-48
45. Goldman L (1995) Cardiac risk in noncardiac surgery: an update. Anesth Analg 80: 810-820
46. Detsky AS, Abrams HB, Forbath N, et al (1986) Cardiac assessment for patients undergoing noncardiac surgery: a multifactorial clinical risk index. Arch Intern Med 146: 2131-2134
47. Shah KB, Kleinman BS, Sami H, et al (1990) Reevaluation of perioperative myocardial infarction in patients with prior myocardial infarction undergoing noncardiac operations. Anesth Analg 71: 231-235
48. American College of Cardiology/American Heart Association Task Force on Practice Guidelines (1996) Guidelines for perioperative cardiovascular evaluation for noncardiac surgery. Circulation 93: 1278-1317
49. Mitchell CK, Smoger SH, Pfeifer MP, et al (1998) Multivariate analysis of factors associated with postoperative pulmonary complications following general elective surgery. Arch Surg 133: 194-198
50. Ebert TJ, Kharasch ED, Rooke GA, et al (1997) Myocardial ischemia and adverse cardiac outcomes in cardiac patients undergoing noncardiac surgery with sevoflurane and isoflurane. Anesth Analg 85: 993-999
51. Mangano DT, Borowner WS, Hollenberg M, et al (1990) Association of perioperative myocardial ischemia with cardiac morbidity and mortality in men undergoing noncardiac surgery: the Study of Perioperative Ischemia Research Group. N Engl J Med 323: 1781-1788
52. Voelker R (1995) Anesthesia-related risks have plummeted. JAMA 272: 445-446
53. Lagasse RS, Steinberg ES, Katz RI, et al (1995) Defining the qualitity of perioperative care by statistical process control of adverse outcomes. Anesthesiology 79: 422-434
54. Christopherson R, Beattie C, Frank SM, et al (1993) Perioperative morbidity in patients randomized to epidural or general anesthesia for lower extremity vascular surgery: perioperative ischemia randomized anesthesia Trial Study Group. Anesthesiology 79: 422-434
55. Sorensen RM, Pace NL (1991) Mortality and morbidity of regional versus general anesthesia. Anesthesiology 75: A1053
56. Marx GF, Mateo CV, Orkin LR (1973) Computer analysis of postanesthetic deaths. Anesthesiology 39: 54-58
57. Farrow SC, Fowkes FGR, Lunn JN, et al (1982) Epidemiology in anesthesia. II. Factors affecting mortality in hospital. Br J Anaesth 59: 834-841
58. Holland R (1987) anesthetic mortality in New South Wales. Br J Anaesth 59: 834-841
59. McQuay HJ, Carroll D, Moore RA (1988) Postoperative orthopaedic pain: the effect of opiate premedication and local anesthetic blocks. Pain 33: 291-295
60. Salomaki TE, Leppaluoto J, Laitinen JO, et al (1993) Epidural versus intravenous fentanyl for

reducing hormonal, metabolic, and physiologic responses after thoracotomy. Anesthesiology 79: 672-679

61. Jayr C, Thomas H, Rey A, Farhat F, et al (1993) Postoperative pulmonary complications: epidural analgesia using bupivacaine and opioids versus parenteral opioids. Anesthesiology 78: 666-676
62. Galimberti G, Caristi D, Iscra F, et al (1996) Blended anesthesia vs general anesthesia: is blended anesthesia a really cheaper technique in decreasing postoperative costs? Br J Anaesth 76: A227
63. Tuman KJ, McCarthy RJ, March RJ, et al (1991) Effects of epidural anesthesia and analgesia on coagulation and outcome after major vascular surgery. Anesth Analg 73: 696-704
64. Davies MJ, Silbert BS, Mooney PJ, et al (1993) Combined epidural and general anesthesia versus general anesthesia for abdominal aortic surgery. Anaesth Intensive Care 21: 790-794
65. Myles PS, Williams NJ, Powell J (1994) Predicting outcome in anesthesia: understanding statistical methods. Anaesth Intensive Care 22: 447-453

Postoperative Pain Challenge

F. GIUNTA, A. PAOLICCHI

Acute postoperative pain treatment leads to prompt patient recovery and a faster reinstatement in society. Acute Pain Service (APS) outcomes are: patient's comfort and pain relief, morbidity reduction and shorter hospitalization with a faster patient recovery. This project needs a multidisciplinary intervention based on anesthetic and analgesic techniques, which allows faster alimentation and mobilization, and less-invasive surgery [1, 2]. Acute postoperative pain treatment is very important because, when inadequate, hospitalization may be longer and morbidity increased.

At present, in Italy there are few hospitals with an APS, but acute postoperative care is growing and the interest for new therapeutic protocols is clear [3].

Acute postoperative pain has some specific characteristics:

- pain severity and length can be expected
- onset predictable
- controlled by adequate therapy

Moreover acute postoperative pain relief is achieved by a multimodal approach:

- preoperative information
- therapy by fixed protocols
- many postoperative evaluations to check patients' clinical state and to carry out therapeutic corrections, when necessary.

Methods

In our APS we use therapeutic protocols according to the surgery and patients' characteristics. Our protocols are based on different pain stimuli, the patient's clinical state and state of mind, and human and material resources.

The therapeutic strategy, according to the type of surgery, in 4,236 patients observed by APS (February 1998 to July 2001) is shown in Table 1.

Table 1. Pain relief according to type of surgery (PCA = patient-controlled analgesia)

		ANALGESIA %								
KIND OF SURGERY:	PATIENTS TOTAL N°	Ketorolac i.v	Tramadol	Ketorolac+Tramadol continuos infusion	Morphine i.m	Ketorolac+morphine continuos infusion	Ketorolac+morphine i.m	PCA	Epidural	Other FANS
THYROID	950	82,5	8,1	0,6	6,6	0,0	0,5	0,4	0,2	0,9
BREAST	266	74,8	12,0	1,5	6,0	0,0	3,8	0,0	0,0	1,9
MAJOR ABDOMEN	770	11,2	10,8	5,6	9,6	2,3	4,5	23,2	32,6	0,1
MINOR ABDOMEN	917	78,2	9,3	1,1	4,4	0,0	1,4	3,6	1,6	0,4
MAJOR UROLOGIC	457	5,7	4,4	4,8	6,3	7,4	4,6	29,5	37,2	0,0
MINOR UROLOGIC	332	65,1	5,1	0,3	17,2	1,2	3,6	1,2	4,2	2,1
MAJOR TORACIC	87	59,8	10,3	2,3	3,4	0,0	3,4	14,9	5,7	0,0
MINOR TORACIC	55	72,7	9,1	0,0	14,5	0,0	1,8	0,0	0,0	1,8
MAJOR VASCULAR	38	26,3	7,9	0,0	13,2	5,3	7,9	5,3	34,2	0,0
MINOR VASCULAR	57	89,5	1,8	0,0	3,5	0,0	0,0	0,0	0,0	5,3
OBSTETRIC	197	1,5	0,0	0,0	2,0	41,6	0,0	5,6	49,2	0,0

As a pain indicator we used Numerical Verbal Scale (NVS), Visual Analog Scale (VAS) at rest, and Visual Analog Scale on movement. We checked the patients every 3 h from awakening to the 15th postoperative hour, then at the 24th postoperative hour and the 36th postoperative hour. For the first 2,709 patients our aim was to achieve and maintain VAS at rest ≤ 4 with a 5% cut-off. For 1,218 patients from October 2000, our aim was a VAS at rest ≤ 2 with a 5% cut-off.

Table 2. Analgesic protocols used by APS for 4,236 patients

	Ketorolac i.v	Epidural	PCA	Morphine i.m	Ketorolac+morphine i.m	Ketorolac+tramadol continuous infusion
Analgesic protocols	62%	15%	9%	8%	4%	2%

From a clinical point of view, pain relief, when it is achieved, does not completely correspond to patients' well being. In fact when pain is controlled, new symptoms, able to influence the patients' postoperative course, emerge. Discomfort is caused by the patient's disease, there are side effects of the analgesic therapy and problems associated with patients' psychological and clinical state. We have considered clinical disturbances reported by patients as discomfort indicators and consider their treatment necessary for a better recovery.

Discomfort indicators include: shivering, sedation, psychomotor agitation, confusion, humour disturbance, postoperative nausea and vomiting (PONV), insomnia, pruritus, cephalalgia, decubitus pain, cough, dyspnea, pharyngodynia, surgical drain pain, bladder catheter pain, gastric probe pain, vein pain, dysuria, urinary retention, hiccups, paraesthesia, rash, and peristalsis [4].

In order to evaluate the APS quality, at the end of 48 postoperative hours' observation, 412 patients (10% of the sample) completed a questionnaire to obtain information on sex, age, surgery, and analgesia, with six multiple answer questions and free spaces for suggestions and criticisms.

Results

Pain

The fixed aim was not achieved during the first 6 postoperative hours (VAS>4, 14.8% at awakening, 8.2% at 3rd postoperative hour) in the first 2,709 patients even though there was a consistent increase of patients with VAS at rest ≤ 4 (Table 3).

Table 3. VAS values of 2,709 patients after surgery

VAS values	Awakening	3rd h	6th h	9th h	12th h	15th h	24th h	36th h
0	21.8%	26.6%	34%	38.6%	45.3%	54%	63.3%	73.4%
1	7%	11.4%	10.8%	15.9%	16.9%	16.3%	13.9%	14%
2	17.8%	24.9%	25.5%	23.9%	20.8%	8.9%	12.8%	7.2%
3	20.8%	16.4%	17.7%	13.1%	10.7%	5.9%	4.9%	2.8%
4	17.6%	12.4%	7.4%	5.6%	3.2%	2.7%	1.8%	1.7%
5	9%	6%	3%	2%	2%	2%	3%	0.4%
6	3.2%	0.9%	0.9%	1%	0.9%	0.3%	0%	0.6%
7	1.3%	0.5%	0.3%	0.1%	0.1%	0.2%	0%	0%
8	1.1%	0.8%	0.1%	0.1%	0%	0%	0%	0%
9	0.1%	0%	0%	0%	0%	0%	0%	0%
10	0.1%	0%	0%	0%	0%	0%	0%	0%

We then modified the therapeutic strategy in the recovery room with higher opioids doses combined with other drugs with the aim of obtaining a VAS at rest ≤ 2.

In this group of 1,218 patients our aim was soon achieved at patients' discharge from the recovery room (4.1% of patients with VAS > 2 at 3rd postoperative hour) (Table 4).

Table 4. VAS values in 1,218 patients after surgery

VAS values	Awakening A	Awakening D	3rd h	6th h	9th h	12th h	15th h	24th h	36th h
0	34%	40%	46.4%	57%	65.8%	71.5%	75.9%	77.8%	82.3%
1	24.2%	30.8%	34.3%	30.6%	26.8%	20.7%	17.7%	16.7%	13.1%
2	23.7%	23%	15.2%	9.7%	6.2%	5.7%	4.8%	3.4%	3%
3	10.7%	3.6%	2.7%	2%	0.5%	1.2%	0.9%	0.4%	0.2%
4	5%	1.3%	1%	0.4%	0.2%	0.5%	0.6%	1%	1%
5	0.8%	0.4%	0.4%	0.3%	0.3%	0.2%	0%	0.2%	0.4%
6	0.5%	0.5%	0%	0%	0.1%	0.2%	0.1%	0.4%	0%
7	0.7%	0.3%	0%	0%	0%	0%	0%	0.1%	0%
8	0.1%	0.1%	0%	0%	0.1%	0%	0%	0%	0%
9	0%	0%	0%	0%	0%	0%	0%	0%	0%
10	0.3%	0%	0%	0%	0%	0%	0%	0%	0%

Discomfort symptoms

The incidence of symptoms of discomfort reported by patients at awakening is shown in Table 5.

Table 5. Incidence of symptoms of discomfort reported at awakening

	Pharyngodynia	Shiver	Sedation	Ponv	Cough
Discomfort symptoms	26.6%	11.3%	8.7%	7.7%	7.3%

	Cephalalgia	Decubitus pain	Psychomotor agitation	Confusion	Humor disturbance
Discomfort symptoms	5.4%	4.5%	4.4%	1.9%	0.6%

Pain and discomfort symptoms vary in duration and intensity; hence discomfort symptoms need many observations and consequently their treatment must change during the postoperative period.

PONV has a great influence in the postoperative course; its prevention and care allows a faster recovery time; moreover its control in minor surgery (in particular day-surgery) allows faster discharge. A variety of factors have been implicated in PONV, including surgical procedures (laparoscopy > open surgery), type and duration of anesthesia (propofol antiemetic action), patient's characteristics and diseases (female > male, motion sickness), degree of postoperative pain, analgesic postoperative treatment (opioids' emetic action), and so on [5].

In the first 2,709 patients, PONV, as occasional or continuous nausea or vomiting, had an incidence of 8.6% at awakening, 6.2% after 6-12 postoperative hours, 4% after 12-24 postoperative hours, and 2.5% after 36 postoperative hours. In another group of 1,527 patients, more-frequent evaluations show a higher PONV incidence: 9.8% at awakening, 7.8% at 3rd postoperative hour, 7% at 6th postoperative hour, 5.8% at 9th postoperative hour, 3.3% at 12th postoperative hour, 2.5% at 15th postoperative hour, 2.4% at 24th postoperative hour, and 2% at 36th postoperative hour.

Figure 1 shows the trend in discomfort symptoms in 1,527 patients.

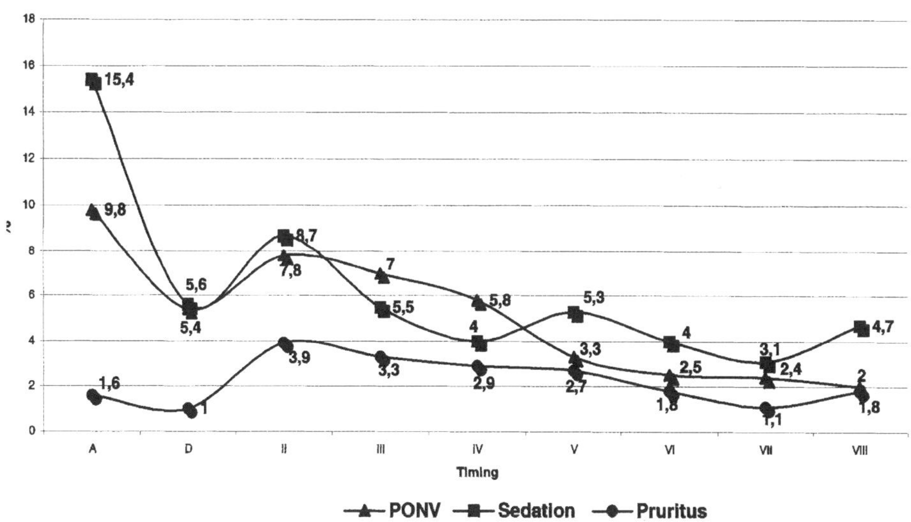

Fig. 1. Postoperative nausea and vomiting (PONV), sedation, and pruritus trends in 1,527 patients

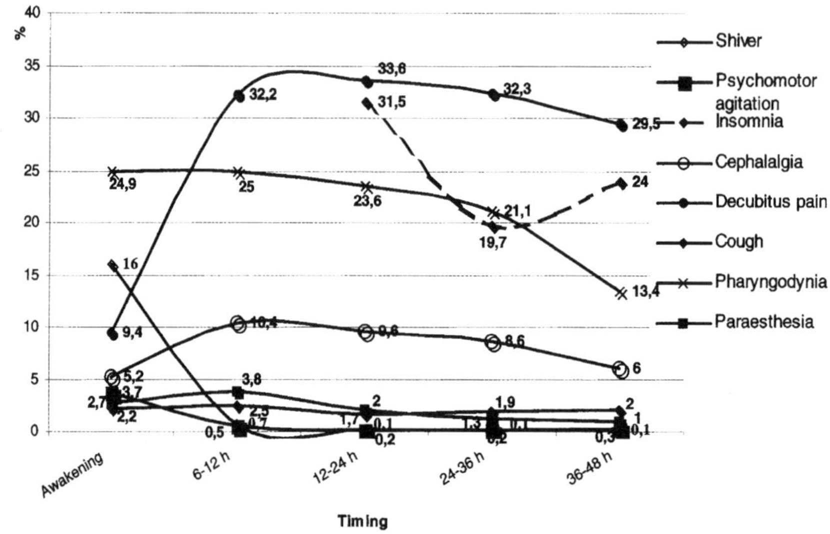

Fig. 2. Other discomfort symptoms in 1,527 patients during the postoperative period

Analgesia, on its own, can cause a lot of side effects; for example epidural analgesia can make mobilization easy, but at the same time has side effects such as pruritus and mean arterial pressure reduction. Pruritus is the most-frequent side effect after analgesia with epidural opioids.

In the same types of surgery with the same blood volume, mean arterial pressure can be different with different postoperative analgesic strategies (Fig. 3).

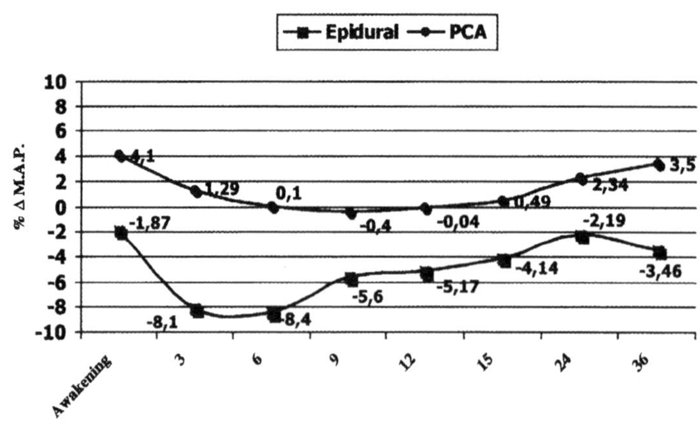

Fig. 3. A study by our Acute Pain Service in 1999 of 174 patients treated with epidural analgesia and 94 patients treated with patient-controlled analgesia (PCA). It shows the different postoperative mean arterial pressure (MAP) trend. Vasodilatation causes lower MAP values in the epidural population

This evidence suggests a different therapeutic approach (volemia control) based on the analgesic strategy [6].

Quality

Quality cycle (Deming's cycle) [7] applied to PONV evaluation suggests new strategies. PONV score systems able to provide an accurate description of this side effect in terms of intensity and length should be implement.

PONV should be directly reported by patients between one evaluation and another

When pain was treated, PONV was the most-frequent symptom reported by patients in a questionnaire at the end of the 48-h observation period. This confirms the importance of the careful evaluation and treatment of PONV during the postoperative period.

This kind of analysis can be applied to other signs. In fact we can identify other relationships among surgical procedures, anesthesia and discomfort symptoms. The patient's discomfort can be reduced by the right behavioral attitude and therapies.

For example neck hyperextension during thyroid surgery often causes cervical pain, which can be reduced by less "extreme" (sweeter) positions; intense shivering during locoregional anesthesia or at awakening after surgery can be reduced by heating systems.

Patients' satisfaction

In the satisfaction portion of the questionnaire, 96% of patients considered themselves "very" or "extremely" satisfied with the assistance received; 81.5% have responded that pain control treatment has been "good" or "very good", 17% "satisfactory", and only 1.5% have not been satisfied. The expectations raised by the anesthesiology visit have been "totally" or "in good part" maintained for 91.5% of the patients, while they have been "partially" fulfilled only for 7.5%. The judgement of the 94% of patients on the anesthesiology group has been near to optimum; the remaining 6% has been satisfied. The most-frequent disturbances reported by patients have been PONV (9%), bed pain (4.9%), cephalalgia (4.1%), pharyngodynia (2.7%), and wound pain (1.7%).

Discussion and conclusions

Discomfort and its treatment widen the remit of the APS to perioperative medicine; in fact good management of volemia, PONV control, shivering control, and evaluation of vital signs are all end-points. The APS aim is not only pain relief, but must facilitate faster mobilization through local and regional analgesic techniques besides traditional drugs.

Low doses of different analgesic drugs (opioids with local anesthetics, α_2-agonist and/or non-steroidal anti-inflammatory drugs) in multimodal or balanced therapy give pain relief with few side effects [8].

Our data show a strict correlation between VAS and NVS for low-intensity levels of pain, but not for VAS values higher than 4; in fact the number of patients who have a "NVS absent" is similar to patients with "VAS 0", patients with "NVS light" correspond to 100% of patients with "VAS 1" and about 50% of patients with "VAS 2" and patients with "NVS bearable" correspond to the rest of patients with "VAS 2" and the 100% of patients with "VAS 3" (Fig. 4).

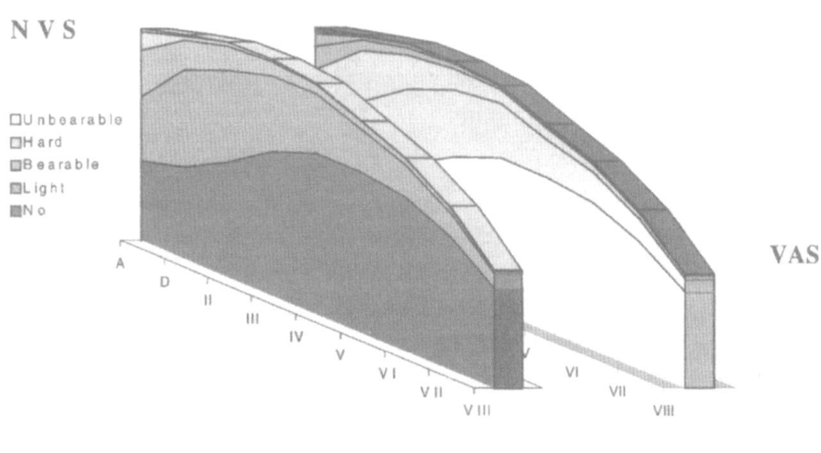

Fig. 4. Visual Analog Scale (VAS) and Numerical Verbal Scale (NVS) values in patients after surgery

As pain and discomfort symptoms are strictly linked to cultural and social conditions, previous experiences, patient's gender, and relationships between patient and health personnel, APS must establish a direct relationship with the patient (pact among patients and the doctor) [9].

Information given to patients preoperatively must become the first means of helping them. Correct preoperative information is necessary to avoid the aura of mystery and the sense of fear linked to surgery, and to reduce the operation to a curative act, eliminating its diagnostic aspect, which often causes patients' anguish. In fact, nowadays, surgery has lost its diagnostic role because diagnosis is often achieved before the operation; so we must help patients to overcome the remaining fear of anesthesia and surgery, which is often unfounded. This means correct preoperative information about every aspect related to the disease (techniques, risks, postoperative symptoms, incidence of side effects, and so on). In other words it is necessary to devote time, sympathy, and attention to patients.

References

1. Kehlet H (1997) Multimodal approach to control postoperative pathophysiology and rehabilatation. Br J Anaesth 78: 606-617
2. Joshi GP (1994) Postoperative pain management. Int Aesthesiol Clin 32: 113-126
3. Bertini, Tagariello V, Rossignoli L (1995) Organizzazione di un servizio di terapia antalgica post-operatoria. In: Nolli M, Albani A, Nicosia F (eds) Il Dolore post-operatorio – Valutazione e trattamento Mosby Doyma Italia, Astra
4. Giunta F, Paolicchi A, Teti G, et al (1999) Matrioska's game: postoperative pain and discomfort – quality valuation. Volume Atti Congresso Second International Meeting Dialogues on Anaesthesia and Intensive Care. Naples, February 4-6: p 22-25
5. White PF (1995) Management of postoperative pain and emesis. Can J Anaesth 42: 1053-1055
6. Paolicchi A, Giunta F, Teti G, De Masi F (1999) Perdurale e PCA in Chirurgia Maggiore. ALR 8 [Suppl]:68
7. Perraro F (1999) Miglioramento Continuo della Qualità dell'Assistenza Sanitaria. Volume Atti Congresso Second International Meeting Dialogues on Anaesthesia and Intensive Care. Naples, February 4-6: p 5-8
8. Hellyer PW (1997) Management of acute and surgical pain. Semin Vet Med Surg (Small Anim) 12:106-114
9. Brydon CW, Asbury AJ (1996) Attitudes to pain relief in adult surgical patients. Anaesthesia 51: 279-281

The Challenge of Postoperative Analgesia

N. RAWAL

Recent surveys show that a large proportion of patients still receive in adequate post-surgical analgesia, this problem is international in character. Analgesia techniques such as patient-controlled analgesia (PCA), spinal opioids alone or in combination with local anaesthetics and other regional analgesia techniques provide superior pain relief as compared to intermittent i.m. injection of opioids. However, these techniques have their own risks and therefore require special monitoring. The first line of defence against serious complications is an organization that provides appropriate education and policies which allow nurses and physicians to safely care for patients. It is increasingly clear that the solution to the problems of postoperative pain management lies not so much in the development of new techniques but in the development of an organization to exploit existing expertise.

Need for acute pain services (APS)

Although national guidelines for managing of postoperative pain have been published in several countries, the impact of these guidelines on patient care is unclear. The available data are not encouraging. In the United Kingdom, 4 to 5 years after publication of professional guidelines, less than half of hospitals surveyed had implemented a key recommendation to introduce an acute pain service (APS). The principal obstacles were financial constraints, newly qualified doctors were still undereducated regarding pain management [1], and pain relief remained inadequate [2]. Similar problems have been identified in the United States [3, 4], Germany [5], and a 17-nation European survey [6]. Reflecting widespread dissatisfaction with pain management in the USA the Joint Commission on Accreditation of Healthcare Organizations (JCAHO) has issued guidelines for hospital-wide improvement of pain management. The key recommendations are shown in Table 1. The JCAHO recommendations have to be implemented from 2001, it remains to be shown how they impact acute pain management in the USA.

Table 1. Joint Commission on Accreditation of Healthcare Organizations (JCAHO) – pain management guidelines*

• Recognize right of patients to pain management
• Assess and record existence, nature and intensity in all patients
• Assure staff competency in pain assessment and management
• Establish policies/procedures for effective pain management
• Educate patients and families about effective pain management
• Address patient needs for symptom management at hospital discharge
Pain is a major public healthcare problem that is treatable and mostly avoidable

*Endorsed by American Pain Society. Pain management standards will be scored from 2001, hospitals must demonstrate one year of compliance for accreditation

An APS using a multi-disciplinary team approach have received widespread acceptance and formal support from many institutions and organizations such as the UK Royal Colleges in 1990 [7], Australian Faculty of Anaesthetists in 1991 [8], US Acute Pain Management Guideline Panel in 1992 [9], International Association for Study of Pain [10] in 1992 and German Society of Anaesthesiologists and Surgeons in 1997 [5]. The key recommendations of the UK working party are shown in Table 2; similar recommendations have been made by other organizations. A recent survey showed that there is a large degree of variation in what is thought to constitute an APS in the UK [11].

Table 2. UK working party* – key recommendations

1. Need for education and training in changing antiquated staff attitudes and practice, together with adequate resources
2. Systematic recording of patients' pain, as with blood pressure/heart rate
3. A named member of staff to be responsible for a hospital policy towards post-operative analgesia, subject to continuous appraisal
4. All major hospitals performing surgery should introduce an acute pain service using a multi-disciplinary team approach with input of medical, nursing, pharmaceutical and psychological expertise. The anaesthetist has a primary role to play
5. There is need for a powerful, safe analgesics and long-acting non-toxic local anaesthetics

* Royal College of Surgeons and College of Anaesthetists, London 1990 [7]

US style APS – time to re-evaluate?

Although the concept of APS was first introduced in Europe [12], APS seems to be better established in the USA. Most major institutions in the USA have anaesthesiology-based APS [13]. The comprehensive pain management teams usually consist of a staff anaesthesiologists, resident anaesthesiologists, specially trained nurses, pharmacists and physiotherapists. Sometimes biomedical and infusion pump dispensing personnel are included. Secretarial and billing personnel are also a part of the US-style APS. Patients under the care of acute pain services are visited and assessed regularly by members of the team. Although pain management is often very satisfactory, the economic costs of such services are high, therefore the benefits are not available to all surgical patients because of reimbursement regulations.

Anaesthesiologist-based APS organization models usually provide "high tech" pain management services. This is not surprising because anaesthesiologists have special expertise in the field of advanced analgesic techniques such as epidural and PCA. Therefore most APS in the USA are essentially PCA and/or epidural based services only. Although the implementation of anaesthesiologist-based APS has had a considerable impact on pain management in surgical wards only a small percentage of patients receive the benefits of such APS. A good APS organization is one which ensures optimal pain management for every patient who undergoes surgery including children and those undergoing surgery on an ambulatory basis. Furthermore, the record of the US-style APS in implementing hospital-wide quality assurance measures such as frequent recording of pain intensity and recording treatment efficacy (VAS before and after treatment) has been generally unimpressive so far. Additionally, the costs of the US-style APS are very high. It is not surprising that such costs are increasingly questioned by health care payers. A downsizing of many APS is taking place in the USA, further reductions are predicted by many. The fee-for-service reimbursement system seems to be reversing the gains made by the introduction of the APS. Increasingly, the PCA services are being taken over by surgeons.

A more important issue with the US-style anaesthesiologist-based APS is a lack of continuity because the anaesthesiologist performing the preoperative evaluation (which includes patient information about proposed postoperative technique) and regional blocks (OR anaesthesiologist) is not the same physician who provides pain management postoperatively (APS anaesthesiologist). To address JCAHO requirements and the issues listed above, perhaps it is time to re-evaluate the role of the APS anaesthesiologist. Since the main aim of the APS is to improve postoperative pain management the APS anaesthesiologist needs to be a part of the OR anaesthesiologist team on a full time basis. This will facilitate co-operation with surgeons which is crucial for the integration of analgesic techniques with postoperative rehabilitation goals established by surgeons. Better feedback regarding efficacy of analgesic techniques in post anaesthesia care unit (PACU), surgical wards and ambulatory surgical units can be expected when the APS anaesthesiologist is full-time in the OR. Regular audit of the APS should be mandatory to identify shortfalls and improve services.

The role of an anaesthesiologist in any APS model is pivotal. However, in the opinion of this author such a role is more effective and professionally more satisfying as a teacher, supervisor, pain expert and performer of regional blocks when this anaesthesiologist is a part of the anaesthesia team rather than part of the geographically and psychologically distant chronic pain management team. Co-operation with chronic pain services will be necessary for "difficult" patients including those with chronic pain and drug abuse problems.

Development of a pain nurse-based acute pain service

It is becoming increasingly clear that simpler and less expensive models have to be developed if the aim is to improve the quality of postoperative analgesia for every patient who undergoes surgery. The organization should also include patients who undergo day-case surgery. Furthermore, in countries with state-financed health services and current budgetary restraints the overstaffed US-style anaesthesiology-based comprehensive, multi-disciplinary postoperative pain control teams appear unrealistic for most institutions.

At Örebro Medical Center Hospital our pain nurse-based anaesthesiologist-supervised model is based on the concept that postoperative pain relief can be greatly improved by provision of in-service training for surgical nursing staff, optimal use of systemic opioids and use of regional anaesthesia techniques and PCA in selected patients. A regular recording of each patient's pain intensity by visual analogic score (VAS) every 3 hours and the recording of treatment efficacy on the vital sign chart are the cornerstone of this model. A VAS above 3 is promptly treated. Surgeon and ward nurse participation are crucial in this organization. A specially trained acute pain nurse (APN) makes daily rounds of all surgery departments. Her duties are described in Table 3. In this organization the treatment of individual patients is based on standard orders and protocols developed jointly by the section anaesthesiologist, chief surgeon and charge nurse of the surgical ward. This gives nurses the flexibility to administer the analgesics when necessary. The section anaesthesiologist has the overall responsibility for pre-, peri- and postoperative anaesthesia care of patients, this includes postoperative pain management. He selects the patients for special pain therapies such as PCA, epidural or peripheral nerve blocks based on the departmental policy of using the "acute pain analgesic ladder" (Fig. 1) and evidence-based protocols. During regular working hours this anaesthesiologist is available for consultation or any emergency, later the anaesthesiologist on-call has the same function. The "pain representatives" from each surgical ward meet four times a year under anaesthesiologist and APN supervision to discuss improvements in APS. In the organization described here the only

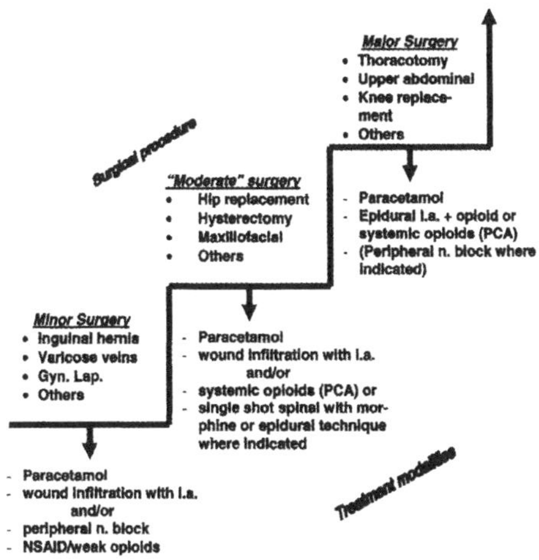

Fig. 1. Acute pain analgesic ladder and evidence based protocols

additional cost is that of the APN. At our hospital about 18 000 – 20 000 surgical procedures are performed each year, our low cost ($2-3 per patient excluding drug and equipment costs) organization is designed to benefit all of these patients. Similar results have been reported from the UK, it was estimated that development of the APS is cost-effective and improves quality of service for patients undergoing surgery [14].

Our organization has been functioning satisfactorily since 1991 and can be easily modified for non-surgical wards [15, 16]. Our latest audit in 1999-2000 has shown that over 95% of the surgical patients were satisfied with their postoperative pain management, received analgesia within 15 minutes and would prefer to have the same analgesic technique again (Table 3).

Table 3. Audit of postoperative pain management at Örebro Medical Center Hospital

300 patients interviewed, Oct 1999 – Feb 2000, elective surgery	
• Personnel assessed pain regularly	90 %
• Patients asked for analgesia if necessary (between pain assessments)	92 %
• Received pain treatment within 15 min	96 %
• Satisfied/very satisfied with pain treatment	90 %
• Would prefer same treatment again	95 %

Role of acute pain nurse

As a result of recent advances in pain management techniques and technology, anaesthesiologists are now offering patients new and highly effective forms of postoperative analgesia. However, it is the responsibility of the trained bedside nurses to deliver these analgesic therapies and to monitor and treat associated adverse effects. Since anaesthesiologists generally have a limited understanding of ward policies an APN can serve as an important link between the anaesthesiologist and bedside nurses.

Specialist nurses with particular training in pain management are increasingly being appointed, frequently as part of an acute pain team or pain management service. They make an invaluable contribution to patient care, bridge the gap between doctors and nurses in their areas of knowledge and responsibility. They can help direct resources, educate nurses and doctors in pain management techniques, give necessary support to the primary nurse and help to initiate and supervise analgesia. Our APN's are nurse anaesthetists with special training in pain management (Table 4).

Table 4. Organization of acute pain services at Örebro Medical Center, Örebro, Sweden

Health care member "pain representative" (named)	**Responsibility**
• Section Anaesthesiologist	Responsible for pre-, peri- and postop care (incl. postop pain) for his/her surgical section
• "Pain representative" ward surgeon	Responsible for mgmt on ward and for active postop rehab program
• "Pain representative" day nurse and "Pain representative" night nurse	Responsible for implementation "Pain representative" night nurse of pain mgmt guidelines and monitoring routines on the ward*
• Acute Pain Nurse (nurse anaesthetist)	• Daily rounds of all surgical wards • Check VAS recording on charts (every patient VAS≤3) • "Trouble-shoot" technical problems (PCA, epidural) • Refer problem patients to Section anaesthesiologist (liaison between surgical ward and anaesthesiologist)
• Acute Pain Anaesthesiologist	Responsible for co-ordination hospital-wide acute pain services and in-service teaching

* Patients are treated on the basis of standard orders and protocols developed jointly by chiefs of anaesthesiology, surgery and nursing sections. Pain representatives (named) meet every three months to discuss and implement improvements in pain management routines.
This organization benefits about 20 000 patients a year VAS≤3, it has been functioning satisfactorily since 1991.

Nurse and patient education

Nurses are in unique position to help patients in pain because they spend more time with them than any other health team member does. As new techniques of pain management are developed, nurses must update their knowledge to provide safe and effective care. Many nurses who are already overwhelmed with new techniques and equipment may react with skepticism and resistance to change in traditional approaches to pain management. Even if it will eventually save nursing time each new technique and piece of equipment such as an epidural and PCA is stressful for the staff until they become familiar with it.

Pain management is influenced by background knowledge, skill and experience of the nursing staff. Many responsibilities for pain management rest with the nurse directly caring for the patient, however many nurses have, in fact, had little formal education on the subject. The nurse on the ward must be informed and confident of the requirements of an analgesic technique. This can be achieved by education and experience in a supportive environment. Protocols should be constructed in conjunction with nursing colleagues and modified as necessary to allow for local nursing practices. Nurse education is widely recognized as an important priority in pain management [17].

Postgraduate training on pain management for practising nurses are increasingly available and education on pain management is becoming more prominent in basic nurse education. Educational devices such as algorithms to guide analgesic administration can lead to substantial improvements in quality of pain relief [1]. The attitude of staff towards pain management has an important influence on the effectiveness of pain relief [2]. The APS is best served by developing a small range of standard analgesic techniques in order to achieve a common level of understanding, familiarity and confidence. It is essential that pain is made visible. Pain should be documented routinely in the patient's notes in a similar way to recording blood pressure or heart rate. This process should be simple and convenient for nursing and the medical staff. Documentation also provides data for audit and facilities review and improvement of care.

Patients are unlikely to be aware of the standard of care they can expect to receive or what they can demand and their attitudes to pain and analgesia are believed to influence strongly the effectiveness of pain relief. Inadequate patient education is associated with a low standard of postoperative pain relief [14]. Patient education is particularly important when drugs are administered by techniques such as patient-controlled analgesia.

Audit of APS

Despite the availability of guidelines and recommendations from multiple pain societies and the advent of postoperative pain services since the late 1980's, recent surveys indicate that a majority of surgical patients experience considerable pain [3]. Such studies suggest that there has been no apparent improvement in postoperative since the first study in 1952 [18].

Studies have shown that the availability of APS per se is no guarantee for effective postoperative analgesia for all patients. Even well-established APS have published data showing a very high incidence of problems with epidural techniques when used on a routine basis on surgical wards. The pain relief for a large number of patients has been unsatisfactory [19-21]. Clearly there is a need for a regular audit of departmental pain management policies to address such issues. Audits should be carried out regularly on the process of pain management, patient experience and cost; the service should be modified according to the outcome. It is essential that pain is regularly evaluated to ensure that it is effectively managed. The minimum standard should be an annual determination of the number of patients in whom the pain score is above the predetermined threshold and identification of reasons for this. The audit method should be developed to meet local conditions. The outcome should be reviewed regularly and the service should be modified to rectify the shortfalls identified. The adverse effects of treatment should also be assessed and documented, and the dose or dose interval should be adjusted accordingly. The main findings of our recent audit (Oct. 1999 – Feb. 2000) of 300 inpatients are shown in Tables 4 and 5.

Table 5. Audit of postoperative pain management at Örebro Medical Center Hospital

300 patients interviewed, Oct 1999 – Feb 2000, elective surgery	
• Paracetamol according to routine	92 %
• Wound infiltration with l.a.	44 %*
• I.V. Opioid (titrated to effect)	53 %
• I.M. Opioid	3 %
• I.V. PCA (*morphine 31, ketobemidone 59*)	30 %
• Epidural (*bupi- + morphine 72, morphine 12, bupi 4*)	26 %
• Peripheral nerve blocks (n=6)	2 %**

* Not used in patients receiving epidural blocks
** Peripheral blocks used more frequently in ambulatory surgery

Future perspectives

Future challenges in postoperative pain management will need to focus on nurse, physician and patient education, specifically targeting attitudes towards pain and expectations. The need for multi-disciplinary APS teams involving anaesthesiologists, surgeons, nurses and other staff to optimize postoperative pain management is not in doubt because an APS addresses important issues such as improvement of quality of analgesia and efficacy and safety of (current and future) analgesic techniques. Any future APS organization will have to include the following: a) Regular pain assessment and documentation ("make pain visible"); b) inclusion of day surgery patients and of children; c) active co-operation with surgeons and ward nurses for development of evidence-based protocols; d) bedside teaching of ward nurses for provision of safe and cost-effective analgesic techniques. These components are relatively non-controversial, the challenge is to incorporate them in an APS model which exploits the full potential of invasive and expensive techniques such as the epidural for aggressive postoperative patient mobilization to improve outcome. The trend towards increased use of peripheral nerve blocks will continue and for many surgical procedures these techniques will replace expensive established methods because they are better than PCA and safer than the epidural [22-25]. For painful ambulatory surgical procedures, the continued development of simple, inexpensive, disposable pump technology will allow safe, incisional analgesia at home [26, 27]. A named member of staff should be responsible for implementing pain management policies in each unit. Patients should be fully informed preoperatively about the range of treatments available and their adverse effects. Patients undergoing day case surgery should have their pain assessed and documented in the same way as inpatients. Day case patients should be given a contact number so that they can discuss their own pain relief needs after discharge and written information about the use of analgesics. A follow-up call on the day after surgery should be mandatory.

The current system of acute pain management often does not integrate pain management with overall perioperative care and postoperative rehabilitation of the patient. The role of co-operation and "team approach" between surgeons, anaesthesiologists, APNs, ward nurses and physiotherapists will become increasingly important. The role of a good APS in developing the cost-effective pain treatment strategies for different surgical procedures cannot be over-emphasized.

Conclusion

The concept of skilled pain therapists collaborating to provide improved postoperative analgesia within the framework of an organized APS appears to be universally applicable. The most obvious components of an acute pain team include anaesthesiologists, surgeons, nurses, and physiotherapists. Protocols encourage consistent standards of safe and effective care and should be used as a framework to individualize treatment. APS models have been described from the USA, the UK, Germany, Switzerland and Sweden. The USA model which consists of anaesthesiologist-based comprehensive pain management teams is quite effective but is too selective and too expensive, it is not transferable to other countries. A pain nurse-based anaesthesiologist-supervised APS in which pain is evaluated in every patient who undergoes surgery has been developed in Sweden. Pain above 3 on the 10 grade visual analogue scale is promptly treated. In this low-cost model the anaesthesiologists' role is teaching and training ward nurses, supervising the APN and selecting patients for special pain therapies such as the epidural, PCA and peripheral nerve blocks. All senior anaesthesiologists (section chiefs) working in the OR are part of this APS.

The means of providing satisfactory analgesia are already present in most hospitals. Careful planning and a multi-disciplinary approach to pain management will ensure that resources are optimally utilized and the quality of pain management is consistently maintained.

References

1. Gould TH, Crosby DL, Harmer M et al (1992) Policy for controlling pain after surgery: effect of sequential changes in management. Br Med J:305:1165-1166
2. Oates JDL, Snowden SL, Jayson DWH (1994) Failure of pain relief after surgery. Attitudes of ward staff and patients to postoperative analgesia. Anaesthesia:49:755-758
3. Warfield CA, Kahn CH (1995) Acute pain management. Programs in US hospitals and experiences and attitudes among US adults. Anesthesiology:83:1090-1094
4. Tittle M, McMillan SC (1994) Pain and pain-related side effects in an ICU and on a surgical unit: nurses' management. Am J Crit Care:3:25-30
5. Wulf H, Neugebauer E, Maier C (1997) Die Behandling akuter perioperativer und posttraumatischer Schmerzen. Empfuhlungen einer interdiszplinaeren Expertenkommission. G. Thieme, Stuttgart, New York.
6. Rawal N, Allvin R and the EuroPain Acute Pain Working Party. (1998) Acute pain service in Europe: a 17-nation survey of 105 hospitals. Eur J Anesth:15:354-363
7. Royal College of Surgeons of England and the College of Anaesthetists Commission on the Provision of Surgical Services. (1990) Report on the Working Party on Pain after Surgery. London, September.
8. National Health and Medical Research Council (Australia). (1998) Management of severe pain, Canberra, Australia.
9. U.S. Department of Health and Human Services. (1992) Acute pain management. Clinical practice guidelines. AHCPR Publications No 92-0032, USA.
10. International Association for the Study of Pain (IASP). (1992) Management of acute pain. A practical guide Task force on acute pain, IASP Publications. Seattle, USA.
11. Windsor AM, Glynn CJ, Mason DG (1996) National provision of acute pain services. Anaesthesia:51:228-231
12. Maier C, Kibbel K, Mercker S, Wulf H. (1994) Postoperative pain therapy at general nursing

stations. An analysis of eight year's experience at an anesthesiological acute pain service. Anaesthesist:43:385-397
13. Ready LB. (1995) How many acute pain services are there in the US and who is managing patient-controlled analgesia? (Letter). Anesthesiology:82:322
14. Kuhn S, Cooke K, Collins M et al (1990) Perceptions of pain relief after surgery. Br Med J:300:1687-1690
15. Rawal N, Berggren L (1994) Organization of acute pain services – a low cost model. Pain: 57:117-123
16. Rawal N. (1999) 10 years of Acute Pain Services: achievements and challenges. Reg Anesth Pain Med;24:68-73
17. Harmer M, Davies KA (1998) The effect of education, assessment and a standardized prescription on postoperative pain management. Anaesthesia;58:424-30.
18. Papper EM, Brodie BB, Rovenstine EA (1952) Postoperative pain, its use in the comparative evaluation of analgesics. Surgery;32:107-109.
19. Ready LB. (1999) Acute pain, lessons learned from 25 000 patients. Reg Anesth Pain Med;24:499-505
20. Cousins MJ, Power I, Smith G. (2000) Pain – a persistent problem. Reg Anesth Pain Med;25:6-21
21. Andersen G, Rasmussen H Rosenstock C et al (2000) Postoperative pain control by epidural analgesia after transabdominal surgery. Efficacy and problems encountered by daily routine. Acta Anaesthesiol Scand;44:296-301
22. Borgeat A, Schappi B, Biasca N, Gerber C (1997) Patient-controlled analgesia after major shoulder surgery: patient-controlled interscalene analgesia versus patient-controlled analgesia. Anesthesiology. Dec;87(6):1343-1347
23. Singelyn FJ, Deyaert M, Joris D et al (1998) Effects of intravenous patient-controlled analgesia with morphine, continuous epidural analgesia, and continuous three-in-one block on postoperative pain and knee rehabilitation after unilateral total knee arthroplasty. Anesth Analg. Jul;87(1):88-92
24. Horlocker TT. (1998) Peripheral nerve blocks – regional anesthesia for the new millennium [editorial]. Regional Anesthesia and Pain Medicine;23(3):237-40.
25. Capdevila X, Barthelet Y, Biboulet P et al (1999) Effects of perioperative analgesic technique on the surgical outcome and duration of rehabilitation after major knee surgery. Anesthesiology. Jul;91(1):8-15
26. Rawal N, Axelsson K, Hylander J et al (1998) Postoperative patient-controlled local anesthetic administration at home. Anesth Analg;86:86-89
27. Rawal N (2000) Patient controlled regional analgesia at home. Tech Reg Anesth Pain Mgmt;4:62-66

The Management of Postoperative Pain. Drugs and Anesthetic Techniques

G. Galimberti

Effective pain relief is very important to treat any patient undergoing surgery. This should be achieved not only for ethical and humanitarian reasons, but also in order to obtain a smoother postoperative course, an earlier discharge from hospital, and a reduction of onset of chronic pain syndromes. In fact, there is now evidence that pain relief has significant physiological benefit. Analgesia for postoperative pain relief has traditionally been provided with widespread use of intramuscolar opioids. However, after surgery, patients frequently experience severe pain and a significant portion receive less than adequate analgesia [1-3]. Furthermore, surveys in the 1980s show that as high as 30%-75% of patients still receive inadequate pain treatment in the postoperative period, in spite of an increasing consciousness of this issue [4-7]. It is remarkable that Smith, in an editorial, asserted "what is so surprising is that, this deplorable state of affairs has persisted and continues to persist in many hospital, despite considerable advances in the pharmacology of analgesic drugs and description of new and improved methods of relieving pain" [8]. Although recent years have seen the widespread use of modern and effective analgesic techniques such as epidural analgesia, postoperative regional blocks and patient-controlled analgesia (PCA) for the relief of postoperative pain, the most frequently used technique in surgical wards still remains intramuscolar opioids prescribed by ward surgeon and administered by ward nurse on an as-needed basis [9]. Multiple reasons for this undertreatment have been identified, but the primary factors appear to be an exaggerated fear of opioid addiction and respiratory depression [1,10]. Another primary cause appears to be the perception that pain is a natural, inevitable accompaniment to illness and disease. Indeed, most patients, physicians, and nurses consider moderate to severe postoperative pain, despite the fact that fear of unrelieved pain is a primary concern of patients before surgery, to be an acceptable consequence of surgical intervention. Pain is invisible on most hospital wards and that is another important factor contributing to undertreatment. Severity of pain is not assessed and consequently it cannot be effectively treated. Thus, one of the most-important changes in improving postoperative pain management is to introduce pain assessment as the fifth vital sign in addition to the traditional four vital signs (temperature, pulse, blood pressure, and respiratory rate). Pain, physiologically, signals the presence of damage or disease within the body. Postoperative pain is the result of surgery but the continuous coming in of nociceptive stimuli during the postoperative period may be deleterious for the patient's outcome [11-13] and may increase the cost of medical care. For example, pain contributes to the perioperative stress response with elevated cathecolamine levels, hypercoagulability, systemic and coronary vasoconstriction, metabolic shifts to the catabolic, protein-wasting state, and immunosuppression. Pulmonary function can also be compromised in patients undergoing abdominal or thoracic surgery, and pain-induced efferent activity is one possible mechanism of postoperative ileus [14]. Postoperative pain is a subjective experience and the need for each patient to reduce or eliminate pain and discomfort is individual. Thus, the management of postoperative pain has to take into account many factors such as clinical factors, patient-related factors, local factors, and organizational factors. Optimal techniques for acute pain management depend on patient co-morbidity, the magnitude of the surgical procedure, and a variety of other factors (previous opioid use, mental capacity, ethnic customs). Analgesia is best provided by a combination of two or more drugs or techniques, with different sites or through different mechanisms of action, or when analgesic effects are synergistic [15].

The recognition that unrelieved pain contributes to perioperative morbidity and mortality has inspired many institutions to develop Acute Postoperative Pain Services (APS) in an attempt to provide more-effective postoperative pain relief [6,13]. It is becoming clear that the solution of the postoperative pain problems lies, over all, in the development of an organization to exploit existing expertise. Nowadays, the implementation of the APS in hospital is strongly recommended by a committee of experts and its role in the management of the quality of postoperative pain relief is increasing year by year.

Physiopathology

Pain is a complex experience, including physiological, psychological, and experiential aspects, which together account for the sensation of pain. According to the definition of pain adopted by the International Association for Study of Pain (IASP), we might define pain as "a subjective and emotional experience associated with actual or potential tissue damage or expressed in terms of such damage". It is obvious that visual analogic scales (VAS) are a very useful tool to evaluate the pain intensity, but cannot express the multiple aspects correlated with the pain experience. The beginning of nociception is generated by nociceptors widely distributed throughout the body, and the signals are then transferred by afferent sensory nerve fibers to the spinal cord and then to the brain. The inflammatory response, consequent of the traumatic damage due to the surgical intervention, is able to unleash and successively amplify a strong and important neurotrasmittors cascade. It is well recognized that an adequate pain relief reduces complications and mortality after major surgery, increasing pulmonary function, chest expansion, effective cough effort, and co-operation with the chest physiotherapist [12, 16]. Also adequate analgesia reduces sympathetic activity, which causes tachycardia, hypertension, increased stroke volume, cardiac work, and myocardial oxygen consumption. The risk of myocardial ischemia or infarction is reduced, as is the risk of deep vein thrombosis, in patients at rest, with platelet aggregation and venous stasis. Furthermore the recent popularity of the fast-tracking anesthesia programs and the increasing number and complexity of day-surgery procedures have increased the need for optimal pain relief. Inadequate analgesia is a major cause of delayed discharge [17-19].

Consequently, postoperative pain is dangerous not only because it is a potent trigger for the stress response involving adverse effects on various organ systems, but also because it may determine a spinal cord hyperexcitability - the so called "wind-up" phenomenon - responsible itself for hyperalgesic and/or spontaneous painful syndromes [20-23]. The "wind-up" mechanism seems to be able to modify the physiological and anatomical neuronal characteristics, through a mechanism called spinal cord "neuroplasticity" and, although the physiopathology is not yet fully understood, it constitutes a sort of neurochemical memory of the pain. In any event, a great contribution to this seems to be related to the intracellular transduction of extracellular signals involving a cascade of phosphorylation-dephosphorylation events leading to modulation of the activity of several different molecules. In fact, repeated nociceptive stimulation determines the release of a variety of excitatory neurotransmitters, such as amino acid glutamate and aspartate, activating *n*-methyl-D-aspartate (NMDA) and alpha-amino-3-hydroxy-5-methyl-4-isoxazoleproprionate (AMPA) receptors located in dorsal horn neurones [24]. NMDA, receptors, in particular, induce the release of substance P and neurokinin A, maintaining the spinal hypersensitivity and potentiating the transmission of nociceptive messages [25]. As a consequence of this receptorial activation, there is at the neuronal level a double action– a quick inflow of calcium (Ca^{2+}) and proto-oncogene transcription. Following repeated sensory stimulation, there are increased gene expressions from some postsynaptic neurones. The c-*fos* and c-*jun* protoncogenes, for example, are part of this cellular program that guarantees synaptic plasticity, i. e., the capacity of neurones to modify their synapses with activity and experience [26]. This activation of transcription factors by synaptic activity might represent the possible link between neurothrophin and neuroplasticity in the developing, as well as the central nervous systems. Consequently, the appearance of new antigens in spinal cord neurones, as a phenotypic expression of the protoncogenes mentioned above, could be the first sign of a structural and chronic modification of protein synthesis providing a persistent track of pain suffered.

During the transition from acute to chronic pain in the dorsal root ganglia and spinal cord, other factors, such as nitric oxide level [27], local blood flow regulation, and the glutamatergic mechanism [28,29], seem to play an important role.

Recently, efforts to improve postoperative pain relief have concentrated on pain preventive regimens directed at decreasing activation of excitatory glutamate receptors of the NMDA subtype. Racemic ketamine blocks NMDA receptor activation in a noncompetitive manner [30,31]. In pain-preventive regimens, subanesthetic-dose i.v. ketamine and dextromethorphan reduced postoperative pain [32,33], and in combination with epidural opioids or local anesthetics, epidural ketamine increased postoperative analgesia [34,35]. The combination of S(+)-ketamine and ropivacaine in epidural anesthesia increases postoperative pain relief when compared with ropivacaine alone in patients undergoing total knee arthroplasty [36]. In contrast, amantadine, another noncompetitive NMDA receptor antagonist, just used in the therapy of Parkinson disease, dementia, and spasticity, at the preoperative dose of 200 mg does not enhance postoperative analgesia in women undergoing abdominal hysterectomy [37]. Over the last decade more attention has been focused on the NMDA receptor because it seems to be involved in the occurrence of opioid-induced hyperalgesia (OIH). It has been observed with the use of very large doses of either i.v. or intrathecal opioids, such as morphine or remifentanil. The mechanistic basis of OIH is unclear, but NMDA receptor activation seems to be a critical step [38,39]. Although the AMPA receptors are involved in nociceptive mechanisms in the spinal cord, the effects of AMPA receptor antagonists are controversial. It is been reported that the AMPA receptor antagonist inhibits the acute first phase [40] but not the tonic second phase [41]. Conversely, it has been observed that the AMPA receptor antagonist reduced the second phase but not the first phase [42]. Other studies have shown that both the first and the second phases are suppressed by the intrathecal [43] and intraperitoneal administration of YM872, a new (α-amino-3-hydroxy-5-methylisoxazole-4-propionic acid receptor antagonist [44].

Clinical factors

The need for analgesia depends in large part on the site of surgery and on the magnitude of the surgical trauma. Generally, thoracic surgery and surgery involving upper abdomen are more painful than surgery on the lower abdomen or on the limbs. Furthermore, the greater the magnitude of surgery, the greater the postoperative discomfort. Surgery involving a body cavity, large joint surfaces, or deep tissues requires more-aggressive and complex pain management techniques to achieve optimal analgesia. Operations on the thorax or upper abdomen may produce profound changes in pulmonary function, an increase in abdominal muscle tone, and an associated decrease in diaphragmatic function. Consequently, the patient will be unable to cough effectively and secretions may lead to lung atelectasis and pneumonia. In addition, pain causes an increase in the sympathetic response of the body, with subsequent increases in heart rate, cardiac work, and oxygen consumption. Prolonged pain has several other effects, such as a reduction of physical activity that can lead to venous stasis and an increased risk of deep vein thrombosis and pulmonary embolism, an alteration of gut and urinary tract motility, which may lead to postoperative ileus, nausea, vomiting, and urinary retention. The choice of analgesic option can be based on the class of surgical procedure (minor, moderate, major), on drug availability, and familiarity with different methods of analgesia.

Minor surgery

Minor surgery (e.g., laparoscopy, arthroscopy, inguinal herniorrhaphy, breast biopsy) produces superficial and minimal surgical trauma, does not need postoperative hospitalization, and traditional analgesic therapy includes oral opioid/acetaminophen or opioid/aspirin combinations. Recent studies suggest that non-steroidal anti-inflammatory drugs (NSAIDs) may be a better choice than opioid combinations following most outpatient surgery. Furthermore, patients receiving NSAIDs have fewer undesirable side effects such as nausea and somnolence than those receiving oral oxycodone/acetaminophen combination [30]. Opioid analgesics are usually not needed after outpatient operations and should be reserved for treatment of breakthrough pain. Infiltration of surgical wound with local anesthetic can also constitute the primary anesthetic technique. For example, inguinal herniorrhaphy can easily be performed with a subcutaneous and subfascial infiltration of local anesthetic (e.g., bupivacaine 0.125-0.25%) in addition an inguinal field block that incorporates blockade of the iliohypogastric and ilioinguinal nerves. The maximum recommended dose of bupivacaine is 175 mg for infiltration (70 ml of 0.25% solution). The wound infiltration provides analgesia for the first 6-12 h and reduces postoperative consumption of systemic analgesics [45].

Intermediate surgery

Patients having intermediate or moderate surgery (e.g., cesarean section, hysterectomy, radical retropubic prostatectomy, appendectomy, total joint replacement) require hospitalization after surgery for management of postoperative pain, postoperative observation, or convalescence. Traditional intramuscular opioid analgesia has been demonstrated to provide inadequate analgesia in most patients and has low patient satisfaction. Although intravenous PCA administered opioids may not reduce morbidity and mortality, there is an improvement of pain scores, patient satisfaction, and a more-constant analgesia [46,47]. Programming a PCA device requires selecting an appropriate intermittent bolus dose, a minimum length of time between doses, and a limit to the hourly dose available. Morphine sulfate, meperidine, and hydromorphone are commonly used in intravenous PCA. High doses of meperidine (600 mg/day) can result in seizures resulting form accumulation of the renally excreted metabolite normeperidine. Thus, meperidine is not recommended for use in patients with high opioid requirements or decreased renal function. Continuous intravenous infusions associated with PCA are almost never indicated in postoperative patients, because this does not improve analgesia but increases opioid side effects and the risk of respiratory depression [48,49]. The addition of parenteral NSAIDs has been demonstrated to decrease requirements for intravenous PCA opioids and to speed recovery of bowel function after surgery [50]. Although single injections of epidural and intratechal opioids can provide better pain relief than intravenous PCA opioids, their role in this patient population remains unclear and requires further study [51]. Finally, infiltration of surgical wounds or blockade of peripheral nerves with local anesthetic can also reduce postoperative pain in this kind of surgery.

Major surgery

Major surgery (e.g., liver or pancreatic resections, bowel resections, thoracotomies, aortic surgery) produces severe trauma, activates a strong stress response, and is associated with significant postoperative morbidity. Intravenous PCA opioids provide better analgesia than intramuscular opioids at rest, but neither reduce postoperative morbidity nor improve convalescence [47]. In contrast, the combination of an epidurally administered opioid and a local anesthetic can provide better analgesia during ambulation, coughing, or activity, can blunt surgical stress response, can improve postoperative pulmonary function, ileus, and decrease the incidence of postoperative thrombosis and thromboembolism, and can, maybe, reduce the incidence of postoperative myocardial ischemia [14]. Epidural analgesic techniques are associated with a low incidence of respiratory depression and the risk is similar to that associated with intramuscular opioids. Nevertheless, epidural analgesic approaches require a higher level of expertise and organizational structure on the part of physicians and nurses than do intramuscular or intravenous opioid analgesic techniques. Thus, patients undergoing major surgery benefit from treatment provided by an Acute Postoperative Service (APS), which can extend 24-h coverage and complete management of the epidural analgesic regimen.

Patient-related factors

Young, healthy patients have a relatively low incidence of major morbidity and mortality after surgery, even if there is inadequate pain management. In contrast, patients with pre-existing co-morbidity, such as unstable angina, can have an increased risk of perioperative morbidity or death as a result of inadequate perioperative pain relief. In this group of patients the risk of postoperative morbidity is quite high [52,53] and they require careful postoperative pain management.

Several factors predict the severity of postoperative pain such as the site and nature of surgery, the nature and intended purpose of the surgery, the patient's fear and anxiety or stories heard from friends and relatives that present the postoperative period in unfavorable way. Adequate time must be allowed to explain the intended operation and the steps that will be taken to ensure pain relief. A clear and friendly explanation in simple terms during the preoperative period will often reduce anxiety and minimize misunderstandings. Clinical studies to date suggest that effective pain therapy can improve the patient's ability to take deep breaths and cough. Similarly, good postoperative analgesia can reduce the postoperative stress response and myocardial ischemia. Nevertheless, larger and more-detailed studies are necessary to determine whether good postoperative pain management can be translated into improvements in patient outcome.

Assessment of pain severity

Pain severity is usually assessed by using rating scales. These methods, either words or numbers, are simple, can be readily understood, and require little in the way of resources and technology. Numerical values can be derived from a visual analogue scale (VAS). Subjects are instructed to indicate the intensity of pain by marking a 100-mm line anchored with terms describing the extremes of pain intensity: no pain at the bottom and worst imaginable pain at the top. A simple numerical rating scale would require the patient to choose a number between 0 and 10 to represent their pain. Another often used measurement of postoperative pain is the five-point verbal pain scale (VPS). It includes the following categories: no pain, mild pain, moderate pain, severe pain, and horrible pain. Also simple questions like "where dose it hurt" and "what does it feel like?" may permit a qualitative evaluation of pain (Table 1).

Table 1. Pain experience history

Child form	Parent form
Tell me about the hurt you have had before	Describe the pain experience your child has had before
Do you tell others when you hurt? If yes, who?	Does your child tell you or others when he/she is hurting?
What do you do for yourself when you are hurting?	How do you know when your child is in pain?
What do you do want others to do for you when you hurt?	How does your child usually react to pain?
What helps the most to take your hurt away?	What works best to decrease or take away your child's pain?
Is there anything special that you want me to know about you when you hurt?	Is there anything that you would like me to know about your child and pain?

The usefulness of these methods have been validated in the setting of chronic pain by several investigators [54-56]. In these settings, the VAS is superior to fixed interval scales, relative pain scales, and verbal reports of pain [57-59]. More recently, the VAS has been used to measure pain in the immediate postoperative period to compare the effect of different analgesic regimens. The VAS it is not easy to use in the postoperative period because of residual anesthesia, blurred vision, or nausea, and several subjects required additional instructions to complete the VAS [60]. In using the VAS for treatment decisions or for the measurement of the effect of pharmacological interventions we have to bear in mind that it has an imprecision of ± 20 mm.

Pharmacology

NSAIDs are the first step in management of pain. They are most useful in alleviating pain from inflammatory conditions. The second step, if pain control is not achieved, is to introduce weak opioid drugs such as codeine or tramadol, together with appropriate agents to minimize side-effects. The final step, if effective pain control is not achieved, is to introduce a strong opioid such as morphine.

Generally, postoperative pain decreases with time and, thus, the need for drugs should cease. Consequently, in the first hours after surgery the pain should be controlled with strong analgesics in combination with local anesthetic blocks and peripherally acting drugs. The second rung on the postoperative pain ladder is the restoration of the oral route to deliver analgesia by using combinations of peripherally acting agents and weak opioids. The final rung is when the pain can be controlled by NSAIDs alone.

Table 2. Unconventional analgesics used in multimodal therapy

1) Adrenergic blockade
    • noradrenaline,
    • guanethidine,
    • phentolamine
2) alpha-2 agonists
    • clonidine
    • dexmedetomidine
3) NMDA antagonists
    • ketamine
    • amantadine
4) Others neuromodulators
    • neurokinin
    • tyrosine kinase receptors
    • sodium channel blockade
    • calcium channel blockade: ziconotide
    • galanin receptor
    • 5HT3 receptor antagonist: alosetron

Since the development of balanced anesthesia, it has become clear that in anesthesia and analgesia, it is better to use more drugs together, with different mechanisms of action, than to use only one This synergistic interaction of the drugs is convenient because it increases the efficiency and safety of the treatment. In fact, the gains from drug and technique combination are twofold, reducing the drug dose and therefore, the side effects. If the mechanism of action is completely separate and the side effects of the drugs and techniques are quite different, it is possible to reduce the total drug dose and, therefore, the incidence and severity of the side effects. Moreover, in the presence of synergism, the final effects are more than simply additive. Thus, at present most anesthesia and analgesia techniques, particularly with high-risk patients, have a multimodal approach in order to reduce afferent input to the spinal cord, to blockade the autonomic response, and to avoid the stress response to surgery. There is evidence that a multimodal analgesic therapy should be chosen to achieve logical drug interactions at the spinal cord. The combination of drugs with different mechanisms of action increase safety and convenience in routine practice. Thus, we can associate opioids and local anesthetics because local anesthetic blocks neuronal sodium channels while opioids act on mu-receptors, probably to open the potassium channels.

NSAIDs and opioids are suggested for minor to moderate pain and combinations of local anesthetics, opioid, and alpha-2 adrenergic agonist for severe pain. NSAIDs analgesia inhibits the cyclooxygenase-dependent prostanoid formation, the intracellular phosphodiesterase, and bradykinin levels. Instead opioids provide effective analgesia through a central mechanism via the opioid receptor.

Recently other unconventional analgesics have been proposed (Table 2). Adrenergic alpha-2 agonists, such as clonidine, are more effective when given epidurally rather than systemically and in association with local anesthetics and/or opioids rather than alone [61]. In addition, clonidine has some side effects such as hypotension, bradycardia, and sedation, probably due to supraspinal mechanisms [62]. For this reason the identification of further adrenergic receptor subtypes offers the possibility to use more-selective and full agonists for the alpha-2 adrenergic receptors, such as dexmedetomidine [63].

Local anesthetics

Regional anesthetic techniques used for surgery, such as local infiltration of incisions with long-acting local anesthetics, blockade of peripheral nerves, and continuous block techniques peripherally or centrally, may have several benefits: reduced blood losses, excellent pain relief, minimal respiratory and cardiovascular effects.

As postoperative pain is multifactorial in origin, it is logical that management should consist of a combination of different approaches in order to achieve the best results. Single infiltration of a surgical wound can provide analgesia for several hours. Further pain relief can be obtained by infusions via a thin catheter. Infiltration of local anesthetics (LA) in the surgical wound, before or at the end of surgery, is a simple and attractive technique, which has been recommended for postoperative pain relief after various surgical interventions [64]. Only with this technique in comparison with a placebo is it possible to observe a significant decrease of postoperative pain at rest, during mobilization, and during cough, together with a reduction in total requirements for supplementary morphine [65]. No clinical differences in postoperative analgesic effects can be demonstrated between ropivacaine and bupivacaine for wound infiltration when they are used in equipotent doses. However, since large volumes of LA are needed, ropivacaine may be preferred because it causes a lower risk of cardiovascular and cerebral side effects than bupivacaine [66]. It has been suggested that "preemptive administration" of incisional LA in addition to general anesthesia may have a greater benefit than spinal anesthesia. This implies that the preemptive administration of LA may have extended effects on postoperative pain due to interference with trauma-induced changes in the peripheral and central nervous systems [67].

Table 3. Local anesthetic for the treatment of acute postoperative pain

Agent	% solution for analgesic blocks	Duration (h)	Max. single dose mg/kg (Total mg in adults)	% solution for infusion	Comments
Lignocaine					
Infiltration	0.5-1	1-2	300	-	Rapid onset.
Epidural	1.5-2	1-2	500	0.3-0.7	Dense motor
Plexus or nerve	0.75-1.5	1-3	500	0.5-1.0	block
Mepivacaine					
Infiltration	0.5-1	1.5-3	400	-	Rapid onset.
Epidural	1-2	1.5-3	500	0.3-0.7	Dense motor
Plexus or nerve	0.75-1.5	2-4		0.5-1.0	block. Longer action than lignocaine
Bupivacaine					
Infiltration	0.125-0.25	1.5-4	175	-	Avoid 0.75%
Epidural	0.25-0.75	2-5	225	0.0625-0.125	in obstetrics.
Plexus or nerve	0.25-0.5	4-24+	225	0.5-1.0	Mainly sensory block at low concentrations. Cardiotoxic after rapid IV injection
Ropivacaine					
Infiltration	0.2	2-6	200	-	Differential
Epidural	0.2-1	0.5-5	200	0.1-0.3	block
Plexus or nerve	0.2-0.75	2-6	225	0.5	(sensory/motor) Reduced cardiotoxicity

Spinal anesthesia provides excellent analgesia for surgery in the lower half of the body, and pain relief can last many hours after surgery. Continuous analgesia using the spinal route has been tried, but epidural analgesia is used more widely.

The use of epidural techniques requires experienced practitioners and specific training nurses for the postoperative pain management of patients in surgical wards. Furthermore, great care must be taken to maintain sterility of the epidural set. Although continuous epidural analgesia with local anesthetics may produce very effective analgesia, they may also produce undesirable and potentially harmful side effects, such as hypotension, sensory and motor block, nausea, and urinary retention. The association of local anesthetic drugs with opioids given centrally may reduce some of these effects. Table 3 lists suggested concentrations, safe maximum doses, and block characteristics of the most widely available local anesthetics.

Non-opioid analgesic

The most commonly used analgesic drugs in hospital around the world are the NSAIDs. These are the main analgesic treatment for mild to moderate pain. NSAIDs have both analgesic and anti-inflammatory actions. Their mechanism of action is predominantly by inhibition of prostanglandin synthesis by the enzyme cyclo-oxygenase, which catalyzes the conversion of arachidonic acid to the various prostaglandins that are the mediators of inflammation.

Table 4. Comparative dosing recommendations for non-steroidal anti-inflammatory drugs (NSAIDs) in management of postoperative acute pain

Drugs	Usual adult dosage	Usual pediatric dosage[a]	Comments
Acetaminophen	650-975 mg/4 h	10-15 mg/Kg per 4 h	Lacks the peripheral anti-inflammatory activity of other NSAIDs
Aspirin	650-975 mg/4 h	10-15 mg/kg per 4 h[b]	The pain-reducing standard against which other NSAIDs are compared; inhibits platelet aggregation; may cause postoperative bleeding
Ibuprofen	400 mg/4-6 h	10 mg/kg per 6-8 h	Brand and generic, oral-suspension and tablet forms available
Ketoprofen	25-75 mg/6-8 h	/	
Meclofenamate	50 mg /4-6 h	/	
Mefenamic acid	250 mg/6 h	/	
Naproxen	550 mg initial dose, followed by 275 mg/6-8 h	5 mg/kg per 12 h	Liquid and tablet forms available
Sodium salicylate	325-650 mg/3-4 h	/	Generic available
Ketorolac	30-60 mg IV or IM initial dose, following by 15-30 mg/6 h; oral dose following IV or IM dosage: 10 mg/6-8 h	/	IV or IM dosing not exceeding 5 days

[a] Drug recommendations for children are limited to NSAIDs for which paediatric dosing experience is available
[b] Contraindicated in the presence of fever or other evidence of viral illness

All NSAIDs work in the same way and consequently there is no advantage in giving more than one at a time. NSAIDs are, in general, more effective for superficial pain (skin, buccal mucosa, joint surfaces, bone) and may be usefully combined with opioids, due to the different mechanism of action. The choice of a NDAIDs should be made on the basis of availability, cost, and length of action (Table 4). All NSAIDs may have side effects, such as antiplatelet action leading to increased bleeding time and the inhibition of prostaglandin synthesis that may produce gastric bleeding and impairment of renal function.

Paracetamol has analgesic and antipyretic properties but little anti-inflammatory effect. It is well absorbed orally and is metabolized almost entirely in the liver. It has few side effects in normal dosage and is widely used for the treatment of postoperative pain. Doses range from a minimum of 500 mg, via oral or anal route, to 4 g daily. After prolonged use, paracetamol causes hepatotoxicity in overdosage by overloading the normal metabolic pathways with the formation of a toxic metabolite.

Weak opioids

The most commonly used weak opioids throughout the world are: codeine, dextropropoxyphene, and tramadol.

Codeine, derived from opium alkaloids, is markedly less active than morphine, has predictable effects, and is effective against mild to moderate pain. Doses range from 15 to 60 mg every 4 h with a maximum dose of 300 mg/day. There is a "roof effect" and, thus, if pain is not responding to maximum dose a stronger drug should be used. It is possible to use with paracetamol.

Dextropropoxyphene is structurally related to methadone but is a relatively poor analgesic. It offers few advantages over codeine and can be used in combination with paracetamol. Doses range from 32.5 mg (in combination with paracetamol) to 60 mg every 4 h, with a maximum dose of 300 mg/day.

Tramadol hydrochloride is a centrally acting, synthetic analgesic that is not derived from natural sources and is not chemically related to opioids. The mechanism of action is not fully understood. The drug, however, appears to have two modes of action. It binds with low affinity to mu-opioid receptors; this blocks pain impulses from reaching the brain, in the same way as opioids. Tramadol, in addition, inhibits reuptake of norepinephrine and serotonin, altering the way the brain monitors pain signals. Tramadol does not inhibit production of prostaglandins, so the risk of gastrointestinal bleeding and renal toxicity is reduced. Clinical studies found that approximately 250 mg tramadol a day, in divided doses, produced pain relief equivalent to that produced by five doses of acetaminophen 300 mg with codeine phosphate 30 mg, five doses of aspirin 325 mg with codeine phosphate 30 mg, or two to three doses of acetaminophen 500 mg with oxycodone hydrochloride 5 mg. The most frequently reported side effects have been dizziness, nausea, constipation, headache, and somnolence. The starting dose for mild and moderate pain is 1 mg/kg. The daily dose recommended is 500 mg or 300 mg in older patients. The onset of analgesia occurs in approximately 20-30 min with a duration of 4-6 h. For patients with creatinine clearance less than 30 ml/min, lengthening the dose interval to 12 h is recommended, with a maximum daily dose of 200 mg. For patients with hepatic cirrhosis, the recommended dose is 50 mg every 12 h. The normal dose may need to be doubled for patients who are also taking carbamazepine.

Strong opioids

Severe postoperative pain requires strong opioids. Early administration will achieve effective analgesic concentrations and make it easier to maintain the therapeutic level of the drug in the blood. When the level of pain relief is satisfactory, the maintanance dose is achieved by regular administration of opioid (Table 5).

Table 5. Comparative dosing recommendations for opioids in management of postoperative acute pain

Drug	Approximate equianalgesic parenteral dose	Recommended starting dose in adults weighing more than 50 kg	Recommended starting dose in children and adults weighing less than 50 kg
Morphine	10 mg /3-4 hs	10 mg /3-4 h	0.1 mg/kg per 3-4 h
Codeine	75 mg /3-4 h	60 mg /2 h	Not recommended
Hydromorphone	1.5 mg/3-4 h	1.5 mg/3-4 h	0.015 mg/kg per 3-4 h
Meperidine	100 mg/3 h	100 mg/3 h	0.75 mg/kg per 2-3 h
Metadone	10 mg /6-8 h	10 mg /6-8 h	0.1 mg/kg per 6-8 h
Oxymorphone	1 mg/3-4 hs	1 mg/3-4 h	Not recommended
Buprenorphine	0.3-0.4 mg/6-8 h	0.4 mg/6-8 h	0.004 mg/kg per 6-8 h
Pentazocine	50 mg/3-4 h	Not recommended	Not recommended

Conventional intramuscular delivery of opioids is a familiar practice and is inexpensive, and the gradual onset of pain relief permits easy assessment of possible overdose. A disadvantage of the method may be that the dose is too large (side effects) or too small (no pain relief). In addition, the injections are painful and the onset of pain relief is delayed while the drug is absorbed. Intravenous administration produces immediate analgesia after surgery. This has the disadvantages of producing fluctuations in plasma concentrations and requiring careful and continuous supervision by dedicated people.

Regional analgesia

In regional analgesia, only a specific area of the body is targeted for pain relief. It involves placing a needle near nerves supplying the area of the body to be operated on and injecting a pain reliever directly into this area (e.g., reconstruction on the hand, bunionectomy, total knee replacement, rotator cuff repair, exploratory laparotomy, thoracotomy). Several different types of regional analgesia are available such as spinal, epidural, and regional block analgesia.

Continuous spinal analgesia

Continuous spinal anesthesia (CSA) has numerous advantages over epidural anesthesia and single-shot spinal anesthesia (SSA), such as the more-obvious end point for catheter placement (cerebrospinal fluid), careful titration of drugs minimizing cardiovascular instability, low doses of local anesthetic with minimal risk of toxicity, prolonging of anesthesia and potential use for postoperative pain relief. On the other hand, it is a time-consuming technique. It is associated with a risk of postspinal headache (PDPH), potential for catheter breakage, and potential serious neurological complications, such as persistent cauda equina syndrome [68,69].

CSA is indicated for lower abdominal and lower surgery in elderly and high-risk patients. CSA is used also in trauma patients, where it is associated with fewer technical problems and faster onset than combined spinal-extradural anesthesia [70], and for long-term analgesia in cancer patients. There are a few published studies on the use of CSA for postoperative analgesia [69,71-74] and only one comparative study with epidural analgesia [75]. Postoperative analgesic regimens have been described for bupivacaine, morphine, and diamorphine infusions. Recently, the infusion of a combination of bupivacaine 1 mg/h and morphine 8 μg/h in patients undergoing hip and knee artroplasty provided similar postoperative pain relief as bupivacaine alone infused at rate of 2 mg/h but with less motor block [76]. Although intrathecal morphine prolongs the postoperative analgesia, it is associated with major side effects, such as delayed respiratory depression and high incidence of nausea and vomiting. There is considerable evidence that the addition of intrathecal midazolam to bupivacaine produces better postoperative analgesia without delaying recovery to ambulation and ability to void [77].

Continuous epidural analgesia

Recent years have seen a growing use of epidural anesthesia and analgesia (EAA). Epidural analgesia involves delivery of anesthetic medication on nerves within the epidural space where a small catheter is placed. Frequently the patient can be given control over this mechanism just as with the i.v. PCA. A so-called walking epidural is used for pain following surgical procedures or pain relief for very early labor. Several studies have demonstrated that epidural analgesia reduces perioperative physiological responses to surgery in addition to providing postoperative pain relief. Furthermore, epidural analgesia is associated with a lower need for prolonged mechanical ventilation and recovery in the intensive postanesthesia care unit, earlier postoperative mobilization, rehabilitation and nutrition, shorter length of total hospital stay, and reduction of costs [78]. Epidural analgesia seems to influence the early postoperative outcome, while long-term survival seems to be dependent on other factors, such as the preoperative patient status and the surgical procedures.

Regional block analgesia

There are a large variety of specific nerve blocks that can be used to ensure comfort postoperatively. Some of these are local infiltration, intercostal nerve block, paravertebral nerve block, and intrapleural analgesia. Each of these techniques has advantages and disadvantages, but all avoid secondary effects of systemic analgesics, such as respiratory depression, unnecessary sedation, and dysphoria. The postoperative pain relief can be obtained by using local anesthetics (lidocaine, bupivacaine) in association with opioid agonists (morphine, buprenorphine) and alpha-2-adrenergic agonists (xylanine, medetomidine). More recently an innovative technique of local anesthetic administration at home has been experienced by many patients who underwent the following surgeries: orthopedic (knee, shoulder, iliac bone graft, maxillofacial, halux valgus), breast augmentation, inguinal hernia, and varicose vein [79]. The technique involves the placement of a multihole, thin (22-gauge) epidural catheter subcutaneously into the surgical wound, subacromially, intraarticularly, or in the axillary brachial plexus sheath. The catheter is connected to a 50- or 100- ml elastomeric (baloon) pump filled with a volume of local anesthetic to provide ten doses for postoperative pain management. When the patients feels pain, the local anesthetic infusion is started by opening the clamp; the patient stops the infusion by closing the clamp after the prescribed time (usually 6 min) or earlier if pain relief is adequate.

Acute Pain Services

Task-force of experts from Australia, United Kingdom, and United States recommend the implementation of Acute Pain Services (APS) as a major instrument for improving the quality of postoperative pain relief. Moreover, several interdisciplinary committees of experts have published guidelines that recommend frequent bedside pain assessment, evaluation of treatment efficacy, and a collaborative interdisciplinary organization for postoperative pain relief [80-82].

The idea of a service dedicated to relieve postoperative acute pain was first introduced in Germany in 1985 [83]; nevertheless the first description of APS was published in 1988 by Ready et al. [84]. In the United States the development of APS proceeded at a remarkable rate so that, nowadays, all major institutions have APS. In Europe, the situation is quite different. In fact, in some countries as United Kingdom [85], Sweden, and Holland the concept of APS has been widely accepted, and dedicated pain services have been established in many locations. In other countries, most hospitals are inadequate in the management of postoperative pain and thus, the treatment of postoperative pain continues to be inadequate. In 1990 a report by a joint working party of the Royal College of Surgeons and College of anesthetists was published, as an attempt to establish APS in all major hospital of the United Kingdom [86]. Within 4 years the percentage of hospitals with some sort of APS increased from 2.8 to 42.7%; hospitals with at least one physician attending to acute pain management increased from 5.7 to 65.2, while hospitals with a dedicated acute pain nurse increased from 2.3 to 39.3%. There was also a significant increase in educational programs for medical and nursing staff about pain relief, and of protocols and guidelines [87].

The main targets of these APS are the frequent pain evaluation by VAS, checking the analgesic treatment, and recording pain at the patient's bedside.

There is still a strong debate about which APS organization is the best in particular to restrict costs. In the literature, several models of APSs are described. At present, the main models are the anesthesiologist-based APS proposed by Ready et al. [84] and used in the United States and the nurse-based anesthesiologist-supervised APS proposed in Sweden by Rawal [7]. In any case, APS are an important tool to improve postoperative pain management and consequently to reduce morbidity, to obtain early alimentation and rehabilitation. The key-points for improving acute pain management are the option for safety and simplicity of analgesic methods in order to accommodate increasing demands of quality assurance in pain and patient satisfaction, the regular measurement and recording of pain at the patient's bedside, and evidence-based decision making, the appropriate choosing of drugs and their route, mode of delivery and, the interdisciplinary approach to the postsurgical patient.

References

1. Cohen FL (1980) Postsurgical pain relief: patients' status and nurses' medication choices. Pain 9: 265-74
2. Maier C, Raetzel M, Wulf H (1994) Audit in 1989 and 1994 of the Department of anesthesiology and Intensive Care, Hospital of Christian -Albrechts-University, Schwanenweg 21, D 24105, Kiel, Germany
3. Neugebauer E, Hempel K, Sauerland S et al (1998) The status of perioperative pain therapy in Germany. Results of a representative, anonymous survey of 1000 surgical clinics. Chirurg 69: 461-466
4. Donovan M, Dillon P, McGuire L (1983) Incidence and characteristics of pain in a sample of medical-surgical inpatients. Pain 30: 69-78
5. Kuhn S, Cooke K, Collins M, et al (1990) Perceptions of pain relief after surgery. BMJ 300: 1687-1690
6. Owen H, McMillan V, Rogowski D (1990) Postoperative pain therapy: a survey of patients' expectations and their experiences. Pain 41: 303-307
7. Rawal N (1994) Organization of Acute Pain Services. Pain 57: 117-123
8. Smith G (1991) Pain after surgery (editorial). Br J Anaesth 67: 232-233
9. Rawal N (1996) Organization of postoperative pain service. In: Gullo A (ed) Anesthesia pain intensive care and emergency medicine. Springer-Verlag Italia, Milan, pp 835-840
10. Weis OF, Sriwatanakul K, Alloza JL, et al (1983) Attitutes of patients, housestaff, and nurses toward postoperative analgesic care. Anesth Analg 2: 70-4
11. Watson A, Allen PR (1994) Influence of thoracic epidural analgesia on outcome after resection for esophageal cancer. Surgery 115: 421-432
12. Yeager MP, Glass DD, Neff RK, et al (1987) Epidural anesthesia and analgesia in high-risk surgical patients. Anesthesiology 66: 729-736
13. Rawal N (1999) Organization of acute pain services. In: Gullo A (ed) Regional anesthesia, analgesia and pain management. Springer-Verlag Italia, Milan, pp 227-234
14. Liu S, Carpenter RL, Neal JM (1995) Epidural anesthesia and analgesia. Their role in postoperative outcome. Anesthesiology 82: 1474-1506
15. Kehlet H (1995) Synergism between analgesic. Ann Med 27: 259
16. Shulman MS, Brebner J, Sandler A (1983) The effect of epidural morphine on postoperative pain relief and pulmonary function on thoracotomy patients. Anesthesiology 59: A192
17. Carli F (1999) Fast-track program for abdominal surgery. In: Gullo A (ed) Anesthesia pain intensive care and emergency. Springer, Milan, pp 211-218
18. Sharrock NE (1999) Fast-track anesthesia and postoperative care: orthopaedic surgery In: Gullo A (ed) anesthesia pain intensive care and emergency. Springer, Milan, pp 219-223
19. Rawal N, Hylander J, Nydahl PA et al (1997) Survey of postoperative analgesia following ambulatory surgery. Acta anesthesiol Scand 41: 1017-1022
20. Kehlet H (1991) The surgical stress response: should it the prevented? Can J Surg 34: 565-567
21. Kehlet H (1989) Surgical stress: the role of pain and analgesia. Br J Anaesth 63: 189-195
22. Biebuyck J (1995) Epidural anesthesia and analgesia. Anesthesiology 82: 1474-1506
23. Coderre TJ, Katz J, Vaccarino AL et al (1993) Contribution of central neuroplasticity to pathological pain: review of clinical and experimental evidence. Pain 52: 259-285
24. Liu H, Mantyh PW, Basbaum AI (1997) NMDA-receptor regulation of substance P release from primary afferent nociceptors. Nature 386: 721-724
25. Harris JA, Corsi M, Quartaroli M et al (1996) Upregulation of spinal glutamate receptors in chronic pain. Neuroscience 74: 7-12
26. Schaible H-G, Jarrott B, Hope PJ et al (1990) Release of immunoreactive substance P in the spinal cord during development of acute arthritis in the knee joint of the cat: a study with antibody microprobes. Brain Res 529: 214-223
27. Curran T, Margan JI (1994) Fos: an immediate-early transcription factor in neurons. J Neurobiol 26: 403-412

28. Meller ST, Gebhart GF (1993) Nitric oxide (NO) and nociceptive processing in the spinal cord. Pain 52: 127-136.
29. Coderre TJ (1993) The role of excitatory amino acid receptors and intracellular messengers in persistent nociception after tissue injury in rats. Mol Neurobiol 7: 229-246
30. Wong HY, Carpenter RL, Kopacz DJ, et al (1993) A randomized, double-blind evaluation of ketorolac tromethamine for postoperative analgesia in ambulatory surgery patients. Anesthesiology 78: 6-14
31. Orser BA, Pennefather PS, MacDonald JF (1997) Multiple mechanisms of ketamine blockade of N-methyl-D-aspartate receptors. Anesthesiology 86: 903-917
32. Øye I, Paulsen O, Maurset A (1992) Effects of ketamine on sensory perception: evidence for a role of N-methyl-D-aspartate receptors. J Pharmacol Exp Ther 260: 1209-1213
33. Aida S, Yamakura T, Baba H, et al (2000) Preemptive analgesia by intravenous low-dose ketamine and epidural morphine in gastrectomy: a randomized double-blind study. Anesthesiology 92: 1624-1630
34. Suzuki M, Tuesda K, Lansing PS, et al (1999) Small-dose ketamine enhances morphine-induced analgesia after outpatient surgery. Anesth Analg 89: 98-103
35. Helmy SAK, Bali A (2001) The effect of the preemptive use of the NMDA receptor antagonist dextromethrophan on postoperative analgesic requirements. Anesth Analg 92: 739-744
36. Himmelseher S, Ziegler-Pithamitsis D, Argiriadou H, et al (2001) Small-dose S(+)-ketamine reduces postoperative pain when applied with ropivacaine in epidural anesthesia for total knee arthroplasty. Anesth Analg 92: 1290-1295
37. Gottschalk A, Schroeder F, Ufer M et al (2001) Amantadine, a N-methyl-D-aspartate receptor antagonist, does not enhance postoperative analgesia in women undergoing abdominal hysterctomy Anesth Analg 93: 192-196
38. Celerier E, Rivat C, Jun Y et al (2000) Long-lasting hyperalgesia induced by fentanyl in rats: preventive effect of ketamine. Anesthesiology 92: 465-472
39. Li X, Angst MS, Clark JD (2001) Opioid-induced hyperalgesia and incisional pain. Anesth Analg 93: 204-209
40. Hunter JC, Singh L (1994) Role of excitatory amino acid receptors in the mediation of the nociceptive response to formalin in the rats. Anesth Analg 174: 217-221
41. Coderre TJ, Melzack R (1992) The contribution of excitatory amino acids to central sensitization and persistent nociception after formalin-induced tissue injury. J Neurosci 12: 3665-3670
42. Simmons RM, Li DL, Hoo KH, et al (1998) Kainate GluR5 receptor subtype mediates the nociceptive response to formalin. Neuropharmacology 37: 25-36
43. Nishiyama T, Gyermek L, Lee C, et al (1999) The spinal and nociceptive effects of a novel competitive AMPA receptor antagonist, YM872, on thermal or formalin-induced pain in rats. Anesth Analg 89: 143-147
44. Hishiyama T, Gyermek L, Lee C et al (1999) The systemically administered competitive AMPA receptor antagonist, YM872, has analgesic effects on thermal or formalin-induced pain in rats. Anesth Analg 89: 1534-1537
45. Harrison CA, Morris S, Harvey JS (1994) Effect of ilioinguinal and iliohypogastric nerve block and wound infiltration with 0.5% bupivacaine on postoperative pain after hernia repair. Br J Anaesth 72: 691-693
46. White PF (1985) Patient-controlled analgesia: a new approach to the management of postoperative pain. Semin Anesth 4: 255-266
47. Ballantyne JC, Carr DB, Chalmers TC, et al (1993) Postoperative patient-controlled analgesia: meta-analyses of initial randomized controlled trials. J Clin Anesth 5: 182-193
48. Schug SA, Torrie JJ (1993) Safety assessment of postoperative pain management by an acute pain service. Pain 55: 387-391
49. Etches RC (1994) Respiratory depression associated with patient-controlled analgesia: a review of eight cases. Can J Anaesth 41: 125-132

50. Parker RK, Holtmann B, Smith I, et al (1988) Use of ketorolac after lower abdominal surgery. Effect on analgesic requirement and surgical outcome. Anesthesiology 80: 6-12
51. Eisenach JC, Grice SC, Dewan DM (1988) Patient-controlled analgesia following cesarean section: a comparison with epidural and intramuscolar narcotics. Anesthesiology 68:444-448
52. Yeager MP, Glass DD, Neff RK, et al (1987) Epidural anesthesia and analgesia in high-risk surgical patients. Anesthesiology 66: 729-736
53. Tuman KJ, McCarthy RJ, March RJ, et al (1991) Effects of epidural anesthesia and analgesia on coagulation and outcome after major vascular surgery. Anesth Analg 73: 696-704
54. Scott J, Huskisson EC (1976) Graphic representation of pain. Pain 2: 175-184
55. Gaston-Johansson F, Gustafsson M (1990) Rheumatoid arthritis: determination of pain chararcteristics and comparison of RAI and VAS in its measurement. Pain 41: 35-40
56. Jensen MP, McFarland CA (1993) Increasing the reliability and validity of pain intensity measurement in chronic pain patients. Pain 55: 195-203
57. Joyce CRB, Autshi DW, Mason RM (1975) Comparison of fixed interval and visual analog scales for rating chronic pain. Eur J Clin Pharmacol 8: 415-420
58. Ohnhaus EE, Adler R (1975) Methodological problems in the measurement of pain: a comparison between the verbal rating scale and the visual analog scale. Pain 1: 379-384
59. Carlsson AM (1983) Assessment of chronic pain. Aspects of the reliability and validity of the visual analog scale. Pain 16: 87-101
60. DeLoach LJ, Higgins MS, Caplan AB, et al (1998) The visual analog scale in the immedaite postoperative period: intrasubject variability and correlation with a numeric scale. Anesth Analg 86: 102-106
61. Armand S, Langlade A, Boutros A, et al (1998) Meta-analysis of the efficacy of extradural clonidine to relive postoperative pain: an impossibile task. Br J Anaesth 81: 126-134
62. Kirno K, Landin S, Elam M (1993) Epidural clonidine depresses sympathetic nerve activity in humans by a supraspinal mechanism. Anesthesiology 78: 1021-1027
63. Dyck JB, Maze M, Haack C, et al (1993) The pharmacokinetics and hemodynamic effects of intravenous and intramuscolar dexmedetomidine hydrochloride in adult human volunteers. Anesthesiology 78: 813-820
64. Ready LB (1990) Acute postoperative pain. In: Miller RD (ed) Anesthesia, 3rd ed Churchill Livingstone, New York, pp 2135-2146
65. Dierking GW, Ostergaard E, Ostergard HT et al (1994) The effects of wound infiltration with bupivacaine versus saline on postoperative pain and opioid requirements after herniorrhaphy. Acta anesthesiol Scand 38: 289-292
66. Erichsen CJ, Vibits H, Dahl JB (1995) Wound infiltration with ropivacaine and bupivacaine for pain after inguinal herniotomy. Acta anesthesiol Scand 39: 67-70
67. Tverskoj M, Cozacov C, Ayache M, et al (1990) Postoperative pain after inguinal herniorrhaphy with different types of anesthesia. Anesth Analg 70: 29-35
68. Horlocker TT, McGregor DG, Matsushige DK, et al (1997) A retrospective review of 4767 consecutive spinal anesthetics: central nervous system complications. Anesth Analg 84: 578-584
69. Denny NM, Selander DE (1998) Continuous spinal anesthesia. Br J Anaesth 81: 590-597
70. Wilhelm S, Standl T, Burmeister M et al (1997) Comparison of continuous spinal with combined spinal-extradural anesthesia using plain 0.5% bupivacaine in trauma patients. Anesth Analg 85: 69-71
71. Bachman M, Laasko E, Niemi L, et al (1997) Intrathecal infusion of bupivacaine with or without morphine for postoperative analgesia after hip and knee arthroplasty. Br J Anaesth 78: 666-670
72. Burckett KR, Denny NM (1991) Initial experience of continuous subarachnoid diamorphine infusion for postoperative pain relief. Reg Anaesth 16: 253-256
73. Niemi L, Pitkamen M, Dunkel P, et al (1996) Evaluation of the usefulness of intrathecal bupivcaine infusion for analgesia after hip and knee arthroplasty. J Anaesth 77: 544-545
74. Niemi L, Pitaken MT, Tuominen MK, et al (1993) Comparison of intrathecal fentanyl infusion with intrathecal morphine infusion or bolus for postoperative pain relief after hip arthroplasty. Anesth Analg 77: 126-130

75. Standl T, Eckert S, Schulte am Esch J (1995) Microcatheter continuous spinal anesthesia in the post-operative period: a prospective study of its effectiveness and complications. Eur J Anaesthesiol 12: 273-279
76. Niemi L, Pitkanen M, Tuominem M (1994) Technical problems and side effects associated with continuous intrathecal or extradural post-operative analgesia in patients undergoing hip artroplasty. Eur J Anesthesiol 11: 469-474
77. Batra YK, Chari P, Dhillon MS, et al (1999) Addition of intrathecal midazolam to bupivacaine produces better post-operative analgesia without prolonging receovery. Int J Clin Pharmacol Ther 10: 519-523
78. Liu S, Carpenter RL, Neal JM (1995) Epidural anesthesia and analgesia. Anesthesiology 82: 1474-1506
79. Rawal N, Axelsson K, Hylander J, et al (1998) Postoperative patient-controlled local anesthetic administration at home. Anesth Analg 86: 86-89
80. American Society of Anesthesiologists Task Force on Pain Management, Acute Pain Section (1995) A practical guidelines for acute pain managements in the peri-operative setting. Anesthesiology 82: 1071-1081
81. Max MB, Donovan M, Portenoy RK (1991) American Pain Society Quality Assurance Standards for Relief of Acute Pain and Cancer Pain, Committee on Quality Assurance Standanrds, American Pain Society, In: Bond MR, Charlton JE, Woolf GJ (eds) Proceedings of the VIth World Congress on Pain. Elsevier, New York, pp 185-189
82. Ready LB, Edwards WT (1992) Management of acute pain. A practical guide. Task Force on Acute Pain, International Associate for the Study of Pain. Seattle
83. Maier C, Kibbel K, Mercker S, et al (1994) Postoperative pain therapy at general nursing stations. An analysis of eight years of experience at an anesthesiological acute pain service. anesthesist 43: 385-397
84. Ready BL, Oden R, Chadwick HS, et al (1988) Development of an anesthesiology-based postoperative pain management service. Anesthesiology 68: 100-106
85. Burstal R, Wegener F, Hayes C (1988) Epidural analgesia: prospective audit of 1062 patients. Anaesth Intensive Care 26: 165-172
86. The Royal College of Surgeons of England and The College of anesthesists (1990) Commission on the Provision of Surgical Services. Report of the Working Party on Pain after Surgery. London: HMSO, London
87. Windsor AM, Glynn CJ, Mason DG (1996) National provision of acute pain services. anesthesia 51:228-231

Postoperative Analgesia in Ambulatory Surgery

N. RAWAL

Recent advances in anaesthetic and surgical techniques along with escalating health costs have resulted in an ever increasing number of surgical procedures being performed on a day-case basis word-wide. The cost-effectiveness of day-case surgery is well recognized. Day-case surgery constitutes 60-70% of all surgery performed in North America in the 1990' s [1], in other parts of the world the numbers are lower. However, as outcome data become available confirming the safety of day-case surgery, it is anticipated that even more procedures will be performed on a day-case basis.

The major advances in anaesthetic techniques include the use of rapidly dissipated anaesthetic agents and increasing use of regional anaesthetic techniques. It is also expected that the diversity and complexity of operations performed in the outpatient setting will continue to increase.

The majority of day-case surgery procedures are associated with a relatively minor surgical trauma so the discharge of these patients is frequently dependent on recovery from anaesthesia. The top priorities of successful outpatient surgery are the four A's of alertness, ambulation, analgesia and alimentation. Excessive fatigue, nausea, vomiting or unrelieved pain will delay discharge; these symptoms are the most common reasons for unanticipated hospital admission. Since the proportion of surgery is changing from inpatient to outpatient, and early discharge and patient satisfaction are important goals, pain management is receiving greater attention.

Severity of pain after day-case surgery

The problem of postoperative pain after the patient is discharged has generally been poorly studied [1]. Postoperative pain is one of the most common complaints after surgery and continues to be a challenge for anaesthesiologists. Contrary to a common belief that day surgery is followed by mild pain, recent studies have shown that undertreatment of pain is common. About 30-40% of discharged outpatients may suffer from moderate to severe pain during the first 24-48 hours [2, 3]. This pain decreases with time but it may be severe enough to interfere with sleep and daily functioning. Lengthy surgical procedures and certain types of operations (orthopaedic, urological, anorectal, hernia repair, breast augmentation, laparoscopic cholecystectomy, ENT, dental) are predictors of severe pain and can be expected to have greater analgesic requirements [2-4].

As in adults most studies of analgesia in paediatric day-case surgery have focused on the immediate postoperative course and largely ignored the risk of post-discharge severe pain at home, when it becomes the responsibility of the parent [5]. Studies have shown that more than 50% of children experience clinically significant pain after discharge.

Impact of pain after day-case surgery

Severe postoperative pain causes extreme discomfort, sleep deprivation and suffering. Along with postoperative nausea and vomiting (PONV) it is the main cause of delayed discharge, contact with the hospital after discharge, unanticipated hospital admission and increased costs. Postoperative pain following day surgery may last several days, this can have implications for return to work and for community health services. Currently a majority of patients undergoing day-case surgery are healthy; however, increasingly elderly patients and those with concurrent disease are being included. The physiological effects of pain may be particularly harmful in patients with ischaemic heart disease or chronic respiratory problems.

The intensity of acute postoperative pain may be important for predicting the development of chronic pain after leg amputation, breast surgery and thoracotomy. In day-case surgery chronic pain is a significant problem after open groin hernia repair, the reported incidence varies from 0-12%. The intensity of early postoperative pain may be an important predictor for development of chronic pain [6].

Changes in children's behaviour have been seen following both day-case and inpatient surgery. The changes are mostly transient but in some children they persist for several weeks, months or even years. A recent multicenter survey showed a 47% incidence of problematical behavioural changes and the main predictors were: age of the child (highest incidence below 3 years of age), pain at home and a previous difficult experience of health care. The authors emphasized the importance of effective prevention and treatment of pain [7]. Postoperative pain also seems to be a clear predictor of PONV in children.

Choice of anaesthetic technique and perioperative analgesia

Safety, fast recovery and minimal postoperative problems are essential in selecting surgical procedures and anaesthesia techniques for day-case surgery. The choice of anaesthetic technique can influence postoperative morbidity at home.

With modern general anaesthesia techniques, recovery after surgery can be both rapid and complete. However, in many day-care patients regional anaesthetic techniques might be preferable. Regional anaesthesia can reduce or avoid the hazards and discomforts of general anaesthesia, including sore throat, airway trauma and muscle pain. Regional anaesthesia, whether by epidural, spinal, peripheral nerve block or field block techniques, offers a number of advantages to outpatients undergoing surgery. These techniques provide analgesia without sedation, earlier discharge and prolonged postoperative analgesia. Local or regional anaesthesia can be used alone, in combination with sedation techniques or as part of a balanced analgesia with general anaesthesia. Decreased requirements of opioids reduce the incidence of postoperative nausea.

A controversial issue in day surgery is whether regional anaesthesia offers significant benefits over general anaesthesia for ambulatory surgery. Literature presents conflicting reports; however, its real place will vary from one institution to another. All general and regional anaesthesia techniques have their own advantages and disadvantages. Surgeon and patient acceptance of the technique, and the expertise of the anaesthesiologist are crucial. It is essential that each facility audit its own complication rates, recovery room times and patient opinions to determine the relevance of regional or general anaesthesia. Day surgery performed under local anaesthesia is often the simplest, safest and cheapest. It is surprising how little sedation patients require if the atmosphere is conducive and the surgeon handles the tissues gently.

Strategies for postoperative pain management

Optimal postoperative pain control for day-case surgery should be effective and safe, produce minimal side effects, facilitate recovery, and be easily managed by patients at home. Analgesia techniques should permit "normal" activities, additional analgesic supplements should be provided to cover any painful activity. Rescue analgesia medication should be provided if the prescribed analgesic is ineffective. It has been shown that the use of pre-packaged take-home analgesics specific to the type of surgery and breakthrough medication can lead to improved pain control, morbidity and sleep [8].

Pain assessment and documentation

Pain intensity must be assessed and reassessed frequently and documented on the bedside chart ("make pain visible"). The day care facility should define a maximum acceptable pain score and train the personnel to promptly treat pain if it is above the defined level. At our institution a hospital-wide policy of keeping pain levels at ≤ 3 on the 10-grade visual analogic score (VAS) has been functioning satisfactorily since 1991 for surgical day-case and in-patients. Pain intensity is assessed and documented every 3 hours for in-patients and at least every hour for day-case surgery patients [9]. It is important to assess pain and efficacy of analgesia at rest and during activity. A practical scheme is to assess pain at rest in early recovery and at rest **and** during activity at and after discharge. In situations where communication is difficult a verbal or observer (nurse) scoring system can be used [10]. After paediatric surgery in small children it may be difficult to determine whether the child is in pain because small children are unable to verbalize their feelings. If a child's pain is treated at home, parents have to estimate the level of pain and therefore need to be informed appropriately. Pain assessment tools have been formulated and validated for parents to use at home [11]. Documentation of pain scores also allows the DSU to perform regular audits to confirm that pain management techniques are not causing problems at home after discharge.

Choice of analgesic drugs after discharge

Oral analgesics are the mainstay of continuing pain control at home and it is important to encourage patients to take analgesics pre-emptively and regularly, starting before the local anaesthetic effect has worn off. For mild pain, simple analgesics such as paracetamol may be sufficient. Patients with mild to moderate pain in day surgery benefit from combinations of NSAID's and weak opioids (most commonly codeine and dextropropoxyphene) in addition to regional or local anaesthesia. The patient response to drugs varies, so rescue analgesia for postoperative pain beyond acceptable levels may be needed. Strong opioids are generally avoided because of their well-known side effects including the risk of respiratory depression.

In general there is a great need for powerful non-opioid analgesics in future day surgery and they may either be prescribed alone or used to reduce the opioid requirements. These drugs intravenously may prove more convenient and less unpleasant than either intramuscular or rectal administration.

Regional techniques at home

Administration of local anaesthetic in the surgical wound is effective and safe but the analgesia lasts only a few hours. We have described a technique using an elastometric balloon pump, which allows the patient to self-administer local anaesthetic analgesia at home [12]. The technique involves the placement of a multihole, thin epidural or Perifix brachial plexus catheters subcutaneously into the surgical wound, subacromially, intraarticularly or in the axillary brachial plexus sheath (depending on surgical site). The catheter is tunnelled 4-5 cm subcutaneously by the surgeon and firmly secured on the skin by sterile tape. Axillary brachial plexus catheters are placed and secured in position by anaesthesiologists. The catheters are introduced 3-5 cm within the sheath and secured to the skin by transparent dressing and tape.

Using an aseptic technique the catheters are connected to a 50 mL or 100 mL elastomeric (balloon) pump with the appropriate concentration and volume of a local anaesthetic drug. The balloon pump is filled with a volume of local anaesthetic to provide 10 doses for postoperative pain management. Postoperatively, when the patient feels pain he starts the local anaesthetic infusion by opening the clamp. The patient stops the infusion by closing the clamp after the prescribed time (usually 6 minutes) or earlier if he is satisfied with the pain relief. When the patient does not need analgesia any further, he removes the tape, pulls out the catheter and discards the pump. In most cases the patient self-administers the first dose in the post anaesthesia care unit (PACU).

Bupivacaine or ropivacaine 0.125 % was used in brachial plexus catheters, in all other catheters a 0.25 % concentration was used. The 0.125 % solution was used to reduce or avoid the risk of possible injury due to excessive motor block. The maximum volume of local anaesthetic allowed for each administration was 2.5 ml for maxillofacial surgery, 5-10 ml for surgical wounds, 10 ml for the remaining procedures. An appropriate pump (50 ml or 100 ml) filled with local anaesthetic to provide 10 doses at home was given to the patient before discharge. The patient was instructed to avoid using the pump more than once every hour. Follow-up consisted of evaluation of pain relief at home, pump function, use of rescue medication and overall satisfaction/dissatisfaction with the technique.

Pain relief was graded good to excellent by 90% of the patients. Onset of analgesia was experienced within 5 minutes, the duration of analgesia after each administration of local anaesthetic varied from 2-8 hours. Patient follow-up did not reveal any infection or any other major problem with the technique, patient satisfaction was very high. To date over 700 patients undergoing a variety of surgical procedures have been treated with PCRA at our hospital without any major complications.

Recent controlled trials have demonstrated the efficacy and safety of an incisional catheter PCRA in patients undergoing Caesarean section, abdominal hysterectomy and inguinal hernia repair. Our controlled comparison between ropivacaine (0.125%) and bupivacaine (0.125%) for axillary brachial plexus PCRA at home demonstrated the feasibility, efficacy and safety of this technique to treat pain outside the hospital. Both drugs provided effective analgesia; however, patient satisfaction was better with ropivacaine PCRA [13]. White cell counts, bacterial culture of the catheter tips or wound inspection has not shown any evidence of infection.

Further studies are necessary to establish the efficacy and safety of this promising new technique of PCRA at home after ambulatory surgery. Studies are also necessary to evaluate the optimal concentration and volume of local anaesthetic and also the possible role of adjuvant drugs. The importance of adequate patient information is emphasized.

References

1. Chung F, Ritchie E, Su J (1997) Postoperative pain in ambulatory surgery. Anesth Analg;85:808-816
2. Beauregaard L, Pomp A, Choinière M (1998) Severity and impact of pain after day-surgery. Can J Anaesth;45:304-311
3. Rawal N, Hylander J, Nydahl P-A et al (1997) Survey of postoperative analgesia following ambulatory surgery. Acta Anaesthesiol Scand;41:1017-1022
4. Jin FL, Chung F (1998) Postoperative pain – a challenge for anaesthetists in ambulatory surgery (Editorial). Can J Anaesth;45:293-296
5. Wolf AR (Editorial) (1999) Tears at bedtime: a pitfall of extending paediatric day-case surgery without extending analgesia. Br J Anaesth;82:319-320
6. Callesen T, Bech K, Kehlet H (1999) Prospective study of chronic pain after groin hernia repair. Br J Surg;86:1528-1531
7. Kotiniemi LH, Ryhänen PT, Moilanen IK (1997) Behavioral changes in children following day-case surgery: a 4-week follow-up of 551 children. Anaesthesia:52:970-976
8. Marquardt HM, Razis PA (1996) Prepacked take-home analgesia for day case surgery. Br J Nurs;5:1114-1118
9. Rawal N (1999) 10 years of acute pain services - achievements and challenges. Reg Anesth Pain Med;24:68-73
10. Rudkin GE (1997) Pain management in the adult day surgery patient. In: Practical anaesthesia and analgesia for day surgery. Bios Scientific Publishers Oxford, UK;Pp 207-210
11. Chambers CT, Reid GJ, McGrath PJ et al (1996) Development and preliminary validation of a postoperative pain measure for parents. Pain;68:307-313
12. Rawal N, Axelsson K, Hylander J et al (1998) Postoperative patient-controlled local anesthetic administration at home. Anest Analg;86:86-89
13. Rawal N, Allvin R, Hallén J et al (2000) Ropivacaine versus bupivacaine for axillary plexus analgesia at home – a controlled trial of PCRA. Int Monitor Reg Anaesth;12:199 (Abs).

Cost-Effectiveness of Postoperative Pain Management

N. RAWAL

It is clear that if postoperative analgesia is improved with surgical wards techniques such as patient-controlled analgesia (PCA), epidural analgesia and peripheral nerve blocks have to be introduced on a routine basis. These techniques provide superior analgesia as compared to i.m. opioids but have their own risks and therefore require special monitoring. Traditional methods of analgesia are not risk-free and the risks have rarely been quantified. While better postoperative pain is relatively easily achievable, there has to be a balance between acceptable risk, perceived benefit and cost-effectiveness.

In general cost issues in pain management have been poorly studied. The main reason seems to be that traditional analgesic techniques, such as oral medications or intramuscular injections, were relatively inexpensive. The introduction of newer (usually expensive) drugs and techniques, such as PCA and the epidural analgesia, has resulted in far greater direct and indirect costs. A thirty-fold range of costs has been shown for different opioids [1]. The diminishing health care budgets have also forced us to evaluate cost-effectiveness of various treatments. In addition to drug costs, the costs associated with route of administration and personnel costs should also be considered. Thus, drugs like morphine and fentanyl are relatively inexpensive but if they are administered epidurally the monitoring costs increase considerably.

Cost-effectiveness of analgesic techniques

Continuous epidural block offers the most effective form of postoperative analgesia. However, due to autonomic block, there may be a profound physiological effect on the patient. Thus a balance must be found between effective analgesia and possible danger. Autonomic dysfunction affects cardiovascular, gastrointestinal and urinary bladder function. Similarly, the advantages of superior epidural opioid analgesia have to be justified in individual cases against the "cost" of greater invasiveness and extended monitoring due to the risk of late-onset respiratory depression. Epidural and intrathecal injections require skill to perform the procedure, have a documented failure rate (especially thoracic epidural) and occasionally may be associated with serious complications. The potential morbidity associated with the epidural technique, epidural catheters and continuous intravenous epidural infusions should also be considered. For patients receiving epidural or intrathecal opioids, there are additional costs of observing these patients in high-dependency units. The use of opioids either i.m. at regular intervals, as continuous intravenous (i.v.) infusions or PCA and the use of potent parenteral non-steroidal anti-inflammatory drugs (NSAID) can provide analgesia less invasively and with a lower rate of complications than spinal opioids. The choice of opioid and technique of its administration will also have cost implications. In a patient-controlled study epidural PCA (PCEA) fentanyl was compared with a single dose epidural morphine for post-caesarean section analgesia. Analgesia was similar but the costs for PCEA fentanyl ($57) were seven times higher than epidural morphine ($7.50) [2]. Similarly, in another controlled trial the average hospital drug cost for PCEA sufentanil ($120) was about 26 times higher than PCEA fentanyl ($4.50), analgesia was similar but dizziness and vomiting were more frequent after sufentanil.

Analgesia techniques and postoperative outcome

Numerous studies have shown that techniques such as i.v. opioid PCA, peripheral nerve blocks and epidural analgesia are superior to conventional i.m. injections of opioids. Patient satisfaction with these techniques is high; however, reduced pain and suffering or good patient satisfaction is not considered sufficient in this age of diminished health care budgets. Therefore, the increased costs of newer analgesic techniques have to be justified in terms of better outcomes such as reduced morbidity and shorter hospitalization. There is no overwhelming evidence that effective postoperative pain relief assures good postoperative outcome. Many studies have demonstrated that epidural local anaesthetic-containing epidural techniques reduce adverse physiologic responses to surgery; however, the true impact of this technique remains controversial. Most studies lack sufficient statistical power to detect clinically significant differences; many studies do not meet the necessary criteria for a randomized, controlled trial [3].

I.V. PCA and outcome

A meta-analysis of 15 randomized, controlled trials involving 800 patients undergoing a variety of surgical procedures showed greater patient satisfaction with I.V. PCA as compared with i.m. opioid injection. This was the only unsurprising advantage of the I.V. PCA: the meta-analysis did not demonstrate any difference in analgesic use, incidence of side effects or hospitalization time [4]. Indeed, even patient satisfaction may not be different if i.m. opioids are administered appropriately. In a recent study, post-hysterectomy analgesia was equally effective with I.V. PCA and i.m. morphine, no significant differences were observed in the incidence of side effects or patient satisfaction. PCA was considerably more costly [5]. Although PCA continues to be the standard of care there is little rationale or scientific evidence that I.V. PCA improves the outcome. The clinical benefits of PCA remain undefined; further studies are necessary to address the issue of cost-effectiveness.

Epidural techniques and outcome

In high-risk patients with poor preoperative pulmonary function, epidural analgesia can be expected to significantly reduce the risk of postoperative pulmonary complications and indeed may be the analgesic technique of choice. In patients with chronic lung disease with copious secretions the epidural block is more effective in increasing VC than it is in normal patients. In these patients, the epidural block may be lifesaving. The only alternative in many patients lies in prolonged postoperative ventilator treatment. However, in many patients the effects of epidural analgesia are not as dramatic as expected. Some improvement in functional residual capacity and vital capacity may be seen; but the results are not consistent, and improvement is limited to the reduction of deterioration rather than restoration of the preoperative values.

A controlled trial comparing i.m. and epidural morphine in grossly obese patients undergoing upper abdominal surgery showed that epidural technique improved postoperative mobilization and pulmonary function and also reduced the incidence of pulmonary complications such as atelectasis and parenchymal infiltrations. Furthermore, the length of hospital stay could be reduced by 2 days [6]. The effects of epidural anaesthesia and postoperative analgesia on postoperative morbidity have been evaluated in a group of high-risk patients undergoing major abdominal, thoracic, or vascular surgery. Patients receiving intraoperative epidural block and postoperative epidural local anaesthetics and/or opioid had decreased postoperative morbidity and improved operative outcome as compared to their counterparts receiving intraoperative general anaesthesia and postoperative parenteral opioid analgesia. This resulted in shorter hospitalization, reduced costs, and lower mortality. Although the study protocol has been criticized, one important conclusion was that the total hospitalization costs were lower in the epidural group ($15,019 versus $ 25,514) [7]. In a study of patients with arteriosclerotic vascular disease undergoing aortic bypass surgery postoperative analgesia was provided either with epidural analgesia or on-demand opioids. In patients receiving epidural analgesia the incidence of thromboembolic, infectious and cardiovascular complications as well as duration of intensive care unit (ICU) stay were significantly reduced [8]. These studies have demonstrated that in high-risk patients undergoing major surgery epidural analgesia using local anaesthetics and/or opioids is the method of choice and is cost-effective. A meta-analysis of randomized, controlled trials to assess the effects of seven analgesic therapies (epidural opioid, epidural local anaesthetic, epidural opioid with local anaesthetic, thoracic versus lumbar epidural opioid, intercostal nerve block, wound infiltration with local anaesthetic, and intrapleural local anaesthetic) on postoperative pulmonary function after a variety of procedures has shown that postoperative epidural pain control can significantly decrease the incidence of pulmonary morbidity. None of the other analgesic techniques had a significant impact on pulmonary outcome [9]. Thus, thoracic epidural with local anaesthetics maintained into the postoperative period can improve pulmonary outcome in high-risk patients. In contrast, the use of this technique in low-risk patients appears to offer minimal pulmonary outcome advantages over I.V. PCA [3].

A crucial aspect of cost-effectiveness of pain management is its potential to prevent chronic pain. A recent survey showed that chronic pain is common after surgical procedures such as amputation, inguinal hernia, breast, lung and gall bladder surgery. One of the most important predictive factors is the intensity of acute postoperative pain. Chronic pain is costly to society in terms of suffering and disability [10]. There is increasing evidence that the epidural technique can prevent or reduce the incidence of post-limb amputation phantom pain and post-thoracotomy chronic pain. Although cost-effectiveness of this treatment has not been studied, the benefits in terms of improved functionality, quality of life, demands on the healthcare systems and costs are obvious.

An important advantage of the thoracic epidural technique in combination with general anaesthesia in major thoracic or abdominal surgery is the significant reduction in postoperative intubation time and requirement of mechanical ventilation. In an uncontrolled study evaluating over 450 surgical cancer patients it has been demonstrated that cost savings of $4,675 could be achieved for each patient managed by the epidural technique, primarily due to decreased ICU time and hospitalization [11]. It is emphasized that the benefits of the epidural technique in the combination approach are lost if the catheter is not sited appropriately, if doses of local anaesthetic are inadequate or if inhalation or opioid anaesthetic doses are not reduced [12].

One reason why improved outcome is difficult to demonstrate is that pain management strategies are not integrated with overall perioperative care and postoperative rehabilitation of the patient. The importance of co-operation and "team approach" between surgeons, anaesthesiologists, APN, ward nurses and physiotherapists is becoming increasingly clear. The role of a good acute pain service (APS) in developing the cost-effective, evidence-based pain treatment strategies for different surgical procedures is crucial.

Peripheral nerve blocks and outcome

Nearly all of the studies evaluating the role of regional anaesthesia and analgesia in perioperative outcomes involve the epidural or spinal techniques. There are few studies on the peripheral nerve block outcome. However, it has been suggested that in this era of cost containment the demonstrated advantages of techniques such as the epidural need to go beyond improved pain scores and opioid sparing. In the absence of concrete information on the benefits it is difficult to introduce such analgesia methods due to concerns about rare but disastrous complications such as neuraxial haematoma which is associated with low molecular weight heparin [13].

Peripheral nerve blocks provide excellent analgesia over a limited field and with minimal systemic effects. The blocks are generally easy to perform, inexpensive and very safe. Peripheral blocks are possible for nearly all kinds of surgery. Even in situations where the block is ineffective for surgery the catheter can often be used for postoperative pain management. The technique is underused both for surgery and postoperative pain treatment. Peripheral nerve blocks have extended the indications for day-case surgical procedures such as major shoulder surgery and knee reconstruction. Comparative studies of interscalene block versus general anaesthesia for day-case shoulder arthroscopic surgery showed that 8 % of the patients receiving general anaesthesia required unanticipated admission versus none in the patients receiving interscalene block [14, 15].

There is increasing evidence from prospective randomized studies that peripheral nerve blocks are better than PCA and safer than the epidural. The influence of 3 different analgesic methods on postoperative pain and rehabilitation was evaluated in patients undergoing total knee arthroplasty. Regional techniques (epidural and 3-in-1 block) provided better pain relief and faster postoperative rehabilitation than I.V. PCA. eripheral nerve block was as efficient as epidural analgesia and was associated with less side effects. The authors concluded that continuous 3-in-1 block should be the analgesic technique of choice [16].

In another comparative study of the effects of 3 analgesic techniques on the surgical outcome and duration of rehabilitation after major knee surgery regional techniques (continuous epidural and continuous femoral) showed significantly better pain scores at rest and during continuous passive motion compared with I.V. PCA morphine analgesia. Long-term follow up showed that the duration of stay in the rehabilitation centre was significantly shorter (10-13 days) in patients who received regional analgesia. Since there were no major differences in analgesia and rehabilitation the authors concluded that the routine use of the continuous epidural technique should be restricted because shortening the hospital stay justifies neither the discomfort of side effects nor the danger of potentially serious complications. In contrast continuous femoral block appears to have all the requirements to become the main choice of regional analgesia following major knee surgery [17].

Two techniques of patient-controlled analgesia, (i.e., patient-controlled interscalene analgesia and I.V. opioid analgesia) were compared to evaluate postoperative pain after major shoulder surgery. The use of patient-controlled interscalene analgesia provided better pain relief than I.V. opioid PCA, as can be expected the technique was also associated with a significantly reduced incidence of side effects such as vomiting and pruritus [18].

Peripheral nerve blocks may be used when the epidural and spinal techniques are avoided for example in anticoagulated and febrile patients because of the serious consequences of neuraxial bleeding or infection. For many surgical procedures these techniques may replace the more invasive and risky techniques such as the epidural and I.V. opioid PCA. Further outcome studies, including those in the ambulatory setting, are necessary to define the role of peripheral nerve blocks and incisional local anaesthetic techniques in influencing postoperative outcome.

Role of simple, inexpensive techniques

Although the traditional method of injecting i.m. opioids on an as-needed basis has been universally condemned as the major cause of inadequate postoperative analgesia, the role of simple analgesic techniques should not be overlooked or underestimated. It should be recognized that with attentive nursing, greater flexibility of administration, better understanding of pharmacokinetics of prescribed analgesics and regular pain scoring i.m. or i.v. opioids and/or non-opioids can provide excellent analgesia. Treatment of pain by opioids remains the most versatile and widely used technique. Injecting of i.m. opioids on-demand represents familiar practice; generations of nurses have used the technique, which may, therefore, be safe because of accumulated experience. Since no special equipment is required, the technique is simple and inexpensive. Gradual onset of analgesia allows observation of gradual onset of possible overdose. The challenge is to organize proper administration of systemic opioids alone (preferably i.v. or through an indwelling subcutaneous butterfly needle) or in combination with non-opioid analgesics.

Organization of acute pain services

It is becoming increasingly clear that cost-effective APS models have to be developed if the aim is to improve the quality of postoperative analgesia for every patient who undergoes surgery. The organization should also include patients who undergo day-care surgery. In countries with state-financed health services and current budgetary restraints the USA-style anaesthesiology-based comprehensive, multidisciplinary postoperative pain control teams are too expensive ($200-300 per patient) and appear unrealistic for most institutions.

The role of a good APS in developing cost-effective treatment strategies for pain management following different types of surgery cannot be over-emphasized. A low-cost model has been described in which every patient's pain is assessed and documented frequently and in which ward nurses, surgeons, physiotherapists and anaesthesiologists work as a team to exploit the potential of analgesic techniques for aggressive mobilization routines to improve outcome [19].

Audit should be carried out regularly on the process of pain management, patient experience and cost, the service should be modified according to the outcome. It is essential that pain is regularly evaluated to ensure that it is effectively managed. The minimum standard should be at least an annual determination of the number of patients in whom pain score is above the predetermined threshold and identification of reasons for this. The audit method should be developed to meet local conditions.

Conclusion

Apart from humanitarian considerations, adequate pain relief can be expected to modulate nociception-induced responses such as metabolic response to surgery, or autonomic and cardiovascular responses which have adverse effects on organ function and muscle spasm. Obvious economic gains can be expected from early ambulation, reduced morbidity and shorter hospitalization in the postoperative period. Early alimentation and the return to a normal living pattern will facilitate patient rehabilitation. Analysis of cost-effectiveness of postoperative pain management has to consider several issues; costs of analgesics, equipment and nursing time; duration of stay in the postoperative care unit, intensive care unit and in the hospital; postoperative morbidity and mortality. The goal of pain relief is to identify for each surgical patient the most cost-effective analgesic method that provides functional pain relief with minimal side effects.

References

1. Zenz MW, Tryba M (1996) Economic aspects of pain therapy. Curr Op Anaesth 5:430-435
2. Miguel R, Timble G (1990) Patient-controlled epidural sufentanil. Reg Anesth 15:35
3. Grass JA (2000) The role of epidural anesthesia and analgesia in postoperative outcome. Anesth Clin North Am 18:407-428
4. Ballantyne JC, Carr DB, Chalmers TC et al (1993) Postoperative patient-controlled analgesia: Meta-analysis of initial randomized controlled trials. J Clin Anesth 5:182-193
5. Choinière M, Rittenhouse BE, Perrault S et al (1998) Efficacy and costs of patient controlled analgesia versus regularly administred intramuscular opioid therapy. Anesthesiology 89:1377--1388
6. Rawal N, Sjöstrand U, Christoffersson E et al (1984) Comparison of intramuscular and epidural morphine for postoperative analgesia in the grossly obese: influence on postoperative ambulation and pulmonary function. Anesth Analg 63:583-592
7. Yeager MP, Glass DD, Neff RK et al (1987) Epidural anesthesia and analgesia in high-risk surgical patients. Anesthesiology 66:729-736
8. Tuman KJ, McCarthy RJ, March RJ et al (1991) Effects of epidural anesthesia and analgesia on coagulation and outcome after major vascular surgery. Anesth Analg 73:696-704
9. Ballantyne JC, Carr DB, deFerranti S et al (1998) The comparative effects of postoperative analgesia therapies on pulmonary outcome: cumulative meta-analysis of randomized, controlled trials. Anesth Analg 86:598-612
10. Perkin FM, Kehlet H (2000) Chronic pain as an outcome of surgery – a review of predictive factors. Anesthesiology 93:1123-1133

11. deLeon-Casasola OA, Lema MJ, Karabella D et al (1994) Epidural analgesia versus intravenous patient-controlled analgesia. Reg Anesth 19:307-315
12. Stevens RA (guest editor) (2000) Combined regional and general anesthesia. Techn Regional Anesth Pain Manage 4:67-105
13. Todd MM, Brown DL (1999) Regional anesthesia and postoperative pain management. Long-term benefits from a short-term intervention. Anesthesiology 91:1-2
14. Brown AR, Weiss R, Greenberg C et al (1993) Interscalene block for shoulder arthroscopy: Comparison with general anesthesia. Arthroscopy 9:295-300
15. D'Állessio JG, Rosenblum M, Shea KP et al (1995) A retrospective comparison of interscalene block and general anesthesia for ambulatory surgery shoulder arthroscopy. Reg Anest 20:62-68
16. Singelyn FJ, Deyaert M, Joris D et al (1998) Effects of intravenous patient-controlled with morphine, continuous epidural analgesia, and continuous three-in-one block on postoperative pain and knee rehabilitation after unilateral total knee arthroplasty. Anesth Analg 87:88-92
17. Capdevila X, Barthelet Y, Biboulet P et al (1999) Effects of perioperative analgesic technique on the surgical outcome and duration of rehabilitation after major knee surgery. Anesthesiology 91:8-15
18. Borgeat A, Schäppi B, Biasca N, Gerber C (1997) Patient-controlled analgesia after major shoulder surgery. Anesthesiology 87:1343-1347
19. Rawal N, Berggren L (1994) Organization of acute pain services - low cost model. Pain 57:17-223

Neurologic Complications in Cardiac Surgery. Is it Predictable?

J.O.C. Auler Jr.

Despite all the progress observed in cardiac surgery in the last decades that have had an influence on the overall decrease of morbid-mortality, neurologic adverse effects presently represent a very important subject. After five decades since the first described reports of cardiopulmonary bypass (CPB), an enormous amount of medical information has been published about this method and the possible adverse effects or complications. As we mentioned adverse cerebral outcome is one of the principal causes of the length of stay and cost of hospitalization after cardiac surgery [1]. The question, based on the available medical information is "Would neurologic undesirable effects be minimized or even predictable during cardiac surgery?" Our aim in this lecture is to review these points and in a didactic meaning focus on cardiac surgery with CPB as an incidence of the nervous system morbidity, its classification according to morbid neurologic outcomes, the risk and mechanisms of neurological injury associated with the surgical procedure and, finally, the intraoperative management that may interfere with reducing cerebral events.

The incidence of nervous system morbidity

The reported incidence of postoperative cerebral complications after cardiac surgery varies extensively as a corollary of study design, if prospective or retrospective, methods and criteria used to assess neurologic injury, type of cardiac surgical procedures as well as the management during CPB. Most of the studies emphasize CAGB (coronary artery bypass grafting) and vary according to different centres from 0.4 to 5.4% with similar variability in the rates of encephalopathy, delirium and confusion [2]. The first question is "Does cardiac surgical population belong in the same group of age and general health status of major risk than the general population undergoing noncardiac surgery?" First of all, it is important to consider that the primary risk factors involved with the incidence of stroke and cognitive disturbances or even permanent intellectual damage in the general population, also define the persons of higher risk for neurologic morbidity in the cardiac surgery patient group. Surgical procedure by itself, including anaesthesia, post operative period either cardiac or noncardiac involves neurologic risk. The European study including 1218 elderly patients submitted to noncardiac surgery demonstrates this point. In that study, a neurocognitive exam was performed before surgery, at hospital discharge, and at 3 months postoperatively. The study showed a 26% incidence of cognitive dysfunction after surgery remained in 10% of the patients 3 months later [3]. In a prospective study 2108 patients underwent elective coronary bypass surgery from 24 US institutions, patients were evaluated for two general categories of neurologic outcome: type I, focal injury, or stupor or coma at discharge; and type II, deterioration in intellectual function, memory deficit, or seizures. The study presented the following results: Negative cerebral outcomes occurred in 129 patients (6.1 %), a total of 3.1 % of patients had type I neurologic outcomes, and 3.0% had type II outcomes. Predictors of type I were proximal aortic atherosclerosis, a history of neurologic disease, and older age, systolic hypertension on admission, pulmonary disease, and excessive consumption of alcohol [4]. Age alone represents an important comorbidity factor for neurologic complications in cardiac surgery. Patients aged over seventy have 4% to 9% incidence of stroke or coma following operation when compared to less than 1% incidence in those under sixty [4].

Based on the data of 24 U.S. medical centres, neurologic complications occur in a mean of 6% of the patients. These adverse effects represent an increase in the rates of mortality (5 to 10 times), as well as an increase in the duration of time spent in the ICU and hospital (4 times).

Classification according to morbid neurologic outcome

Neurological complications of cardiac surgery may involve diverse areas of the brain and may be manifested as a large range of clinical syndromes. A constellation of cognitive disturbances, transient ischaemic attacks, memory deficit, seizures, strokes with permanent deficits or even coma and death as a consequence have been described following cardiopulmonary bypass. In an attempt to facilitate the design and interpretation of the results of the clinical studies, researches have been proposed the following classification in patients undergoing CABG or combined CABG and open-ventricle procedures: type I, cerebral deaths due to strokes or hypoxic encephalopathy, nonfatal strokes, and new transient ischaemic attacks or type II new intellectual deterioration at discharge or new seizures, confusion, memory deficit, without evidence of focal injury [4-5]. According to this classification, Wolman et al. [5] classified 273 patients undergoing combined CAGB and open ventricle procedures with 8.4% of the adverse effects relating to type I and 7.3% of the effects relating to type II. In that report, coincident with the findings of Roach GW and colleagues [4] predictors of type I were correlated to extensive aortic atherosclerosis or thrombus, and type II outcomes were predicted by history of endocarditis, low cardiac output after surgery, presence of dysrhythmias, hypertension and history of excessive alcohol intake [5].

Risk and mechanisms of neurological injury

Although CAGB with CPB is the standard surgical coronary revascularization procedure, off pump CAGB raises a question if CPB may be considered as an independent predictor of cerebral events in coronary artery bypass grafting. The medical literature is polemic [6] whether CPB is or is not considered an isolated risk factor. Taggart et al. [6] proposed to investigate the current impact of CPB on cognitive functioning by comparing neuropsychologic performance at discharge and at 3 months in patients undergoing CAGB with and without CPB. They found similar patterns in early decline and late recovery of cognitive function in patients undergoing CAGB off pump and with pump, suggesting that CPB is not the major cause of postoperative cognitive impairment. In major surgery including cardiac operations it is reasonable to suppose that the contribution of perioperative factors of neurologic risk and outcome may be associated with increased atheroembolic risk, inadequate brain perfusion, anaemia, dysrhythmias, dehydration and disorders of coagulation [7]. Excluding frank neurologic injury due to definite brain lesions, may neuropsychologic impairment after CAGB, with or without CPB, and other types of operations may also attribute to the anaesthetic procedure. Some authors speculate that the neuropsychologic dysfunction after surgery may result in part from anaesthetic dependent cerebral ischaemia or disturbances of cerebral auto regulation [8-9]. In cardiac surgery with CPB the preoperative risk tends to coexist with embolization, hypoperfusion and inflammation, considering the principal factors relating to intraoperative adverse cerebral outcome. Embolic events associated with aortic atheromas, platelet-fibrin, fat, leukocyte aggregates and air bubbles or foreign particle generated in the CPB circuit as well as in the cardiac chambers seem to be the primary cause of cardiac surgery related to brain injury [10-11]. Gaseous microemboli originate from a number of sources during bypass; however, oxygen microbubbles generated by bubble oxygenators have traditionally been the most commonly reported cause. The production of gaseous microemboli by membrane oxygenators is significantly reduced or insignificant; nevertheless, physical damage to the membrane material or elevated transmembrane pressure may permit bubble formation on the blood side. Regarding the type of oxygenator, the warming and rewarming of blood during bypass alter the characteristic solubility of gases allowing bubbles to be released directly into patients circulation [7]. Utilizing the transcranial Doppler technique to detect cerebral air bubbles during open heart valve operations van de Linden and Casimir-Ahn [12] observed spread emboli during the insertion of the aortic cannula, at the start of CPB, and after the declamping of the aorta with the heart beating while empty. Thus, this study indicates that meticulous deairing before declamping the aorta, a short period of filling of the beating heart before final closure of aorta or vent, associated with reduction of cerebral blood flow by hyperventilation, may decrease the incidence of cerebral emboli. Macro and micro nongaseous emboli represent another important source of embolization causing brain damage, and may consist of platelet-fibrin microaggregates, atheroma or fat. The importance of aortic atheroembolism has been emphasized by Kats and colleagues [13] who found that the incidence of stroke was 25% in patients with a mobile plaque of the aortic arch when compared with 2% in those with a fixed plaque. The severity of aortic atheromatous disease increases with age, almost 80% in the eighth decade [13]. Patients with a previous cerebrovascular disease such as a stroke or TIA or even asymptomatic but with documented atheromatous disease in the extracranial cerebral arteries are more at risk of a perioperative stroke [4]. Besides age, both hypertension and diabetes are independent risk factors for neurologic complications following cardiac surgery. Even though there are no convincing data showing that the mean arterial pressure during CPB is a primary determinant of brain injury, regional hypoperfusion during CPB represents additional risks in diabetics, hypertensive or in the presence of extensive atherosclerotic disease patients. In that situation a narrowing of cerebral penetrating arteries occurs, with reduced collateral flow, and altered capacity of autoregulation. All these circumstances favour either increased risk of embolization or regional hypoperfusion [7].

The systemic inflammatory response linked with CPB have been studied and are characterized by the following: release of cytokines in response to activation of the coagulation; fibrinolytic and complement cascades; liberation of free radicals; and hydrogen peroxide and proteolytic during leukocyte degranulation. The endothelial dysfunction correlated to inflammatory response may contribute to brain injury, otherwise insignificant insults may be transformed into clinically important consequences [14].

Genetic susceptibility has recently been hypothesized in an attempt to explain the different outcomes in patients belonging to the same group of clinical risk, and investigations have been focusing on the S100 protein. The protein has been suggested as a promising marker for cerebral injury during cardiac operation [15]. The S100 protein is usually not present in plasma, but can be detected after stroke, subarachnoidal haemorrhage, head trauma, and CPB [16]. Jonsson et al. [17] aimed to characterize the S100 release pattern after CPB in 5,15 patients submitted to CABG. They measured the S100 protein at the end of CPB and after 5,15, and 48 hours and determined the mean of the cerebral outcome clinical examination. Their data showed that the early release of the S100 protein was associated with age and CPB time, but not with cerebral outcome. The late release of the S100 protein showed a correlation with cerebral complications and predictors for such outcome [17]. The S100 protein seems to be an indication for the severity of a brain injury, but does not provide precise information on the anatomical distribution of the injury and its clinical impact [18].

In conclusion, in adults post cardiac surgical neurological adverse effects occur due to a variety of concentrated and coexisting neurologic risk factors. The factors include age, gender, low cardiac output due to severity of cardiac disease, previous cerebrovascular disease, diabetes mellitus and genetic susceptibility, and education level. Other aspects such as duration of CPB, cerebral embolization, aortic atheromatous disease, temperature, characteristics of perfusion, temperature, hyperglycemia and acid base management are controversal. The reduction in neurologic morbidity depends on the application of risk stratification and technical and pharmacological interventions [18].

Intraoperative management that may interfere in reducing cerebral events

Presently, cardiac surgery requiring CPB has a significant risk of neurologic complications. As previously mentioned, stroke (1 to 9%), and neurocognitive disorders (10 to 60%) immediately after surgery are high risk indicators with 5-20% remaining at hospital discharge. Although postcardiac brain injury occurs due to the occurence of a number of neurologic risks, interventions capable of potentially reducing neurologic morbidity should be considered. Arrowsmith et al. [18] summarised neuroprotective interventions in two categories: physical and pharmacological. Physical can be defined as interventions during surgery. The most important physical interventions beside expeditious surgery and CPB, can be listed as follow: temperature, mean arterial pressure, glucose and carbon dioxide management. The role of temperature in neurologic outcome came about after several studies, all of them showing that hypothermia during CPB may confer some degree of "brain protection". Martin et al. [19] (1994) compared assigned patients undergoing CPB in two groups, 35 degrees centigrade or higher or 28 degrees centigrade or lower. The results showed a threefold greater incidence of neurologic morbidity in the warm group [19]. Another controversial point elicits controversies is related to the perfusion pressure during CPB. Although there is a general consensus that 50 mmHg (MAP) is a mean arterial pressure for cold CPB, some groups advise a mean arterial pressure higher than 70 mmHg. Gold et al. [20] compared cardiac and neurologic outcome in two groups of patient randomly assigned to a low (50-60 mmHg) or high (above 80mmHg) MAP. The follow-up (six months) showed significant low levels of neurologic and cardiac complications in the group with higher arterial pressure [20]. Nevertheless not all data are in agreement, but considering that the current surgical population is increasing in age and "neurologic risk" it maybe cautious to assume that patients will benefit from maintaining a mean arterial pressure in the autoregulatory brain perfusion range during CPB (i.e., minimal 50 mmHg or above). Although the control of glucose and acid–base based on pH strategy has been highlighted by several studies but its influence on the neurological outcome is not proven to be significant [18].

Efforts to reduce neurologic morbidity related to cardiac surgery vary in multiple directions. In an experimental study to verify the quantification and distribution of cerebral emboli during CPB in the swine, Plochl and Cook [21], demonstrated that cerebral embolization is determined by the level of $PaCO_2$ during the risks of embolization (e.g., aorta cannulation, starting of CPB, and the restarting of the heart beat after aorta declamping). In CPB practice, reductions in $PaCO_2$, by hyperventilation, causing cerebral vasoconstriction, may reduce the risk of brain injury [21]. Other practical interventions during CPB, which minimize embolic risk in the atherosclerotic aorta have led to the use of epiaortic ultrasonography to guide the aorta management, cannula insertion, clamping and declamping [22]. Transesophageal echocardiography has been largely used to monitor the deairing of cardiac chambers and the localization of the plaques of aorta atherosclerotic disease to guide aortic interventions [23].

In the CPB circuit several modifications (e.g., arterial line filters, hollow fiber oxygenators, better material biocompatibility) have been recently introduced to reduce neurologic risks due to inflammatory reactions, embolic phenomena, and others [7].

Finally, pharmacological interventions have been proposed in an attempt to reduce "cerebral risk" associated with cardiac surgery. These agents can be classified as depressors of neuronal activity, inhibitors of ischaemic pathway and anti-adhesive when considering metabolic suppression, barbiturates and recently propofol have been considered. Controversial data from different studies of cardiac surgery related to a possible neuroprotective effect promoted by the barbiturates, disregard this agent as "protective" in the routine practice of cardiac surgery. The introduction of propofol re-established as the potential neuroprotective agent in cardiac surgery. Also controversial is the burst suppression effect of propofol, perhaps having a role in reducing cerebral metabolism during CPB. Souter et al. [24] reported that propofol does not promote an improvement on cerebral oxygen venous saturation during rewarming, when a burst suppression at end of CPB is present. Calcium antagonists are the main inhibitors of the cellular ischaemic pathway. A clinical trial employing nimodipine in valvar replacement was reported by Legault and colleagues [25]. Their double-blind prospective trial was terminated because of lack of efficacy and significant adverse effects. Anti-adhesive agents represent a new strategy for leukocyte inhibition, endothelial protection, inhibition of excitatory amino acid receptor antagonists ect. with the potential to control inflammatory reaction. Anti-adhesive agents also promote some degree of organic, including brain during cardiac surgery with CPB. In conclusion, the significant risk of neurologic adverse effects during cardiac surgery explains the new interests in protective strategies. Neuromonitoring such as electroencephalogram, transcranial Doppler, near infrared spectroscopy, jugular bulb oxyhemoglobin saturation and possible others, will probably have the same importance as the traditional respiratory and cardiovascular monitoring during cardiac operation.

References

1. Tu JV, Mazer CD, Levinton C et al (1994) A predictive index for length of stay in the intensive care unit following cardiac surgery. Can Med Assoc J 151:177-185
2. Mangano DT (1995) Cardiovascular morbidity and CABG surgery – a perspective: epidemiology, costs, and potential therapeutic solutions. J Cardiol Surg 10(Suppl):366-368
3. Moller JT, Cluitmans P, Rasmussen LS et al (1998) Long term postoperative cognitive dysfunction in the elderly. Lancet 351:857-861
4. Roach WG, Kanchuger M, Mangano MC et al (1996) Adverse cerebral outcomes after coronary bypass surgery. N Engl J Med 335:1857-1863
5. Wolman RL, Nussmeier NA, Aggarwal A et al (1999) Cerebral injury after cardiac surgery: identification of a group of extraordinary risk. Stroke 30:514-522
6. Taggart DP, Browne SM, Halligan PW, Wade DT (1999) Is cardiopulmonary bypass still the cause of cognitive dysfunction after cardiac operations. J Thorac Cardiovasc Surg 118(3):414-420
7. David JC (2000) Neurologic effects. In: Gravllee PG, Davis FR, Kursz M, Utley RJ (eds) Cardiopulmonary bypass: principle and practice. 2th ed. Lippincott Williams & Wilkins, Philadelphia, pp 404-424

8. Klafta JM, Jacny JP, Yong CJ (1995) Neurological and psychiatric adverse effects of anaesthetics: epidemiology and treatment. Drug Safety 13:281-295
9. Williams–Russo P, Sharrock NE, Mattis S et al (1995) Cognitive effects after epidural *vs* general anesthesia in older adults. JAMA 274:44-50
10. Blauth CI, Cosgrove DM, Webb BW et al (1992) Atheroembolism from the ascending aorta. An emerging problem in cardiac surgery. J Thorac Cardiovasc Surg 103:1104-1112
11. Blauth CI (1995) Macroemboli and microemboli during cardiopulmonary bypass. Ann Thorac Surg 59:1300-1303
12. van der Linden J, Casimir-Ahn H (1991) When do cerebral emboli appear during open heart operations? A transcranial Doppler study. Ann Thorac Surg 51:237-241
13. Katz ES, Tunick PA, Rusinek H (1992) Protruding aortic atheromas predict a stroke in elderly patients undergoing bypass: experience with intraoperative transesophageal echocardiography. J Am Coll Cardioll:104:70-77
14. Hill GE (1996) The inflammatory response to cardiopulmonary bypass. Int Anesthesiol Clin 34:95-108
15. Johnsson P (1996) Markers of cerebral ischemia after cardiac surgery. J Cardiothorac Vasc Anesth 10:120-126
16. Zimmer DB, Cornwall EH, Landar A (1995) The S100 protein family, history, function, and expression. Brain Res Bull 37:417-429
17. Jönsson H, Johnssn P, Alling C et al (1998) Significance of serum S100 release after coronary artery bypass grafting. Ann Thorac Surg 65:1639-1644
18. Arrowsmith JE, Grocott HP, Reves JG (2000) Central nervous system complications of cardiac surgery. Br J Anesth 84:378-393
19. Martin TD, Craver JM, Gott JP et al (1994) Prospective, randomized trial of retrograde warm cardioplegia: myocardial benefit and neurologic threat. Ann Thorac Surg 57:298-304
20. Gold JP, Charlson ME, Williams-Russo P et al (1995) Improvement of outcomes after coronary artery bypass. A randomized trial comparing intraoperative high versus low mean arterial pressure. J Thorac Cardiovasc Surg 110:1302-1311
21. Plochl W, Cook DJ (1999) Quantification and distribution of cerebral emboli during cardiopulmonary bypass in the swine. The impact of CO_2. Anesthesiology 909:183-190
22. Wareing TH, Davila-Roman VG, Barzilai B et al (1992) Management of the severely atherosclerotic ascending aorta during cardiac operations. A strategy for detection and treatment. J Thorac Cardiovasc Surg 103:453-462
23. Hartman GS, Yao FS, Bruefach MIII et al (1996) Severity of aortic atheromatous disease diagnosed by transesophageal echocardiography predicts stroke and other outcomes associated with coronary artery surgery: a prospective study. Anesth Analg 83:701-708
24. Soulter MJ, Andrews PJ, Alston RP (1998) Propofol does not ameliorate cerebral venous oxyhemoglobin desaturation during hypothermic cardiopulmonary bypass. Anesth Analg 86:926-931
25. Legault, Furberg CD, Waggenknecht LE et al (1996) Nimodipine neuroprotection in cardiac valve replacement: report of an early terminated trial. Stroke 27:593-598

Myocardial Revascularization with Laser

J.O.C. Auler, L. A. Dallan, S. Almeida de Oliveira

Laser is abbreviation for Light Amplification by the Stimulated Emission of Radiation, i.e., light intensified by the stimulated emission of the radiation. It can be defined as electromagnetic radiation which manifest itself as monochromatic light, therefore waves in the same length and the same ondulatory phases which, for that reason, add up energy.

Because of these properties laser carries almost the maximum energy to a luminous radiation. The light amount of energy provides laser with a huge capacity for destruction when it interacts with any material. This destructive capacity depends on the type of laser, the distance between the source and the material, the means of transmission, the angle of incidence, the time of exposure, the composition and the color of the material with laser effects.

Types of laser beams

The first device for the amplification of the short waves by stimulated emission of radiation was made in 1951, at Columbia University (U.S.A.) based on the Theory of Relativity. At present, there are over 2000 different types of lasers, that can be grouped in:

- Gaseous: helio-neon, Krypton, neodymium, yttrium (alluminium) garnet (YAG), argon, CO_2 and others.
- Liquid: mercury, ammonia, chemical dyes and others.
- Solid: ruby, sapphire and others.

The difference among them is their wave length. The shorter the wave-length the stronger its action. Laser beams can be continuous or pulsating. Their power is expressed in watts (W), and they vary from deciwatts (10^{-1}) to megawatts (10^6).

Interaction between laser beams and biological tissue, cellular or organic substance destruction by laser is made by photocoagulation (coagulation necrosis), burn (leaving charred remains), liquefaction (leaving liquid remains), or vaporization. Beside the spot hit by the radiation, the energy of the laser beam is absorbed only by a thin layer of the tissue adjacent to it. The thickness of this layer depends on the type of laser, on the power used and on the time of the application. Therefore, when high power is used (>400 W), or when the laser beam is applied for fractions of a second, this layer does not practically exist [1].

Use of laser beams in medicine

Laser beams have been initially used in ophthalmology, and was experimentally studied as a photocoagulative in animal's retina. Nevertheless, it was only from 1970 that this process became prevalent through its commercialization and ample diffusion. Its introduction in urology and neurosurgery was almost simultaneous and started around 1979.

Use of laser beams in the cardiac muscle

In 1981 Mirhoseini & Cayton [2] proposed the use of the laser beams to create transmyocardial canals. These authors used a CO_2 laser of 450W, in a model of acute myocardial ischaemia, by means of a occlusion of the anterior interventricular ramification of the left coronary artery in dogs. They observed absence of mortality in the dogs treated with laser and a death rate of 83% in the control group. After two years, Mirhoseini et al. [3] reported the use of this technique on a patient submitted to classical myocardium revascularization. The anterior interventricular ramification of the left coronary artery was occluded and the anterior left ventricle (LV) wall was hypokinetic. Laser beams were applied to this cardiac wall which presented a post-operative improvement in its contractility.

Okada et al. [4] used a CO_2 laser (85W) to create six orifices in the anterior left ventricle of a 55-year-old patient suffering from laser ray application, access to the heart is either made by means of a small thoracotomy carried out in the 4th or 5th left intercostal space, similar to the slightly invasive surgery employed in cases of isolated surgeries, or through a sternotomy when surgery is accompanied by traditional myocardium revascularization.

Okada et al. [4] report angina, refractory to clinical treatment. The authors also report significant clinical improvement nine months after the surgery.

Since 1988, a highly-powered CO_2 laser beam (800W) has been developed in San Francisco Heart Institute, California (U.S.A.). This laser, synchronized to the electrocardiogram, was able to penetrate the cardiac wall with a simple pulse. The possibility of creating a canal in about 40 ms has eliminated the need of cardiac arrest to make it.

Since 1990, this CO_2 laser has been used in human hearts while they are beating and aiming the transmyocardial revascularization. During this period, over 4,000 procedures using laser beams have been carried out in more than eighty Services of Cardiac Surgery. In February 1998 the Heart Institute of Hospital das Clínicas of FMUSP first used the TMRL with a CO_2 laser [5].

Comparative studies with CO_2 laser

The use of laser beams was approved by the American Food and Drug Administration (FDA) in September (1990) to carry out comparative clinical studies. Since then, several protocols have been established, rigorously observed, which can be grouped up in the following three phases:

Phase I

This phase has tried to assess the procedure safety with transmyocardial revascularization laser (TMRL) in the beating heart [6].

Phase II

The target in Phase II has been to assess the efficiency of TMRL in patients suffering from angina pectoris class III and IV, refractory to treatment with drugs and non liable to myocardial revascularization through surgery or angioplasty.

Phase II was carried out in eight Centres of Cardiac Surgery and was performed on 201 non randomized patients. The surgery death rate was 9%, and angina showed a reduction in at least two classes in 74% of the patients. ($p<0.05$) [7].

Phase III

Phase III started in 1995 and its aim was to prove, in a randomized way, the safety and efficiency observed wit the TMRL in phase II [6].

A prospective study was carried out in 192 patients in 12 Cardiac Surgery Centres of reference. The target was to compare the results obtained with the use of laser beams, to the ones obtained with drug treatment in patients suffering from a angina pectoris, III and IV degrees, non liable to classical surgical treatment or angioplasty.

The death rate was 3.3% (3/91) of the patients in the randomized group that received TMRL. Unstable angina was a major factor of mortality during the two weeks previous to surgery. Old age and a low fraction of cardiac output had no influence in the perioperative mortality. The clinical success was defined by the reduction of, at least, two classes in the angina degree. A significant reduction in the symptoms of angina ($p<0.005$) was presented by 72% of the patients belonging to the TMRL group after a period of 12 months when compared to only 13% of the patients in the clinically treated group . Moreover, 30% of the patients in the TMRL group haven't presented any type of angina from the moment of the surgical procedure and onward. After 12 months, the perfusion in the left ventricle defined by Thalium scintilography improved in 19% of the TMRL group and worsened in 17% of the TM group ($p<0.05$).

The clinical investigation of phase III confirmed, in a randomized way, the results found after studying phase II. It also proved to be a safe and efficient method for the treatment of this specific group of patients.

Use of laser beams in patients suffering from refractory angina. The clinical treatment with drugs based on nitrates, beta blockers and calcium channels antagonists was complemented by the introduction of two direct procedures of myocardial revascularization grafts surgically carried out on the coronary arteries and coronary transluminal angioplasty. In spite of such advances, patients with intractable angina and in the final stages of coronary arterial disease can still be observed in clinical practice even after all traditional therapeutic including surgery methods have been exhausted [8].

Indirect methods for myocardial revascularization

Before concluding that the myocardium could be directly nourished with blood supplied from the left ventricle, it should be taken into account that a revision accomplished in comparative anatomy found that the heart of reptiles receives oxygenated blood from multiple channels originating from the myocardial cavity [9].

Based on such findings, Sen et al. suggested "snake heart" surgery. This procedure involves transmyocardial acupuncture in ischaemic areas of the heart of animals resulting in a reduction of the infarcted area as well as prolonging life [10].

This study takes on more importance when one considers that in the embryo phase the human heart is directly supplied with blood flown from the left ventricle through a broad net of capillaries. However, there is usually a regression of these capillaries with the further development of the coronary arteries.

It can be considered that Vineberg´s proposed surgery of 1946, describing the implantation of one or both internal thoracic arteries in the core of myocardial musculature has unquestionably been the most successful in this phase. What could have been inferred from this surgery was a difference in the myocardial circulation, in relation to other organs, that provided a new vascular formation. Implanted grafts established clear-cut connections with the coronaries by means of these newly created vessels [11].

Criticism based on the channels that were obtained through needle-made acupuncture by Sen et al. [10] referred that the lengthy scarification carried out in the cardiac tissue could eventually jeopardize the effectiveness of the procedure. The use of laser rays was then contemplated as an alternative method in considering the possibility of alleviating the fibrotic process. Recent use of laser rays as a MR method has had a noticeable development, even before the scientific foundations of such technology had been sufficiently recognized. This has probably happened in consequence of the satisfactory results obtained in several studies encompassing selected groups of patients who, though previously submitted to different surgical procedures, had eventually undergone a TMRL surgery. Not only had they survived but also their angina condition was relieved.

Options for the type of laser

In relation to other types of lasers the CO2 laser was the better choice due to certain advantages concerning its performance on tissues. Apart from being the most powerful the CO2 laser is emitted through continuous waves as opposed, for instance, to the holmium: YAG laser that is emitted through wave pulses [12].

Cardiac arrhythmias caused by laser ray application

Based on the necessity for multiple pulses to create a transmyocardium channel is related to cardiac arrhythmias. At the beginning of their experimental studies, Mirhoseini et al. [13] have demonstrated that laser activation, in the course of myocardial cells repolarization (during the "T" wave of the electrocardiogram), increased the incidence of arrythmogenic disorders that were followed by a decrease in cardiac output.

This problem has been circumvented in our study by a synchronic activation of the laser rays with the "R" wave (depolarization) of the electrocardiogram. We have noticed an incidence of 2% of intra-surgery arrhythmias in our patients. Kadipasaolu et al. found similar results when using the TMRL [14] together with the CO_2 laser. This study detected 15% of ventricular arrhythmias in pigs when laser rays were synchronic to the T wave while only 3% of arrhythmias were detected when laser rays had been synchronic to the "R" wave.

Previous myocardium revascularization

Our study revealed that 68.8% of patients receiving TMRL had been previously submitted to one or more cardiac surgeries, apart from innumerous PTCA procedures. These data are similar to data described in literature where approximately 90% of patients had already been revascularized and 50% of them had been previously submitted to PTCA [1].

Occlusions or stenoses can eventually occur in previously implanted grafts some years after myocardium revascularization, or even in consequence of evolution developed in the coronary arterial disease, that gives origin to an additional ischaemic process to the myocardium. Therefore, another potential TMRL use is for patients to be submitted to surgeries for the purpose of a new myocardium revascularization.

Anaesthesia, surgical access and postoperative care

Once patients scheduled for laser procedure represent class II or signs of angina and heart failure anaesthesia requires extensive haemodynamic monitoring, including transesophageal echocardiography. A transesophageal echocardiography is relevant not only for the monitoring of the ventricular function but also for visualizing the performance of the micro air bubbles in the left ventricule cavity, consequent to the dispersion of the laser ray heat when in touch with blood, that offers the assurance of its penetration into the cavity. For laser ray application, access to the heart is either made by means of a small thoracotomy carried out in the 4th or 5th left intercostal space, similar to the slightly invasive surgery employed in cases of isolated surgeries, or through a sternotomy when surgery is accompanied by traditional myocardium revascularization. This is relevant in that the laser initial proposition is based on the certainty that channels created from the ray-beam, though closed on the surface, still maintain a certain communication between the cavity and the sinusoidal plexus for the transport of oxygenated blood. With the exception that laser does not cause an immediate improvement in cardiac function, but can worsen it due to traumatic oedema, postoperative care does not demand special consideration.

Experience of the Heart Institute – InCor of Hospital das Clínicas

From February 1998 to February 2001, 50 patients were submitted to TMRL in the hospital; 36 (72%) of the patients were male within an average age group of 59.7 years. In the same period, more then 2,000 patients were submitted for traditional revascularization which makes the selection of this procedure a concern.

TMRL was exclusively carried out in 64% of the patients and only 36% of the patients underwent laser and traditional myocardium revascularization.

Number of Channels

At the beginning of our study the highest possible number of channels allowed by the epicardium and only the neighbouring areas of vessels and coronary arteries and also the previous grafts were left intact. The question arises from the maximum possible number of channels allowed in each area until the injured tissue does not overcome TMRL benefits. A majority of surgeons currently give preference to the execution of one channel to each square centimetre of myocardium surface [25]. In the first half of the patients in our series the average of effective myocardium perforations was 29.8 pulses per patient, but in the second half of the patients the rate dropped to 18.1.

Laser ray power

When the laser ray pulse makes contact with the heart its power is transferred to myocardium. Absorption of this power by tissue water produces vapour consisting of air bubbles. The phase from the liquid state to a gaseous state provokes a volumetric expansion that, in turn, opens spaces in the core of the tissue and creates the channels. TMRL was first initiated with 25 to 30 joules of power, until the intensity increased or diminished depending on the success achieved in the creation of channels which are evident by a transesophageal echocardiography [14].

Angina pectoris

In our study the improvement in angina pectoris symptoms with the use of TMRL is easily seen. After a 12-month period of follow-up, approximately 87.8% of patients (Canadian Cardiovascular Society Angina) moved from class III or IV to class 0, 1 or II ($p<0.0001$) of angina. Furthermore, angina had altogether disappeared in 66.6% of these patients. Considering that the success in this procedure is limited to a two degrees reduction in the angina classification [7], patients in our study achieved a rate of success rate of 87.8% after twelve month period of TMRL ($p<0.0001$).

According to this aspect, our results are in agreement with literature. The conclusion of phase III of the multi-centre study comparing TMRL to clinical treatment by means of a prospective and randomized study in 192 patients, revealed the reduction in the degree of angina among 72% of the patients belonging to the TMRL group as compared to only 13% of the patients assisted with clinical treatment ($p<0.05$). On the other hand, 30% of the patients in the clinical treatment group had their angina symptoms aggravated and several of them were submitted to TMRL [1]. The criteria orienting the change of the groups was not only supported by a mere failure of the clinical therapy but comprised patients with a history of acute myocardium infarct followed by a post-infarct angina or who had developed a pattern of unstable angina exclusively controlled through intravenous medication. Such instability has inclusivly contributed to the higher-rate of per-surgery mortality of 17% in the case of patients who changed the group as compared to 4% of the initial TMRL group. Thirty two percent of our patients reduced their use of anti-ischaemic therapy. In phase III of the multi-centre study the reduction was 48% for the TMRL group whilst only one patient of the clinical treatment group received reduced medication.

Quality of life

There was a significant improvement in the quality of life in our group of patients ($p=0.0001$) after TMRL. The return of the patient to household chores and to social and working activities was also considered. Results obtained have reinforced the clinical advantages offered by TMRL to patients either with obstructive and diffuse coronary arterial disease or who have had exhausted all traditional therapeutic treatments for angina.

Mortality rate

In our study, 3 (6.0%) premature deaths were observed, 2 of them intra-hospital and 1 after the hospital discharge as a consequence of pulmonary infection and septic shock which had occurred within 30 days after the procedure.

Occurrence of infarct was not confirmed in two of the patients who died in the initial phase, due to the following reasons: one of the patients exhibited a low cardiac output and the death of the second patient occurred when extubated a few hours after surgery, caused by a sudden and irreversible cardiac arrest.

The above results are in accordance with literature where risks of immediate death are referred to instabilities occurring in clinical manifestations. Such risks would therefore be higher when TMRL was carried out in the proximity of acute cardiac events. A study performed by March [16] shows immediate deaths in 27% of patients submitted to surgery within one to seven days after episodes of unstable angina and then the rate dropped to 16% when the interval was situated around 8 to 14 days and to 1% in patients within an interval longer than 15 days. Although 8 patients had been diagnosed with unstable angina, only one in our series was in the emergency unit under the use of intravenous heparin and nitroglycerin.

In the medium term evolution, 2 deaths related to myocardium infarct occurred in the 12th and 14th month after surgery.

Myocardial perfusion

In the evaluation of the method, changes occurred in myocardial perfusion with TMRL representing a subject of considerable relevance. In his evaluation of results, Horvarth [1] noticed through analysis performed with thallium 201, in phase III of a multi-centre comparative study, improvements in the LV perfusion of 19% of the patients after 6 to 12 months of the TMRL procedure whereas in the group under clinical treatment 17% of the patients had had their condition worsened in relation to the pre-surgery period. The majority of patients who had had their conditions improved with myocardial perfusion exhibited a concurrent improvement in their class of angina. Another evaluation [17], using tomography with positron emission, confirmed the general improvement in the myocardial perfusion after TMRL. However, such improvement was more noticeable in the subendocardial region as compared to the subepicardial region. Nevertheless, all authors did not unanimously achieve the same results. Hillis & Lange [18] consider negligibly consistent, or even no evidences of improvements in myocardial perfusion after TMRL. Failure to demonstrate alterations occurred in the perfusion of the left ventricle could be related more to the poor sensibility of the radioisotope exams made by the authors than to the absence of a patent effectiveness.

Comparative studies carried out in our series, through Sestamibi.99mTc during dipyridamole stress, revealed an improved myocardial perfusion only in patients who had had TMRL associated with myocardium revascularization.

Function of the left ventricle

Medium and long-term conclusive studies covering the function of the left ventricle after TMRL are not yet available. Donovan et al. [19] carried out an echocardiographic study under dobutamine stress in patients submitted to TMRL and demonstrated that after six months after the procedure patients with refractory angina were capable of reducing abnormalities in the motility of the ischaemic cardiac wall and of improving the tolerance induced by the dobutamine stress. Estimate of the LV function, obtained from our casuistic through magnetic resonance and echocardiography, enabled the assertion that post-surgery EF was slightly higher ($p = 0.0382$) than pre-surgery.

Stages of channel evolution

Thermal injury

Two stages can be considered in the evolution of channels obtained through TMRL. The first phase is characterized by a thermal injury produced on the tissues bordering the channel. Considering that patients submitted to TMRL also harbour a refractory angina and different degrees of myocardium commitment it is advisable that channels are created with the minimum amount of muscular necrosis. In this sense, we believe that CO_2 utilization was beneficial to our patients once it has been known that this high-powered laser inflicts minor injuries when compared to others.

Cicatrization

The second phase of the process of channel creation is related to the cicatrization. In this period, the migration of the fibroblasts is important for the production of sufficient collagen in that the exertion of significant tensile force stimulates the remodelling of the channel.

There is a consensus that thermal coagulation of the muscle, followed by a concurrent exposition of interstitial collagen during the process of channel creation, gives origin to a bordering thrombogenic surface. From this moment on, the period of time necessary for its eventual occlusion is controversial.

The aftermath of channels

Supposition that TMRL makes trans-myocardial channels remains pervious and supplying oxygenated blood directly from the left ventricular cavity has opened way for controversies. The functioning mechanism of these channels presupposes:

1) That channels are patent.
2) That channels establish communications between the endocardium and the sinusoidal myocardial plexus.
3) That oxygenated blood passes through such communications from the left ventricule to the arteriolar system.

In the first place, the actual existence of myocardial sinusoids has been questioned. Recent studies [20] expostulate that sinusoidal plexus described by Wearn in 1993 [21] would be a mere dehydration artifact. Furthermore, it has been mentioned that such structures, restricted to foetal circulation, would later undergo a process of atrophy after the delivery period followed by the substitution of coronary epicardial arteries and by the intra-myocardium arterial-capillary system [22].

Another remaining argument inquires how would the transference of blood from the LV to the myocardium be physiologically possible through a pressurised gradient. The first arising dilemma would be how to adequately estimate the measure of the myocardium tension. When an evaluation is carried out with the use of micro-manometers, intra-myocardium systolic pressure is invariably higher than the LV pressure, however, a reversion of results was noticed when opened collapsible catheters were used. Frazier et al. [22] succeeded in the measure of this gradient with the use of up-to-date pressure transducers and admitted the potential existence of a positive gradient in the direction of the lumen-endocardium that would provide the necessary driving power for whatever eventual flow of blood that had originated from TMRL. Reinforcing such findings, recent studies [23] carried out through high definition echocardiogram revealed evidences that contrast injected into the left ventricule of patients submitted to TMRL moved directly towards the myocardium wall during the systolic phase of the cardiac contraction. Studies developed in our patients with the use of magnetic resonance similarly revealed that, in the majority of cases, contrast (gadolinium) injected in the venous system initially contrasted with the epicardium of the left ventricule roaming in a later phase towards the endocardium. Only a single patient exhibited a reversed flow, i.e., from the endocardium to the epicardium. Such scrutiny reinforces the hypothesis of a medium term occlusion of channels. It is however doubtful that blood flows through the channels immediately after they are installed as we had the opportunity of noticing in the intra-surgery period of TMRL through the flush of blood that surfaced the heart after laser was discharged. Nevertheless, what will happen to the channels in the future has not yet been satisfactorily clarified.

Necropsy studies

In human beings morphological data concerning the patent of channels is limited to the description of isolated cases in patients whose death occurred in different periods after TMRL and their contribution for definitely elucidating the dilemma is negligible. In the analysis made in the heart of a patient who died 2 hours after TMRL, with CO_2 laser, Lutter et al. [24] verified that all 15 installed channels were pervious and with the interior spared from the presence of fibrin or thrombus.

Sigel et al. [25] observed controversial findings in necropsies performed in 3 patients similarly submitted to TMRL. Periods between surgeries and deaths were respectively 24 hours, 10 days and 3 weeks. Histological examination carried out in the patient whose death occurred in the first day revealed well individualized channels whereas in the patient who died 10 days later the channel borders had also remained distinctly recognizable. However, in the last case well marked channels were crammed with granulation tissue and fibrosis. Summers et al. [26] documented the case of a 60-year old patient who died in a car accident 261 days after a TMRL angina treatment with 31 myocardium perforations. This patient had had an asymptomatic evolution in accordance with reports registered in the several ambulatory returns. Necropsy later revealed an extensive scarification of the epicardium and no patent channels were noticed in the macroscopy or in myocardium histology. On the other hand, Cooley et al. [27] described the case of a patient who had likewise died 3 months after TMRL and whose necropsy identified nine channels perpendicularly oriented towards the epicardium surface with a diameter of approximately 20 to 70 μm, encircled by fibrous conjunctive tissue and containing red blood cells. Considering the hypothesis of an eventual occlusion of the channels, it remains to be discussed what justification exists for the unquestionable clinical improvement noticed in patients.

Neoangiogenesis

In studies developed with laboratory animals or in necropsies, frequent findings of angiogenesis stimulation by means of a myocardial application of laser have been recently emphasized. The presence of granulation tissue represented by fibrosis, neo-vascular formation and lymphomononuclear inflammatory infiltrate observed in the heart of a patient deceased 14 months after TMRL confirms our hypothesis. Several works [16] have evidenced that TMRL is capable of stimulating angiogenesis in the ischaemic myocardium. This presupposes the hypothesis that the myocardium injury created by channels provokes a local inflammatory response that, on the other hand, liberates cytokines and growth factors and stimulates the reception of these same factors. Evidences that TMRL unleashes a process of vascular growth can only be found after the second or third weeks after the procedure followed by a further progressive development after this period [28].

Myocardial denervation

Myocardial denervation has been suggested as a potential mechanism for the TMRL relieve of angina. Experimental works developed in dogs by Sundt & Kwong [29] concluded that TMRL, using Holmium: YAG laser, is capable of destroying the cardiac nervous fibers. With the use of bradykinin in areas of animals heart treated with laser authors concluded for the presence of some interference in the function of cardiac afferent nerves through losses observed in homodynamic responses. Such hypothesis is based on the possibility of the angina pain transmission by afferent sympathetic fibers and on the knowledge about the existence of post-ganglial sympathetic fibers situated on the surface of the epicardium. This would justify the silent myocardial ischaemia frequently noticed in diabetic patients who usually exhibit an autonomic neuropathy that gives origin to the concept that the relieve of the patients symptoms is not bound to an improvement of the myocardial perfusion with TMRL but to the fact that patients become "liberated from angina pain" because of denervation. Thus liberated from angina symptoms patients would run a higher exposition to the risks of ischaemia that would lead to an increased number of myocardium infarcts or sudden deaths. Such risks, however, have not been confirmed in several studies carried out in different centres.

Revascularization associated with TMRL

We believe that TMRL higher potential is related to its utilization associated with myocardium revascularization. Among the several studies that have been developed in this field, a prospective and randomized multi-centered study should be emphasized comparing direct surgery for coronary artery revascularization, as an isolated procedure, against the same technique used in association with TMRL (holmium: YAG laser). In this study 221 patients [30] with one or more viable myocardium areas, but to a certain extent inadequate to the treatment with systemic-coronary grafts, were identified for traditional surgery procedures. Patients were randomized in two groups: patients of the first group received grafts in areas where arteries were susceptible of revascularization, and were supplemented with a laser discharge on non-viable areas. The second group received exclusively grafts in viable areas whilst territories inadequate for revascularization were left intact. The rate of in-hospital mortality was similar in the two groups (8.8% and 8.4% respectively). The after surgery death rate, however, was significantly lower in the group submitted to revascularization associated with TMRL (0.9%) than in the group in which isolated surgery had been performed heading to the conclusion that TMRL, in the condition of a supplementary method for traditional surgery, apart from offering assurance to procedures, also decreased mortality rate in patients non susceptible of a thorough revascularization by means of an isolated traditional surgery.

Percutaneous laser

A number of patients bearing refractory angina have recently received a holmium: YAG laser treatment through percutaneous cardiac catheterization. This method creates partial channels originated from the patient endocardium [1]. Activation of laser on the surface of the left ventricle creates a channel with an approximate depth of 6mm, therefore the myocardium wall thickness should be over 8mm. A multi-centre study was performed comparing patients using percutaneous laser associated to traditional medication with patients receiving an isolated medication treatment, reporting classes of angina were significantly lower in the laser group [30]. Galli et al. [31] described this procedure in 15 patients in whom an average of 13 channels were opened by ischaemic territory. According to authors, a remarkable alleviation was noticed in the angina symptoms. In spite of the fact that this procedure does not create transmural channels, discussions concerning this method superposes the ones previously carried out about the use of holmium: YAG laser in which its pulsatile characteristic predisposes to more significant injuries to the myocardium tissue neighbouring the channels.

Future perspectives

Considerable expectations therefore exist concerning the therapeutic procedures of laser rays for an increasing group of patients in advanced stages of obstructive coronary disease for whom some spark of hope have lately started to glow. Isolated or associated with conventional surgery, TMRL is capable of providing satisfactory results for this selected group of patients. In our studies, we have had the opportunity of verifying a substantial decrease in the angina symptoms as well as an increased improvement for the practice of exercises.

We believe that TMRL future paths should be drawn towards procedures designed to improve angina symptoms, with a minimally possible invasive consequence, and simultaneously associated with a significant reduction of undesirable effects. Improvements in the percutaneous application of laser rays, comprising catheters transmitting high-powered lasers capable of freely sailing in the interior of the LV, or through thoracoscopy interventions, have been included in this forefront.

References

1. Horvath KA (1999) Transmyocardial laser. In: Franco K, Verrier ED (eds) Advanced therapy in cardiac surgery. BC Deker, Saint Louis, pp 129-134
2. Mirhoseini M & Claiton MM (1981) Revascularization of the heart by laser. J Microsurg 2:253-260
3. Mirhoseini M, Fisher JC, Clayton M (1983) Myocardial revascularization by laser. Lasers Surg Med 3:241-245
4. Okada M, Ikuta H, Shimizu K et al (1986) Alternative method of myocardial revascularization by laser: experimental and clinical study. Kobe J Med Sci 32:151-161
5. Oliveira SA, Dallan LAO, Lisboa LA et al (1999) Revascularização transmiocárdica com laser de CO_2: experiência clínica inicial. Arq Bras Cardiol 72:441-450
6. March RJ & Klontz B (1999) Transmyocardial laser revascularization. In: Cohen, Mack, Fonger & Landreneau (eds) Minimally invasive cardiac surgery. Quality Medical Publishing, Chicago, pp 329-336
7. Horvath KA, Cohn LH, Cooley DA (1997) Transmyocardial laser revascularization; results of a multicenter trial with transmyocardial laser revascularization used as sole therapy for end-stage coronary artery disease. J Thorac Cardiovasc Surg 113:645-654
8. Schoebel FC, Frazier OH, Jessurun GA (1997) Refractory angina pectoris in end-stage coronary artery disease: evolving therapeutic concepts. Am Heart J 134:587-602
9. Horvath KA, Smith WJ, Laurence RG et al (1995) Recovery and viability of an acute myocardial infarct after transmyocardial laser revascularization. J Am Coll Cardiol 25: 258-263
10. Sen PK, Daulatran J, Kinare SG et al (1968) Further studies in multiple transmyocardial acupuncture as a method of myocardial revascularization. Surgery 64:861-870
11. Vineberg AM (1946) Development of anastomosis between coronary vessels and transplanted internal mammary artery. Can Med Assoc J 55:17-19
12. Jansen ED, Frenz M, Kadipasaoglu KA et al (1997) Laser tissue interaction during transmyocardial laser revascularization. Ann Thorac Surg 63:640-647
13. Mirhoseini M, Muckerheide M, Clayton MM (1982) Transventricular revascularization by laser. Lasers Surg Med 2: 187-198
14. Kadipasaoglu KA, Sartori M, Masai T et al (1999) Intra-operative arrhythmias and tissue damage during transmyocardial laser revascularization. Ann Thorac Surg 67:423-431
15. Mueller XM, Bettex D, Tevaerai HT et al (1998) Acute effects of transmyocardial laser revascularization on left-ventricular function; a haemodynamic and echocardiographic study. J Thorac Cardiovasc Surg 46:126-129
16. March RJ (1999) Transmyocardial laser revascularization with the CO_2 laser: one year results of a randomized, controlled trial. Semin Thorac Cardiovasc Surg 11: 12-18

17. Hovarth KA, Mannting F, Cummings N et al (1996) Transmyocardial laser revascularization: operative techniques and clinical results at two years. J Thorac Cardiovasc Surg 111:1047-1053
18. Hillis LD & Lange RA (1999) Transmyocardial LASER revascularization. N Engl J Med 341:1075-1076
19. Donovan CL, Landolfo KP, Lowe JE et al (1997) Improvement in inducible ischemia during dobutamine stress echocardiography after transmyocardial laser revascularization in patients with refractory angina pectoris. J Am Coll Cardiol 30:607-612
20. Tsang JC & Chiu RC (1995) The phantom of "myocardial sinusoids": a historical reappraisal. Ann Thorac Surg 60:1831-1835
21. Wearn JT, Mettier SR, Klumpp TG et al (1933) The nature of the vascular communications between the coronary arteries and the chambers of the heart. Am Heart J 9:143-164
22. Frazier OH, Kadipasaoglu KA, Cooley DA (1998) Transmyocardial laser revascularization: does it have a role in the treatment of ischemic heart disease? Tex Heart Inst J 25:24-29
23. Berwing K, Bauer EP, Strasser R et al (1997) Functional evidence of long-term channel patency after transmyocardial revascularization. Circulation 96(suppl 1):I-564. (abstract)
24. Lutter G, Schwarrzkopf J, Lutz C et al (1998) Histologic findings of transmyocardial laser channels after two hours. Ann Thorac Surg 65:1437-1439
25. Sigel JE, Abramovich CM, Lytle BW et al (1998) Transmyocardial laser revascularization: three sequential autopsy cases. J Thorac Cardiovasc Surg 115:1381-1385
26. Summers JH, Henry AC, Roberts WC (1999) Cardiac observations late after operative transmyocardial laser "revascularization". Am J Cardiol 84:489-490
27. Cooley DA, Frazier OH, Kadipasaoglu KA et al (1994) Transmyocardial laser revascularization with the CO_2 laser: anatomic evidence of long-term channel patency. Tex Heart Inst J 21: 220-224
28. Roethy W, Yamamoto N, Burkhoff D (1999) An examination of potential mechanics underlying transmyocardial laser revascularization induced increases in myocardial blood flow. Semin Thorac Cardiovasc Surg 11:24-28
29. Sundt 3rd TM, Kwong KF (1999) Clinical experience with the holmium: YAG laser for transmyocardial laser revascularization and myocardial denervation as a mechanism. Semin Thorac Cardiovasc Surg 11:19-23
30. Allen KB, Fudge Tl, Selinger Sl et al (1997) Prospective randomized multicenter trial of transmyocardial revascularization versus maximal medical management in patients with class IV angina. Circulation 96 (suppl 1):564 [abstract]
31. Galli M, Zerboni S, Politi A et al (1999) Percutaneous transmyocardial revascularization with holmium laser in patients with refractory angina: a pilot feasibility study. G Ital Cardiol 29:1020-1026.

Advances in Anaesthesia Techniques for Children

A. Sarti, R. Scarpa, S. Banti

Anaesthesiology is an ever-changing field. New drugs and techniques are continuously developed and considered for the anaesthetic plan, in a continuum of perioperative clinical practice, whether outpatient or inpatient. The use of regional anaesthesia techniques in children has increased dramatically. Local anaesthetics, once not considered by most anaesthetists for children anaesthesia, have become a valuable weapon even for the pediatric anaesthesiologist. Regional analgesia is most commonly used in conjunction with light general anaesthesia or sedation in pediatrics, although in certain circumstances a regional anaesthetic alone may be the preferred technique [1]. Combined general and regional anaesthesia is currently the most frequent routine technique used for children in many countries. Supplementing a general inhalation or intravenous anaesthetic with a central or peripheral nerve block results in pain-free awakening and excellent postoperative analgesia without the side effects of opioid drugs. The nervous blockade can be performed either before surgery or at the end of surgery, before the awakening. Performing the blockade at the end of surgery may prolong postoperative analgesia. As the block is performed after the induction of anaesthesia, but before the beginning of surgery, the use of intravenous or inhalation drugs is required for the maintenance of the anaesthetic. Consequently, the awakening results pain-free, quick, and smooth. Rarely, if ever, an anaesthetic should be performed without using some kind of local or regional analgesia. Indeed, even if a regional block is not feasible or desirable, it is possible to take advantage of the EMLA cream for intravenous cannulation or of the wound infiltration for postoperative analgesia. Paracetamol or even better the association of paracetamol and codeine is effective for pain control for minor and moderate surgery. These analgesics should be administered prior to surgery or, if a local or regional technique has been added, at the end of surgery by the rectal route for pre-emptive analgesia. Wound infiltration is definitely safe,, easy, and very useful for early postoperative analgesia. This simple technique, which is greatly underused and undervalued, has virtually no contraindication, except a known documented previous undesired reaction to local anaesthetic agents. It allows the anaesthesiologist to gain time in order to plan and realize the postoperative pain treatment. For the anaesthetist, who is not familiar with regional analgesia techniques, wound infiltration is the best way to increase the quality of postoperative analgesia with no risks unless toxic doses of the local anaesthetic agent are injected.

The combination of a general inhalation anaesthetic given by a laryngeal mask plus a peripheral block (ileoinguinal-hypogastric block) is gaining popularity for many routine surgical procedures at the groin area below the umbilicus, such as inguinal hernia repair or correction of an undescended testis. Alternatively, the anaesthetic can be induced and maintained with an intravenous drug, such as propofol. In this case, because of the lack of analgesic properties of propofol, it may be better supplementing the propofol sedation with an analgesic agent such as ketamine prior to the blockade, or with a central block, such as a *caudal block* or a *spinal block*, where a basic covering of the general anaesthesia is not necessary.

The sacral intervertebral epidural block may be an alternative of caudal or low lumbar epidural block. During childhood the sacral intervertebral spaces may be punctured with a technique similar to the one used for a lumbar epidural blockade. The main advantage is that most anaesthetists, who do not know the caudal technique, are familiar with the loss of resistance technique to find the epidural space. The spinal cord ends at a lower level into the spinal canal in infants and young children, compared to the adult patients. At S1-S2 level there is definitely no risk of punctioning the spinal cord even if a dural tap is a possible complication at this level [2].

Inhalation anaesthetic agents

Nothing is more elusive than finding the ideal inhalation anaesthetic agent. However, sevoflurane and desflurane solve some of the problems associated with halothane and isoflurane anaesthesia. Sevoflurane is certainly a welcome addition to the care of pediatric patients, particularly in terms of a more rapid and acceptable induction of anaesthesia. The smell is acceptable to most children, the uptake of the drug is quick, and there is less metabolism than with halothane. There is little doubt that the gaseous induction is more rapid and that the increase in the inspired sevoflurane concentration proceed faster than with halothane. A quick induction, not longer than that obtained by an injection of thiopental or propofol is reached by using a high initial concentration of sevoflurane (8%) in 66% nitrous oxide for most children. This method is very useful for those children who might struggle during the traditional mask induction of anaesthesia. The anaesthesia circuit is filled with 66% nitrous oxide and the maximum concentration of the halogenated agent. The mask is applied to the face as the child pauses in full exhalation and then is asked to produce a full inspiration.

The effects on the cardiovascular system of sevoflurane are less than those caused by halothane [3, 4], but sevoflurane seems to have more profound effects on respiration [5]. The effects of sevoflurane on the central nervous system are similar to those of isoflurane. The major concerns with sevoflurane relate to potential nephrotoxicity due to formation of toxic metabolites and elevated levels of inorganic fluoride with prolonged administration [6]. Another concern is the case of generalized but clinical silent seizure-like EEG activity observed rarely in both normal children and children with seizure disorders [7]. A higher incidence of emergence agitation has been reported with sevoflurane compared to halothane even with adequate analgesia [8].

The author's own practice is to use sevoflurane with 66% nitrous oxide for the induction of the anaesthetic and then change to isoflurane and oxygen-air (plus an opioid drug if a regional blockade is not feasible) for maintenance during the procedure, to avoid the issue of potential toxicity of sevoflurane and to save money.

Desflurane is very pungent in terms of airway irritation and it is not recommended for the gaseous induction of anaesthesia in pediatric patients [9]. This agent provides a very stable maintenance period, easily altered depth of anaesthesia and rapid awakening, because of a blood-gas partition coefficient similar to that of nitrous oxide.

Intravenous agents

Propofol has gained popularity in pediatric anaesthesia both for induction and for maintenance. This highly lipophilic drug is rapidly distributed in highly perfused organs, accounting for its quick onset. It is rapidly redistributed and metabolized in the liver and other organs, such as kidney and lung, accounting for its rapid recovery [10]. An advantage of propofol is the lower incidence of nausea and vomiting associated with its use for induction and maintenance [11]. The brief pharmacodynamic action accounts for the need of frequent small boluses or constant infusion to maintain a stable plane of sedation. Propofol seems particularly suited for induction of anaesthesia and for short-term infusions in the operating room and for a variety of non-operating room procedures because of the ease of controlling the depth of sedation as well as rapidity and the quality of recovery. In the author's opinion propofol sedation, either as intravenous induction and subsequent boluses or as continuous infusion, depending on the length of the procedure, gives the best technique for radiological non-painful procedures, such as CT and NMR imaging. Other advantages of propofol are the lower incidence of laryngospasm in comparison to thiopental, better preservation of airway patency further improved by the chin-lift manoeuvre, and better condition for a laryngeal mask insertion when compared with thiopental [12, 13]. The major drawback is the pain-associated injection, which can be diminished by using large veins and by concomitant or even better previous injection of lidocaine 0.5 mg/Kg. Metabolic acidosis and fatal myocardial failure have been reported in children in the intensive care environment with long-term propofol infusions [14, 15]. Even if this association is still debatable and the clinical importance of these case reports needs careful re-evaluation, in the author's opinion it is wise to limit the use of this agent for short-term sedation (hours) in children anaesthesia and intensive care and to avoid this drug for sedating neonates and infants.

Midazolam has almost replaced diazepam in pediatric anaesthesia. This water-soluble benzodiazepine offers significant advantages. Solubility in water eliminates the pain on intravenous injection. The elimination half-life is much shorter compared with diazepam. This drug is suitable as a continuous infusion both in the operating room and in the intensive care unit [16]. Oral midazolam has become the most used premedication for children in many centres. This drug can be administered also nasally, rectally, and intramuscularly. There is some evidence suggesting that the amnestic properties of midazolam may be superior to those of diazepam [16]. It is important to remember that because of different fat solubility, it takes three times longer for intravenous midazolam to achieve a peak central nervous system effect (almost 5 minutes) when compared with intravenous diazepam [17]. Waiting enough time between doses and continuous clinical observation and monitoring are therefore paramount.

Opioid drugs

Morphine is still the most used opioid drug by continuous infusion or intermittent boluses for postoperative pain management in children. Fentanyl is the most commonly used opioid supplement for general anaesthesia in the pediatric population. All other newer opiates are more expensive. Alfentanil is a fentanyl analogue whose main advantage is the lower lipid solubility and smaller volume of distribution compared with fentanyl [18]. Sufentanil has been used in children undergoing cardiac surgical procedures. The elimination of this drug is not affected by renal or liver failure but it is briskly altered by variations in hepatic blood flow [18]. Remifentanil is the newest synthetic opioid. An ester linkage allows very rapid metabolism by blood and tissues esterases. Thus, metabolism is not affected by hepatic or renal function. Unlike all other opioids, there is no increase in the duration of effect with increasing doses or duration of infusions. Indeed, the rate of its metabolism is so rapid that the plasma concentration curve during constant infusions is virtually flat. This translates into the ability to rapidly increase or decrease the opioid effect. However, at the end of the anaesthetic a longer acting opioid or a regional block is necessary so that the child wakes up pain-free. This opioid is considered the opioid of choice for critically ill infants and children in whom prolonged postoperative ventilation is not desirable [19].

Myorelaxants

Although succinylcholine has still the most rapid onset and the briefest duration of action of all muscle relaxants, its use for routine surgical procedures has greatly declined, because of many well-known side effects. In the author's opinion, according to other authors [20] succinylcholine must now be considered an emergency drug for immediate control of the airway and for treatment of severe laryngospasm. Even for a rapid control of the airway, such as in rapid-sequence endotracheal intubation, no data prove that succinylcholine may be safer than a rapid onset competitive muscle relaxant such as rocuronium [21]. Comparable intubating conditions 30 seconds after administration of succinylcholine (1.5 mg/Kg) and rocuronium (1.2 mg/Kg) following thiopental have been demonstrated in a recent trial [21]. With both drugs the need for ventilation prior to intubation was avoided in this study [22]. However, with rocuronium there is the disadvantage that the duration of its neuromuscular block may exceed the duration of the planned surgical procedure because the clinical duration of this relaxant agent is similar to that of vecuronium.

Mivacurium is a short-acting nondepolarizing relaxant, which turned out to be very useful for brief surgical procedures requiring endotracheal intubation in children, such as adenoidectomy and tonsillectomy. The recovery times in children are around 30% faster than those observed in adult patients [23]. The neuromuscular blockade of mivacurium is twice as long as that of succinylcholine, but only 40% as long as atracurium or vecuronium. Thus, the muscle blockade lasts enough for completion of most brief routine procedures in children. A potentiation of the neuromuscular effect of mivacurium occurs in the presence of halogenated agents, more pronounced with sevoflurane and isoflurane than with halothane [23].

Cisatracurium, a stereoisomer of atracurium, is three times more potent than atracurium, with a similar duration of action [24]. The higher potency of cisatracurium has some advantages: its histamine-releasing effects are minimal, no bronchospasm occurs and there are no changes in heart rate and blood pressure. Pancuromium is still used for cardiac surgery in association with high-dose fentanyl or sufentanil. The vagolitic effect of this neuromuscular agent counteracts the vagotonic effect of the opioid and its muscle relaxant properties counteract the narcotic-induced chest wall rigidity.

Local anaesthetics

Ropivacaine, like levobupivacaine is a levo enantiomer with a higher threshold for cardiac and neurologic toxicity compared to bupivacaine [25]. Ropivacaine is also considered to have a lesser degree of motor blockade for equianalgesic potency, but there still are conflicting data in this regard. Ropivacaine has been reported to produce a denser blockade of A delta and C fibers than bupivacaine when low concentrations are used [26]. Clinical well-controlled studies in children do not report any detectable motor-sensor differential. Some trials in infants and children report a longer duration of analgesia with ropivacaine, compared to bupivacaine, despite the use of lower potency solutions [27].

Cuffed tracheal tubes, laryngeal mask airway and cuffed oropharyngeal airway

For children under 7-8 years of age the use of uncuffed tracheal tubes is generally recommended. Recently, cuffed tracheal tubes have been proposed for young children [28]. The advantage of cuffed tubes is claimed to be the lack of the necessity to change to a bigger tube when there is excessive air leakage around the first selected uncuffed tube placed into the trachea, but the majority of the pediatric anaesthesiologists still advocate the use of uncuffed tubes under 7-8 years of age [29].

The use of the laryngeal mask airway (LMA) has increased dramatically in pediatric anaesthesia. This device has become a standard alternative for airway management in many types of surgical cases. It is suggested that LMA can be used for any case in which spontaneous ventilation is planned. In comparison to the face mask, the advantages of the LMA are that the anaesthetist's hands are free for other tasks and there is a decrease of pollution in the operating room environment [30]. LMA for controlled ventilation has been reported in adults and children, but this practice is still controversial because of concerns of possible air insufflation into the stomach and the consequent risk of regurgitation [31]. The trauma of the intubation can certainly be avoided with LMA. This is particularly important when repeated procedures are necessary over a short period of time or in the presence of a reactive airway. Another clear advantage of LMA compared to endotracheal intubation is that a larger bronchoscope may be used for flexible bronchoscopy [32]. However, since the LMA is a supraglottic device, the risk of a laryngospasm is still present and the protection against regurgitation and pulmonary aspiration of gastric content is obviously lacking.

The cuffed oropharyngeal airway (*COPA*) is an oral airway with an inflatable cuff around it and an adapter at its proximal end for connection to the anaesthesia circuit [33]. Even if there are no pediatric sizes available, the 8-cm size has been used in small children. The possible advantages over the use of the LMA are not yet clear and more research is needed to establish the role of this new device in children. The COPA has also been used as an aid for fiberoptic intubation [34].

References

1. Bouchut JC, Dubois R, Foussat M et al (2001) Evaluation of caudal anaesthesia performed in conscious ex-premature infants for inguinal herniotomies. Pediatr Anaesth 11: 55-58
2. Busoni P, Sarti A (1987) Sacral intervertebral epidural block. Anesthesiology 67:993-995
3. Lerman J. Sikik N, Kleinman S et al (1994) The pharmacology of sevoflurane in infants and children. Anesthesiology 80:814-824
4. Ariffin SA, Whyte JA, Malins AF et al (1997) Comparison of induction and recovery between sevoflurane and halothane supplementation of anaesthesia in children undergoing outpatient dental extractions. Br J Anaesth 78:157-159
5. Brown K, Aun C, Stocks J et al (1998) A comparison of the respiratory effects of sevoflurane and halothane in infants and young children. Anesthesiology 89:86-92
6. Eger EI 2d, Ionescu P, Laster MJ et al (1997) Baralyme dehydration increases and soda lime dehydration decreses the concentration of compound A resulting from sevoflurane degradation in a standard anesthetic circuit. Anesth Analg 85: 892-898
7. Komatsu H, Taje S, Endo S et al (1994) Electrical seizure during sevoflurane anaesthesia in two pediatric patients with epilepsy. Anesthesiology 81:1535-1537
8. Mazurek AJ, Przybylo HJ, Martini DR et al (1999) Emergence patterns following sevoflurane and halothane anesthesia in children. Anesthesiology 91: A 1299
9. Mannion D, Casey W, Doherty P (1998) Desflurane in paediatric anaesthesia. Pediatric Anaesthesia 4: 301-306
10. Reber A, Wetzel SG, Schnabel K et al (1999) Effect of combined mouth closure and chin lift on upper airway dimensions during routine magnetic resonance imaging in pediatric patients sedated with propofol. Anesthesiology 90:1617-1623
11. Habre W, Sims C (1997) Propofol anaesthesia and vomiting after myringoplasty in children. Anaesthesia 52:544-546
12. Harling DW, Harrison DA, Dorman T et al (1997) A comparison of thiopental-isoflurane

anaesthesia vs. propofol infusion in children having repeat minor haematological procedures. Paediatr Anaesth 7:19-23
13. Bahndla HP, Smith DE, Kiernman MP (1997) Laryngeal mask airway facilitated fiberoptic broncoscopy in infants. Can J Anaesth 44:1242-1247
14. Strickland RA, Murray MJ (1995) Fatal metabolic acidosis in a pediatric patient receiving an infusion of propofol in the intensive care unit: Is there a relationship ? Crit Care Med 23: 405-409
5. Parke TJ, Stevens JE, Rice AS et al (1992) Metabolic acidosis and fatal myocardial failure after propofol infusion in children: Five case reports. Br Med J 305: 613-616
16. Nottermann DA (1997) Sedation with intravenous midazolam in the pediatric intensive care unit. Clin Pediatr 36: 449-454
17. Tolia V, Fleming SL, Kaufman RE (1990) Randomized, double blind trial of midazolam and diazepam for endoscopic sedation in children. Dev Pharmacol Ther 14:141-147
18. Scholz J, Steifath M, Schulz M (1996) Clinical pharmacokinetics of alfentanil, fentanyl and sufentanil: An update. Clin Pharmacokinet 31:275-292
19. Lynn AM (1996) Remifentanil: The pediatric anaesthetist's opiate ? Paediatr Anaesth 6:433-435
20. Goudsouzian NG (1995) Recent changes in the package insert for succinylcholine chloride: Should this drug be contraindicated for routine use in children? Anesth Analg 80: 207-208
21. Goudsouzian NG (2001) Muscle relaxants in children. In: Coté CJ, Todres ID, Ryan JF, Goudsouzian NG (eds) A Practice of Anesthesia for Infants and Children. WB Saunders Company, Philadelphia, pp196-215
22. Mazurek AJ, Rae B, Hann S et al (1998) Rocuronium versus succinylcholine: Are they equally effective during rapid-sequence induction of anesthesia ? Anesth Analg 87:1259-1262
23. Meretoja OA, Wirtavuori K, Taivainen T et al (1996) Time course of potentiation of mivacurium y halothane and isoflurane in children. Br J Anaesth 76: 235-238
24. Belmont MR, Lien CA, Quessy S et al (1995) The clinical pharmacology of 51W89 in patients receiving nitrous oxide/opioid/barbiturate anesthesia. Anesthesiology 82:1139-1145
25. Thomas JM, Schug SA (1999) Recent advances in local anesthetics: Long acting amide enantiomers and continuous infusions. Clin Pharmacokinet 36:67-83
26. Markham A, Fauls D (1996) Ropivacaine: A review of its pharmacology and therapeutics use in regional anesthesia. Drugs 52: 429-449
27. Ivani G, Lampugnani E, Torre M et al (1998) Comparison of ropivacaine with bupivacaine for paediatric caudal block. Br J Anaesth 81:247-248
28. Tu HN, Saidi N, Leiutaud T at al (1999) Nitrous oxide increases endotracheal cuff pressure and the incidence of tracheal lesions in anesthetized patients. Anesth Analg 89:189-190
29. Wheeler M, Coté JC, Todres ID (2001) Pediatric Airway. In: Coté CJ, Todres ID, Ryan JF, Goudsouzian NG (eds) A Practice of Anesthesia for Infants and Children. WB Saunders Company, Philadelphia, pp 79-120
30. O'Hare K, Kerr WJ (1998) The laryngeal mask as an antipollution device. Anaesthesia 53:51-54
31. Ismail-Zade IA, Vanner RG (1996) Regurgitation and aspiration of gastric contents in a child during general anaesthesia using the laryngeal mask airway. Pediatr Anaesth 6:325-328
32. Bandhla HP, Smith DE, Kiernan MP (1997) Laryngeal mask airway facilitated fiberoptic bronchoscopy in infants Can J Anaesth 44:1242-1247
33. Brimacombe J, Berry A (1998) The cuffed oropharyngeal airway for spontaneous ventilation anaesthesia. Clinical appraisal in 100 patients. Anaesthesia 53:1074-1079
34. Greenberg RS, Kay NH (1999) Cuffed oropharyngeal airway (COPA) as an adjunt to fiberoptic tracheal intubation. Br J Anaesth 82:395-398

Pain Management in Children

P. Busoni, A. Messeri

In a 1983 report Mather and Mackie stated that children were particularly likely to be denied management which satisfactorily relieved pain [1]. More recently, it has been reported that, even though improvements have been obtained, it is still a challenge to optimize the postoperative pain management of children [2]. Children tend to receive less analgesia than adults and the drugs are often discontinued sooner. Therefore management of pain in children tends to be inadequate in many circumstances. It is not simply true that potent analgesics are dangerous when used in children because of the risk of side effects and addiction. Furthermore, neonates and young children are particularly unfortunate, even if there is no evidence to support the idea that pain is less intense due to their developing nervous system. Pain sensitivity of neonates may be more profound than that of older individuals because their nervous system may be less effective at blocking painful stimuli than that of adults. [3]

It is now well established that failure to manage pain adequately can have immediate deleterious physiological, biochemical, and behavioural effects. These include significant fluctuation in heart rate, blood pressure, intra-cranial pressure, blood oxygen levels, and stress hormone levels, as well as increase in sleep disturbances, agitation and crying. There is also growing evidence that unmanaged pain can have longer-term consequences.

As with all pain, successful management depends upon identification and treatment of all the contributing factors, in particular fear and anxiety. Pain assessment presents a major challenge, especially in those patients who cannot explain how they feel and who cannot understand the relationship between the treatment and the pain. Several attempts have been made to develop observational scales that could be useful in assessing pain. The Children's Hospital of Eastern Ontario Pain Scale (CHEOPS) is an example, and some validation data suggest it is useful for assessing pain by observing behaviour [4].

The Smiley Analog Scale consists of a series of faces with various expressions ranging from sad to happy. The child is asked to select a face that depicts how he or she feels. A Color scale has also been used with younger children, where the child selects a color to indicate the intensity of pain. These systems of patient reports have some usefulness, depending on the age of the child, but are not useful when the child has acute pain.

Self reporting becomes easier when children are 6 years of age and older, where a Visual Analog Scale (VAS) can be used. This technique uses a 10 cm line, with the words "No Pain" on one end and "Worst Pain Possible" on the other end. The patient is asked to make a mark on the line indicating the intensity of pain. A variation of this technique asks the patient to rate pain intensity by selecting a number from 0-10, 0 being no pain and 10 indicating the worst possible pain. However, in many circumstances, assessing simple factors such as whether or not the children are asleep, crying, relaxed, tense or are responding to their parents may be useful to create a cumulative pain score for the purpose of studying postoperative pain management techniques.

Management of pain in children needs to be handled more actively than adults. Greater efforts should be made to anticipate pain. Children cannot be relied upon to ask for analgesia as an adult might do. It may be better to establish a schedule of regular analgesia. The route of administration will depend on the drug to be used, the severity of the pain and the likely side effects. Drugs are best taken orally if possible but the rectal route may be more tolerable if vomiting is a problem. The parental route (by injection) should be used if the drug selected can only be given by that method or where other method has failed. The intravenous route should be used rather than Intramuscular injections because the injection itself can be very painful.

Perioperative and postoperative pain management

Available local anaesthetic creams can be applied under an occlusive dressing to produce an anaesthesia for the skin up to an hour. These may enable painless placement of venous catheters or allow infiltration of the area with local anaesthetic. These creams should not be used rectally, directly on the wound or on mucous membranes. EMLA should be used with caution in infants under 3 months of age or in patients who are taking sulphonamides or other methaemoglobin inducing medications.

A lignocaine gel can be used to provide analgesia following circumcision and after repair of lacerations. Application of bupivacaine and adrenaline on the open wound towards the end of surgery provides excellent analgesia. Topical local anaesthesia, such as eye drops, can be used to provide analgesia following ophthalmic surgery.

Many procedures associated with the relief of pain can be painful. The performances of regional blockades, wound infiltration and the placement of intravenous or subcutaneous lines and catheters may be carried out without discomfort or resistance whilst the patient is anaesthetized. Infiltration of a local anaesthetic agent into the wound before wakening can reduce pain for long periods. Bupivacaine instillation before closure of small wounds is also very effective. A continuous infusion of 0.25% bupivacaine through a small cannula at a rate of 1-3 mLs /hour provides a simple, safe and effective method of analgesia at the donor site of the skin graft or iliac crest bone graft.

Subcutaneous injection of local anaesthetic is as painful as a bee sting. This is due to the low pH, which is necessary for the long-term preservation of the anaesthetic solution. Adding 1 cm of bicarbonate to the anaesthetic solution makes the infiltration painless.

Regional anaesthesia undertaken while the child is under general anaesthesia can give prolonged control of pain and avoid or reduce the use of opioids. Ilioinguinal and iliohypogastric nerve blocks are excellent methods for analgesia after hernia repair and orchidopexy. The procedure is easy, and 0.4 mL/kg of 25% bupivacaine will provide long-lasting pain relief after surgery. Circumcision and hypospadias operations may be carried out with nerve block of the penis.

Regional anaesthetic techniques with either a caudal or lumbar epidural catheter may also be used for postoperative pain control. The use of epidural narcotics has become an increasingly frequent technique because it provides a long-lasting analgesia.

Non-Steroidal Anti-Inflammatory Drugs (NSAIDs) along with local anaesthesia are the mainstay of postoperative pain relief among the paediatric population. However, use of these agents is not recommended for children under one year of age due to the possibility of immature renal function and hepatic metabolism. Aspirin should not be given to children under 12 years of age because of the association with Reye's syndrome. Probably the most used NSAID in children is ibuprofen. This is available as a suspension or a syrup and should be given up to a dose of 20 mg/kg/day. Diclofenac is also popular and is given up to 3 mg/kg/day.

Paracetamol is a very safe and effective analgesic in children including infants and neonates. It can be given as an oral suspension in a dose of 15 mg/kg to a maximum of 60 mg/kg in 24 hours. Slightly higher doses (20 mg/kg) are needed if this drug is used rectally as absorption is less reliable.

Opioids are the mainstay of management in most forms of acute severe pain, such as postoperative pain, post traumatic pain etc. The term *opioid* is used to describe this group of drugs whose action is "morphine-like". *Opiate* refers to phenanthrene alkaloids, such as morphine and codeine, which are derived from opium, an extract of poppy seeds [5]. Other synthetic opioid drugs, such as meperidine, methadone, and the phenylpiperidines (fentanyl and its analogues) are structurally different from morphine, though acting in similar way. The term narcotic should be avoided because of its negative associations and imprecision.

In neonates the opioid clearance is reduced. Children who are 6 months old are no more susceptible to respiratory depression than adults but in children the titration against the pain is even more important.

Codeine is effective by mouth for mild to moderate pain and is usually taken in combination with paracetamol. This drug is not suitable for intravenous use as it can produce severe drops in blood pressure and apnoea. Doses of codeine syrup ranging from 0.5-1 mg/kg can be given orally or by intramuscular injection every 4 hours. As a suppository 1 mg/kg of codeine can be given every 4 hours.

Morphine is the drug of choice for children who are inpatients. Morphine given intravenously is the prefered route, however other routes can be used. A dose of approximately 0.05 mg/kg is effective in many patients for providing pain relief. Side effects (as with all opioids) include itching, urinary retention, histamine release, nausea or vomiting .

The recommended oral doses of morphine range from 200-400μ/kg taken every hour. Subcutaneous or intramuscular routes consists of 100-150 μ/kg taken every 4 hours. Intravenous doses of 50-100μ/kg are taken over a 30 minute period as a loading dose and then 5-40 μ/kg taken every hour.

Numerous synthetic drugs, such as fentanyl, sufentanil, and alfentanil are now available, although these agents generally are not labelled for use in small children. These drugs are advantagous because they are quite potent, and are more receptor specific than older opioids, possibly causing less side effects. Synthetic drugs do not release histamine to the same extent as morphine and meperidine. Since they are short acting, they are given by continuous infusion for long term pain relief.

Children as young as five years of age can use PCA satisfactorily. This is one of the rare circumstances where a background infusion may be of some benefit, as children rarely remember preoperative instructions immediately upon waking.

PCA doses consist of: background infusion with 4μ/kg of morphine taken every hour. If needed, a repeated dose of 10-20 μ/kg is given as well as a 5-15 minute lock-out. A four hour dose limit is advisable and should be calculated after the patient's response is assessed (usually around 400 μ/kg).

The use of methadone is recommended during postoperative pain relief to avoid repeated intramuscular injection. The recommended dose of methadone is 0.2 mg/kg [6].

Procedural pain

The management of acute pain and anxiety in children undergoing therapeutic and diagnostic procedures outside the operating room has substantially developed in the last years. [7] Skilled and well trained personnel is mandatory. Monitoring is also an important part of management. The most effective monitoring during sedation is close, continuous observation of the patient. Patients are at highest risk for complication during the first 5 to 10 minutes after the intravenous administration of medication and during the period immediately after the end of the procedure [7]. All the patients must be monitored until they are no longer at risk for cardiorespiratory depression.

A wide range of shorter-acting agents with multiple routes of administration now available are:

1. *Chloral Hydrate* (PO: 25-100 mg/kg: repeated dose of 25-50 mg/kg after 30). It is mainly used during MR or CT procedures, when only an immobile child is what is needed. In fact, this drug has no analgesic properties. Glycinemia without ketosis is a strict contraindication.
2. *Midazolam* (IV: 0.05-0.1 mg/kg; PO: 0.5-0.75 mg/kg). It is commonly used for sedation in children during procedures. The effects can be reversed with the antagonist *flumazenil* (0.02 mg/kg dose)
3. *Barbiturates* (Pentobarbital 1-6 mg/kg). They are widely regarded as the drugs of choice to facilitate diagnostic imaging in children three years of age or older.
4. *Fentanyl* (IV: 1.0 μg/kg/dose). It is preferred because its action has faster onset and shorter duration and limited histamine release.
5. *Ketamine* (IV: 1- 1.5 mg/kg dose slowly over a period of 1-2 min. IM: 4-5 mg/kg). It preserves upper-airway muscular tone and protective airway reflexes. Dysphoric emergences reactions are rarely noted in children.

Finally, non pharmacological therapy may be helpful in children. It includes distraction techniques, watching videos, music and hypnotic therapy.

Chronic pain management

Chronic pain in children can be caused by a number of factors, although cancer is the most frequent cause of severe pain [8]. The cancer mass itself can produce pain by tissue distention or infiltration. Inflammation due to infection, necrosis, or obstruction can also cause pain. Bone pain in children with cancer is caused by infiltration of the periosteum, pathologic fractures, tumour growth of surrounding tissues, or stimulation of the nerve endings in the endosteum by chemical agents released from the diseased bone. These chemical agents include prostaglandin, bradykinin, substance P and histamine. Bone marrow infiltration with malignant cells causes pain described as dull, aching, or penetrating, and can be generalized to one or more areas, or localized. Tissue distention, infiltration or inflammation may cause a generalized dull, throbbing pain. Visceral organ pain may be poorly localized because the nociceptors that transmit pain messages back to the brain are not well established. Obstruction of major organs can cause the onset of acute, severe pain. For example, tumours found in the retroperitoneum may result in obstruction of a ureter, causing acute onset of sharp, localized pain that is similar to the pain caused by appendicitis. Children with nerve invasion often experience weakness, numbness, or paresthesias. A child with a spinal cord tumour may complain of muscle spasms, back pain and heaviness in the lower extremities. These children may also develop urinary retention or incontinence [9].

Cancer treatment related pain in children occurs from the three commonly used treatment modalities: surgery, chemotherapy, and radiation therapy. Children undergoing surgery for excision of a primary tumour experience postoperative pain and are at risk for secondary infection that may lead to additional pain. Chemotherapeutic agents can also be a cause of pain during treatment [10].

Vincristine, a plant alkaloid, is most commonly associated with peripheral neuropathies, characterized by dysesthetic pain that presents as a burning sensation, causing pain upon light contact with the skin . Mucositis is a common side effect of chemotherapy, often seen in children receiving anthracyclines (i.e., daunorubicin), alkylating agents (i.e., cyclophosphamide), antimetabolites (i.e., methotrexate), and epipodophyllotoxins (i.e., VP-16), and after receiving preparative regimens for bone marrow transplantation. Radiation therapy to the head and neck area is associated with severe mucositis in children. Post radiation pain may occur in certain body regions, caused by fibrosis or the scarring of connective tissues and secondary injury to the nerve structures. Other treatment-related side effects that cause pain include: skin reactions from radiation therapy; abdominal pain from vomiting, diarrhoea, or constipation; and infections such as, typhlitis, cellulitis, or sinusitis [11].

The management of chronic pain includes a pharmacological treatment [12] always combined with a non-pharmacological approach.

Pharmacological treatment

NSAIDs / Acetaminophen

Non-steroidal anti-inflammatory drugs (NSAIDs) have analgesic, anti-pyretic, and anti-inflammatory activity. NSAIDs act peripherally to provide analgesic effects by interfering with the synthesis of prostaglandin, through the inhibition of cyclooxygenase (COX). There are two isoenzymes of COX; COX-1 and COX-2. The COX-1 isoform is expressed primarily in the kidney, gastrointestinal tract and on platelets. In contrast, the COX-2 isoform is found in low levels in tissues, but is induced during inflammation. By selectively inhibiting the COX-2 isoform, prostaglandin pathways are influenced, decreasing pain and inflammation and avoiding the toxicities of the inhibition of COX-1. Most NSAIDs are non selective inhibitors of COX.

There are now two selective COX-2 inhibitors available. However, little is known about the side effects and the paediatric data for dosing is limited.

The side effects of nonselective NSAIDs include decreased platelet aggregation, gastric irritation, and the potential for renal toxicity with long term use. Children with low platelet counts or who are neutropenic should be monitored carefully when taking nonselective NSAIDs for pain relief. The nonselective NSAID choline magnesium trisalicylate does not interfere with platelet aggregation, but its use should be avoided in children with platelet counts less than 20,000 or with active bleeding [9]. Acetaminophen has similar analgesic and antipyretic effects to the NSAIDs, but does not provide an anti-inflammatory effect.

Acetaminophen does not affect platelet function or irritate the stomach, but hepatic toxicity can occur with high doses of acetaminophen (i.e., >75 mg/kg/day or 4 g/day).

Acetaminophen preparations are available with the opioid drugs of codeine, oxycodone and hydrocodone. These combination drugs are beneficial for mild to moderate pain that does not respond to acetaminophen or NSAIDs alone. When using acetaminophen in combination with codeine or hydrocodone, it is important not to exceed the maximum daily dose of the acetaminophen component of the drug. If pain increases or persists beyond the maximum dosage of a combination preparation, switching to a stronger opioid agent would be the next step in managing a child's pain. NSAIDs are limited to a ceiling dose when increasing the dose only produces toxicity and no pain relief.

Opioids

Opioids bind with certain receptors (Mu, Kappa, Delta) in the Central nervous system (CNS) and peripheral tissues to provide analgesic effects. Mu receptors are located in the CNS and provide central analgesia, but also play a role in the development of respiratory depression, physical dependence and withdrawal symptoms. The greatest concentration of kappa receptors are located in the cerebral cortex and substantia gelatinosa of the dorsal horn. Kappa receptors are responsible for the level of analgesia in the spinal cord and the brain, but have less of a role in physical dependence and withdrawal. Delta receptors are concentrated in the substantia gelatinosa of the dorsal horn and have a primary effect upon spinal and supraspinal analgesia.

Mu-agonist drugs are the most commonly used class of opioids, and include drugs such as morphine, fentanyl, and codeine. The analgesic effect of these drugs have no maximum dosage and dosing is limited only by the presence of unmanageable side effects [13]. Meperidine also falls into the class of Mu-agonists. However, meperidine is not recommend as an analgesic drug, due to its short duration of action and the accumulation of a toxic metabolite *normeperidine*, which causes undesirable CNS side effects, including seizures, at low doses of the drug. *Meperidine should not be used for chronic pain control in children.* Opioids can be given orally, rectally, as subcutaneous or intravenous infusions, intramuscularly, transdermally, and directly into the CNS via epidural/caudal/intrathecal injection, depending on the drug. The most common side effects of opioid analgesia in children are constipation, sedation, pruritus, and nausea or vomiting. Respiratory depression is the most frequently cited concern of health care providers although it has a relatively rare occurrence. The risk of respiratory depression decreases significantly when children are on opioid analgesics for prolonged periods of time. When mild respiratory suppression occurs it is easily managed by awakening the child, giving oxygen, and decreasing further opioid doses by 25%.

Non-pharmacological pain interventions

Non pharmacological interventions in the management of pain have been found to be highly effective for some children and for some procedures [14]. These techniques are easy to learn and should be used when possible to give the child some control in the management of pain. The examples given for distraction, muscle relaxation, and guided imagery are easy techniques to learn and can be used with young children. Additional interventions requiring specialized training include therapeutic touch and acupressure. However, nonpharmacologic interventions are an adjunct to, not a substitute for, pharmacological interventions.

Distraction

Distraction is used to focus the child's attention away from the pain. For children, simple distraction techniques can be very effective in decreasing pain. Simple measures such as looking at books, blowing bubbles, and counting are favorite distraction techniques for children. Touch can be an important distraction technique by stroking, patting and rocking infants as well as children who are in distress.

Deep breathing is the easiest technique to use with young children. The child is instructed to take a deep breath through the nose and blow it out through the mouth. Making a conscious effort to count the child's respiration focuses attention on the breathing. For school aged children, asking them to hold their breath during a painful procedure transfers their focus to their breathing and not on the procedure. Asking children to "blow away their pain" has also been discussed as an effective distraction technique [15].

Parents should be taught distraction measures and encouraged to hold their children for comfort as much as possible. Parent coaching gives them a way to participate in decreasing their child's pain and also may provide some benefit in decreasing parent anxiety and worry.

Guided imagery

Guided imagery engages the child by focusing on a pleasant activity, providing distraction from the pain, or changing the perception of the painful experience. Imagery is used to give the child the opportunity to imagine being in a more pleasant situation. Effective use of imagery involves all of the child's senses. When imagining a favorite place the child is asked to feel the warmth all around, see the colors, smell the odors, and hear the sounds. This helps the child create a clear scene in their mind. It is important to stress that every child needs a favorite place to go that is safe. This safe place provides a means of escape. Children often like to imagine they are watching a favourite television show or movie. The child can be involved in this type of imagery by asking him to discuss what is happening on the television show like a cartoon. He can sometimes imagine being a particular character in the cartoon.

References

1. Mather L, Mackie J (1983) The incidence of postoperative pain in children. Pain 15:271-282
2. Kart T, van der Laan K, Crombach J et al (1996) Postoperative pain management in children has been improved, but can be further optimized. Eur J Padiatr Surg 6:259-264
3. Golianu B, Krane EJ, Galloway Ks et al (2000) Pediatric acute pain management. Pediatr Clin North Am 47:559-587
4. McGrath PJ, Johnson G, Goodman JT et al (1985). CHEOPS: A behavioural scale for rating postoperative pain in children. Advances in Pain Research and Therapy 9:395-402
5. Martin WR (1984) Pharmacology of opioids. Pharm Review 35:285-323
6. Berde CB, Stehna NF, Holzman RS et al (1987) Pharmacokinetics of methadone in children and adolescents in the postoperative period. Anesthesiology 67:A519
7. Krauss B, Green SM (2000) Sedation and analgesia for procedures in children. NEJM 13: 938-945
8. APS – American Pain Society (1999) Principles of analgesic use in the treatment of acute pain and cancer pain, (4 th ed.). Glenview, IL, American Pain Society.

9. Collins JJ and Berde CB (1997) Management of cancer pain in children. In PA Pizzo and DG Poplack (Eds), Principles and Practice of Pediatric Oncology, 3rd ed, (pp. 1183-1199). Philadelphia: Lippincott-Raven.
10. Foley KM (1996) Controlling the pain of cancer. Sci Am 275(3),164-165.
11. McCaffery M and Pasero C (1999) Pain: A Clinical Manual, 2nd ed. St. Louis: Mosby.
12. Taketomo CK, Hodding, JH and Kraus DM (1998) Pediatric dosage handbook, 4th ed, 1997-1998.Hudson, Ohio: Lexi-Comp.
13. Leahy S, Hockenberry-Eaton M and Sigler-Price K (1994) Clinical management of pain in children with cancer: selected approaches and innovative strategies. Cancer Practice 2(1), 37-45.
14. Broome ME, Bates TA, Lillis PP and McGahee TW (1990) Children's medical fears, coping behaviors, and pain perceptions during a lumbar puncture. Onc Nurs Forum 17(3), 361-367.
15. French GM, Painter EC, and Coury DL (1994) Blowing away shot pain: A technique for pain management during immunization. Pediatrics, 93(3), 384-388.

How Can Anesthetists Modify Stress Response during Perioperative Period?

V. Novak-Jankovič, V. Paver-Eržen

During his daily routine, the anesthetist as a specialist of perioperative medicine deals with injured and surgical patients who are under huge stress. The essential task of an anesthetist is not only providing anesthesia and analgesia, but maintaining vital functions, such as circulation and respiration. The anesthetist has to be familiar with the pathophysiology of the neuroendocrine stress response to trauma and surgery and also with the drugs and anesthetic techniques that can diminish any negative consequences. Stress is defined as a state of disharmony or threatened homeostasis provoked by psychological, environmental, or physiological stress [1]. Stress response or general adaptive response refers to the biochemical and physiological adaptation made by an organism, presumably to allow for improved survival after injury [2]. Stress response is adaptive for injury "in the wild". Stress response developed allowing injured animals to survive by metabolizing their own stored body fuels [3]. However stress response after surgical injury is potentially harmful to the patient and can result in a poor postoperative outcome [4, 5].

The pathophysiology of the stress response

Surgical injury, trauma or infection of a tissue induce an acute inflammatory reaction with excessive mediator release. This cumulative homeostatic process is known as inflammation, and the immediate set of reactions induced is known as the acute-phase response. Activated macrophages release cytokines that initiate the accumulation of inflammatory cells. The liver is responsible for determining the level of essential metabolites provided to the organism during the critical stages of stress, such as acute-phase plasma proteins. They include the increase of C-reactive protein, fibrinogen, α_2-macroglobulin, and the decrease of albumin and transferrin. The acute-phase response subsides in 24 – 48 h, and within a few days the organism returns to normal function. However, this normal pathway can be prolonged and can convert to the chronic phase of inflammation [6]. The response to injury is initiated by somatic and autonomic nerve impulses and the release of cytokines – activated messengers of the immune system. After major surgery the main cytokines released are interleukin-1, tumor necrosis factor-α, and interleukin-6. The blood-brain barrier is lacking in the area of the preoptic nucleus of the hypothalamus, and the cytokines therefore pass from the circulation to the brain [7]. Within minutes of an acute stress, corticotropin-releasing factor (CRF) appears in the paraventricular nucleus and is secreted through the hypothalamic-pituitary-hypophyseal portal venous plexus to the anterior pituitary gland. CRF then induces secretion of proopiomelanocortin, which is subsequently cleaved to form adrenocorticotropic hormone (ACTH). ACTH stimulates the adrenal gland. Activation of the hypothalamic–pituitary–adrenal axis occurs with consecutive release of stress hormones ACTH, human growth hormone (HGH), antidiuretic hormone (ADH), β-endorphin, prolactin, cortisol, and glucagon. During major surgical stress, a pulsatile release of CRF occurs [8]. CRF affects the sympathetic nucleus in the brain stem locus coeruleus, so sympatho-adrenal activation occurs with an increased secretion of catecholamines from the adrenal medulla and a release of noradrenaline from presynaptic nerve terminals. The net effect of the neuroendocrine response to surgery is an increased secretion of the catabolic hormones. Cortisol and the catecholamines increase glycogenolysis and gluconeogenesis; peripheral utilization of glucose is decreased, so blood glucose concentrations increase. Increased cortisol concentrations stimulate protein catabolism. Triglycerides are metabolized by lypolysis to glycerol and free fatty acids. Lypolysis is stimulated by catecholamines, HGH, and cortisol. ADH stimulates water retention and aldosterone stimulates sodium reabsorption [4, 9]. Corticosteriods, endorphins, and catecholamines in general suppress immune system functions. Corticosteroids have anti-inflammatory and anti-allergic effects by decreasing metabolism of arachidonic acid, decreasing cytokine and immunoglobulin production, and decreasing lymphocyte count. A bidirectional communication, "cross talk", exists between the immune and neuroendocrine system [10]. Hormonal, metabolic, and immune stress responses can result in a poor postoperative outcome.

The influence of surgical procedures of the neuroendocrine stress response

The more invasive the surgical procedure, the greater the release of stress hormones occurs. A ninefold increase of adrenaline in arterial concentrations was found in response to cardiopulmonary bypass in men [11]. In orthotopic liver transplantation, β-endorphin release was increased [12]. Postoperative congestive heart failure and renal insufficiency are associated with greater intraoperative catecholamine levels during abdominal and thoraco-abdominal aortic reconstruction [13]. Hormonal and metabolic responses to cardiac surgical operations in neonates are extreme, and are associated with a high hospital mortality rate [5]. Undesirable aspects of the stress response to surgery can be minimized by the use of certain anesthetic techniques.

The effects of anesthesia on the stress response to surgery

General anesthesia

High doses of opioids can reduce or prevent the hormonal and metabolic responses to the stress of surgery [14]. Morphine administered intravenously in large doses prior to skin incision inhibits the initial endocrine metabolic response to open heart surgery [15]. In a randomized trial, preterm babies undergoing ligation of a patent ductus arteriosus had lower concentrations of stress hormones and a lower incidence of circulatory and metabolic complications in the fentanyl group than the non-fentanyl group [16]. In cardiac surgery, the neonates who received high-dose sufentanil had a significantly reduced concentration of stress hormones and a decreased incidence of sepsis, metabolic acidosis, disseminated intravascular coagulation, and postoperative deaths compared with the halotan morphine group [17]. High-dose fentanyl anesthesia prevented the increases in blood glucose, plasma cortisol, and plasma HGH concentrations prior to cardiopulmonary bypass [18].

It has been demonstrated that etomidate-induced suppression of cortisol biosynthesis results in a blockade of 11-β-hydroxylase in the adrenal gland, mediated by the imidazole radical of etomidate. Cortisol and aldosterone are depressed by etomidate, but the clinical relevance is minimal after a single bolus injection [19]. The blockade of the adrenal cortex by chronic use of etomidate is dangerous, and has been associated with increased mortality in intensive care units [20]. In oral premedication, midazolam has significantly suppressed the adrenaline and cortisol concentrations in patients undergoing intraocular surgery [21]. It was shown that propofol produces a fall in the ACTH response to electroconvulsive therapy when compared with thiopentone, possibly via a reduction in central noradrenergic activation [22]. In patients undergoing coronary artery bypass graft, propofol infusion significantly reduced cortisol, adrenaline, and noradrenaline concentrations [23]. Ketamine used as the sole anesthetic agent significantly activated the sympatho-adrenergic system with increased plasma concentrations of catecholamines [24]. Adams et al. [25] demonstrated that inhalational anesthetic agents halothane, enflurane and isoflurane can in a similar manner reduce plasma levels of adrenaline, noradrenaline, ADH, ACTH, and cortisol in patients undergoing orthopedic surgery [25]. Sevoflurane anesthesia has been recommended for removal of insulinoma because it is considered to suppress the spontaneous release of insulin [26]. $Alpha_2$ adrenoceptor agonists have a number of neuroendocrine effects and can diminish the stress response to trauma and surgery [27, 28]. They inhibit the secretion of ACTH and reduce the secretion of cortisol, catecholamines, vasopressin, and other hormones during surgery [29-31]. They can also reduce the postoperative adrenergic response to surgery [32, 33]. They act as centrally acting sympatholytic agents and inhibit the stress responses mediated by the sympathetic nervous system. $Alpha_2$ adrenoceptor agonists inhibit presynaptic release of noradrenaline in the spinal dorsal horn. They depress the activity of the neurons and the release of substance P [34]. The use of the $alpha_2$ adrenoceptor agonist: clonidine, dexmedetomidine and mivazerol in every day anesthetic practice is becoming more and more popular because they induce anxiolysis, analgesia, improve intraoperative hemodynamic stability, and reduce anesthetic requirement [35].

In our study we have demonstrated that clonidine can modulate the immune stress response to thoracic surgery. It decreased the total number of leukocytes and segmented neutrophil and lymphocyte count at the end of surgery. The effects were more pronounced when clonidine was given epidurally than intravenously [36].

Regional anesthesia

Blockade of afferent neural impulses from the site of surgical injury by epidural analgesia can suppress the endocrine and metabolic stress response to surgery [37]. High thoracic epidural anesthesia combined with general anesthesia attenuates postoperative myocardial ischemia and the perioperative stress response to cardiopulmonary bypass and cardiac surgery [38]. Combined epidural and light general anesthesia decreased cortisol and β-endorphin levels, and thereby attenuated the stress response in open heart surgery patients [39]. Thoracic epidural anesthesia depressed the sympathetic response, presumably by blocking afferent sympathetic pathways. However it did not attenuate an increase in cortisol, one of the hypothalamic-pituitary-adrenal stress hormones during carbon dioxide laparoscopic cholecystectomy. This action may be due to the inability of epidural anesthesia to block phrenic nerves that can convey noxious surgical stimulation to the central nervous system [40]. Epidural analgesia extending from T4 to S5 with bupivacaine reduced the cortisol and metabolic stress response to subumbilical surgery [41], but not to upper abdominal surgery [42]. Thoracic epidural blockade failed to suppress adenocortical response in upper abdominal and thoracic surgery, since the vagal afferent pathway is not affected [43]. Epidural analgesia has prevented postoperative lymphopenia and granulocytosis in women undergoing abdominal hysterectomy [44].

Surgical outcome

There has been a great deal of interest in the modification of the stress response with respect to the potential beneficial effects on surgical outcome [3]. The first study on this topic suggesting that postoperative epidural opioid use may decrease patient mortality was by Yeager et al [45] in 1987. The results of this study showed that intraoperative epidural anesthesia with local anesthetics followed by postoperative epidural narcotic analgesia in high-risk patients significantly decreased patient mortality, cardiac failure, infections, hospital and physician costs. The study did not address the question of whether the improved outcome was the result of intraoperative or postoperative factors [45]. A second study confirming the role of epidural opioid analgesia in improving outcome after major vascular surgery was reported by Tuman et al [46] The rates of cardiovascular, thrombotic, infectious, and overall postoperative complications, as well as duration of intensive care unit stay, were significantly reduced in patients who had received general anesthesia combined with postoperative epidural analgesia compared with those who had received general anesthesia with on-demand narcotic analgesia [46]. Raggi et al [47] have shown that a combination of the epidural technique using local anesthetics intraoperatively and morphine postoperatively offers many advantages. These benefits include inhibition of the surgical stress response, decreased cardiorespiratory depression, blood loss, intubation time, and pulmonary infection, thromboembolism, hyperglycemia, hypertensive response, nitrogen sparing, prevention of immunosuppression, and enabled earlier ambulation and hospital discharge [47].

A retrospective analysis of patients who underwent coronary artery bypass graft surgery has shown that combined general and thoracic epidural anesthesia had a lower incidence of arrhythmias, respiratory complications, and decreased time to tracheal extubation compared with the general anesthesia group [48].

Patients having received combined general and epidural anesthesia emerged from anesthesia faster, with less pain on awakening, had better psychomotoric functions, and were less drowsy in the early postoperative period compared with general anesthesia [49].

Mortality was significantly lower in the subarachnoid anesthesia group by 14 days after repair of fractured neck of femur compared with the general anesthesia group. However, at the end of 2 months the mortality rate was similar in both groups [50].

Despite evidence that regional anesthesia may be associated with fewer perioperative complications than general anesthesia, most studies that have compared cardiac outcome after general or regional anesthesia have not shown major differences. Bode et al [51] reported that patients who underwent peripheral vascular surgery were randomly assigned to receive general, epidural, or spinal anesthesia. The choice of anesthesia did not significantly influence cardiac morbidity and overall mortality in that study [51].

Although epidural anesthesia and analgesia may improve the outcome in a high-risk patient population, potential benefits in a low-risk population remain poorly defined, because of the low rate of morbidity in these patient groups. Significant beneficial effects of epidural analgesia have been observed only for intermediate outcomes, not for ultimate patient outcome. Future studies require formation of multicenter study groups and necessitate enrolment of thousands of patients [52].

When individual trials are unable to produce significant results, it is often due to insufficient number of patients. Meta-analyses are a useful tool for combining the data from multiple trials to increase the number of patients. The meta-analyses of Ballantyne et al [53] have shown that epidural opioids compared with systemic opioids result in a significant decrease in the incidence of atelectasis, pulmonary infection, and of pulmonary complications overall.

Regional anesthesia has distinct advantages over general anesthesia in terms of surgical outcome; abdominal surgery has less-prolonged ileus, the incidence of deep venous thrombosis is reduced by regional anesthesia in patients having lower extremity surgery without thromboprophylaxis, the patients with cardiac disease probably do better with the lower catecholamine levels associated with the use of regional anesthesia, pulmonary function is improved by postoperative epidurals in patients having intraabdominal and intrathoracic procedures, etc. However, regional anesthesia is not a panacea, but in the right patients and the right situations it can improve surgical outcome [54].

Early enteral nutrition started not later than 24 h after admission to the intensive care unit has been demonstrated to have a positive effect on intestinal permeability and the development of multiple organ failure in patients with multiple injury [55].

Multimodal approach to control postoperative pathophysiology and rehabilitation

Positive effects of certain anesthetic techniques (e.g., epidural anesthesia and analgesia) in decreasing postoperative morbidity and mortality remain open to professional discussion despite many field research studies supporting their use. A more-complex, multimodal approach to perioperative treatment is widely accepted and recommended by many [56].

The results of Moiniche et al [57] suggest that a combined approach of optimal pain relief with balanced analgesia, enforced early mobilization, and oral feeding may reduce the length of convalescence and hospital stay after colonic operations. Brodner et al [58] demonstrated that recovery after abdominothoracic esophageal resection may be improved by the introduction of intraoperative thoracic epidural analgesia, patient-controlled postoperative epidural analgesia, earlier extubation, and early mobilization of the patient. In this study, patients regained gut function earlier, showed less catabolism, rapid efficient spontaneous ventilation, and with earlier mobilization, a shorter stay in the intensive care unit.

The multi-modal approach to improve postoperative outcome has been proposed. This implies a revision of the entire surgical care program (anesthesia, analgesia, surgical nursing, surgical care), according to recent scientific data [59].

References

1. Black PH (1994) Central nervous system-immune system interactions: psychoneuroendocrinology of stress and its immune consequences. Antimicrob Agents Chemother 38:1-6
2. Speight KL (1993) Perioperative stress response suppression in cardiothoracic surgery. In: Grevlee, Rauck (eds) Pain management in cardiothoracic surgery. Lippincott, Philadelphia, pp 169-199
3. Desborough JP (2000) The stress response to trauma and surgery. Br J Anaesth 85:109-17.
4. Weissman C (1990) The metabolic response to stress: an overview and update. Anesthesiology 73:308-328
5. Anand KJS, Hansen DD, Hickey PR (1990) Hormonal-metabolic stress responses in neonates undergoing cardiac surgery. Anesthesiology 73:661-670
6. Baumann H, Gauldie J (1994) The acute phase response. Immunol Today 15:74-80
7. Black PH (1994) Immune system-central nervous system interactions: effects and immunomodulatory consequences of immune system mediators on the brain. Antimicrob Agents Chemother 38:7-12
8. Calogero AE, Norton JA, Sheppard BC, et al (1992) Pulsatile activation of the hypothalamic-pituitary-adrenal axis during major surgery. Metabolism 41:839-845
9. Bessey PQ, Watters JM, Aoki TT, et al (1984) Combined hormonal infusion simulates the metabolic response to injury. Ann Surg 200:264-281
10. Blalock JE (1989) A molecular basis for bidirectional communication between the immune and neuroendocrine systems. Physiol Rev 69:1-30

11. Reves JG, Karp RB, Buttner EE, et al (1982) Neuronal and adrenomedullary catecholamine release in response to cardiopulmonary bypass in man. Circulation 66:49-55
12. Acosta F, Diaz J, Moreno J, et al (1995) Relationship between β-endorphin release and surgical stress in orthotopic liver transplantation. Transplant Proc 27:2303
13. Roizen MF, Lampe GH, Benefiel DJ, et al (1987) Is increased operative stress associated with worse outcome? Anesthesiology 67:3A
14. Bovill JG, Sebel PS, Stanley TH (1984) Opioid analgesics in anesthesia: with special reference to their use in cardiovascular anesthesia. Anesthesiology 61:731-755
15. Brandt MR, Korshin J, Prange Hansen A, et al (1978) Influence of morphine anesthesia on the endocrine-metabolic response to open-heart surgery. Acta Anaesth Scand 22:400-412
16. Anand KJS, Sippell WG, Aynsley-Green A (1987) Randomised trial of fentanyl anesthesia in preterm babies undergoing surgery: effects on the stress response. Lancet 31:243-247
17. Anand KJS, Phil D, Hickey PR (1992) Halothane-morphine compared with high-dose sufentanil for anesthesia and postoperative analgesia in neonatal cardiac surgery. N Engl J Med 326:1-9
18. Walsh ES, Paterson JL, O'Riordan JBA, et al (1981) Effect of high-dose fentanyl anesthesia on the metabolic and endocrine response to cardiac surgery. Br J Anaesth 53:1155-1165
19. Vanacker B, Wiebalck A, VanAken H, et al (1993) Quality of induction and adrenocortical function. A clinical comparison of etomidate-lipuro and hypnomidate. anesthesist 42:81-89
20. Adams HA, Hempelmann G (1991) The endocrine stress reaction in anesthesia and surgery-origin and significance. Anasthesiol Intensivmed Notfallmed Schmerzther 26:294-305
21. Kiefer RT, Weindler J, Ruprecht KW (1998) The endocrine stress response after oral premedication with low-dose midazolam for intraocular surgery in retrobulbar anesthesia. Eur J Ophthalmol 8:239-245
22. Child CSB (1993) anesthesia and the endocrine response to surgery. Curr Anesth Crit Care 4:13-18
23. Ng A, Tan SSW, Lee HS, et al (1995) Effect of propofol infusion on the endocrine response to cardiac surgery. Anaesth Intensive Care 23: 543-547
24. Adams HA (1997) Endocrine reactions following S-(+)-ketamine. anesthesist 46 [Suppl 1]:S30-S37
25. Adams HA, Russ W, Leisin M, et al (1987) Inhalation anesthetic agents and endocrine stress response during surgery. A comparison of halothane, enflurane and isoflurane. anesthesist 36:159-165
26. Holdcroft A (2000) Hormones and the gut. Br J Anaesth 85:58-68
27. Helbo-Hansen S, Fletcher R, Lundberg D (1986) Clonidine and the sympatico-adrenal response to coronary artery by-pass surgery. Acta anesthesiol Scand 30:235-242
28. Eisenach JC, DeCock M, Klimscha W (1996) Alpha 2-adrenergic agonists for regional anesthesia. Anesthesiology 85:655-674
29. Quintin L, Roudot F, Roux C, et al (1991) Effect of clonidine on the circulation and vasoactive hormones after aortic surgery. Br J Anaesth 66:108-115
30. Kallio A, Koulu M, Scheinin H, et al (1988) Acute effects of medetomidine, a selective alpha 2-adrenoceptor agonist, on anterior pituitary hormone and cortisol secretion in man. Acta Endocrinol (Copenh) 119:11-15
31. Masala A, Satta G, Alagna S, et al (1985) Effect of clonidine on stress-induced cortisol release in man during surgery. Pharmacol Res Commun 17:293-298
32. Dorman T, Clarkson K, Rosenfeld BA, et al (1997) Effects of clonidine on prolonged postoperative sympathetic response. Crit Care Med 25:1147-1152
33. Ellis JE, Drijvers G, Pedlow S, et al (1994) Premedication with oral and transdermal clonidine provides safe and efficacious postoperative sympatholysis. Anesth Analg 79:1133-1140
34. Eisenach J, Detweiler D, Hood D (1993) Hemodynamic and analgesic actions of epidurally administered clonidine. Anesthesiology 78:277-287.
35. De Kock M (1996) Alpha-2 adrenoceptor agonists: clonidine, dexmedetomidine, mivazerol. Curr Opin Anesthesiol 9:295-299

36. Novak-Janković V, Paver-Eržen V, Bovill JG, et al (2000) Effect of epidural and intravenous clonidine on the neuro-endocrine and immune stress response in patients undergoing lung surgery. Eur J anesthesiol (EJA) 17:50-56
37. Stenseth R, Bjella L, Berg EM, et al (1994) Thoracic epidural analgesia in aortocoronary bypass surgery II. Effects on the endocrine metabolic response. Acta anesthesiol Scand 38:834-839
38. Loick HM, Schmidt C, VanAKen H, et al (1999) High thoracic epidural anesthesia, but not clonidine, attenuates the perioperative stress response via sympatholysis and reduces the release of troponin T in patients undergoing coronary artery bypass grafting. Anesth Analg 88:701-709
39. Chae BK, Lee HW, Sun K, et al (1998) The effect of combined epidural and light general anesthesia on stress hormones in open heart surgery patients. Surg Today 28:727-731
40. Aono H, Takeda A, Tarver SD, et al (1998) Stress responses in three different anesthetic techniques for carbon dioxide laparoscopic cholecystectomy. J Clin Anesth 10:546-550
41. Kehlet H, Brandt MR, Hansen AP, et al (1979) Effect of epidural analgesia on metabolic profiles during and after surgery. Br J Surg 66:543-546
42. Naito Y, Tamai S, Shingu K, et al (1992) Responses of plasma adrenocorticotropic hormone, cortisol, and cytokines during and after upper abdominal surgery. Anesthesiology 77:426-431
43. Bromage PR, Shibata HR, Willoughby HW (1971) Influence of prolonged epidural blockade on blood sugar and cortisol responses to operations upon the upper part of the abdomen and the thorax. Surg Gynecol Obstet 132:1051-1059
44. Rem J, Brandt MR, Kehlet H (1980) Prevention of postoperative lymphopenia and granulocytosis by epidural analgesia. Lancet 9:283-284
45. Yeager MP, Glass DD, Neff RK, et al (1987) Epidural anesthesia and analgesia in high risk surgical patients. Anesthesiology 66:729-736
46. Tuman KJ, McCarthy RJ, March RJ, et al (1991) Effects of epidural anesthesia and analgesia on coagulation and outcome after major vascular surgery. Anesth Analg 73:696-704.
47. Raggi R, Dardik H, Mauro AL (1987) Continuous epidural anesthesia and postoperative epidural narcotics in vascular surgery. Am J Surg 154:192-197
48. Turfrey DJ, Ray DAA, Sutcliffe NP, et al (1997) Thoracic epidural anesthesia for coronary artery bypass graft surgery. Effects on postoperative complications. anesthesia 52:1090-1113
49. Handley GH, Silbert BS, Mooney PH, et al (1997) Combined general and epidural anesthesia versus general anesthesia for major abdominal surgery: postanesthesia recovery characteristics. Reg Anesth 22:435-441
50. McKenzie PJ, Wishart HY, Smith G (1984) Long-term outcome after repair of fractured neck of femur. Comparison of subarachnoid and general anesthesia. Br J Anaesth 56:581-585
51. Bode RH, Lewis KP, Zarich SW, et al (1996) Cardiac outcome after peripheral vascular surgery. Comparison of general and regional anesthesia. Anesthesiology 84:3-13
52. Liu S, Carpenter RL, Neal JM (1995) Epidural anesthesia and analgesia. Their role in postoperative outcome. Anesthesiology 82:1474-1506
53. Ballantyne JC, Carr DB, deFerranti S, et al (1998) The comparative effects of postoperative analgesic therapies on pulmonary outcome: cumulative meta-analyses of randomized, controlled trials. Anesth Analg 86:598-612
54. Ballantyne J (2001) Does regional anesthesia improve outcome after surgery. Refresher course lectures. 9th ESA Annual Meeting, Gothenburg, pp 41-50
55. Kompan L, Kremžar B, Gadžijev E, et al (1999) Effects of early enteral nutrition on intestinal permeability and the development of multiple organ failure after multiple injury. Intensive Care Med 25:157-161.
56. Kehlet H (1997) Multimodal approach to control postoperative pathophysiology and rehabilitation. Br J Anaesth 78:606-617
57. Moiniche S, Bulow S, Hesselfeldt P, et al (1995) Convalescence and hospital stay after colonic surgery with balanced analgesia, early oral feeding, and enforced mobilisation. Eur J Surg 161:283-288.
58. Brodner G, Pogatzki E, Van Aken H, et al (1998) A multimodal approach to control postoperative

pathophysiology and rehabilitation in patients undergoing abdominothoracic esophagectomy. Anesth Analg 86:228-234
59. Kehlet H (2000) Accelerated postoperative recovery. Book of proceedings. 12th World Congress of anesthesiologists. Montreal, Canada, pp 200

OBSTETRICS

Trends in Obstetric Anaesthesia

G. Lyons

In this chapter I shall be discussing those aspects of practice that are changing. For many of us these are uncontrollable trends of an epidemiological nature, evolution in society, rather than revolution in clinical practice. Changes in society are likely to make a greater impact on practice than the introduction of new drugs or equipment. To illustrate these points I have drawn on international, national and local data.

Maternal mortality

Maternal mortality is frequently used as an indicator of standards of care, and data can be used to make comparisons between countries. Two potential difficulties with this are that national collections of statistics vary significantly in quality, and that international definitions are not always used. In Italy, [1] haemorrhage is responsible for most maternal deaths, whilst in the UK, thromboembolism is the greatest killer. Deaths from haemorrhage occur in the hospital and are easily notifiable, whilst deaths from thromboembolism tend to be scattered, risking underreporting.

In the UK, maternal deaths from anaesthesia have almost disappeared, at 0.5 per million births, 1:300,000 caesarean sections approximately [2]. The developed world has broadly similar data. With the decline in the number of anaesthesia related deaths, the effectiveness of mortality data to inform and influence practice has diminished. Attention is turning to the use of 'near-miss' reporting, and the incidences of severe obstetric morbidity to evaluate current standards of care. A recent case controlled study estimated the incidence of severe obstetric morbidity at 12 per 1000 deliveries. Risk factors for morbidity were; age more than 34, non white ethnic group, hypertension, previous postpartum haemorrhage, emergency caesarean section, antenatal admission to hospital, multiple pregnancy, social exclusion, and iron or anti depressant therapy. Most events were in conjunction with haemorrhage and pre-eclampsia [3].

The admission of intensive care by obstetric patients is another indicator of morbidity. One of the difficulties with this index is that the scope of intensive care varies greatly, from elevated high dependency care to multi organ support. It is not surprising that there is a tenfold difference in admission rates reported, from 0.1% to1% [4]. The causes of admission to intensive care mirror the causes of maternal death, without thromboembolism. The collection of critical incident, near-miss and severe morbidity data is likely to become a widespread practice.

General anaesthesia

General anaesthesia in obstetric practice is a risk factor for both mortality and morbidity. In the UK, nearly all maternal anaesthetic deaths occur in relation to general anaesthesia. Hawkins et al, in the USA, estimated the relative risk ratio of general to regional anaesthesia for the years 1985 to 1990, at approximately 17 :1 [5]. An Australian survey of 61,000 deliveries showed that the risk of intensive care admission due to a complication of general anaesthesia was 1:932, compared with 1:4177 for regional anaesthesia, when provided for delivery [6]. In the developed world the trend has been for an increasing use of regional anaesthesia. Madej et al showed that the introduction of spinal anaesthesia reduced the requirement for emergency general anaesthesia [7]. In St James' University Hospital, general anaesthesia is used in 5% of caesarean sections, but for the St Luke's and Roosevelt Hospital in New York, the figure is 1%. The decline of general obstetric anaesthesia has meant that University Hospitals are no longer able to teach general anaesthesia for caesarean section [8]. As yet there is no evidence to suggest that lack of experience with general anaesthesia is, in itself, a cause of morbidity. This is despite the increasing incidence of complexity in cases. As general anaesthesia is used less often, the women receiving general anaesthesia tend to have proportionately more comorbidity [9].

Caesarean section

The developed world is seeing an increase in demand for caesarean section, the world's commonest operation. In the private sector, with the highest rates, economic factors are responsible, but maternal choice and defensive medicine are both putting pressure on upward rates. In our unit, in twenty years the incidence of caesarean delivery has risen from 8% to 25%. Although the birth rate in our city is declining slowly, the climbing incidence of caesarean delivery has doubled the work of obstetric anaesthetists, and quadrupled the risk of morbidity [3]. There is no accepted approach for controlling the numbers of caesarean sections performed, perhaps because not everybody agrees that it is undesirable [10].

One additional pressure towards operative delivery is the trend for women to delay their first baby. Collis et al showed that the risk of intervention increased with each decade of reproductive life. For women over the age of 34, the chance of an uncomplicated vaginal delivery was 40%. Unsurprisingly, increasing age was also associated with greater use of epidural pain relief in labour [11].

Complex cases

Diets of fast food, sweet drinks and snacks, together with a less active lifestyle have bred a generation of obese children, who are now in their reproductive years. Women who deliver in St James' are shorter and heavier than women who deliver in Rome. Obesity makes all forms of anaesthesia more demanding.

Medical advances in congenital heart disease, cystic fibrosis and childhood cancer, mean that more children live to reproductive age. With their transplanted organs, failing organ function and iatrogenic disabilities, they make occasional but taxing demands on the both manual dexterity and clinical judgement of the Obstetric Anaesthetist [12]. In societies where recreational drug use is rife, abuse increases risk of intervention, and complicates pain relief and venous access [13].

Changes in society are more likely to increase demands upon obstetric anaesthesia than the reverse. Maintaining high standards in the face of a more complex workload can have its difficulties. Improving standards goes a step further in that it often requires a change in practice.

Antenatal assessment

A relatively recent change in practice has been the setting up of Anaesthetic Antenatal Clinics. In the UK such clinics are likely to see mainly high risk women, particularly those with medical disorders. In France there is a well established system because the law requires that all pregnant women are seen by an anaesthetist before delivery. The clinic can be used to predict which women are most likely to require operative delivery, and promote early regional block in labour, for this group. The same can be done for problems with intubation. This policy reduces the need for emergency general anaesthesia [14]. Outside France, the Anaesthetic Antenatal Clinic is not universal, and tends only to occur where interested individuals have made a special effort.

Smaller needles

The severity of post dural puncture headache decreases in proportion to the gauge of the needle used. The adoption of pencil point needles will also reduce the risk of post dural puncture headache, but only for a given gauge. If a change to a pencil point needle is accompanied by a reduction in gauge, then significant improvements in morbidity can be made. Reported incidences for post dural puncture vary greatly, but our experience was that despite several new needles, the epidural blood patch rate was always in the region of 5%. Changing to a 27 gauge pencil point needle reduced the blood patch rate to 0.2-0.3%. Others describe a similar incidence of headache with this needle [15]. The arguments for reducing the gauge of spinal needles are the same for the Tuohy, but there is no evidence that the trend in spinal anaesthesia has affected epidural practices. Exchanging a 16 gauge Tuohy needle for an 18 gauge needle reduced the need for epidural blood patch following inadvertent dural puncture, from 80% to 50%, in our unit.

Epidural pain relief in labour

Availability of epidural pain relief in labour varies greatly, depending on the unit. In France, the overall rate is 48% and in the UK it is 24%. Data from Italy suggests that the availability and uptake is on the increase [1].

Traditional epidural services relied on bolus administration, and then continuous infusions. Patient controlled epidural analgesia is associated with reductions in dose and fewer analgesic interventions [16], and is very gradually becoming more popular, despite the need for specialized equipment. The use of needle through needle combined spinal and epidural analgesia appears to have reached a steady state. In a few units it is the routine procedure and in many others it is used occasionally. The trend is to use higher volumes of more dilute epidural local anaesthetic with added opioid, to achieve better analgesia but with less motor block. Higher volumes of more dilute local anaesthetic often achieve reductions in dose to the levels associated with tests of intravenous and subarachnoid injection. Because of this some anaesthetists argue that test dosing has become irrelevant, and that the main dose can also serve as test dose. A few units have dispensed with test dosing as a result, but the arguments have, so far, only made a small impact on practice. Because doses of local anaesthetic used to provide analgesia are now so small, the case for safer local anaesthetics has become irrelevant. The rationale for the use of either ropivacaine or levobupivacaine is much stronger for epidural anaesthesia than it is for analgesia. The debate regarding the claimed benefits of these drugs continues around the relationship of potency to toxicity, and a wealth of conflicting data.

Conclusion

Maternal mortality due to anaesthesia is falling, due to greater uptake of regional blockade and improving standards. Alternative markers for monitoring standards are required. The demand for analgesia for labour and anaesthesia for delivery continues to increase. The population is tending to survive more serious childhood illnesses, getting more obese, and having babies later in life. These factors combine to increase both the volume and complexity of obstetric anaesthetic practice. Anaesthetic antenatal assessment, smaller needles for regional blockade and lower dose drug regimes for epidural pain relief in labour are all considered to reduce risk of morbidity.

References

1. Capogna G (2000) Obstetric anaesthesia practices in Italy. In: Reynolds F (ed) Regional analgesia in obstetrics. Springer, London, pp 39-41
2. Report on confidential enquiries into maternal deaths in the United Kingdom 1994-1996 (1998) Why mothers die. Her Majesty's Stationery Office, London
3. Waterstone M, Bewley S, Wolfe C (2001) Incidence and predictors of severe obstetric morbidity: case control study. Br Med J 322: 1089-1093
4. Robinson A P C, Lyons G (1999) Morbidity and mortality from obstetric anaesthesia in the 1990s. Curr Opin Anaesthesiol 12: 277-281
5. Hawkins J L, Gibbs C P, Orleans M et al (1997) Obstetric anesthesia workforce survey. 1981 versus 1992. Anesthesiology 87: 135-143
6. Stephens I D (1991) ICU admissions from an obstetric hospital. Can J Anaesth 38: 677-681
7. Madej T H, Jackson I J B, Wheatley R G et al (1993) Assessing introduction of spinal anaesthesia for obstetric procedures Quality in Health Care 2: 31-34
8. Johnson R V, Lyons G, Wilson R C et al (2000) Training in obstetric general anaesthesia is a vanishing art. Anaesthesia 55: 179-183
9. Tsen L C, Pilsner R, Camaan W R (1998) General anesthesia at a tertiary care hospital 1990-1995: indications and implications Int J Obs Anesth 7: 147-152
10. Leitch C R, Walker JJ (1994) Caesarean section rates Br Med J 308: 133
11. Collis R E, Sewell J M A, Mapleson W W (2000) Analysis of maternal age and social class on risk of obstetric intervention and obstetric anaesthetic requirements Br J Anaesth 86: 311P
12. Gorton H, Wilson R C, Robinson A P C et al (2000) Survivors of childhood cancers: implications for anaesthetists Br J Anaesth 85: 911-913
13. Birnbach D J, Van Zundert A (1997) Drug abuse in the pregnant woman. In: Russell I F, Lyons G (eds) Clinical problems in obstetric anaesthesia. Chapman and Hall, London, pp 221-228
14. Hamza J, Ducot B, Dupont X et al (1995) Anaesthesia consultation can decrease the need for general anaesthesia for emergency caesarean section in parturients with difficult airway. Br J Anaesth 74: A353
15. Schneider M C, Schmid M (2000) Post dural puncture headache. In: Birnbach D J, Gatt S P, Datta S (eds) Textbook of obstetric anesthesia. Churchill Livingstone, New York, pp 487-503
16. Van der Vyver M J, Halpern S J, Joseph G (2001) Patient controlled epidural analgesia vs continuous infusion for labor pain: a meta-analysis. Anesthesiology 94: 1 A71

Inhalation Anesthesia for Cesarean Section

C. MELLONI

There is no doubt that today regional analgesia is considered the method of choice for cesarean section. This can be ascribed to the superior safety for the mother, fetus, and newborn offered by the regional analgesia [1]. This has led to a recent article with the title "Training in obstetric general anesthesia: a vanishing art? [2].

However,, there are still indications for general anesthesia (GA). Listed below are the indications, advantages and disadvantages of GA versus of regional anesthesia.

Clinical situations in which GA may be more appropriate than regional anesthesia include the following:

1. Hypovolemia or hemorrhage
2. Severe, acute fetal distress – some question this indication, believing that comparable results can be obtained with regional anesthesia
3. Patient refusal of or inability to co-operate for regional anesthesia
4. Certain forms of heart disease that cannot tolerate hypotension (e.g., aortic stenosis, Eisenmenger's syndrome)
5. Anesthesia personnel are inexperienced in providing regional anesthesia
6. Any instance when regional anesthesia is contraindicated (e.g., sepsis, coagulopathies, infection at the site, etc.)

Advantages:

The advantages of GA can be listed as follows:

1. Asleep and unaware
2. Total pain relief
3. Little risk of drug depression when administered properly
4. Optimum operating conditions

The disadvantages include:

1. Asleep and unaware
2. Husband less likely to be allowed in the operating room (OR)
3. Drug depression of fetus
4. Stress response to intubation

5. Increased postoperative morbidity
6. Cardiovascular changes of intubation
7. Aspiration
8. Difficult intubation

Although there are many individual variations on how to provide general anesthesia for cesarean section, usually the process is accomplished in a manner similar to that outlined below:

1. Atropine 0.4-0.6 mg or glycopyrrolate 0.2-0.3 mg IM or IV
2. Antacids or H_2 blockers: because particulate antacids may produce rather extensive histological and physiological derangement in case of aspiration, 30 ml of a clear nonparticulate antacid such as 0.3 M sodium citrate is preferred. Cimetidine, ranitidine, or omeprazole may be used in place of the acids for elective Cesarean section. However, H_2 blockers would not antagonize the gastric content already present inside the stomach.
3. Left uterine displacement (LUD): the uterus impinges on the inferior vena cava and aorta during the latter months of pregnancy preventing cardiac return and reducing cardiac output; hence, it is mandatory to avoid the so--called aortocaval compression, both for maternal and fetal reasons. This is usually accomplished with a combination of the lateral tilt of the surgical bed and a small pillow placed below the right hip, although special devices have been developed and used with success.
4. Induction versus uterine incision - delivery interval (I-D): recent data indicate that it is not the induction of anesthesia to delivery interval that matters, but rather the uterine incision- delivery interval (UI-D). As this interval increases, low Apgar scores increase. Optimum time is less than 90 s. Between 90 and 180 s, the outcome of the newborn may be compromised, and after 180 s the newborn is at high risk. During this uterine incision- delivery interval, difficulties occor with the operation and there is excessive manipulation of uterine vessels. The surgical incision decreases the vascular supply to the placenta, and this in turn jeopardizes the fetus, and consequently the neonate.
5. Preoxygenation is always a good idea; only 4-5 large breaths may be necessary, but the maximum rise in the maternal pAO_2 is only attained with at least 5 min of oxygen breathing100%.
6. Precurarization inhibits succinylcholine-induced muscle fasciculations, which in turn raise intragastric pressure. However, during fasciculations, pressures above the lower esophageal sphincter rise as much as intragastric pressures, thus minimizing risk from the increased intragastric pressure. Also, pregnant patients appear to fasciculate very little following suc-

cinylcholine, and fasciculations give a clear indication of when to intubate the patient.

7. Thiopental, 3-4 mg/kg, or ketamine 1 mg/kg: both of these agents have been used extensively as induction agents and have very little, if any, effect on the newborn. Ketamine provides its own analgesia, is associated with less awareness and recall, and produces no greater and perhaps even less cardiovascular response than thiopental. Propofol 2-2.5 mg/kg is being used more frequently.
8. Cricoid pressure - a simple maneuver to prevent regurgitation of stomach contents. It should always be applied immediately following the induction dose of the hypnotic and not released until the endotracheal tube (ETT) is known to be in place and the cuff is inflated.
9. Succinylcholine, 1-1.5 mg/kg - this drug does not cross the placenta at levels that are clinically significant.
10. Intubation - a neuromuscular blockade monitor is very helpful in determining proper time for the initial attempt.
11. Checking the correct ETT placement: monitoring of end tidal $C0_2$ by capnography or mass spectrometry can be particularly helpful, and is most reliable. The tube must be in place before the operation begins: bilateral auscultation of the chest assures the proper positioning of the ETT in the trachea.
12. Nitrous oxide/oxygen in a 50-50 mixture: safe for mother and fetus.
13. Halothane 0.5%, enflurane 0.5-1.0%, isoflurane 0.75%, sevoflurane 0.5--1%, desflurane 2.5% is started immediately following intubation. These agents provide analgesia and hypnosis, decreasing the state of awareness. At these concentrations they do not promote uterine bleeding. If beta--mimetics have been given to prevent premature labor or ameliorate fetal distress, halothane should be avoided because the danger of serious arrhythmias is greater.
14. Succinylcholine drip or a competitive muscle relaxant at low dosage is administered if coughing and bucking occur before the delivery of the infant or where maintenance of muscular relaxation is helpful.
15. Once the infant is delivered, the volatile agent can be continued, or discontinued with administration of a potent analgesic such as fentanyl, and provision of additional hypnosis with repeated boluses or a continuous infusion (propofol)
16. Oxytocin is given as an IV infusion (10-20 units/l); a bolus is better avoided, since it can produce marked vasodilatation and hypotension.
17. Extubation - The patient is extubated awake, when she is responsive to oral command as well as being completely recovered from whatever muscle

relaxation was used. Aspiration not only occurs at the time of induction of anesthesia, but also during emergence.

18. Recovery room - The patient is taken to an appropriately staffed and equipped recovery room.
19. Failed intubation - A plan is necessary and drills for failed intubation should be frequently practised, because mother and fetus oxygenation is vital, and hypoxia constitutes the most-frequent cause of serious morbidity and mortality.

As can be seen from the scheme outlined above, there are still controversies and differences in practice among practitioners. Inhalation anesthesia is administered mainly for the purpose of decreasing or avoiding maternal awareness. Moir [3] reported no maternal awareness if 0.5% halothane was added to 50% nitrous oxide; Crawford [4] used 0.1% methoxyflurane and claimed a marked reduction in the incidence of intraoperative awareness. Nevertheless, intraoperative awareness was still observed by others [5, 6]. The pain and discomfort thresholds in late pregnancy are reported to be higher [7], and consequently, anesthetic requirements are reduced in parturients by 25%-40%. These combine with reduced functional residual capacity and increased cardiac output to favor a faster induction of inhaled anesthesia [8]. However, there must be sufficient wash-in and transfer time to allow the inhaled anesthetics to reach the target sites and provide analgesic effects. Nitrous oxide has a low blood/gas partition coefficient and consequently a fast induction time; however, when used alone, even at concentrations of 75%, it does not guarantee sufficient analgesia for surgery [9]. The halftime of blood-brain equilibration of thiopental is 1-2 min [10]; therefore, even the transfer of thiopental from blood to the effect or site in the central nervous system is not instantaneous [11].

Furthermore, thiopental is a hypnotic that provides very little or no analgesia. Therefore the depth of GA currently provided for Cesarean section is inadequate at the time of surgical incision.

The recent introduction of sevoflurane and desflurane in the anesthetists' aramamentarium improves the situation. They rapidly equilibrate between inspired and expired air due to low blood solubilities, similar to that of nitrous oxide. Gambling et al [12] compared sevoflurane 1% and isoflurane 0.5% in a 50% nitrous oxide and oxygen mixture for maintenance, in terms of maternal and neonatal outcomes. They compared neonatal outcome in both groups with a cohort of patients delivered by Cesarean section using spinal anesthesia with 1.5 ml hyperbaric bupivacaine 0.75 and 10 μg fentanyl. Intraoperative hemodynamic variables and perioperative adverse events were recorded. Neonatal data included Apgar scores at 1 and 5 min, umbilical artery gas analysis, neurological adaptive capacity scores (NACS) at 2 and 24 h, and a modified neonatal behavioral assessment scale (NBAS) at 24 h. Sevoflurane and isoflurane at equi-anesthetic concentrations [0.46 minimal alveolar concentration (MAC)/h] were associated with similar blood pressure and heart rate changes during the operation. Blood loss, uterine tone, and perioperative complications were not problematic and were similar with the two drugs. No differences were seen in emergence times or in the time to discharge from the recovery room. Similarly, the level of postoperative comfort was the same in both groups. Comparing the general and the spinal anesthetic groups, no differences could be detected in neonatal outcome. Fluoride concentrations were modestly increased above preoperative levels in maternal and umbilical blood samples after sevoflurane administration. The authors concluded that there are no significant differences between sevoflurane 1% and isoflurane 0.5% for maintenance of GA during cesarean birth.

A second and important reason for the administration of volatile agents during cesarean section is the attenuation of the metabolic and endocrine responses to pain and stress associated with surgery. Nociceptive stimulations trigger a cascade of reactions, leading to sympathetic over-activity and resulting in increased oxygen consumption and catabolism. Uterine vasoconstriction resulting from increased catecholamines may compromise uteroplacental blood perfusion and the status of the infant [13]. Furthermore, intraoperative awareness and pain perception may lead to a phobia of surgery and doctors, or even result in traumatic neurosis in the mother [14, 15].

Obviously, a patient undergoing surgery should be adequately anesthetized and shielded from pain, stress, and other nociceptive stimuli. Nevertheless, ever since the advent of muscle relaxants, the traditional respiratory pattern and muscle responses have been precluded as indicators of anesthesia depth. Thiopental can decrease the plasma catecholamine levels, as well as subsequent hemodynamic responses, but may not eliminate the stress itself. Furthermore, parturients during labor generally have various degrees of anxiety, fear, or painful uterine contractions that also influence plasma catecholamine concentrations. The correlations between stress, catecholamine levels, and hemodynamic responses in cesarean section are often poor, and do not reflect the real picture because of the great variation of the background [16]. However, the administration of volatile agents at low concentrations has been associated with a reduction in maternal (and fetal) catecholamine levels and improvement in utero-placental perfusion.

In order to evaluate depth of anesthesia, computerized electroencephalography (EEG) has been utilised. This now includes various time intervals to map each waveform in relation to its frequency, amplitude, and time of occurrence, thus making the interpretation of EEG much less complicated than it once was. When blood oxygen and carbon dioxide tensions remain constant, thiopental produces a characteristic progression of EEG changes [17]. Stimulation can induce arousal reactions that are accompanied by an increase in EEG frequency. Bispectral EEG monitoring with its resultant bispectral index (BIS) has been recently proposed for monitoring depth of anesthesia. In many reports BIS monitoring has been shown to correlate well with depth of anesthesia. Recently its usefulness has been confirmed in obstetrics. Weyns et al [18] compared either 4 mg/kg thiopental or 2 mg/kg propofol given over 20 s, with suxamethonium (1.5 mg/kg) given to facilitate endotracheal intubation, and maintenance by inhalation of 50% nitrous oxide in oxygen. Time to delivery (min 5.5, SD 1.8 min) and hemodynamic or respiratory parameters were similar between the two groups. At time of delivery there was a statistically significant difference in BIS index (propofol m 72, SD 13; thiopental m 83, SD 9), while there was no correlation between BIS at delivery and neonatal Apgar scores at 1 and 5 min. Therefore propofol seemed to offer better depth of anesthesia than thiopental, without adversely affecting neonatal Apgar scores.

The usefulness of BIS was confirmed in another study [19] where isoflurane was compared with propofol plus fentanyl after delivery of the infant; both techniques gaved a satisfactory depth of anesthesia, but uterine contraction was considered poor in 25% of women under isoflurane 0.5 MAC.

However, when the BIS was evaluated as a measure of sedation, there were problems in the definition of terms (sedation) and in the correlation between loss of consciousness and other indicators [20, 21]. Kearse et al [21] analyzed the relationship between the BIS readings and conscious processing of information during propofol sedation and hypnosis. They could not identify a gradual, continuous descent from alertness to varying stages of vigilance, inattention, and unresponsiveness, but found that the volunteer simply did or did not respond to commands. Leslie et al [22] reported that the BIS predicted propofol-induced suppression of learning during regional anesthesia. They found that the slopes of the isoflurane curve reflecting the relationship were different from those of propofol or midazolam, and no logistic relationship could be derived for alfentanil [23]. Therefore it seems at present wise to concur with Kissin [24] that BIS is "most promising as a monitor of unconsciousness.", but since " The BIS is an empirical index derived statistically from a database which included many, but not all, types of anesthetics and the combinations, when the BIS is used with new drug or new patient population that was not in original database, it must be revalidated."

A recent study investigated the relationship of SEF with recall [25]. Responsiveness to verbal commands was recorded every minute in the period from the induction of anesthesia to the delivery of the newborn using the Tunstall isolated forearm technique and correlated with the SEF90 value. The patients were randomized to receive either thiopentone 4 mg/ kg or ketamine 1 mg /kg for induction of anesthesia. Before the administration of succinylcholine a tourniquet was applied to the free arm, and inflated to 200 mmHg to maintain motor function to one arm. The EEG recordings started 5 min before induction and were performed throughout anesthesia. The incidence of responsiveness to verbal commands was lower in the ketamine group (24%) where the average SEF90 was 12.0 ± 3 Hz, than in the thiopentone group (52%), where the average SEF90 was 18.09 ± 3 Hz ($p = 0.01$). The results suggest that SEF values of 8.6 Hz were sufficient to avoid responsiveness to verbal commands. These levels of EEG activity could be recommended, but may not be applicable to obstetrics.

Since EEG monitoring is certainly not routine in the field of obstetric anesthesia, the assessment of adequacy still depends on clinically relevant signs [26, 27]. Because our main concern is whether or not the mothers are feeling pain during surgery, we rely on the patient herself to signal her ability to hear or perceive pain, rather than on indirect signs. Currently, the nearest we have to a "gold standard" is the use of the isolated forearm technique to directly communicate with the subject [28].This technique is unreliable after 20 min, as ischemic paralysis occurs [29].

Moir's study [3] and most others [30] on the adequacy of anesthesia or intraoperative awareness, have depended on recall. However, recall is but one measure of memory and is therefore not reliable as a test of awareness or wakefulness [31]. Even with the aid of hypnosis, only a fraction of the events that occurred under anesthesia may be available for recall, although they may be remembered in other ways [32]. In the study of King et al [33] no patient showed any recollection of noxious stimulation or auditory information presented to them intraoperatively, but most did show evidence of awareness and pain perception at the time. This demonstrated that intraoperative awareness or pain perception may occur without recall. This could be due to spontaneous memory decay, or retrograde amnesia induced by the drugs used after the delivery [26, 34]. The ability to hear and process information may not be totally suppressed even during deep anesthesia [26, 35, 36].

Other studies have reported that patients did learn nonverbal responses to intraoperative suggestions [31, 37]. Nevertheless, insufficient anesthesia should be differentiated from awareness with adequate anesthesia. The detection of awareness as well as pain perception in paralyzed patients under light general anesthesia and the adequacy of anesthesia is a balance between the depressing effects of the drugs and the stimuli presented to the patient.

Awareness itself is not the important issue, because patients calmly undergo surgery with regional blocks or even analgesia and local infiltration. Many mothers want to be awake to experience the birth of their children. Rather, the issue is that the patient has experienced pain, yet cannot call for help. A memory of being conscious may not be as traumatic as one of actually feeling pain. The unconscious storing of a traumatic memory may well act as a chronic psychological irritant [37]. When the benefits of light GA are desired for the infant, it may be prudent to protect the mother from perceiving pain and stress. Moreover awareness during GA is a frightening experience, which may result in serious emotional injury and post-traumatic stress disorder. Recently an in-depth analysis of cases from the database of the American Society of Anesthesiologists Closed Claims Project explored the contribution of intraoperative awareness to professional liability in anesthesia [38]. Awareness claims accounted for 79 (1.9%) of 4,183 claims in the database, including 18 claims for awake paralysis, i.e., the inadvertent paralysis of an awake patient, and 61 claims for recall during GA, i.e., recall of events while receiving GA. The majority of awareness claims involved women (77%), younger than 60 years of age (89%), American Society of Anesthesiologists physical class I—II (68%), who underwent elective surgery (87%). Most (94%) claims for awake paralysis represented substandard care involving errors in labeling and administration, whereas care was substandard in only 43% of the claims for recall during GA ($p<0.001$). Claims for recall during GA were more likely to involve women [odds ratio (OR) = 3.08, 95% confidence interval (CI) = 1.58, 6.06] and anesthetic techniques using intraoperative opioids (OR = 2.12, 95% CI = 1.20, 3.74), intraoperative muscle relaxants (OR = 2.28, 95% CI = 1.22, 4.25), and no volatile anesthetic (OR = 3.20, 95% CI = 1.88, 5.46).The data were not addressed specifically to obstetric patients, but they clearly demonstrate the dangers of light anesthesia and awareness, with the possibility of legal action.

A recent study [39] investigated the incidence of explicit memory (i.e., conscious recall) and implicit memory (e.g., improved memory test performance in the absence of conscious recall) during emergency cesarean sections with consistently light levels of hypnosis. Words were presented via headphones, and the BIS was recorded throughout surgery. Memory for the presented words was tested after recovery with a word-stem completion test. Using both parts of the process dissociation procedure allowed separation of explicit and implicit memory. In the "inclusion" part of the process dissociation procedure, patients are asked to complete word stems, if possible, with the corresponding words recalled from the intraoperative presentation. In the "exclusion" part, patients are instructed to avoid the words presented intraoperatively and to use other words instead. In the absence of recall, patients are asked to use the first word that comes to mind. The mean BIS during word presentation was 76.3 ± 3.0. On average, the 24 patients were able to make correct inclusion-exclusion decisions. In the inclusion part, hit rates, i.e., the probability of responding with a word presented during surgery, were higher than base rates (0.37 vs. 0.31), whereas in the exclusion part hit rates were lower (0.23 vs. 0.28). Importantly, the patients made these inclusion-exclusion decisions without being able to consciously recall the words presented during surgery. The study concluded that if words are presented at relatively light levels of anesthesia, patients are able to control their inclusion-exclusion decisions. This weak form of explicit memory can occur in the absence of conscious recall. It is unclear at the moment how to avoid this problem, since induction-delivery times tend to be shorter. It should be noted that the anesthesia administered to these patients was "light", consisting of thiopental 4 mg/kg, succinylcholine 100 mg, nitrous oxide 50% and isoflurane 0.2% end tidal, with morphine and nitrous oxide 70% added after delivery.

Although the prevention of maternal awareness is a major reason for the administration of inhalatory agents, it should not be forgotten that minimal fetal and consequently neonatal depression is also important. Therefore the rate of uptake of the inhalatory agents by mother and fetus should be compared in order to choose the best balance between protection against light anesthesia and the danger of neonatal depression. Dwyer et al [40] studied 23 patients undergoing cesarean section who received either 0.5% halothane or 0.8% isoflurane to supplement nitrous oxide–oxygen anesthesia. The rate of uptake of the agents by the mother and fetus was investigated by measuring partial pressures in maternal arterial (pa) and fetal umbilical venous (puv) blood. Isoflurane uptake by the mother was more rapid than halothane; at delivery, mean Pa of isoflurane as a fraction of the inspired partial pressure (pI) was 0.44 compared with 0.35 for halothane; mean puv as a fraction of maternal pa at delivery was 0.71 for both agents; thus placental transfer was the same for both agents. Consequently mean puv/pI was greater for isoflurane (0.32) than halothane (0.26) The rate of uptake of isoflurane by the mother during cesarean section was more rapid than halothane. The rate of uptake by the fetus from the mother was the same for halothane and isoflurane, so that fetal partial pressure as a fraction of the inspired partial pressure was greater for isoflurane than halothane. This should be the same for the less-soluble anesthetics, such as sevoflurane and desflurane, so that fetal equilibration should be faster but at the same time emergence should be faster. Uptake of isoflurane is more rapid than halothane because of its lower blood–gas partition coefficient . Blood partial pressures of both agents increased rapidly. The smallest arterial partial pressure of isoflurane in any patient after administration of 0.8% isoflurane for 5 min was 0.23%. Taking into account the reduction in anesthetic requirements in pregnancy , this partial pressure of isoflurane is equivalent to that found by Chortkoff et al [41] to prevent recall in volunteers when combined with 40% nitrous oxide . It is not surprising therefore that this technique is adequate to prevent awareness during cesarean section.

Other studies have measured rate of uptake of isoflurane and halothane during cesarean section. McCrirrick et al [42] measured arterial isoflurane concentrations, which, if converted to partial pressures using blood–gas partition coefficients measured by Gibbs et al [43], correspond to pa/pI values of 0.62 and 0.64 after 5 and 10 min of isoflurane administration, respectively . Tunstall and Hawksworth [44] measured blood halothane concentrations, which, if corrected to blood partial pressures, correspond to pa/pI ratios of 0.41 and 0.49 after 5 and 10 min of halothane administration, respectively. Uptake of isoflurane and halothane by the fetus from maternal blood occurred at the same rate; puv/pa ratios for the two agents at delivery were identical. Volatile agents are highly lipid soluble and cross the placenta freely, so that puv approached pa. As pa/pI was significantly greater for isoflurane than halothane at delivery, puv/pI was also significantly greater for isoflurane than halothane.

The puv/pa ratios noted are comparable with those reported for nitrous oxide by Marx et al (0.79)[45] and Hay (0.71) [46]. Stengeret al [14] found a puv/pa ratio of 0.91 for nitrous oxide after prolonged anesthesia (mean duration 35 min); Latto and Waldren [47] measured maternal and fetal blood concentrations of halothane at delivery after administration of 0.65% halothane. When these concentrations were converted to partial pressures using the blood–gas partition coefficients measured by Gibbs, et al [43], the puv/pa ratio was 0.49. Tunstall and Hawksworth [44] found a mean puv/pa ratio of halothane at delivery of 0.75. Stenger et al [14] found that puv/pa ratios correlated with the duration of administration of nitrous oxide and the same positive correlation was found between puv/pa and duration of administration of halothane ($p<0.05$), but not isoflurane.

Blood–gas partition coefficients are significantly less in the newborn infant than in adults, so that elimination of volatile agents should be rapid when respiration has been established. Fetal washout was not measured but Apgar scores were satisfactory in all infants at 5 min after delivery, suggesting that volatile agents are rapidly eliminated by the fetus. Elimination of enflurane by the neonate occurs rapidly and, as isoflurane has a lower blood solubility, it should be eliminated even more rapidly.

Although there is lack of published scientific evidence, there is no reason for not applying the same reasoning to sevoflurane and desflurane.Desflurane has been used by Navarro [48] in Germany; desflurane 2.5% was compared with isoflurane 0.5% in a randomized study comparing maternal and newborn effects with epidural anesthesia. Fifty patients under GA were randomly designated to receive either desflurane 2.5% or isoflurane 0.5% maintained in a 50-50% nitrous oxide and oxygen mixture. Twenty-five patients were assigned to receive epidural anesthesia using 15 ml ropivacaine 7.5 mg/ml with fentanyl 100 μg. Intraoperative hemodynamic changes, blood loss, and maternal awareness were recorded. Apgar scores at 1 and 5 min, neurological adaptive capacity scores (NACS) at 2 and 24 h and umbilical vein blood gas analysis were performed to assess neonatal outcome. Intraoperatively, heart rate and blood pressure changes were similar in both desflurane and isoflurane groups at 0.4% MAC. Blood loss and arterial blood gas analysis were not problematic and did not differ significantly between the three groups. In the desflurane group, the patients were more easily awakened and were more co-operative compared with the isoflurane group. The patients were interviewed about intraoperative awareness 24 and 48 h after the operation. None of them reported awareness during the operation. Similarly, the level of postoperative comfort was the same in both groups. Comparing GA with epidural anesthesia, no differences could be detected in neonatal outcomes. The study indicated that the one significant difference between desflurane 2.5% and isoflurane 0.5% anesthesia for cesarean section is the rapid recovery with desflurane, which makes it an attractive alternative to other inhalation anesthetics available to obstetric anesthesiologists. Considering the physical characteristics of sevoflurane, the same considerations may apply, with the added bonus of the possibility of gaseous induction, being non irritant [49].

All inhaled anesthetics cross the placenta; fetal uptake depends on uterine blood flow, the solubility of the drug in fetal blood, and the fetal distribution of the drug. Once across the placenta, there is rapid distribution to highly perfused fetal organs, such as the brain, liver, and kidneys. Uptake of drugs with lower blood –gas partition is more rapid, but for the same reason even washout should be faster.

In conclusion, we propose that the current sequence of GA for abdominal delivery should be modified to always include a potent inhalation agent to provide sufficient analgesia before the skin incision. This could be achieved by use of the least-soluble potent inhalatory agents desflurane and sevoflurane. The current practice of allowing surgery to start immediately after endotracheal intubation does not provide adequate analgesia at the time of skin incision during cesarean section. This may cause detrimental effects to both the mother and the newborn. When GA is indicated, besides informing the patient of the possibility of intraoperative awareness, it would probably be preferable to include some drugs that provide analgesia among the induction agents [50] or to perform a local anesthetic infiltration along the site of skin incision before induction of GA.

The only serious drawback of the inhalation agents is linked to their well-known effects on uterine activity; at the same MAC, they all exhibit significant uterine relaxant properties and these effects are most feared in obstetrics where following delivery the uterine musculature should promptly contract in order to exert a antihemorrhagic action. Blood loss has been correlated with GA and inhalation techniques, because halogenated agents decrease uterine muscle tone in a dose-related manner [51-54]; however at low MAC values these concerns have not been substantiated and generally in the immediate post-partum period the uterus has been able to respond to oxytocin administration [55]. However since uterine bleeding is slightly increased even at low MAC values [56-58], in order to avoid any problems and according to many published studies that demonstrated more blood loss following inhalation anesthesia than with intravenous analgesics and hypnotics, my suggestion is to stop the vapor during delivery, washing out the circuit with a high fresh gas flow and switching to a intravenous analgesic hypnotic combination immediately following delivery of the baby. Nitrous oxide can be continued since it has no effects on myometrial contractility.

Newborn condition after cesarean section performed under GA is comparable to that with regional techniques [59];however in the largest study performed to date, including 3,940 deliveries between 1975 and 1983, the multivariate analysis demonstrated that the risk of poor neonatal outcome following cesarean section was greater following GA than regional anasthesia [60].

The factors associated with low 1-min Apgar scores were:
primiparity, grand multiparity, antepartum disease (preeclampsia, diabetes mellitus, maternal heart disease, RH isoimmunization, early antepartum hemorrhage), presence of fetal distress, low gestational age, use of narcotics during labor, breech presentationm, nonelective ceseran section, and administration of GA.

However, it is difficult to draw definitive conclusions about neonatal outcomes due to the wide differences in anesthetic techniques and the concomitant risk factors; for instance duration of anesthesia has been reported to be a critical factor, with Apgar scores inversely related to duration of anesthesia [14]; the importance of direct uterus manipulation has been already described.

References

1. Hawkins JL, Koonin LM, Palmer SK, Gibbs CP (1997) Anesthesia related deaths during obstetric delivery in the United States.Anesthesiology 86:277-284
2. Tsen LC, Camann W (2000) Training in obstetric general anesthesia: a vanishing art? Anesthesia 55:179-183

3. Moir DD (1970) Anesthesia for Caesarean section; an evaluation of a method using low concentration of halothane and 50 per cent of oxygen. Br J Anaesth 42:136-142
4. Crawford JS (1971) Awareness during operative obstetrics during general anesthesia. Br J Anaesth 43:179-82
5. Tunstall ME (1979) The reduction of amnesic awakefullness during Caesarean section. anesthesia 34:316-319
6. Bergstrom H, Bernstein K (1968) Psychic reaction after analgesia with nitrous oxide for Cesarean section. Lancet II:541-542.
7. Cogan R, Spinnato JA (1986) Pain and discomfort thresholds in late pregnancy. Pain 27:63-68
8. Palahniuk RJ, Shnider SM, Eger El II (1974) Pregnancy decreases the requirement for inhaled anesthetic agents. Anesthesiology 41:82-83
9. Roizen MF, Horrigan RW, Frazer BM (1981) Anesthetic doses blocking adrenergic stress and cardiovascular responses to incision: MAC BAR. Anesthesiology 54:390-398
10. Stanski DR, Hudson RJ, Homer TD et al (1984) Pharmacodynamic modelling of the thiopental anesthesia. J Pharmacokinet Biopharm 12:223-240
11. Bihrer M, Maitre PO, Hung OR, et al (1992) Thiopental pharmacodynamics. I. Defining the pseudo-steady state serum concentration-EEG effect relationship. Anesthesiology 77: 226-236
12. Gambling DR, Sharma S, White P, et al (1995) Use of sevoflurane during elective cesarean birth: a comparison with isoflurane and spinal anesthesia. Anesth Analg 81:90–95
13. Schnider SM, Bichl DE (1980) The effects of maternal stress and general anesthesia on plasma catecholamine and uterine blood flow in the pregnant ewe. In: Sten L, (eds) Intensive care of the newborn. III. Masson, New York, pp 31-35
14. Stenger VG, Blechner JN, Prystowsky H (1969)A study of prolongation of obstetric anesthesia. Am J Obstet Gynecol 103:901-907
15 Latto IP, Waldron BA (1977) anesthesia for Caesarean section: analysis of blood concentrations of halothane using 0.2% or 0.65% halothane with 50% nitrous oxide in oxygen. Br J Anesth 49:371-378
16 Zaloga GP (1988) Catecholamine in anesthetic and surgical stress. Int Anesth Clin 26:187-98
17. Bihrer M, Maitre PO, Hung OR, et al (1992) Thiopental pharmacodynamics. I. Defining the pseudo-steady state serum concentration-EEG effect relationship. Anesthesiology 77: 226-236
18. Weyns H. De Deyne C, Corneillie M.et al (1999) Is there a correlation between maternal BIS at delivery comparing propofol and thiopental and neonatal apgar scores? Br J Anaesth 82:160-161
19. Tsai PS, Huang CJ, Hung YC, Cheng CR (2001) Effects on the bispectral index during elective caesarean section: a comparison of propofol and isoflurane. Acta anesthesiol Sin 39:17-22
20. Chemik DA, Gillings D, Laine H, et al (1994) Validity and reliability of the observer's assessment of alertness/ sedation scale: study with intravenous midazolam. J Clin Psychopharmacol 10: 244-251
21. Kearse LA Jr, Rosow C, Zaslavsky A, et al (1998) Bispectral analysis of the electroencephalogram predicts conscious processing of information during propofol sedation and hypnosis. Anesthesiology 88:25-34
22. Leslie K, Sessler DI, Schroeder M, Walters K (1995) Propofol blood concentration and the bispectral index predict suppression of learning during propofol/epidural anesthesia in volunteers. Anesth Analg 81:1269-1274
23. Glass PS, Bloom M, Kearse L, et al (1997) Bispectral analysis measures sedation and memory effects of propofol, midazolam, isoflurane, and alfentanil in healthy volunteers. Anesthesiology 86:836-847
24. Kissin I (2000) Depth of anesthesia and bispectral index monitoring Anesth Analg 90:1114-1117
25. Gaitini L, Vaida S, Collins G, Somri M, Sabo E (1995) Awareness detection during Caesarean section under general anesthesia using EEG spectrum analysis Can J Anaesth 42:377-381
26. Ghoneim MM, Block RI (1992) Learning and consciousness during general anesthesia. Anesthesiology 76:279-305

27. Griffith D, Jones FG (1990) Awareness and memory in anesthetized patients. Br J Anaesth 65:603-605
28. Jessop F, Jones JG (1991) Conscious awareness during general anesthesia–what are we attempting to monitor? Br J Anaesth 66:635-637
29. Breckenridge JL, Aitkenhead AR (1983) Awareness during anesthesia: a review. Ann R Coll Surg Engl 65:93-96
30. Brice DD, Hetherington RR, Utting JE (1970) A simple study of awareness and dreaming during anesthesia. Br J Anaesth 42: 535-542
31. Breckenridge JL, Aitkenhead AR (1983) Awareness during anesthesia: a review. Ann R Coll Surg Engl 65:93-96
32. Goldmann LK (1988) Information processing under general anesthesia: a review. J R Soc Med 81:224-227
33. King H, Ashley S, Brathwaite D, et al (1993) Adequacy of general anesthesia for cesarean section. Anesth Analg 77:84-88
34. Dundee JW, Wilson DB, (1980) Amnesia action of midazolam. Anesthesia 35:459-462
35. Bethune DW, Ghosh S, Gray B, et al (1992) Learning during general anesthesia: implicit recall after methohexitone or propofol infusion. Br J Anaesth 69:197-199
35. Block RI, Ghoneim MM, Sum Ping ST, Ali MA (1991) Human learning during general anesthesia and surgery Br J Anaesth 66: 170-178
36. Bennett HL, Davis HS, Giannini JA (1985) Non verbal response to intraoperative conversation. Br J Anaesth 57:174-179
37. Blacher RS (1984) Awareness during surgery. Anesthesiology 61:1-2
38. Domino KB; Posner KL., Caplan R, Cheney F. (1999) Awareness during anesthesia : a closed claims analysis. Anesthesiology 90:1053-1061
39. Lubke GH, Kerssens C, Gershon RY, Sebel PS (2000) Memory formation during general anesthesia for emergency cesarean section.Anesthesiology 92:1029-1034
40. Dwyer R,Fee JPH, Moore J (1995) Uptake of halothane and isoflurane by mother and baby during Caesarean section. Br J Anaesth 74:379-383
41. Chortkoff BS, Bennett HL, Eger EI II (1993) Does nitrous oxide antagonize isoflurane-induced suppression of learning? Anesthesiology 79:724-732
42. McCrirrick A, Evans GH, Thomas TA (1994) Overpressure isoflurane at Caesarean section: a study of arterial isoflurane concentrations. Br J Anesth 72:122-124
43. Gibbs CP, Munson ES, Tham MK (1975) Anesthetic solubility coefficients for maternal and fetal blood. Anesthesiology 43:100-103
44. Tunstall ME, Hawksworth GM (1981)Halothane uptake and N2O concentration; arterial halothane levels during Caesarean section. anesthesia 36:177-182
45. Marx GF, Joshi CW, Orkin LR (1970) Placental transmission of nitrous oxide. Anesthesiology 32:429-432
46. Hay DM (1978) Nitrous oxide transfer across the placenta and condition of the newborn at delivery. Br J Obstet Gynaecol 85:299-302
47. Latto IP, Waldron BA (1977) anesthesia for Caesarean section: analysis of blood concentrations of halothane using 0.2% or 0.65% halothane with 50% nitrous oxide in oxygen. Br J Anesth 49:371-378
48. Navarro EM (2000) Desflurane-general anesthesia for cesarean section compared with isoflurane and epidural anesthesia. Anasthesiol Intensivmed Notfallmed Schmerzther 35:232-236
49. Schaut DJ (1997) Sevoflurane inhalation induction for emergency caesaren section in a parturient with non intraveous access. Anesthesiology 86:1392
50. Gin T, Warwick D, Ngan Keeet et al (2000) Alfentanil given immediately before the induction of anesthesia for elective cesarean delivery. Anesth Analg 90:1167-1172
51. Naftalin NJ, Phear WPC, Goldberg AH (1975) Halothane and isometric contractions of isolated pregnant rat myometrium. Anesthesiology 42:458-463

52. Naftalin NJ, McKay DM, Phear WPC, Goldberg AH: (1977)The effects of halothane on pregnant and nonpregnant human myometrium. Anesthesiology 40:15-19
53. Munson ES, Maier WR, Caton D (1969) Effects of halothane, cyclopropane and nitrous oxide on isolated human uterine muscle. J Obstet Gynaecol Br Commonw 76:27-33
54. Munson ES, Embro WJ (1977) Enflurane, isoflurane, and halothane and isolated human uterine muscle. Anesthesiology 46:11 14
55. Marx GF, Kim YI, Lin CC, Halevy S, Schulman H (1978) Postpartum uterine pressures under halothane or enflurane anesthesia. Obstet Gynecol 51:695-698
56. Piggott SE, Bogod DG, Rpsen M, Rees GAD, Harmrer M (1990) Isoflurane with either 100% oxygen or 50% nitrous oxide in oxygen for cesarean section.Br J Anaesth 65:325-329
57. Thirion A-V, Wright RG, Messer CP, Rosen MA, Shnider SM (1988) Maternal blood loss associated with low dose halothane administration for cesarean section. Anesthesiology 69:A693
58. Gilstrap LC, Hauth JC, Hankins GDV, Patterson AR (1987) Effect of type of anesthesia on blood loss at cesarean section. Obstet Gynecol 69:328-332
59. James FM, Crawford JS, Hopkinson R (1977) A comparison of general anesthesia and lumbar epidural analgesia for elective cesarean section.Anesth Analg 56:228-233
60. Ong BY, Cohen MM, Palahniuk RJ (1989) Anesthesia for cesarean section:effects on neonates.Anesth Analg 68:270-275

Principles of Epidural Dosing in Labour

G. LYONS

Choice in local anaesthetic dosing extends to three variables: mass, concentration and volume. These interact and can be manipulated to achieve a desired effect. Decisions also have to be made regarding choice of local anaesthetic, the addition of other analgesic drugs, and the mode of administration. The issues can be considered in terms of best practice, understanding failure, and adopting the best solution.

Yau et al investigated six cocktails of bupivacaine and fentanyl for pain relief in labour. They gave 8mL boluses of plain bupivacaine, and with fentanyl 50μg or 100μg, for both 0.125% and 0.25%. The group receiving plain bupivacaine 0.125% was abandoned because there were too many failures. There were no differences in terms of analgesia or duration between the remaining groups [1]. Does this mean that bupivacaine 0.125% is not strong enough for labour analgesia? Is the dose of fentanyl unimportant? Why does fentanyl improve analgesia in the 0.125% groups, but not the 0.25% groups? An analysis of the principles of dosing can answer theses questions.

The analgesic band

Although there may be some evidence that epidural local anaesthetics are active in the dorsal horn of the cord, conduction blockade of the nerve root is the principle action. Epidural administration produces a band of analgesia with definable upper and lower limits. Bromage and Covino, pioneers of epidural anaesthesia, experimented with varying doses of lidocaine, and found that the size of the band in terms of dermatomes was proportional to the mass of local anaesthetic administered. The concentrations of lidocaine used tended to be greater than those that might be used for analgesia today [2]. The concept that dermatomal spread is solely dependent on dose now needs qualification. Columb et al gave 150mg chloroprocaine in varying dilutions using a sequential allocation technique to women in labour. When the concentration fell below

0.5%, failures of analgesia started to occur [3]. This suggests that dose is not the sole arbiter of block, and that an adequate concentration is necessary before an administered dose can be effective.

Differential block

Nerve roots carry a range of fibers with afferent and efferent functions. These fibers differ in terms of size, speed of conduction, and myelination according to their function. The fattest and fastest fibers are Aa motor fibers, and the slowest and smallest are unmyelinated C pain fibers. The ideal goal in labour would be to block all nociceptive afferent transmission while sparing all fibers with non-nociceptive functions. A high, anaesthetic concentration will block all afferent and efferent functions, with dense analgesia and motor block, but for lower concentrations, the degree of differential nerve block is controlled by local anaesthetic concentration [4]. The larger the fiber, the greater is the distance between nodes of Ranvier. As the distance between the nodes increases, so does the concentration of local anaesthetic required to block conduction. By reducing concentration it is possible to achieve differential nerve block according to a hierarchy of nerve fiber size (Table 1).

Table 1. Hierarchy of nerve fibers, sizes, characteristics and functions. Cm is the minimum concentration of local anaesthetics required to block conduction at two nodes of Ranvier.

Class	A-alpha	A-beta	A-gamma	A-delta	B	C
Function	Motor	Touch, pressure	Proprioception	Pain, temp	Preganglionic autonomic	Pain, temp
Myelin	+++	++	++	++	+	-
Diameter (μm)	12-20	5-12	5-12	1-4	1-3	0.5-1
Speed (m/sec)	70-120	30-70	30-70	12-30	1-3	1-2
Cm/ onset time	6th	5th	4th	3rd	2nd	1st

The goal in labour is to block C and Aδ pain fibers but leave Aα motor fibers intact. Because the fast motor fibers have a higher blocking concentration, a selective sensory block is achievable. The traditional teaching is that B sympathetic fibers are blocked first, and this would create difficulties if all women with selective sensory blockade suffered from postural hypotension. Clinical experience suggests otherwise. Breen et al found that 92% of women receiving an epidural cocktail of bupivacaine/fentanyl/epinephrine were comfortable,

68% could walk, 17% had evidence of motor block and 9% had postural hypotension [5]. This infers that unmyelinated C pain fibers are blocked first, and that many women do not have complete B sympathetic block.

The *visceral* pain of the first stage of labour may be C fiber mediated, and the *somatic* pain of the second stage might have a greater component of Aδ fibers. Capogna et al have shown that advancing labour increases the analgesic requirement [6]. One explanation of this would be increasing Aδ recruitment as the foetal head descends. More support for this comes from the use of intrathecal opioids, which are more effective at treating pain mediated through C than Aδ fibers. Intrathecal opioids in labour are effective during the first stage, but not for the second [7]. For all these reasons, use of low concentrations of epidural local anaesthetic combined with opioid in the first stage, should allow painless mobility.

Addition of opioids

Many anaesthetists add opioid to their epidural local anaesthetic without a clear rationale. Examination of the dose – response curve for bupivacaine indicates that the EC95 for bupivacaine will lie between 0.12% and 0.14% [8]. The closest concentration in clinical use that corresponds to this is 0.125% bupivacaine. For this concentration and all higher concentrations it should be possible to achieve satisfactory first stage analgesia without recourse to opioid.

Increasing doses of epidural fentanyl decrease the concentration of epidural bupivacaine required for analgesia in a dose dependent manner [9]. The rationale for adding fentanyl then becomes clear. Bupivacaine of 0.125% or higher will produce a degree of motor blockade, so to achieve motor sparing analgesia, a lesser concentration is required. Without fentanyl, this will not be adequately effective.

There are other beneficial effects. The addition of epinephrine to lidocaine extends both the spread of the analgesic band and the duration of analgesia, and similarly, the addition of opioid will also increase the duration of analgesia [2]. Smith et al have shown that in women receiving equianalgesic mixtures of plain bupivacaine and bupivacaine with added fentanyl, the addition of fentanyl can increase the spread of the analgesic band [10]. This is despite the bupivacaine/fentanyl mixtures having lower concentrations, and therefore smaller doses of bupivacaine. Adding opioid allows a reduction in concentration, which produces differential block. Without an increase in volume, this also means a reduction in dose, but if fentanyl increases the size of the analgesic band, analgesia may be maintained at the lower dose. The role of fentanyl is to promote differential block with separation of sensory and motor effects, with analgesia maintained despite a reduced dose of local anaesthetic.

Role of volume

Epidural drugs require a fluid vehicle to achieve adequate spread to nerve roots, and this is one of the least researched aspects of epidural dosing. Experience suggests that anaesthetists are more conservative with volume than with dose, but evidence suggests that dose produces more problems than volume. The concentration of local anaesthetic required to block conduction is indirectly proportional to the length of nerve that it bathes. This phenomenon is known as *decremental block* [4]. If this is true, the use of dilute concentrations of local anaesthetic will be more effective if given in a large volume. Lyons et al measured the median effective analgesic volumes (EV50) for plain bupivacaine 0.125% and 0.25%, at 13.2mL and 9.2mL respectively. In clinical terms, these volumes probably correspond to EV60-70. The respective doses of bupivacaine were 17mg and 23.1mg. This difference was significant. By increasing the volume by 50%, and halving the concentration, it was possible to achieve a dose reduction of 25% without any sacrifice of analgesia [11]. This supports the concept of decremental block in clinical practice, and points to beneficial effects from giving higher volumes.

Understanding failures

It is now clear that the reason for failure of analgesia in the study of Yau et al was due to the 8mL bolus volume of 0.125% bupivacaine. This approaches half of the EV50 for that concentration and was clearly too small to be effective. The EV50 of 0.25% bupivacaine is 9.2mL, and is close to the volume used in this study, but the analgesia was sufficient. It is harder to show differences when the groups are small.

We can also understand why adding fentanyl made no difference to the analgesia provided by 0.25%, and why there was no difference between the groups of fentanyl. Clinically successful epidural analgesic solutions produce satisfactory analgesia in a high proportion of patients. Once a low pain score has been achieved, adding more local anaesthetic, fentanyl or more fentanyl, will not further improve satisfaction. Only when failures of analgesia occur are we able to make comparisons of analgesic efficacy.

Assuming that all epidurals are correctly placed, failures occur because either the analgesic band does not include the requisite nerve roots, or there is a source of pain outside the expected distribution. For the first stage of labour this must be from T11 to L2. High volume, low concentration bupivacaine with fentanyl generally produces an analgesic band that extends from T10 to L3/4, and this meets the requirements for first stage analgesia. A small number of women with the foetus in the occipito-posterior position experience pain outside the first stage distribution, and although the analgesic band is in place, from the bedside the epidural appears to be a failure [12]. Extension of the band to achieve analgesia requires an increase in dose that is probably best accomplished by increasing the concentration, and the density of the block. The penalty will be greater motor blockade.

The high volume low concentration approach can also be inadequate as the second stage approaches. The same remedy can be adopted.

Methods of administration

Bolus administration is associated with tachyphylaxis, but in clinical practice with bupivacaine, this is rarely seen. Continuous infusion is associated with a gradual onset of a denser block [13].

Conclusion

If the goal of analgesia in labour is selective blockade that spares motor function, then low concentration local anaesthetic supported by opioid is the best solution. The addition of opioid will extend the limits of the analgesic band. A higher bolus volume will allow some reduction in dose, and improve safety. The onset of the second stage may require a higher concentration of local anaesthetic. The lower limit of the analgesic band is often in the region of L3/4, and if the source of pain is sacral in origin, the epidural will appear to fail. The analgesic band can be extended by increasing the dose.

References

1. Yau G, Gregory MA, Gin T et al (1990) The addition of fentanyl to epidural bupivacaine in the first stage of labour. Anaesth Int Care 18: 532-535
2. Cousins MJ, Bromage PR (1988) Epidural neural blockade. In: Cousins MJ, Bridenbaugh PO (eds) Neural blockade in Clinical Anaesthesia and Pain Management. Lippincott, Philadelphia, pp253-360
3. Columb MO, Lyons G, Naughton NN et al (1997) Determination of the minimum local analgesic concentration of epidural chloroprocaine in labor. Int J Obs Anesth 6: 39-42
4. Fink BR (1992) Towards the mathematization of spinal anesthesia. Reg Anesth 17: 263-273
5. Breen TW, Shapiro T, Glass B et al (1993) Epidural anesthesia for labor in an ambulatory parturient. Anesth Analg 77: 919-924
6. Capogna G, Celleno D, Lyons G et al (1998) Minimum local analgesic concentration of epidural bupivacaine increases with progression of labour. Br J Anaesth 80: 11-13
7. Mather LE (1994) Opioid analgesic drugs. In: Nimmo WS, Rowbotham DJ, Smith G (eds) Anaesthesia 2nd ed. Blackwell, Oxford pp 132-165
8. Columb MO, Lyons G (1995) Determination of the minimum local analgesic concentrations of epidural bupivacaine and lidocaine in labor. Anesth Analg 81: 833-837
9. G Lyons, M O Columb, L Hawthorne et al (1997) Epidural pain relief in labour: bupivacaine sparing by epidural fentanyl is dose dependent Br J Anaesth 78:493-497
10. Smith P S, Robinson APC, Wilson RC et al (2001) Analysis of dermatomal spread of equi-potent extradural analgesia in 76 labouring women receiving either plain local anaesthetics solutions or local anaesthetic and fentanyl. Int J Obs Anesth 10: 232
11. Lyons G, Gorton H, Robinson APC et al (2001) Comparison of minimum local analgesic volumes of two concentrations of epidural bupivacaine. Anesthesiology 94: 1A, A60
12. Benhamou D, Hamza J, Frizelle H (1997) Failure of regional anaesthesia in obstetrics. In: Russell IF, Lyons G (eds) Clinical problems in obstetric anaesthesia. Chapman and Hall, London pp244-247

Epidural, Spinal, or Combined Spinal Epidural for Cesarean Section

I.F. RUSSELL

Epidural, spinal or combined spinal epidural (CSE), which should we use for cesarean section? Factors that may influence the decision include the time available, the presence of a working epidural, the mother's previous experience, the likely duration of surgery, and the presence of maternal pathology especially cardiac, neurological, or previous back surgery. While such factors are often considerations, usually the technique used is entirely due to anesthetist preference.

In the United Kingdom, regional anesthesia now accounts for over 75% of cesarean section anesthetics [1-3]. Of these regional anesthetics, 61% were single-shot spinals, 28% were epidurals, and 11% were CSEs [1]. The distribution of these blocks is very different between elective and emergency cesarean sections, an indication of the different requirements between these two situations. For elective surgery under regional anesthesia, the distribution of the blocks was 78% spinal, 4% epidural, and 18% CSE. For emergency surgery it was 47% spinal, 48% epidural, and 5% CSE [1].

An interesting observation in this survey [1] was the failure rate of the chosen regional anesthetic technique. The overall failure rate (i.e., when the original block was converted to another anesthetic technique) for epidurals was 7.1%, for CSEs was 2%, and for single-shot spinals was 1.9% [1]. Failure of regional anesthesia accounted for 10% of the general anesthetic cases and there was a wide variation [1] among the units. In the 120 units which took part in the survey, the incidence of failed blocks requiring conversion to general anesthesia varied from 0 to 88% [1]. Of the failed blocks, some 32% were converted to general anesthesia intraoperatively [1]. This wide variation in the incidence of failed blocks and the fact that 32% of the failures were not detected until surgery was underway implies that there may have been difficulty in obtaining an adequate level of block in some cases, and that the method used to test the block was not reliable in others. Irrespective of which regional anesthetic technique is to be used, it is important to test the block with a reliable method before surgery starts, as this will afford the opportunity to augment a poor block or to initiate an alternative regional technique on an elective basis, rather than have general anesthesia forced upon us as the only option in the middle of surgery.

Assessment of the block

It is suggested that the height of block for a pain-free cesarean section should be T4 [4] but until recently there was no guidance on how this level should be assessed. The different modalities used to test the block (cold sensation, sharp pin prick, touch) can give very different impressions of the block height. There is a zone of differential block at the cranial end of a spinal or epidural anesthetic such that, on average, cold sensation indicates a block two dermatomes higher than sharp pin prick, and sharp pin prick is in turn two dermatomes higher than touch [5, 6]. However, in any one individual patient, knowing the level of block to sharp pin prick or cold does not enable the level of block to touch to be estimated as there may be up to ten dermatomes difference between sharp pin-prick and touch sensations in individual patients. [5-8]. Figures 1 and 2 illustrate the variations between the levels of sharp pin prick and touch in

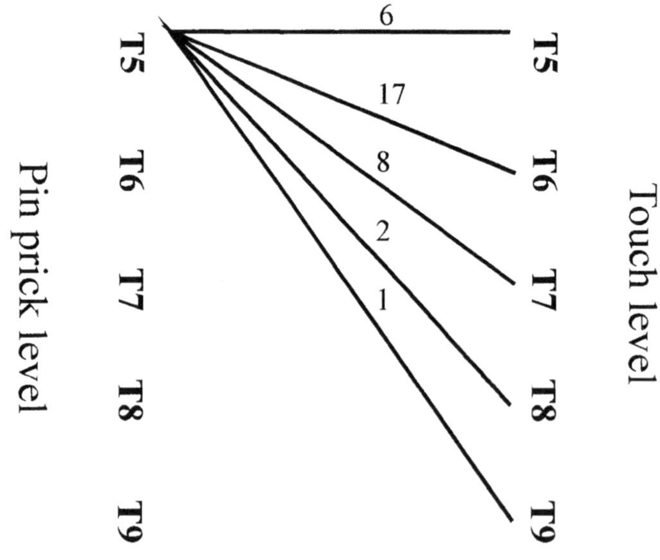

Fig 1. The variation in the levels of anesthesia (touch sensation) when the level of analgesia (sharp pin prick sensation) was T5 – as assessed at the time of delivery in 34 women. The numbers in the middle of the transverse/oblique lines indicate the number of women with that relationship between pin prick and touch levels. The data in this figure were obtained from the original raw data as used in reference [7]

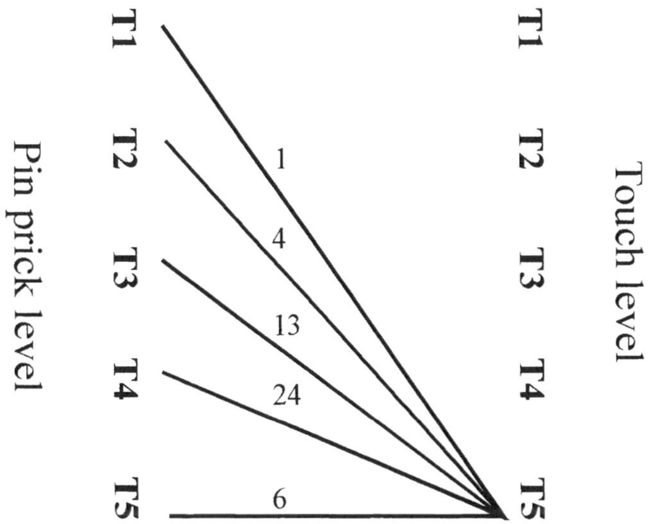

Fig 2. The variation in the levels of analgesia (sharp pin prick sensation) when the level of anesthesia (touch sensation) was T5 – as assessed at the time of delivery in 48 women. The numbers in the middle of the transverse/oblique lines indicate the number of women with that relationship between pin prick and touch levels. The data in this figure were obtained from the original raw data as used in reference [7]

patients who had either a block to pin prick or a block to touch at T5 at delivery of the baby [7].

For many years it has been recognized that some regional anesthetics are more effective than others despite the same level of block to cold or sharp pin prick [9-12] and perusal of the published literature reveals wide variations in the proportion of successful blocks between different studies, all of which have the same high levels of block to cold or sharp pin prick. Figure 2 illustrates this variation in successful blocks: all patients included in the studies in Fig. 3 had a level of block to at least T4 as assessed by sharp pin prick. It is quite clear that the proportion of successful blocks is very different, both within and across the individual studies. Several authors have shown that touch is a more-reliable modality to use for testing a block [16-18], and recent obstetric anesthesia text books now acknowledge this fact and indicate that the block to touch sensation should extend up to include T5 [19, 20].

Since the majority of United Kingdom anesthetists use cold sensation to test the adequacy of their block [21], it is perhaps not surprising that surgery may be started with an inadequate density of block in a proportion of cases, and that general anesthesia will be required to complete surgery. There is, of course, an

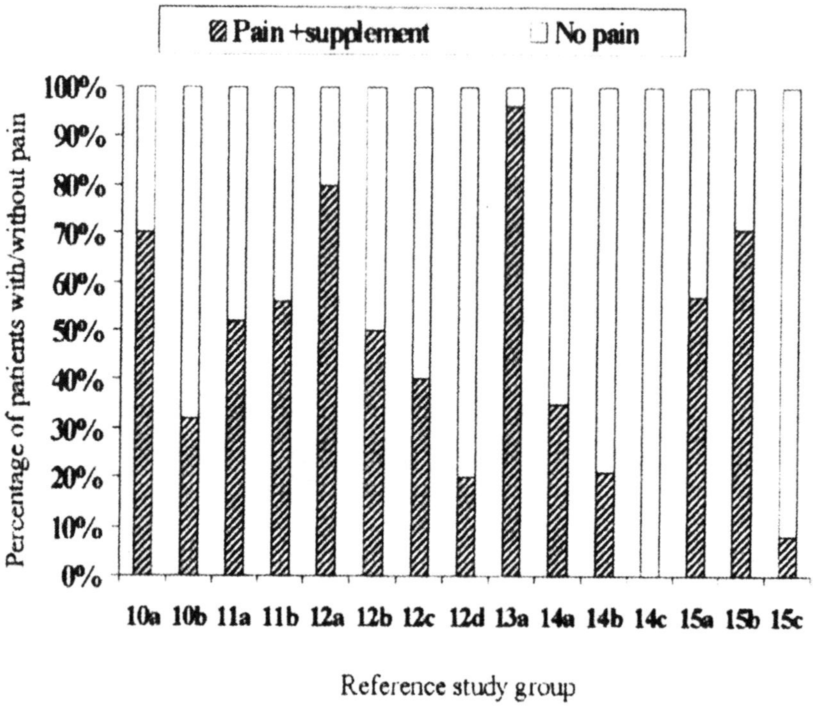

Fig. 3. Six studies involving different spinal anesthetic techniques in which no intrathecal narcotics were used. All women in these studies had a block to pin prick assessed as T4 or above. The numbers below the columns refer to the specific reference and the letters to the group within that reference

apparent contradiction inherent in the above discussion: the vast majority of cesarean sections are performed successfully when cold or sharp pin prick are used to assess the block – does this not indicate that testing with these sensations has merit? Despite the success rates for regional anesthesia, there is no evidence that testing with cold or sharp pin prick has significant predictive value. Most spinal or epidural blocks are successful because anesthetists have developed a technique with a low failure rate – as Oyston says, "*If you give the right dose of the right drug into the right place, the block* ***WILL*** *work. Testing is hardly necessary, and I often omit it.*"[22]. This statement would appear to have some support [21]: 12% of anesthetists rarely or never check the upper dermatomes of their regional block and 68% rarely or never assess the lower level [21]. Unless these anesthetists have very high failure rates, then they must have developed regional anesthetic techniques that work despite being inadequately or never assessed.

Epidural anesthesia

The major disadvantage of initiating an epidural for any cesarean section is the time required, but if a working epidural is already in situ then this disadvantage disappears. Indeed, the presence of a working epidural catheter puts spinal and CSE anesthesia at a significant disadvantage – these may now take longer to initiate than topping up the epidural to achieve an adequate block. It has been suggested that this advantage of epidural analgesia should be put to good use [23]. These authors [23] found that 87% of emergency cesarean sections could be predicted, thus giving anesthetic staff the opportunity to establish epidural analgesia for labor pain relief and the epidural could then be used to "prepare" the patient for surgery before the final decision to operate has been taken.

To obtain the maximum advantage from a working epidural in the emergency situation an appropriate top-up regimen must be used. In the past, slow careful top-up regimens were used and these led to a very slow onset of block, sometimes taking in excess of 60 min before satisfactory anesthesia could be obtained [24, 25] and often theoretically toxic doses of local anesthetics were administered [24]. In addition, with these slow top-up techniques, many women still needed intra-operative supplements – 40% in one study [26]. Over the years there has been a gradual refinement of techniques to reduce the time required to achieve surgical anesthesia and improve the efficacy of the epidural. In general these techniques involve topping up the epidural with the woman in a lateral position using various local anesthetic drug mixtures that include lipid-soluble narcotics, such as fentanyl, sufentanil, or alfentanil and often other drugs such as epinephrine or bicarbonate [25-35]. A regimen in which the complete dose is given over 2–3 min achieves a very rapid onset [32, 35]. Price et al. [32] also showed that the same final block height (to cold) was obtained irrespective of the initial starting block level when 20 ml of lidocaine 2% with epinephrine 1: 200,000 was given. Most of these drug mixtures are not available commercially so care must be taken to ensure that none of the drugs being mixed contain preservatives. The mixtures are best made up immediately before use as there are few data on their stability.

The top-up regimens described above were studied either for elective cesarean section or for topping-up a labor epidural that was unsupplemented with narcotics. Today, women usually receive a low-dose bupivacaine/fentanyl mixture during labor, and a recent study [36] found no difference in the onset time of various mixtures when topping-up the epidurals in these women. In addition, it takes time to prepare the mixtures – up to 4 min for some of them – and this could offset any small saving in time [37]. Thus further studies are needed to evaluate various top-up regimens in women who have already received low-dose epidurals with added narcotic.

With our own top-up regimen [lidocaine 2% (20 ml), fentanyl 100 μg and 1/200,000 epinephrine] given in the labor room during shaving and catheterization, women undergoing emergency cesarean section, even for prolapsed cord, are almost invariably ready for surgery before the surgical team. But there are those who believe that topping-up an epidural rapidly in a labor room, away from full anesthetic monitoring and resuscitation facilities, is an unsafe practice, and certainly there are anecdotal reports of women developing total spinal anesthesia in this situation who then have to be rushed to the operating theater for endotracheal intubation. However, if a patient is moved to the operating theater before topping-up her epidural then often the delay is such that there is no time for the epidural to be topped-up and general anesthesia has to be used. It is then debatable which policy is likely to place a patient at greater risk. If it is felt necessary to transfer patients to the operating theater before topping up the epidural, then it is important that as soon as the decision is made to deliver the baby by emergency cesarean section the mother is immediately moved to theatre – before shaving, catheterizing, obtaining consent, and all the other things that can lead to significant delay.

The importance of a good epidural top-up regimen is illustrated by a recent study [38]. These authors [38] audited 100 consecutive cases where a patient had her epidural topped-up for an emergency cesarean section. They noted that 30% of women received a theoretically toxic dose of local anesthetic drugs, 17% required intravenous or inhalation supplementation during surgery, and in 5% the epidural top-up failed and general anesthesia was induced. They suggest that perhaps it is time to reconsider the place of epidural top-ups and made the proposal that induction of spinal anesthesia may be a safer and more-reliable choice for emergency cesarean section, even in the presence of a functioning epidural. This was a surprising suggestion and stimulated an audit of our own practice. We too examined the records of our last 100 women whose epidural had been topped-up for emergency cesarean sections. We noted 4 complete failures where an apparently effective block for labor could not be extended for cesarean section and, because of time limitations, general anesthesia was used. None of our remaining 96 cases required intra-operative supplementation of any kind, nor did any receive theoretically toxic doses of local anesthetics. It would seem likely that this difference in outcomes is a reflection on the efficacy of the different top-up regimens used – our lidocaine/adrenaline/fentanyl mixture versus the incremental top-up regimen used by Cole et al. [38] (10 ml of 0.5% bupivacaine followed by up to 10 ml lidocaine followed by 3 mg diamorphine). Apart from those cases in which there is a total failure of the epidural and time is of the essence, there are few indications for general anesthesia when a patient with a functioning epidural in situ requires emergency cesarean section. If time is limited and no epidural catheter is in place then, if regional anesthesia is to be used, the choice lies between spinal or CSE.

Spinal anesthesia

Spinal anesthesia is the method of choice in the United Kingdom: some 61% of all regional blocks for Caesarean section in the United Kingdom are now single-shot spinals [1]. There is debate about the best position to use for induction of spinal anesthesia. Many anesthetists find the sitting position technically easier, but it must be remembered that gravity may affect the distribution of a hyperbaric solution and thus the need for intraoperative supplementation. Induction of spinal anesthesia in the right lateral position has been shown to have fewer failures than the left lateral [39, 40]. However, Inglis et al. [41] found no difference in the efficacy of spinals induced in the sitting or right lateral positions but they required intraoperative supplements in a large number of women in both groups: 35% and 38%. This high requirement for supplementary analgesia would seem to indicate some subtle differences between the right lateral technique as used by Inglis et al. [41] and that used in our own hospital. Examination of our published data [42-45] and an audit of the last 150 personal (or personally supervised) spinals for elective cesarean section indicates that no woman required any intra-operative supplements. Further, analysis of additional data from a three-center study of 681 spinal cesarean sections [46] in which our unit took part also showed there was a significant difference in the need for intra-operative supplements between the sitting and right lateral induction positions (8% vs. 17%, $P < 0.002$), but there was no statistical difference between the sitting and left lateral positions. General anesthesia was required in 0.8% of the right lateral spinals, 1% of the sitting spinals, and 1.4% of the left lateral spinals [46]. The effects of posture can also be observed when the "Oxford" position is used: the Oxford position is the left lateral position but with three pillows under the head and a 3-l polyinfusor bag placed under the shoulder to create an upward (lateral) curve of the vertebrae in the thoracic region [47]. Stoneham et al. [47], in a comparison of the Oxford position with the sitting position found that 3.3% of the women in both groups required intraoperative supplements, knife-to-skin occurred more quickly in the sitting group than in the "Oxford" position group (28 min versus 32 min) but there was no difference in the time to delivery (36 min v 40 min). The need for analgesia and the time intervals from spinal injection to skin incision or to delivery of the baby are very different from our experience: no need of supplementary analgesia, 10 - 12 min spinal injection to skin incision time, 16 - 17 minspinal injection to delivery time [44, 45]. By 40 min the vast majority of our cesarean sections are complete!

On the few occasions when a sitting spinal is indicated, the author ensures that the patient is seated so that her right shoulder is towards the head of the table and immediately on completion of the spinal injection she is instructed to lie down on her right side while an assistant brings the legs up onto the table. This reduces to an absolute minimum the time sent in the sitting position after the intrathecal injection. She is then turned from the right lateral to the supine wedged position.

Addition of opioids

The addition of lipid-soluble opioids such as fentanyl or sufentanil contributes considerably to the efficacy of spinal anesthesia, but these drugs are too short-acting to confer much pain relief in the postoperative period other than for the first 2 h [48-50]. Morphine significantly reduces the need for postoperative analgesia, but morphine is poorly lipid soluble and has a slow onset, so its contribution to intra-operative analgesia is minimal [49-51]. Studies of intrathecal morphine have been contradictory. Some have found the intra-operative effects of morphine to be no better than placebo [49, 51] and another found morphine to be no worse than fentanyl [50]. These contradictory results may be due to differences in the anesthetic technique. The two studies described which found morphine no better than placebo [49, 51] induced spinal anesthesia in a sitting position, while Sibilla et al. [50] used the left lateral position. If the sitting position results in a less-effective local anesthetic block than the lateral position, then to ensure a good block the intrathecal narcotic would need to make a greater contribution to the anesthetic effect. It may be that with its slow onset morphine is unable to make this effective intra-operative contribution. Another drawback to intrathecal morphine is the fact that it has a very prolonged half life in the spinal fluid, and as such there is always the potential for late-onset respiratory depression. In those countries where it is legally available, the pharmacokinetic profile of diamorphine makes it the drug of choice for adding to spinal anesthetic solutions. It has a rapid onset of action and makes a significant contribution to intra-operative analgesia [52], its half-life in the cerebrospinal fluid (CSF) is measured in minutes [53], but it has a duration of action similar to morphine [45, 54]. Unlike morphine, diamorphine is taken up rapidly into neural tissue and fixed there, so there are good theoretical reasons why delayed respiratory depression should not occur.

Combined spinal epidural

Of the three techniques, CSE is by far the most expensive. The commercial needle kits and extra drugs required add around £8.00 to the basic cost compared with a single-shot spinal. Like a single-shot spinal, to produce the best results from CSE it is important that one has a clear understanding of how the spread of the spinal component of CSE may be affected by the position used for induction and the time spent in that posture after the spinal injection. It is also important to remember that CSE is a generic term that encompasses several different techniques: needle through needle, two needle same interspace, two needle different interspace. All of these may vary as to whether the spinal injection is given before the epidural catheter is inserted or the epidural catheter is inserted and then the spinal injection is administered. In addition, there are three different basic designs of needle through needle CSE kits - one of these has a double-barrelled needle [55], which enables the epidural catheter to be inserted first.

The optimum distance the spinal needle should protrude beyond the tip of the epidural needle is debatable [56], but it will be different depending on whether a midline or paramedian approach to the epidural space is used. It is surprising that even with a "guide" needle in the epidural space it is still possible to fail with the spinal injection component. There are several reasons for this failure of the spinal component.

1. The spinal needle may be angled too far laterally and miss the dura. This could be due to the direction of the epidural needle per se or to the extra bend given to the spinal needle as it exits the bevelled tip of the epidural needle. This problem can be overcome by ensuring the bevel of the epidural needle is facing axially before penetrating the ligamentum flavum, then any extra bend given to the spinal needle will at least ensure it does not deviate from the midline. Usually the bevel will face cranially as this is the direction in which most of us hope the epidural catheter will go. If this is the case then we need to remember that the spinal needle will be going even more cranially and could be encroaching on the conus of the cord. Special epidural needles with a "back eye" allow the spinal needle to pass straight ahead rather than having to negotiate the curve of the bevel of the epidural needle.
2. If the spinal needle is too short it may not reach the dura. Alternatively, the elasticity of the dura may allow it to stretch and become tented up over the tip of the spinal needle. On occasions the dura is so elastic that it may not be pierced until it is trapped against the surface of a vertebral body. In this case then both anterior and posterior layers of dura will be penetrated

simultaneously and no CSF will be aspirated [57]. Occasionally, the elastic resistance of the dura can be perceived by the operator and in this case asking the patient to give a small cough while holding the needle stationary, or using a very small stabbing motion, will promote penetration of the dura by the needle.

In terms of the efficacy of the initial spinal injection, problems arise with any technique where the spinal injection is given before the epidural catheter is inserted - because of the time required to thread the epidural catheter. During this "epidural insertion" time the spinal anesthetic drug will be under the influence of gravity, and thus the position of the patient is important, then after re-positioning the patient to a supine wedged position the slope of the spinal canal will affect distribution of the spinal anesthetic. These positional effects can be seen in studies using the "Oxford" position and the sitting position. Both the sitting position [58] and the Oxford position [59] limit the spread of the initial spinal injection to the extent that some of the advantages of spinal anesthesia are negated and the epidural catheter becomes a necessity. Thompson [60] presented data from some published and unpublished studies indicating that on a regular basis a top-up via the epidural catheter was a necessity for some 25% of CSE cases. In a randomized study it was shown that 39% of CSEs performed in the sitting position required an epidural top-up compared with 4% induced in a lateral position [58]. Similarly, 28% of women required an epidural top-up when the Oxford position was used for induction [59]. Since the failure rate of a single-shot spinal is only between 1 and 2 %, the 25% need for an epidural supplement to enhance the block from the spinal component of a CSE indicates significant restriction of the spread of the spinal component of a CSE. However, it seems some CSEs work very adequately. Another study comparing lateral and sitting induction techniques for a CSE found no difference in the onset of the block between the positions [61]. The most likely reason for the findings of Yun et al. [61] are that their patients were placed in a supine position within 3 min, whereas patients in the Oxford position may have been in a lateral position for at least 7 min [60]. Also, patients in the study of Yun et al. [61] were excluded from analysis if it took longer than 3 min to attain the supine wedged position. The problems related to delay in passing the epidural catheter can be eliminated if a CSE technique is used whereby the epidural catheter is inserted first before the spinal anesthetic is given. This will provide all the usual advantages of a spinal with the epidural catheter as a backup.

The main advantage of CSEs using the sitting or Oxford position lies in the fact that the spinal anesthetic spread is inhibited - the slower onset of the block results in a lower incidence of hypotension [58]. Again, as with speed of onset of the block, Yun et al. [61] found the opposite – they found a greater incidence and more-severe hypotension in the group who had their CSE induced in the sitting position compared with the lateral inductions.

While CSE in general is claimed to provide the advantages of a spinal with the flexibility of an epidural, and that the deficiencies in the spinal can be covered by the epidural and vice versa, the published data do not altogether support these assertions. As discussed above, often the CSE technique inhibits the spread of the spinal, such that the epidural catheter is frequently required for topping up the anesthetic – in some ways this is like buying an expensive sports car and then driving with one foot on the brake much of the time! If failure of the epidural and spinal components of the CSE are truly independent then the overall failure rate for a CSE (i.e., when general anesthesia is required) should be the product of the epidural failure rate and the spinal failure rate. For elective cesarean sections the spinal failure rate was 1% and the epidural failure rate 3% [1]. Thus the CSE failure rate should have been 0.01 X 0.03 – i.e., around 0.03%. The fact that the actual failure rate for CSE was 0.5% [1] (16 times greater than the theoretical failure rate) suggests that when performing a CSE the failure of the spinal and epidural components are not independent. It is also notable that in terms of total conversion to another anesthetic technique there was no difference between spinal and CSE. The total requirement for spinal anesthesia conversions was 1.9% (to general anesthesia, CSE, or epidural); the total requirement for CSE anesthesia conversions was 2% (to general anesthesia, spinal, or epidural) [1].

While there may be some added benefit of using a spinal and an epidural together, we should not forget that the combination may also result in synergistic effects as regards the complications. With CSE the relatively large doses of drugs intended for the epidural space have even more chance of going astray! When injecting drugs into the epidural space after a CSE it must be remembered that the hole in the dura may lead to somewhat unpredictable effects – sometimes many hours after the original dural puncture. This has led to unexpected cases of respiratory arrest when narcotics are injected into the epidural space [62, 63] or total spinals when an epidural is topped-up. Care is required when topping-up the "failed" spinal component of a CSE. A volume of fluid, even saline alone, in the epidural space can cause a significant rise in spinal anesthetic levels [64-68]. Thus a careful incremental top-up technique is essential to ensure that no unexpected sudden extension of the spinal component occurs.

While CSE has its very strong proponents, it is used for only 9% of cesarean sections in the United Kingdom [1]. Compared with a single-shot spinal, CSE anesthesia is prone to the unexpected [62–68] and, despite being more complicated and expensive, offers no advantage in terms of neonatal outcomes [69].

Unless there are specific indications (e.g., controlling the unpredictable spread of spinal anesthesia in a very obese patient, where the duration of surgery is expected to be prolonged, where there is a need for flexible postoperative analgesia, where there is a requirement for a slow onset of block to enable careful control of blood pressure), there seems little other than personal preference to support their routine use.

Both spinals and CSEs have been implicated in a number of cases of neurological damage [70-73]. This seems to be due to an inability of anesthetists to identify the appropriate lumbar interspace before inserting spinal needles [74, 75]. On only 15% of occasions was L3/4 correctly identified, the remainder of the time it was wrongly identified 1 - 4 spaces higher [75]. Reynolds [71] believes that, in the long hiatus when spinal anesthesia was not practised to any extent in the United Kingdom, anesthetists became "gung ho" in their choice of interspace for insertion of an epidural needle. With epidural anesthesia, the whole spinal canal may be used with relative safety. With the re-introduction of spinal anesthesia and the development of CSEs, many anesthetists seem to have forgotten that it is inadvisable to enter the spinal canal above the termination of the cord and continue to use the intervertebral spaces they would use for epidural anesthesia thereby risking damage to the conus of the spinal cord. As a rule of thumb, the conus never overlaps Tuffier's line in normal individuals [76], so if all attempts at spinal or CSE are no higher than Tuffier's line then the cord should be safe in normal individuals.

Conclusion

Epidural anesthesia is generally accepted as having the highest failure rate of the three types of regional anesthetic [1, 77]. However, a good epidural is just as effective as a good spinal or CSE in terms of patient comfort [78]. Provided anesthetists are aware of the advantages and disadvantages of a particular regional anesthetic technique and use the advantages to good effect while taking the appropriate action to minimize or eliminate the disadvantages, especially testing the block adequately, then there may be little to chose between the various regional anesthetic techniques. Which technique is used will depend on such factors as the time available, maternal choice, anesthetist choice, proposed duration of surgery, and cost.

References

1. Shibli KU, Russell IF (2000) A survey of anaesthetic techniques used for caesarean section in the UK in 1997. Int J Obstet Anesth 9:160-167
2. Khor LJH, Jeskins G, Cooper GM, et al (2000) National obstetric anaesthetic practice in the UK 1997/1998. Anaesthesia 55:1168-1172
3. NHS Maternity Statistics, England:1995-96 to1997-98 http://www.doh.gov.uk/public/sb0114.htm.
4. Datta S, Alper MH (1980) Anesthesia for cesarean section. Anesthesiology 53:142-160
5. Brull SJ, Greene NM (1989). Time-courses of zones of differential sensory blockade during spinal anesthesia with hyperbaric tetracaine or bupivacaine. Anesth Analg 69:342-347
6. Brull SJ, Greene NM (1991) Zones of differential sensory block during extradural anaesthesia. Br J Anaesth 66:651-655
7. Russell IF (1995) Levels of anaesthesia associated with intra-operative pain at caesarean section under spinal or epidural block. Int J Obstet Anesth 4:71-77
8. James KS, Stott SM, McGrady EM, et al (1996) Spinal anaesthesia for caesarean section: effect of Sprotte needle orientation. Br J Anaesth 77:150-152
9. Pan P, Lin Z-F, Lim J, et al (1989) The optimal does of hyperbaric tetracaine spinal anaesthesia for caesarean section. Acta Anaesth Sin 27:349-352
10. Pedersen H, Santos A, Steinberg E, et al (1989) Incidence of visceral pain during cesarean section: the effect of varying doses of spinal bupivacaine. Anesth Analg 69:46-49
11. Alahuhta S, Kangas-Saarela T, Hollmén AI, et al (1990) Visceral pain during caesarean section under spinal and epidural anaesthesia with bupivacaine. Acta Anaesth Scand 34:95–98
12. Hirabayashi Y, Saitoh K, Fukuda H, et al (1995) Visceral pain during caesarean section: effect of varying dose of spinal amethocaine. Br J Anaesth 75:266 -268
13. Santos A, Pedersen H, Finster M, et al (1984) Hyperbaric bupivacaine for spinal anesthesia in cesarean section. Anesth Analg 63:1009-1013
14. Choi HD, Ahn HJ, Kim MH, et al (2000) Bupivacaine-sparing effect of fentanyl in spinal anesthesia for cesarean section. Reg Anesth Pain Med 25:240-245
15. Choi HD, Park NK, Cho HS, et al (2000) Effects of epidural injection on spinal block during combined spinal and epidural anesthesia for cesarean section. Reg Anesth Pain Med 25:591-595
16. Rocco AG, Raymond SA, Murray E, et al (1985) Differential blockade of touch, cold, and pinprick during spinal anesthesia. Anesth Analg 64:917-923
17. Russell IF (1995) Levels of anaesthesia and intraoperative pain at caesarean section under regional block. Int J Obstet Anesth 4:71-77
18. Liu S, Kopacz DJ, Carpenter RL (1995) Quantitative assessment of differential sensory nerve block after lidocaine spinal anesthesia. Anesthesiology 82:60-63
19. Norris MC (1999) Spinal anesthesia for cesarean delivery. In: Norris MC (ed) Obstetric anesthesia, 2nd edn. Lippincott Williams and Wilkins, Philadelphia p 428
20. Yentis SM, Brighouse D, May A, et al (2001) Analgesia, anaesthesia and pregnancy. Saunders, London pp 92-96
21. Bourne TM, deMelo BA, Bastianpillai BA et al (1997) A survey of how British obstetric anaesthetists test regional anaesthesia before caesarean section. Anaesthesia 52:901-903
22. Oyston J. A Guide to Spinal Anaesthesia for Caesarean Section for Anaesthetists & Anesthesiologists. http://www.virtual-anaesthesia-textbook.com.
23. Morgan BM, Magni V, Goroszenuik T (1990) Anaesthesia for emergency Caesarean section. Br J Obstet Gynaecol 97:420-424
24. Crawford JS (1984) Principles and practice of obstetric anaesthesia, 5th edn. Blackwell Scientific Publications, Oxford
25. Moir DD, Thorburn J (1990) Factors modifying epidural block for Caesarean section. In: Reynolds F (ed) Epidural and spinal blockade in obstetrics. Ballière Tindall, London pp 151-159
26. Dutton DA, Moir DD, Howie HB, et al (1984) Choice of local anaesthetic drug for extradural

caesarean section: comparison of 0.5% and 0.75% bupivacaine and 1.5% etidocaine. Br J Anaesth 56:1361-1368
27. Laishley RS, Morgan BM (1988) A single dose epidural technique for caesarean section: a comparison between 0.5% bupivacaine plain and 0.5% bupivacaine with adrenaline. Anaesthesia 43:100–103
28. Norton AC, Davis AG, Spicer RJ (1988) Lignocaine 2% with adrenaline for epidural caesarean section: a comparison with 0.5% bupivacaine. Anaesthesia 43:844–849
29. Howell P, Davies W, Wrigley M, et al (1990) Comparison of four local extradural anaesthetic solutions for elective caesarean section. Br J Anaesth 65:648-653
30. Noble DW, Morrison LM, Brockway MS, et al (1991) Adrenaline, fentanyl or adrenaline and fentanyl as adjuncts to bupivacaine for extradural anaesthesia in elective caesarean section. Br J Anaesth 66:645–650
31. Fernando R, Jones HM (1991) Comparison of plain and alkalinised local anaesthetic mixtures of lignocaine and bupivacaine for elective extradural caesarean section. Br J Anaesth 67:699–703
32. Price ML, Reynolds F, Morgan BM (1991) Extending epidural blockade for emergency caesarean section. Evaluation of 2% lignocaine with adrenaline. Int J Obstet Anesth 1:13–18
33. Clarke V, McGrady E, Sugden C, et al (1994) Speed of onset of sensory block for elective extradural caesarean section: choice of agent and temperature of injectate. Br J Anaesth 72:221–223
34. Gaiser RR, Cheek TG, Gutsche BB (1994) Epidural lidocaine versus 2-chloroprocaine for fetal distress requiring urgent cesarean section. Int J Obstet Anesth 3: 208 - 210
35. Gaiser RR, Cheek TG, Adams HK, et al (1998) Epidural lidocaine for cesarean delivery of the distressed fetus. Int J Obstet Anesth 7:27-31
36. Lucas DN, Ciccone GK, Yentis SM (1999) Extending low-dose epidural analgesia for emergency Caesarean section. A comparison of three solutions. Anaesthesia 54:1173-1177
37. Lucas DN, Borra PJ, Yentis SM (2000) Epidural top-up solutions for emergency Caesarean section: a comparison of preparation times. Br J Anaesth 84:494-496
38. Cole P, Dresner M, Stockwell J, et al (2001) Anaesthesia for emergency caesarean section in women already receiving epidural analgesia. Int J Obstet Anesth 10:214
39. Sprague DH (1976) Effects of position and uterine displacement on spinal anesthesia for cesarean section. Anesthesiology 44:164-166
40. Russell IF (1987) The effect of posture during induction of subarachnoid analgesia for Caesarean section. Right versus left lateral. Br J Anaesth 59:342-346.
41. Inglis A, Daniel M, McGrady E (1995) Maternal position during induction of spinal anaesthesia for caesarean section: a comparison of right lateral and sitting positions. Anaesthesia 50:363-365
42. Russell IF, Holmqvist ELO (1987) Subarachnoid analgesia for caesarean section. A double-blind comparison of plain and hyperbaric 0.5% bupivacaine. Br J Anaesth 59:347-353
43. Graham D, Russell IF (1997) A double-blind assessment of the analgesic sparing effect of intrathecal diamorphine (0.3 mg) with spinal anaesthesia for elective caesarean section. Int J Obstet Anesth 6:224-230
44. Husaini SW, Russell IF (1998) Volume preload: lack of effect in the prevention of spinal-induced hypotension at caesarean section. Int J Obstet Anesth 7:76–81
45. Husaini SW, Russell IF (1998) Intrathecal diamorphine compared with morphine for postoperative analgesia after Caesarean section under spinal anaesthesia. Br J Anaesth 81:135-139
46. Hopkinson JM, Samaan AK, Russell IF, et al (1975) A comparative multicentre trial of spinal needles for caesarean section. Anaesthesia 52:1005-1011
47. Stoneham M, Eldridge J, Popat M, et al (1999) Oxford positioning technique improves haemodynamic stability and predictability of block height of spinal anaesthesia for elective Caesarean section. Int J Obstet Anesth 8:242-249
48. Shende D, Cooper GM, Bowden MI (1998) The influence of intradural fentanyl on the characteristics of subarachnoid block for caesarean section. Anaesthesia 53:706-710
49. Sghirlanzoni S, Attanasio A, Della Grazia L, et al (1995) Spinal anaesthesia for elective caesarean

section: comparison of three different anaesthetic solutions. 14th Annual European Society of Regional Anaesthesia Congress, Prague. The International Monitor September: 89
50. Sibilla C, Albertazzi P, Zatelli R, et al (1997) Perioperative analgesia for caesarean section: comparison of intrathecal morphine and fentanyl alone or in combination. Int J Obstet Anesth 6:43-48
51. Swart M, Sewell J, Thomas D (1997) Intrathecal morphine for caesarean section: an assessment of pain relief, satisfaction and side effects. Anaesthesia 52:373-375
52. Kelly MC, Carabine UA, Mirakhur RK (1998) Intrathecal diamorphine for analgesia after caesarean section. A dose finding study and assessment of side-effects. Anaesthesia 53:231-237
53. Moore A, Bullingham R, McQuay H, et al (1984) Spinal fluid kinetics of morphine and heroin. Clin Pharmacol Ther 35: 40-45
54. Barkshire K, Russell R, Burry J, et al (2001) A comparison of bupivacaine-fentanyl-morphine with bupivacaine-fentanyl-diamorphine for caesarean section under spinal anaesthesia. Int J Obstet Anesth 10:4-10
55. Eldor J, Guedj P, Gozal Y (1992) Combined spinal-epidural anesthesia using the CSEN. Anesth Analg 74:169-170
56. Wildsmith JAW (1998) Problems with combined spinal epidural anesthesia (editorial). Reg Anesth 23:388-389
57. Zarzur E (1998) The posterior epidural space depth. Reg Anesth 23:108-109
58. Patel M, Samsoon G, Swami A, et al (1993) Posture and the spread of hyperbaric bupivacaine in parturients using the combined spinal epidural technique. Can J Anaesth 40:943-946
59. Westerbrook JL, Donald F, Carrie LES (1992) An evaluation of a combined spinal/epidural needle set utilising a 26 gauge, pencil point needle for caesarean section. Anaesthesia 47:990-992
60. Thompson KD (2001) The use of spinal epidural anaesthesia for elective caesarean section is a waste of time and money. Int J Obstet Anesth 10: 30-32
61. Yun EM, Marx GF, Santos AC (1998) The effects of maternal position during induction of combined spinal-epidural anesthesia for cesarean delivery. Anesth Analg 87:614-618
62. Greenhalgh CA (1996) Respiratory arrest in a parturient following intrathecal injection of sufentanil and bupivacaine. Anaesthesia 51:173-175
63. Myint Y, Bailey PW, Milne BR (1993) Cardiorespiratory arrest following combined spinal epidural anaesthesia for Caesarean section. Anaesthesia 48:684-686
64. Budd A, Russell IF (1987) The influence of an epidural fluid challenge on spinal anaesthesia. Obstetric Anaesthetists Association, Spring Meeting, Hull, p 20
65. Blumgart CH, Ryall D, Dennison B, et al (1998) Mechanism of extension of spinal anaesthesia by extradural injection of local anaesthetic. Br J Anaesth 69:457-460
66. Stienstra R, Dahan A, Alhadi BZR, et al (1996) Mechanism of action of an epidural top up in combined spinal epidural anesthesia. Anesth Analg 83:382-386
67. Mardirosoff C, Dumont L, Lemédioni P, et al (1998) Sensory block extension during combined spinal and epidural. Reg Anesth Pain Med 23:92-95
68. Takiguchi T, Okano T, Egawa H, et al (1997) The effects of epidural saline injection on analgesic level during combined spinal and epidural anesthesia assessed clinically and myelographically. Anesth Analg 85:1097-1100
69. Thorén T, Holmström B, Rawal N, et al (1994) Sequential combined. spinal epidural block versus spinal block for cesarean section: effects on maternal hypotension and neurobehavioural function of the newborn. Anesth Analg 78:1087-1092
70. Rajakulendran Y, Rahman S, Venkat N (1999) Long-term neurological complication following traumatic damage to the spinal cord with a 25 gauge Whitacre spinal needle Int J Obstet Anesth 8:62-66
71. Reynolds F (2000) Logic in the safe practice of spinal anaesthesia. Anaesthesia 55:1045-1046
72. Reynolds F (2001) Damage to the conus medullaris following spinal anaesthesia. Anaesthesia 56:238-247
73. Parry H (2001) Spinal cord damage. Anaesthesia 56:290.

74. Van Gessel EF, Forster A, Gamulin Z (1993) Continuous spinal anesthesia where do spinal catheters go? Anesth Analg 76:1004-1007
75. Broadbent CR, Maxwell WB, Ferrie R, et al (2000) Ability of anaesthetists to identify a marked lumbar interspace. Anaesthesia 55:1122-1126
76. Hogan QH (1994) Tuffier's line: the normal distribution of anatomic parameters. Anesth Analg 78:194-195
77. Vegfors M, Cederholm I, Gupta A, et al (1992) Spinal or epidural anaesthesia for elective caesarean section? Int J Obstet Anesth 1:141-144
78. Patel M, Craig R, Laishley R (1006) A comparison between epidural anaesthesia using alkalinized solution and spinal (combined spinal/epidural) anaesthesia for elective caesarean section. Int J Obstet Anesth 5:236-239

Do We Need a Test Dose for Epidural Anaesthesia and Analgesia in Obstetrics?

G. CAPOGNA, M. CAMORCIA

The most important complication of epidural analgesia and anaesthesia is the unrecognized accidental misplacement of either the intravascular or subarachnoid epidural catheter.

If a large volume of local anaesthetic is injected in the subarachnoid space severe hypotension, loss of consciousness and complete paralysis develop over a period of 5-10 minutes following the injection and may last several hours.

Massive intravascular injection of local anaesthetic will result in dose dependent systemic local anaesthetic toxicity, with central nervous system symptoms, seizures and cardiovascular collapse.

The ideal method for excluding intravenous or subarachnoid misplacement of an epidural catheter is controversial.

Intravascular injection

In the obstetric population the risk of unintentional epidural vein cannulation is higher than in the non pregnant population due to dilated epidural veins. Blood vessel puncture occurs in 9% to 20% of obstetric patients [1,2] and intravenous placement of an epidural catheter occurs in approximately 5% of obstetric patients [3].

Correctly placed epidural catheters may migrate into epidural veins or in the subarachnoid space [4].

For this reason, a test dose should be given not only before the initial therapeutic dose, but also before each top-up dose when an intermittent epidural technique is used [5-9].

Aspiration

Careful observation and gentle aspiration of the needle or catheter may identify a vast majority of accidental intravascular misplacement.

Norris et al. demonstrated a sensitivity of 97.9% and a specificity of 100% in detecting intravascular catheter placement with aspiration [10, 11]

Although a false negative aspiration test may occur in over 30% of the single-holed epidural catheters, this is reduced to about 0.4% with multi orifice catheters [3, 11].

The practice of withdrawing an intravenously placed catheter until blood is no longer aspirated has been criticized as being unreliable since the chance of a false negative aspiration test increases. In fact, although blood can no longer be aspirated, the catheter may still be intravenous [11]. For this reason it is probably better to replace such a catheter rather than to try to reposition it.

Incremental injection

The local anaesthetic should be administered in divided doses, each of which serves as its own test dose by relying on the development of subjective symptoms [9]. Theoretically, if small injections are used, the patient will report subjective symptoms before blood local anaesthetic concentration reaches the threshold for seizures- system toxicity [12].

Epinephrine

Epinephrine was the first agent used to identify intravenous misplacement of the epidural catheter and it quickly became established as the cornerstone of the intravenous test dose, although a large number of alternative agents have been investigated since.

In 1981 Moore and Batra [13] described for the first time the cardiovascular effects of 15 μg of epinephrine when injected intravenously in sedated non pregnant patients. They reported the use of intravenous 15 μg of epinephrine mixed with one local anaesthetic suitable to test for subarachnoid injection in a series of 175 surgical patients.

In all but three of these patients the pulse rate increased unmistakably and transiently in the first 60 seconds after injection. The average heart rate increased of approximately 30 beats per minute, with the initial increase occurring at 20 seconds and the heart rate returning towards normal by 60 seconds.

They used the 15 μg dose in order to mimic the administration of 3 ml of a local anaesthetic solution containing 1:200,000 epinephrine.

They demonstrated that the pulse changes are evanescent and then the technique of counting the pulse for 15 seconds is not likely to be reliable in detecting changes that last less than a minute. For this reason, they stressed the need for recording the heart rate with an electrical beat-to-beat calculation by ECG.

They concluded that the ideal test dose should include a dose of 15 μg of epinephrine and a local anaesthetic that would result in a rapid evidence of spinal anaesthesia.

Subsequent studies by Guinard et al. [14] determined the sensitivity of an epinephrine-containing an epidural test dose, as well as its lowest effective dose in healthy non pregnant volunteers. They concluded that 10 μg of epinephrine is the lowest effective dose and that this agent is 100% sensitive in detecting intravascular injection.

The efficacy of the epinephrine test dose in patients treated with β-blockers has been questioned.

In fact, isolated case reports have suggested that β-blockers interfer with epinephrine testing [15, 16].

Guinard et al. [14] confirmed that the presence of acute β-blockade with either a specific [β1] or a non specific (esmolol or propanolol) agent makes the heart rate changes an unreliable indicator of intravascular injection of epinephrine. In fact, propanolol blockade actually resulted in a bradycardia after epinephrine, probably secondary to transient hypertension produced by an unopposed alpha-adrenergic effect of epinephrine. The systolic blood pressure did increase consistently, by 15 mm of Hg, in the presence of both specific and non specific β-blocker agents. Hypertension may be the only reliable indicator of intravascular injection in this population although it has been reported to last only 2 minutes [14].

Parturients

The efficacy of an epinephrine containing epidural test dose in labouring patients has been questioned because of the wide variability in maternal heart rate in pregnancy [17].

Some anaesthesiologists argue that the epinephrine-containing test dose lacks specificity because the maternal response to the drug cannot be distinguished from other causes of tachycardia during labour (pain during uterine contractions) [18-20].

Catwright at al. [20] administered a test dose containing bupivacaine but not epinephrine to100 labouring women. Twenty-four percent of the patients had an increase in heart rate greater than 20 beats per minute and 12% had an increase greater than 30 beats per minute following the injection of the test dose. This would produced a false positive rate of 12% if 30 beats per minute were chosen as the criterion for positivity and a false positive rate of 24% if 20 beats per minute criterion would have been adopted. In addition to this study 14% of the women had contractions during the test period associated with heart rate changes.

The authors concluded that the interpretation of the epinephrine test dose for obstetric patients is difficult because of the poor specificity of the test.

Chesnut et al. [19] reported similar results, showing that 5 out of 10 patients in labour had a spontaneous increase in heart rate of more than 25 beats per minute during a 15 minute observation period before and after the injection of a test dose.

Leighton et al. [17] also demonstrated that the heart rate variability associated with labour makes the standard test dose inaccurate.

Different results were obtained by Van Zundert et al. [9] who used a test dose of 12.5 mg of bupivacaine plus 12.5 μg of epinephrine in two groups of healthy labouring women. They noted a short lived (5 seconds) increase in the maternal heart rate and in the systolic blood pressure soon after injection of the test dose. Unfortunately this study was not randomized, nor double blinded.

Leighton et al. [17] has shown that the heart rate variability associated with labour makes the interpretation of the epinephrine containing test dose inaccurate. In this study they injected 15 μg of epinephrine intravenously in 10 labouring women but only 5 had an increase of heart rate (30 beats per minute from baseline) occurring within 2 minutes and lasting at least 15 seconds. However, they were able to obtain a higher degree of reliability using retrospectively a more complicated peak-to-peak analysis of heart rate changes. This method is based on the detection of a positive maternal tachycardic response of 10 beats per minute over the maximum maternal heart rate measured during the 2 minutes preceding the epinephrine containing a test dose injection. This technique is cumbersome and is not 100% effective; furthermore during peak-to-peak calculations, they could identify only nine out of ten epinephrine injections.

Colonna-Romano [21] confirmed these findings using a baseline to peak criteria assessed in absence of uterine contractions within a minute after a test dose of 10-15 μg of epinephrine.

The safety of epinephrine containing a test dose

Many anaesthesiologists have expressed several concerns regarding the use of an epinephrine containing a test dose in labouring women because it may have adverse effects on the mother or the foetus by producing a reduction in uterine blood flow from α receptor mediated constriction of the uterine artery or of uterine contractions [18, 22, 23] .

In animal models, epinephrine infusion has shown to reduce uterine artery blood flow in the guinea pig [8] and produce deleterious effects in the sheep foetus [22]. In one study, Leighton et al. [17] demonstrated signs of foetal distress in two of ten patients (one with bradycardia and another with late decelerations) following intravenous epinephrine injection.

Youngstrom et al. [24] noted that the intravenous injection of 15 μg of epinephrine did not worsen the foetal condition in acidotic foetal lambs.

Also, Abboud et al. [25] reported that the inclusion of epinephrine in the therapeutic doses used for labour analgesia does not have deleterious effects on the foetus and even reduces the incidence of maternal hypotension.

Any transient effect of epinephrine on uterine blood flow likely represents a less severe insult than systemic local anaesthetic toxicity. Furthermore, the decrease in uterine blood flow is comparable to that which occurs during a uterine contraction.

There is also concern about the possibility of unintentional intravascular epinephrine injection exacerbating the hypertension associated with pre-eclampsia [26].

Heller and Goodman [27] have reported the safe use of epinephrine containing solutions in four pre-eclamptic patients, although none of these involved intravascular injections.

Alternative test dose

Local anaesthetic

Before the 1980's local anaesthetic drugs themselves were used as a test dose to produce subjective signs of early toxicity when injected intravasculary [28].

The signs of central nervous system (CNS) irritability, produced by subtoxic doses of local anaesthetic, include lightheadedness, ringing or buzzing in the ears, perioral tingling, abnormal taste, altered hearing, and drowsiness.

The dose required is larger than the doses necessary to produce subarachnoid anaesthesia, and thus, the standard test dose is insufficient.

The volume used in the traditional test dose (3 ml of the anaesthetic solution) is not sufficient to identify intravascular placement. Furthermore, premedication with sedatives such as benzodiazepines may reduce the sensitivity of this test. Clinical trials on the injection of 100 mg of chlorprocaine [29], 100 mg of lidocaine [30] or 25 mg bupivacaine [12] have shown to be reliable indicators of intravascular injection in unmedicated volunteers.

At the present time the use of subtoxic doses of local anaesthetics does not seem a reliable standard procedure for testing an epidural catheter.

Isoprotenerol

The role of isoprotenerol as an alternative marker of intravascular catheter placement during epidural anaesthesia has been recently questioned.

Isoproterenol, a pure β-adrenergic agonist, produces a $\beta_1$mediated tachycardia and a $\beta_2$mediated vasodilatation with a baroflex induced additional tachycardia as opposed to the bradycardia seen with epinephrine.

Leighton et al. have suggested isoproterenol to be a reliable marker of intravascular injection [31]. They reported that, although the chronotropic response to β-adrenergic stimulation is reduced in term parturients, 5 μg of isoprotenerol produced a significant increase of 15 beats per minute in the maternal heart rate when compared with a saline injection, but that the complicated peak-to-peak analysis of the heart rate was required to detect the change reliably.

These results were confirmed in a randomized trial, studying the haemodynamic effects of an intravenous injection of 5 mg of isoprotenerol in 60 non labouring women at term [32]. In these patients, injection of 5 μg of isoprotenerol consistently increases both maternal heart rate and uterine blood flow.

Studies in pregnant sheep have shown either a minor or no reduction in uterine blood flow and a more consistent heart rate increase than what is seen with the use of epinephrine [23,33].

Ephedrine

Cherala and Greene [34] described the use of ephedrine in the test dose using hypertension as the clinical indicator.

They demonstrated that 15 mg of ephedrine is a reliable indicator of intravascular injection, but this detection requires the complicated peak-to-peak analysis to demonstrate systolic blood pressure changes.

The heart rate analysis alone is not reliable and this makes clinical application difficult because of the need for a long baseline analysis and careful determination of blood pressure.

Air

In 1989 Leighton et al. [35, 36] reported the use of air as an effective marker of intravenous located epidural catheter. The authors demonstrated that 1 ml of air injected into an epidural vein clearly produces audible changes in heart rate sounds monitored with a precordial Doppler stethoscope.

There is some concern that even small bubbles may have the potential to cross a patent foramen ovale and produce systemic embolic lesions.

Another problem is that the correct placement of a precordial Doppler on the chest of a pregnant woman having contractions may represent some challenges that will increase the likelihood of a false negative result.

Fentanyl

The use of 100 μg of fentanyl has been suggested to verify proper epidural catheter placement [37]. Based on prompt appearance of dizziness, drowsiness, and sedation as key findings, the fentanyl effect was more consistently identified after intravenous than epidural administration with a sensitivity of 100% and a specificity of 95%.

However, this dose is considered excessive by many anaesthetists and further investigation is needed.

Test dose and low concentration labour analgesia

The appearance of the symptoms produced by subtossic doses of local anaesthetic are not very useful in labouring patients when diluted doses of local anaesthetic are now commonly used. When very diluted solutions of local anaesthetic are used for labour analgesia the inadvertent intravenous injection will not produce significant signs of systemic toxicity, but merely leads to a failed block [11, 38-40].

If no analgesic effects are noted after an epidural bolus for labour analgesia accidental intravascular injection of the local anaesthetic solution should also be considered.

Subarachnoid injection

The risk of accidental dural puncture and subarachnoid catheter misplacement is described as being as high as 0.6-2.7% in the obstetric population [41]. The intrathecal injection of epidural doses of a local anaesthetic has been estimated to be 2/1000 epidural anaesthetic procedures [42].

Furthermore, correctly placed epidural catheters may migrate into epidural veins or the subarachnoid space [43].

As with the intravenous testing, a subarachnoid accidentally placed catheter can be often diagnosed by gentle aspiration and careful observation of any resulting aspirate. Unfortunately, like the intravenous testing, reliance on aspiration for cerebrospinal fluid alone is hazardous because of false negative results [3, 21].

Assessment of temperature, glucose content or protein content may identify the presence of cerebrospinal fluid and therefore subarachnoid misplacement of an epidural catheter [44].

The use of a multi orifice catheter is likely to enhance the reliability of the aspiration test.

An ideal subarachnoid test dose should allow easy identification of the epidural catheter misplacement an in few minutes without causing total spinal anaesthesia and haemodynamic compromise.

In their original paper describing the components of an effective test dose, Moore and Batra combined 15 μg of epinephrine with a number of different local anaesthetics in a dose that would rapidly result in spinal anaesthesia [13].

Abraham et al. [45] showed that 1.5% hyperbaric lidocaine (2 or 3 ml) produces sensory anaesthesia after epidural injection, but not before three minutes. In contrast, the same drug injected into the subarachnoid space produces sensory changes to pinprick in the S2 dermatome within two minutes. Thus adequate testing requires specific evaluation of pinprick appreciation in the S2 dermatome at two minutes following the test dose injection.

Lidocaine has been commonly used in America, as test dose of up to 45 mg (3 ml of 1.5%) producing a spinal block in few minutes. However, excessively high spinal blocks have been reported with such doses in parturients. [41, 47, 48].

Conversely, in some cases, block may be delayed in onset, giving a false negative result.

Hyperbaric solutions if injected intrathecally, typically produce a rapid onset of sacral analgesia with some evidence of motor block. Unfortunately, the hyperbaric solution described by Abraham is not available commercially. In a study of older, non pregnant patients receiving continuous spinal analgesia for surgery, Colonna-Romano and Lingaraju [48] used the commercially available test dose consisting of 45 mg of lidocaine plus epinephrine (without dextrose). The authors concluded that the best methods for detecting intrathecal injection is an assessment of motor function (straight leg raising) four minutes after the test dose injection. The application of these data to pregnant patients is unclear. Richardson et al. [46], described the rapid onset (1 to 3 minutes) of high levels of spinal anaesthesia with motor block and hypotension in five parturients who had received a test dose that included 45 mg of lidocaine plus 15 μg of epinephrine (without dextrose). This solution is slightly hypobaric at body temperature. Thus the upright posture of these parturients during the injection may have contributed to the high levels of spinal anaesthesia.

Bupivacaine in doses between 7.5 mg (3 ml of 0.25%) and 15 mg (3 ml of

0.5%) is the standard agent used to test for intrathecal placement in the UK.

A block to C3 could be due to the introduction of 15 mg of intrathecal bupivacaine, and both cranial nerve involvement and total spinal block have been reported [49-51].

Conclusions

Labour analgesia

There is now a common belief that the upright position and walking in labour are important to the progress and outcome of labour. Low-dose epidural analgesia and CSE may allow maternal ambulation. A standard lidocaine test dose may affect ambulation producing a motor block [52]. For this reason a lidocaine containing test dose is not often used in labour analgesia.

If no analgesic effects are noted after an epidural bolus accidental intravenous injection of the local anaesthetic solution should be suspected. If early and rapid effective analgesia is noted, inadvertent intrathecal injection should be taken into consideration. Recent studies suggest that standard low-dose loading boluses of 10-15 ml of 0.0625% - 0.10% bupivacaine with opioids added are in themselves suitable test doses [53-55]. No studies are available on the safety and reliability of ropivacaine and levobupivacaine as test doses for labour.

In addition, future studies should be directed to determine how to test an epidural catheter after a CSE analgesia or before an emergency caesarean section in a parturient with an epidural catheter already in place.

Evaluating the risks and benefits and the reliability of an epinephrine test dose in parturients, it seems prudent to include 15 mg of epinephrine as a part of a standard test dose procedure until a better alternative is found. In all cases, continuous electronically monitoring of heart rate and intermittent blood pressure determination before and immediately after the injection is necessary to detect accidental intravenous administration.

Caesarean section

The standard test dose for a caesarean section is 30-45 mg of lidocaine or 7.5-15 mg of bupivacaine with 15 mg of epinephrine. No studies are available on the safety and reliability of ropivacaine and levobupivacaine as test dose for caesarean section. Intravenous ropivacaine and levobupivacaine has been inadvertently administered without complications and published as case-reports in obstetric [56] and non obstetric patients [57]. A safe and readily detectable spinal block in non-obstetric patients was produced by 3 ml of subarachnoid consisting of 0.25% ropivacaine [58,59]. However, the safe subarachnoid dose for these agents is not known.

Recommendations

- No perfect dose exist.
- Observe for the passive return of blood or cerebral spinal fluid (CSF) while positioning the catheter.
- Carefully aspirate for at least 10 seconds with a 5 mL syringe to the 3rd ml mark [60].
- Observe again for the passive return of blood or CSF through the catheter.

Labour

- Do not use lidocaine if walking analgesia is desired.
- The use of epinephrine is controversial.
- Each epidural bolus must be tailored as a test dose.
- Administer the test dose after uterine contraction.
- If no analgesic effects are noted after an epidural bolus accidental intravenous injection of the local anaesthetic solution should be suspected.
- If early and rapid effective analgesia is noted, inadvertent intrathecal injection should be taken into consideration.

Caesarean section

- Administer 45 mg of lidocaine with epinephrine 1:200,000.
- Wait for at least 3 minutes.
- Observe for the occurrence of a sensory sacral block [61].
- Observe for the occurrence of any leg motor block (Bromage criteria).
- Observe for the occurrence of transient and sudden maternal tachycardia (ECG, SaO_2).

References

1. Mannion D, Walker R, Clayton K (1991) Extradural vein puncture: An avoidable complication. Anaesthesia; 46: 585-7
2. Verniquet AJW (1980) Vessel puncture with epidural catheters. Anaesthesia; 35: 660-2
3. Kenepp NB, Gutsche BB (1981) Inadvertent intravascular injections during lumbar epidural anaesthesia (letter). Anesthesiology; 54: 172-3
4. Reynolds F (1988) Epidural catheter migration during labour [letter]. Anaesthesia;43:6
5. Ravindran RS, Albrecht W, McKay M (1979) Apparent intravascular migration of an epidural catheter. Anesth Analg; 58: 252-3
6. Seeling W, Heinrich W (1984) Unexpected intravenous penetration of an epidural catheter. Reg Anaesth; 7: 137-9
7. Robson JA, Brotsky JB (1977) Latent dural puncture after lumbar epidural block. Anesth Analg; 56: 725-35
8. Hartrick CT, Pither CE, Pai U et al (1985) Subdural migration of an epidural catheter. Anesth Analg; 64: 175-8
9. Van Zundert A, Vaes L, Soetens M et al (1987) Every dose given in epidural analgesia for vaginal delivery can be a test dose. Anesthesiology; 67: 436-40
10. Norris MC, Ferrembach D, Dalman H, et al (1998) Does epinephrine improve the diagnostic accuracy of aspiration during labor epidural analgesia? Anesth Analg, 88: 1073-1076
11. Norris MC, Fogel ST, Dalman H, et al (1998) Labor epidural analgesia without an intravascular "test dose". Anesthesiology; 88: 1495-1501
12. Abouleish E, Bourke D (1984) Concerning the use and abuse of test doses for epidural anesthesia. Anesthesiology;61:344-5
13. Moore DC, Batra MS (1981) The components of an effective test dose prior to epidural block. Anesthesiology; 55: 693-6
14. Guinard JP, Mulroy MF, Carpenter RL, Knopes KD (1990) Test dose: optimal epinephrine content with and without acute beta adrenergic blockade. Anesthesiology;73:386-92
15. Popitz-Bergetz F, Datta S, Ostheimer GW (1988) Intravascular epinephrine may not increase heart rate in patients receiving metoprolol. Anesthesiology; 68: 815-816
16. Soni V, Peeters C, Covino B (1981) Value and limitations of test dose prior to epidural anesthesia. Reg Anesth; 6: 23-25
17. Leighton BL, Norris MC, Sosis M et al (1987) Limitation of epinephrine as a marker of intravascular injection in laboring women. Anesthesiology;66:688-91
18. Chestnut DH, Weiner CP (1986) Monitoring maternal heart rate during epidural injection of a test dose containing epinephrine. Anesthesiology; 64: 839-40
19. Chestnut DH, Owen CL, Brown CK et al (1988) Does labor affect the variability of maternal heart rate during induction of epidural anesthesia. Anesthesiology; 68: 622-5
20. Cartwright PD, McCarroll SM, Antzaka C (1986) Maternal heart rate changes with a plain epidural test dose. Anesthesiology; 65: 226-8.
21. Colonna-Romano P, Lingaraju N, Godfrey SD, Braitman LE (1992) Epidural test dose and intravascular injection in obstetrics: sensitivity, specificity, and lowest effective dose. Anesth Analg; 75: 372-376
22. Hood DD, Dewan DM, James III FM (1986) Maternal and fetal effects of epinephrine in gravid ewes. Anesthesiology; 65: 610-603
23. Markus MAE, Vertommen JD, Van Haken UH, Wouters PF (1996) Hemodynamic effects of intravenous isoproterenol versus epinephrine in the chronic maternal fetal sheep preparation. Anesth Analg; 82: 1023-1026
24. Youngstrom P, Hoyt N, Veille JC et al (1990) Effects of intravenous test dose epinephrine on fetal sheep during acute fetal stress and acidosis. Reg Anesth; 15: 237-241
25. Abboud TK, Sheik-ol-Eslam A, Yanagi T et al (1985) Safety and efficacy of epinephrine added to bupivacaine for lumbar epidural analgesia in obstetrics Anesth Analg; 64: 585-591

26. Zuspan FP, Nelson GH, Ahlquist RP (1964) Epinephrine infusion in normal and toxemic pregnancy. Am J Obstet Gynecol; 90: 88-98
27. Heller PJ, Goodman C (1986) Use of local anesthetics with epinephrine for epidural anesthesia in preeclampsia. Anesthesiology; 65: 224-226
28. Marx GF (1984) Cardiotoxicity of local anesthetics- the plot thickens. Editorial. Anesthesiology; 60: 3-5
29. Grice SC, Eisenach JC, Dewan DM, et al (1987) Evaluation of 2-Chlorprocaine as an effective intravenous test dose for epidural anesthesia. Anesthesiology; 67:A627
30. Roetman Kj, Eisenach JC (1988) Evaluation of lidocaine as intravenous test dose for epidural anesthesia. Anesthesiology; 69: A669
31. Leighton BL, De Simone CA, Norris MC, Chayen B. (1989) Isoproterenol is an effective marker of intravenous injection in laboring women. Anesthesiology; 71: 206-209
32. Markus MA, Vertommen JD, Van Aken H et al (1997) Hemodynamic effects of intravenous isoproterenol versus saline in parturient. Anesth Analg; 84: 1113-1116
33. Norris MC, Arkoosc VA, Knobler R (1997) Maternal and fetal effects of isoproterenol in the gravid ewe. Anesth Analg; 85: 385-388
34. Cherala SR, Greene R (1990) Ephedrine as a marker of intravascular injection in laboring parturients. Reg Anesth; 15:15
35. Leighton BL, Norris MC, DeSimone CA et al (1990) The air test as a clinically useful indicator of intravenously placed epidural catheters. Anesthesiology; 73: 610-13
36. Leighton BL, Gross JB (1989) Air: an effective indicator of intravenously located epidural catheters. Anesthesiology; 71: 848-51
37. Yoshii WY, Miller m, Rottman RL et al (1993) Fentanyl for epidural intravascular test dose in obstetric. Reg Anesth; 24: 17-23
38. Marcus MAE, Vertommen JD, Van Aken H et al (1999) The effects of adding isoproterenol to 0.025% bupivacaine on the quality and duration of epidural analgesia in laboring parturients. Anesth Analg; 86: 749-752
39. Cascio MG, Gaiser RR, Camann WR et al (1996) Comparative evaluation of different infusion rates of ropivacaine (2 mg per ml) for epidural labor analgesia. Reg Anesth Pain Med; 23: 548-553
40. Gautier PE, De Kock M, Van Stemberge A, et al (1999) Intrathecal ropivacaine for ambulatory surgery Anesthesiology; 91: 1239-45
41. Richardson MG, Lee AC, Wissler RN (1996) High spinal anesthesia after epidural test dose administration in five obstetric patients. Reg Anesth; 21: 119-23
42. Dawkins CJM (1969) An analysis of the complications of extradural and caudal block. Anaesthesia; 24: 554-63
43. Reynolds F (1988) Epidural catheter migration during labour [letter]. Anaesthesia; 43: 69
44. el- Behesy Ba, James D, Koh KF, Hirsch N (1996) Distinguishing cerebrospinal fluid from saline used to identify the epidural space. Br J Anaesth; 77: 784-5
45. Abraham RA, Harris AP, Maxwell LG et al (1986) The efficacy of 1.5% lidocaine with 7.5% dextrose and epinephrine as an epidural test dose for obstetrics. Anesthesiology; 64: 116-119
46. Richardson MG, Wissler RN (1996) Unexpected high spinal block in obstetrics. Br J Anaesth; 77: 806
47. Palkar NV, Boudreaux RC, Mankad AV (1992) Accidental total spinal block: a complication of an epidural test dose. Can J Anaesth: 39: 1058-60
48. Colonna-Romano P, Padolina R, Lingaraju N et al (1994) Diagnostic accuracy of intrathecal test dose in epidural analgesia. Can J Anaesth; 41: 572-574
49. Fine PG, Wong KC (1984) Cranial nerve block after test dose through catheter in a pre-eclamptic. Can Anaesth Soc J; 31: 565-567
50. Stonham J, Moss P (1983) The optimal test dose for dose for epidural anesthesia. Anesthesiology; 58: 389-90
51. Russel IF (1985) Inadvertent total spinal for cesarean section. Anaesthesia; 40: 199-200

52. Roccaforte JD, Susser L, Lax L et al (1998) Should a test dose of lidocaine with epinephrine be used with the "Walking Epidural" technique? Anesth Analg; 86:S385
53. Vucevic M, Russell IF (1992) Spinal anaesthesia for caesarean section: 0.125% plain bupivacaine 12 ml compared with 0.5% plain bupivacaine 3 ml. Br J Anaesth; 68: 590-595
54. Van Zundert AA, De Wolf AM, Vaes L et al (1988) High volume spinal anesthesia with bupivacaine 0.125% for cesarean section. Anesthesiology; 69: 998-1003
55. Cox M, Lawton G, Gowrie-Mohan S et al (1995) Let us re-examine the safety of midwifes epidural top-ups. Anaesthesia; 50: 750-751
56. Morton CPJ, Bloomfield S, Magnusson A et al (1997) Ropivacaine 0.75% for extradural anaesthesia in elective caesarean section: an open clinical and pharmacokinetic study in mother and neonate. British Journal of Anaesthesia; 79: 3-8.
57. Kopacz, DJ, Allen, HW (1999) Accidental intravenous levobupivacaine. Anesth Analg; 89: 1027
58. van Kleef JW, Veering BTh, Burm AG (1994) Spinal anesthesia with ropivacaine: a double-blind study on the efficacy and safety of 0.5% and 0.75% solutions in patients undergoing minor lower limb surgery. Anesthesia and Analgesia; 78: 1125-1130.
59. Wahedi W, Nolte H, Klein P (1996) Ropivacaine in spinal anesthesia. Anaesthetist; 45: 737-744
60. Odejinmi OD, Yentis SM (2001) Defining an aspiration test for identifying accidental intrathecal placement of epidural catheters. Intern J Obstet Anesth; 10:224 PD17
61. Collis R, Daoud Z (2000) Assessment of S1 motor block for the rapid detection of accidental intrathecal injection of bupivacaine. Intern J Obstet Anesth; 9: 206 P20

Complications in Obstetric Anesthesia

C. MELLONI

In the general organization of this article we will be limited to the complications deriving or related to the administration of obstetric anesthesia, therefore excluding those related to maternal diseases or complicating maternity, like preeclampsia, eclampsia, Hellp syndrome, pulmonary embolism, and so on.

Again, side effects of techniques are not be covered, e.g., hypotension following spinal or epidural anesthesia, sympathetic block, etc., would be considered physiological responses to regional analgesia and are excluded.

Therefore the main topics to be discussed are: mortality, difficult intubation, and complications from regional anesthesia, including spinal, epidural hematoma, headache, cauda equina syndromes, peripheral nerve palsy, blood loss, and coagulopathies.

Maternal mortality

Maternal mortality associated with anesthesia has decreased from 37 per million at the first Confidential Enquiries (1970-1972) [1] to less than 1 at the last report (1994-1996) [2], and there is no doubt that this achievement has been the result of a combination of factors. First, the shift from general anesthesia (GA) to regional, since the risk associated with GA has not decreased [3]. Interestingly, the fatality rate during cesarean section per million of regional anaesthetics has decreased even further from 8.6 for the years 1979-1984 to 1.9 in the years 1985-1990 [4, 5].

The ratio between mortality attributed to regional/general anesthesia has always been in favor of regional since the very first reports [6]; for instance, 1 death was ascribed to epidural against 12 attributed to GA in New York in the years 1979-1981; this trend became more evident over the years when examining the pattern of maternal mortality associated with anesthesia: for England/ Wales 1970-1978 there were 68 deaths attributed to GA, 40 inhalation of gastric contents, and 28 intubation problems, against 7 deaths from regional anesthesia;

for England / Wales 1985-1987 there were 7 deaths from GA, 5 failed intubations and 1 aspiration, against 1 following a regional anesthesia technique.

The ASA closed claim project studying the malpractice claims against anesthesiologists [7] has demonstrated that the complications associated with regional anesthesia are generally less serious and hence involve lower payments than those following GA (91,000 U.S. $ vs. 220,000 U.S. $).

The single most-important complication following regional anesthesia and leading to a malpractice suit is neonatal damage, following maternal convulsions from systemic administration; the malpractice claim quoted before [7] lists 9 damages over 13 regional anesthetics under scrutiny; convulsions occupy 10% of obstetric claims against 1% of all claims, and 83% of cases were associated with severe damage to mother and newborn: 95% (18/19) happened during attempted epidural and in many of these cases faults of technique were recognized, including the lack of a epinephrine test dose. Similarly, in the conclusions from the CEMDUK 1988-1990 [5], there was evidence of substandard care in 50% of all deaths.

The main causes of mortality have been always linked to airway problems, with or without inhalation of gastric content as an aggravating factor; hence the following chapter will deal with the problem of failed intubation.

Failed intubation

Failure to pass the tracheal tube into the trachea has been the more common cause of maternal mortality attributed to GA, with the resultant hypoxia and/or aspiration pneumonias as consequences and leading causes. Failure to intubate the trachea in obstetric patients occurs up to eight times more commonly in the obstetric population, with an incidence as high as 1 in 250 [8], and difficult intubation occurs in around 6% of cases [9]. There are good anatomical and physiological reasons for this: these patients are young, have full dentition, engorged breasts, and less space anteriorly to the neck and chest because of that, disturbing the co-ordinated movement of the hand applying cricoid pressure and that holding the laryngoscope handle. Since total body water is increased in pregnancy, even the water content of the laryngeal and pharyngeal tissued is increased, and laryngeal edema is an early complication of upper respiratory tract infections and pre-eclampsia. A degree of laryngeal edema is probably a normal effect of late pregnancy, and might account for the deteriorating Mallampati view during pregnancy [10], which may worsen even further in labor [11].

However, there are other factors, less well recognized, which almost certainly play a major part in the problem, and these may be listed as "organizational". In the United Kingdom, and probably in many other countries, two-thirds of emergency general anesthetic cesarean sections are conducted outside 'office hours' usually by a trainee. Lack of experience is often exacerbated by the hurried, almost chaotic referral of the patient with 'fetal distress', leaving little time for assessment and increasing the fear factor, which can be very disruptive of calm, skilled implementation of practice. The universal adoption of the left lateral tilt position to minimize aorto-caval compression means that cricoid pressure can mistakenly be applied in a 'backward and left', rather than 'backward and right' direction, thus hiding the laryngeal inlet behind the laryngoscope blade; this is more likely if the whole body is tilted by rotating the table top rather than just the abdomen by inserting a wedge.

The obvious way to avoid a failed intubation is not to use GA; the gradual realization of this truism has led to a remarkable shift towards regional anesthesia for cesarean section in many countries, including the United Kingdom [12] and United States [13]. However, the GA rate can be reduced still further. The commonest reason for GA is perceived lack of time for a regional block, but several studies have shown that these emergency cases can be predicted [14] and that, even if they present late, there is usually enough time to establish an adequate spinal block de novo or to top-up an epidural block. Mixed obstetricians and anesthesiologists rounds, continuous exchange of clinical information, prenatal visits, etc have been suggested as helpful.

Assessment of the airway should be carried out on all patients prior to cesarean section, whatever the choice of anesthetic technique. A rapid check list should at least include the following: [15]:

- Mouth opening – the inter-incisor gap is at least 5 cm (three fingers);
- Pharyngeal wall – the posterior pharyngeal wall can be seen during visual examination during a full mouth opening
- Jaw – the patient can move her lower incisors anterior to the upper incisors
- Neck – the patient can flex / extend her neck through at least 90°
- Weight – the actual weight is not more than 90 kg
- Airway edema – there is no history of pregnancy-induced hypertension, upper respiratory tract infection, stridor, voice change

A single abnormal test should signal caution and two or more should preclude GA; if regional anesthesia is contraindicated, then awake intubation should be considered.

The other assessment that should be made at this point is an estimation of the urgency of the procedure; this will enable the anesthetist to determine what action to take if intubation fails:

Grade 1 – mother's life depends on completion of surgery

Grade 2 – maternal pathology makes alternative regional technique unsuitable
Grade 3 – severe fetal distress – no recovery between contractions
Grade 4 – mild to moderate fetal distress – good recovery between contractions
Grade 5 – elective / failure to progress / maternal distress

Equipment should include at least various tools for dealing with a difficult intubation, including a choice of handles and blades (a short-handled laryngoscope, a McCoy laryngoscope), a gum-elastic bougie, laryngeal mask airway (LMA) of 3 and 4 sizes, a choice of Guedel (including the cuffed oropharyngeal airway (COPA), Combitube or VBM tube, and cricothyrotomy kit. A flexible fiberbronchoscope would be useful, but since it requires considerable skill in order to be used in difficult situations, especially urgent, it is my personal opinion that this is not strictly necessary; again, since no expertise can be acquired with all instruments, it would be wise to be proficient in at least a couple of options, practising often on normal patients and elective cases.

Anesthetists should undergo regular 'fire-drill' simulations of difficult intubation and assistants should be taught the proper application of cricoid pressure, which could be released at intervals.

Simple but crucial tips should be reiterated: good head position, keeping the patient's arms out of the way, full pre-oxygenation, waiting for the relaxant to take effect, not persisting in intubation attempts after failing.

Managing failed intubation

Many algorithms have been described, and the exact sequence of events is probably less important than following these principles:

1. Maintain oxygenation at all costs
2. Maintain protection from aspiration unless such protection interferes with oxygenation
3. Wake the patient up unless grade 1 or grade 2/3 with good airway

Iatrogenic KO due to administration of oxytocics

Methylergonovine and ergonovine are ergot derivatives that may interact with vasopressors causing severe maternal hypertension and cerebrovascular accidents; they are also emetics (in about 10-20% of patients) and may constitute a danger in patients with unprotected airways; the recommendation is to dilute them in a bottle of normal saline (250-500 ml) and administer them at a rate compatible with the therapeutic efficacy, avoiding push intravenous injection.

15-Methyl prostaglandin $F_2\alpha$ is a very effective uterotonic agent that may be administered i.m or directly into the myometrium, but may result in bronchospasm and alteration of the ventilation/perfusion ratio.

Oxytocin possesses a marked but transient direct relaxing effect on vascular smooth muscle; therefore its rapid administration is never recommended, and it should always be infused in a slow-running continuous infusion; since it can exhibit an antidiuretic effect, it could lead to water intoxication in cases of prolonged administration and infusion of excessive volumes of fluid.

Blood loss

Obstetrics is a field of ever-changing situations and massive blood loss can occur, generally because of uterine rupture, uterine atony, and placenta accreta, and therefore even today massive hemorrhage constitutes one of the leading causes of maternal mortality (see references of the CEMDUK); severe coagulopathies may follow and complicate the issue (references of CEMDUK).

Blood salvage has been used with success and no apparent clinical problems [16, 17], and the technique may save patients refusing homologous transfusion; however, whether the reinfused red cell suspension contained a clinically significant amount of amniotic fluid is unknown and this may contribute to disseminated intravascular coagulation.

The anesthesiologist should always be on the lookout for blood loss; at the earliest suspicion, large-bore catheters, an indwelling central venous pressure monitor, arterial line, urine output monitoring, typing and crossmatching for blood, and frequent monitoring of blood volume, hemoglobin and hematocrit and coagulation status should be performed. A protocol should be followed in case of major blood loss, and expert counseling sought from the very beginning, because it may be necessary to obtain advice from experts from quite different fields, like immunology, transfusion, coagulation, resuscitation, nephrology, and so on. In the dramatic instances of the anesthetic management of obstetric hysterectomy, patients could be safely treated under continuous epidural, because none of the cases encountered required intraoperative induction of GA, but regional anesthesia for the patient at risk of major blood loss should answer the following questions:

- Will the patient remain comfortable during prolonged surgery?
- Will operating conditions remain optimal for potentially difficult surgery?
- Will anesthesia-induced sympathectomy exacerbate hypotension during intraoperative hemorrhage?

- Can the patient protect her airway during potentially difficult abdominal surgery, hemorrhage, and hypotension?

Inadvertent intrathecal injection - inadvertent intravenous injection

Inadvertent intrathecal injection of the epidural dose is a relatively frequent event, as high as 0.5-2% of all cases; the consequences of high block and possible airway compromise are clear and constitute one of the major drawbacks of the otherwise well-suited technique of epidural analgesia and anesthesia for obstetrics.

The intravenous injection of local anesthetic may cause seizures and cardiac, arrest, and has been entirely attributed to the epidural attempt, since the subarachnoid dosage is so low that even in case of accidental i.v. injection it is very doubtful it may cause major complications.

These last two complications constitute probably the most-important reasons why spinal subdural administration has became the most-popular and probably the safest way to provide anesthesia for cesarean section and vaginal operative delivery, beside lower anesthetic preparation times and higher success rates [19]. Other technical advantages include faster onset, more reliable and predictable anesthesia, less technical difficulties because of the clear end point of cerebrospinal fluid (CSF) appearance. This is not to say that epidural is an unsafe technique; certainly if an epidural has been placed during labor and is working well it should be used. Epidurals still maintain an important place for elective cesareans in selected cases, when slow onset and careful control of block height are desirable. Moreover, leaving an epidural catheter in situ and administering either intermittent or continuous narcotic plus or minus low dose local anesthetic for many hours is the preferred method of postoperative pain relief in many centers [20].

Headache

Postdural puncture headache (PDPH) represents a frequent complaint in obstetrics. It is reported in up to 39% of cases following spinal anesthesia [21] with varying incidence. Chadwick et al. [22], analyzing malpractice claims, listed headache as the third most-common complication, and it is important to note that such claims resulted in payment in 56% of cases. The headache is not always self-limiting, not always benign, and may be accompanied by serious complications, ranging from visual and auditory disturbances to subdural hematoma.

The pathophysiology of PDPH remains largely unknown. However, there is direct and indirect evidence pointing to CSF leakage at the site of the dural puncture as the causative factor, suggesting that this CSF leakage results in a decrease of the cushion protective effect of the CSF itself on the brain. This decreased volume of fluid brings about a decline in intracranial pressure and consequently causes a descent of the brain when the upright position is assumed, exerting traction on the pain-sensitive intracranial structures; this working hypothesis has stood the test of time. Since the upright position facilitates drainage of the CSF towards the lower epidural space, the shift of the fluid towards the lumbar regions causes brain descent and exerts traction on the brain and meninges, and increases pain, producing the typical postural headache caused by traction on pain-sensitive intracranial structures localized to venous sinuses and dural and cerebral arteries. Pain arising from above the tentorium cerebelli is transmitted via the trigeminal nerve to the frontal region, while pain from below the tentorium is transmitted via the vagus and upper cervical nerves to the occipital region and the neck. Reflex cerebral vasodilatation to compensate for a loss of CSF volume may also cause pain similar to migraine headache.

Secondary to the decreased CSF volume, a rupture of the veins may occur as the brain retracts form the dura resulting in a subdural hematoma [23]; traction on cranial nerves from decreased CSF volume is probably the mechanism leading to the occasional cranial palsies.

The clinical features of PDPH should be more clearly defined, because to date there are no universally agreed definitions [24], from the practical point of view, PDPH could be suspected when:

- it appears within the first 1-7 days after a procedure involving a possible dural puncture, intentional or unintentional, as may happen during attempted epidural
- the typical pain is nuchal/occipital but may be frontal, bifrontal, and extend to the neck, shoulders, and is exacerbated by the assumption of the sitting or upright posture
- the symptomatology lasts longer than 24 h and/or prostrates the patient
- other useful characteristics include, but are not limited to, aggravation by coughing or straining, alleviation by lying down, absence in the supine position and reappearance in case of head elevation.

Symptomatology could vary from very mild to severe, and be accompanied by systemic symptoms like loss of appetite, general malaise, neck stiffness, nausea, vomiting, photophobia, and other neurological signs, such as III, IV, VI, VIII cranial nerves palsies, causing diplopia, tinnitus, bilateral hypoacusia. If severe symptoms persist, the patient is incapacitated and confined to bed and unable to leave the hospital, attend to a child, and so on. Usually the symptomatology resolves spontaneously in a few days, but more-severe morbidity and even mortality have been reported [25, 26]. These are the reasons why any patient with PDPH should receive prompt and effective treatment.

There are at least eight cases of spontaneous hematoma following PDPH following unintentional dural puncture. Diagnosis was made between 8 and 42 days; one death is reported and one other patient had a permanent disability with visual deficits [27, 28].

Factors influencing PDPH

The main factors influencing PDPH depend from the characteristics of the population (patients), the characteristics of the needle, and the factors that depend on the operator (anesthesiologist) [29, 30]. As far as population is concerned, we know already that the obstetric patient constitutes the group at risk because of young age and, of course, female sex. Bearing down efforts at the time of delivery were not a factor in the frequency of PDPH [31].

Needle size and tip design

There is abundant evidence that both needle size and tip design impact the incidence of PDPH. The meta-analyses by Halpern and Preston [32] of 450 articles outlines that there is a reduction in PDPH when (a) a small spinal needle is used compared with a large needle of the same type and (b) when noncutting spinal needles rather than cutting needles are used, The pencil-point needles, like the Whitacre needle, are likely less traumatic to the longitudinal fibers of the dura, separating them, and thus producing a smaller rent with reduced CSF leakage compared with cutting needles. Lambert et al. [33] reported that the rate of PDPH with the 25-gauge Whitacre needle was about half (1.2%) the rate with the 27-gauge cutting needle (2.7%).

The known relationship between PDPH and needle size has prompted the use of extremely fine auge needles 29/32 g, but their use was associated with a high failure rate [34-37]. Among the possible causes were reported the lack of feel, the longer waiting time for the first appearance of CSF at the needle hub, and the greater difficulty of local anesthetic injection.

Because of the well-perceived danger of PDPH after unintentional dural puncture during an attempted epidural and because the incidence of wet tap tends to be higher during the training curve, in case of unintentional wet tap during epidural performance it has been suggested to switch the technique to a continuous spinal in an attempt to reduce the frequency of PDPH. However, continuous spinal analgesia for labor and delivery does not decrease the incidence and severity of headache after dural puncture [38]; while prophylactic blood patch may not be warranted following headache with small-gauge, non-cutting needles for subarachnoid anesthesia, after large-gauge, unintentional dural puncture, prophylactic epidural administration of both saline and blood deserves consideration, as both will reduce the subsequent incidence of PDPH. It is difficult to determine the impact of prophylactic saline or blood administration on the need for subsequent epidural blood patch, because, very often, patients who would benefit from recommended epidural blood patch refused, despite having moderate to severe headache [39].

Bevel direction and angle of insertion

The dura mater has been described as a longitudinally organized fibroelastic membrane [40]; in vivo, the dura is preloaded and subject to longitudinal tensile stresses; a transversely directed needle bevel would cut more fibers than a longitudinally oriented bevel. Thus, with a transverse cut, the borders would tend to be pulled open, resulting in a greater CSF leak; instead, a hole oriented parallel to this tension will tend to close.

Norris et al. [41] investigated unintentional dural punctures occurring during the identification of the epidural space in 1,558 women, and the level of the epidural needle was randomly oriented either parallel or perpendicular to the longitudinal dural fibers during epidural cannulation. Accidental dural puncture occurred in 41 women (2.63%): 20 with the needle bevel oriented perpendicular and 21 with the needle bevel inserted parallel to the longitudinal dural fiber. In those experiencing unintentional dural puncture, 70% (14 of 20) developed PDPH in the perpendicular group, yet only 24% (5 of 21) suffered PDPH in the longitudinal group ($p < 0.005$) These data suggest that the orientation of the epidural needle is not a factor in avoiding an accidental dural puncture, but is crucial in diminishing the resultant PDPH. Moreover, in the series reported by Norris et al. [41] a curative blood patch was required in only 4 cases in the parallel group, while it was deemed necessary in 10 cases in the perpendicular group. A different study indicated that in laboring parturients and in the hands of anesthesiology residents, catheter insertion with the needle orifice oriented cephalad was associated with the greatest initial success and the fewest complications [42]. It has been suggested that the relatively oblique paramedian approach to the extradural, and therefore the subarachnoid space, may result in less leakage of CSF through the dura mater after withdrawal of the needle [43]; an oblique angle of penetration theoretically creates a flap valve that tends to seal the perforation in the dura, but important clinical studies substantiating this point are lacking. It is of some interest to note that the choice of the air or saline approach in the loss of resistance identification of the epidural space does not impact on the frequency and severity of headache, even if most headaches after dural puncture with air presented a rapid onset and a short duration, most probably as a consequence of the injection of intracranial air [44].

Number of punctures

There are few reports addressing whether multiple dural punctures impact the frequency of PDPH; some did not find any association between number of punctures and incidence of headache [45, 46], while others [47] confirmed the assumption that repetition of dural puncture increases the risk of PDPH; unfortunately specific data in the obstetric population are lacking, but it seems reasonable to infer that, being a population at risk for the development of PDPH, repeated dural punctures will be followed by an increase in PDPH.

Differential diagnosis

When analyzing perioperative headaches, it is frequently assumed that any headache occurring in the early postoperative period is an anesthesia-related headache. Therefore, anesthesiologists often deal with the differential diagnosis of postoperative headache. It is important when creating the differential to bear in mind two clinical complications that must be considered: aseptic meningitis and bacterial meningitis. Although beyond the scope of this review, not every headache after spinal anesthesia should immediately be attributed to PDPH causes [48], but all possible differential diagnoses should be considered in order to avoid the dramatic consequences of the more-serious complications, notably meningitis.

Treatment

There is consensus that a patient's position in the early hours after spinal anesthesia does not influence the progress of PDPH, but it just delays the onset of the PDPH if it develops. Another purpose of bed rest is to alleviate the PDPH symptoms, especially in the more-severe cases, and to prevent further complications resulting from "traction" and rupture of bridge meningeal veins caused by decreased CSF pressure.

Symptomatic therapy for PDPH includes psychological support, bed rest, hydration, nonopioid analgesics, and other historical maneuvers, e.g., tight abdominal binders and forced fluid intake of 3 l/day or more in a double-blind, placebo-controlled trial, intravenous caffeine (300-500 mg) also produced short-term symptomatic relief of PDPH [49]. This supportive treatment does not reverse the natural process of PDPH, except as it allows time to help alleviate the headache.

The loss of CSF through the dural puncture site with resultant intracranial hypotension demands therapy directed at restoring the subarachnoid pressure relationships. Administration of an epidural blood patch is believed to form a "patch" over the meningeal hole, thereby minimizing the ongoing CSF leak while the meningeal rent heals [50]. Gormley [50] reported use of an extradural, autologous blood injection to "patch" the hole in the dura in 1960, and the first series of patients treated was published by Carrie [51]. Since then, the technique has been used safely and successfully, symptoms being relieved within 1-24 h in 85-90% of patients; 90% of patients who fail an initial blood patch will respond to a second patch, and extensive experience has been gained. The amount of blood used for PDPH treatment has increased continually from 2-3 ml up to 18-20 ml; the progress of extradural blood patches in five patients was followed with magnetic resonance imaging [52] from 30 min to 3 h after the patch; the blood markedly compressed the thecal sac producing a mass effect over four to five vertebral levels. Previous data with radioactive blood had shown a mean spread of six segments upward and three segments caudally. This mass effect probably is responsible for the rapid increase in CSF pressure and the fast alleviation of headache. After 7 h, there is no compression effect and the blood adheres thinly to the dural sac, extending further cephalad and caudad. The epidural blood patch also extends into the subarachnoid space and extensively into the subcutaneous fat of the back. The authors speculate that this extensive subcutaneous hematoma is responsible for the backache reported in 20%-35% of patients after epidural blood patch. These authors recommend slowly injecting up to 20 ml of blood at or below the level of the previous spinal puncture. If the patient feels discomfort or pain during injection, the volume should be reduced.

Timing of blood patch has raised a hot debate: prophylactic blood patch, in a nonrandomized observational study did not decrease the frequency of headache or the need for a subsequent therapeutic blood patch [53], so that it appears reasonably safe to delay the blood patch until 48 h after dural puncture, maximizing success rate [54] and most probably avoiding unnecessary interventions. In the meantime medical therapy should be instituted.

Other treatment methods for refractory disabling PDPH include epidural injections of saline (30-50) ml [55], but the method is less effective than epidural blood patch [56], dextran (20-30 ml) [57], or systemic administration of caffeine, sodium benzoate [58], sumatriptan (Imigran, Glaxo Wellcome, 50/100 mg, supp 25 mg, parenterally 6 mg) [59, 60], a serotonin type -Id receptor agonist (that produces vasoconstriction of dilated cerebral vasculature, which contributes to the severity of headaches), and theophylline [61]. The use of a fibrin glue patch has also been tested in an in vitro model [62]. Collier [63] described the anecdotal use of long-acting adrenocorticotropic hormone (ACTH) to effectively relieve PDPH in six patients, and recently [63], the use of a single intravenous infusion of ACTH, 1.5 U/kg in 250 ml of normal saline, has been reported to provide effective relief in two cases of PDPH. Physical methods include bedrest and abdominal binders; psychological support is of great importance.

Neurological complications

There is ample evidence that a large proportion of neurological complications are completely unrelated to anesthetic care; nevertheless, lay opinion tends to infer some kind of iatrogenic causation in cases of adverse neurological outcome whenever anesthesia has been administered. Such a point of view particularly applies to regional anesthesia because of its high visibility, as pointed out by Bromage [65]. Since neuraxial regional anesthesia plays a major part in obstetric practice and, thus, is being offered to increasing numbers of parturients as the most-effective technique for labor pain relief due to its unmatched and still growing popularity, some adverse effects and even minor complications related to regional anesthesia are to be expected statistically, despite the very low risk of severe injuries; unfortunately accurate data on the frequency of certain complications are not available as the denominators (i.e., number of procedures performed) are unknown. Furthermore, many complications may be missed due to underreporting or failure of recording. Obviously, clinical audits reporting neurological complications, which are based on comprehensive data collection, are rare. Therefore, case reports and anecdotal accounts still may have quite a strong formative influence on anesthetic risk assessment and public opinion, and subsequent decision making.

A considerable proportion of neurological complications can be attributed to a variety of nonanesthetic causes: among these are preexisting medical conditions such as polyneuropathy, postinfectious neuritis, collagen and vascular disorder, multiple sclerosis (which can worsen during pregnancy and parturition, and thus mimic complications otherwise attributed to regional anesthesia), spontaneous epidural abscess, or hematoma.

More importantly, obstetric causes can be directly responsible for a variety of neurological injuries, since during the descent through the maternal pelvis, the fetal head may produce a compression injury of the lumbosacral trunk or the femoral, obturator, lateral cutaneous nerves, and common peroneal nerve, thus resulting in transient postpartum neurological dysfunction with an approximate prevalence of 1 in 2,100 - 4,000 [65], without forgetting the minor sequelae [66], represented as dorsalgia in 14%, headache 4%, paresthesias 2.7%, bladder incontinence in 15%, and dysuria in 4% (Birmingham, UK, 11,701 questionnaires on 30,096 deliveries).

A prospective study on the occurrence of obstetric palsies of the lower limbs revealed that among 34 Nigerian women with signs of neurapraxia, foot drop was the most-frequent presenting feature (88%), followed by femoral neuropathy (26%) and spastic paraparesis (15%). Only in 76% of patients was complete recovery observed. By a similar mechanism, the blades of forceps may also cause direct trauma to the nerves and thus produce paresthesias or transient neurological deficits; these effects were described long before regional anesthesia was implemented in obstetric care [67]. Injuries of peripheral nerves may occasionally arise from direct external pressure; pressure on the area of the common peroneal nerve may occur in the lithotomy position by inappropriate use of stirrups, as well as by prolonged squatting, and produce foot drop [68, 69].

A recent well-conducted audit [70] examined all 48,066 deliveries of the North West Thames region during 1 year; 19 neurological disturbances were discovered, with 2 hypoxic cerebral damages, 1 following a cardiac arrest in a patient with cardiomyopathy and subsequent death, and 1 tetraparesis following hemorrhage; 5 patients complained of nervous root damages in different areas; Bell palsy, cervical, L5 prolapsed disc, sciatic neuritis exacerbation, 1 foot drop (spontaneous delivery under nitrous oxide analgesia of a large baby via a small pelvis). In 3 cases peripheral nerve palsies were found (lateral popliteus, ulnar, meralgia parestetica). In 5 cases medical preexisting diseases were identified (2 space-occupying lesions,1 sclerosis multipla,1 diabetic neuropathy,1 meningitis).

The most-serious occurrence of anterior spinal artery syndrome due to vascular occlusion to the cord by the fetal head is extremely rare, but in a minority of women the major blood supply to the conus medullaris originates from branches of the internal iliac arteries instead of the artery of Adamkiewicz, and these constitute a high-risk subgroup for ischemic cord injury.

Anesthesia-related peripheral neurological injury ranges from mild and transient functional impairment to severe and permanent injury; the reported incidence varies from 0.008 to 0.36%:

- Crawford [71] (1985) 4 /27,000

- Ong et al. [72] (1987) 34 /9,403
- Holdcroft and Hibbard [73] (1990) 43 /505,000
- Scott and Tunstall [74] (1995) 38 /108,133
- Holdcroft et al. [75] (1995)1 /13,007
- Puech et al. [76] (1999)1 /10,995

Compression of the spinal cord by space-occupying lesions (hematoma, abscess) often develops quite insidiously but, in the worst case, can result in paraplegia if prompt diagnosis and urgent surgical decompression are not done [77-80]; this condition is to be differentiated from coincidental spinal disc prolapse [81]. Neurotoxicity resulting in permanent neurological injury (cauda equina syndrome) has been attributed to chemical contamination, antioxidants (sodium bisulfite), and overdoses of local anesthetics (lidocaine).

In order to calculate the relative risk of complications associated with obstetric regional anesthesia, the case reports are not helpful, but we need large well-conducted prospective or retrospective studies; from some of these, including approximately 505, 000 obstetric epidurals [82, 83], a few serious events can be found, because of over 108 events only 5 gave permanent sequelae; 1 case of bilateral subdural hematoma after accidental dural puncture, 1 quadriplegia due to thrombosis of a cervical hemangioma, 1 paraplegia of unknown origin, 1 abscess, and 1 subdural hematoma evacuated with success. Events of lesser magnitude included 5 cranial nerve palsies, 38 peripheral neuropathies, and 60 acute reactions. Epidural analgesia was considered to have contributed to postpartum neurological sequelae in 1 of 13,000 parturients, while the overall incidence of prolonged postpartum neuropathy was 1 in 2,530 deliveries [84, 85]. From the above-mentioned studies an overall incidence between 1/2,500 and 1/100,000 serious sequelae of regional anesthesia for obstetrics can be derived; while the risk of epidural abscess has been estimated between 1:500,000 [74] and 1:27,000 [71] during labor and 1:75,000 for epidural. A large survey of the literature discovered 45 cases quoted in Medline [Schneider, unpublished work]; such a large variability cannot be explained, but certainly these data call for better-conducted prospective studies.

The risk of epidural abscess in patients receiving epidural anesthesia and/or analgesia has not shown any relationship with systemic or localized infection in obstetrics [86]: of 10,047 deliveries, 319 cases of chorioamniniotis were identified and 100 had blood cultures taken on the day of delivery, 8 consistent with bacteremia. Of the 319 patients, 293 received a regional anesthetic, in 43 patients antibiotics were administered prior to needle or catheter placement. No patient in the study, including those with documented bacteremias, had infectious complications. In addition, mean temperatures and leukocyte counts in patients with blood cultures taken showed no significant differences between bacteremic and nonbacteremic groups. Therefore the authors continued to administer spinal and epidural anesthesia in patients with suspected chorioamnionitis because the potential benefits of regional anesthesia outweigh the theoretical risk of infectious complications.

Since so many studies failed to clearly identify maternal risk factors for maternal morbidity and mortality, we read with great interest the most-recent article by Panchal et al. [87]. The authors found that patients who died were significantly more likely to be African-American (60.7% versus 33.3%, OR=5.4, 95% CI=2.83-10.1, P<0.001), rather than racial category other than African-American or white (OR 12.2), cesarean section (60.0% versus 26.7%, OR=5.3, 95% CI=3.10-8.98, P<0.001), delivering in a minor teaching hospital (OR 3.1), and being transferred from another hospital (OR 6.2). Maternal mortality ratio for women <34 years was 13.9 compared with 23.9 with advanced maternal age.

Similarly, Endler et al. [88] underlined obesity, emergency surgery and hypertension as the most-important factors related to maternal mortality; since cesarean section is a well-recognised risk factor, one approach toward complication reduction could be to decrease the percentage of cesarean sections over all births; however, over the last decades there has been a marked increase in the number of cesareans performed (in the US, 5% in 1970, 25% in 1988, and 21% in 1995). The current cesarean rates are thought to be too high, but it seems very difficult to reduce, because some reasons for the increase in rate include the fact that:

- women are having fewer children and expect them to be perfect
- obstetricians rightly fear litigation in the event of poor neonatal outcome
- cesarean section is now a low-risk procedure for mother and baby

It is highly probable that maternal mortality (and hence at least the most-serious morbidity) goes underreported; Panchal et al. [87] demonstrated an overall death ratio of 16.4, i.e, at least twice of that reported by the CDC [89]. Most probably the discrepancy reflects the fact that some statistics derive from analyses of maternal death certificates, while in the State of Maryland the data derived from an anonymous database called the Uniform Health Discharge Data Set (UHDDS),where deliveries occurring in hospital are mandatorily reported. Therefore, for the same reasoning, even the definition of maternal death could be different, since it may cover different time spans following or preceding delivery.

Conclusions

The data presented in this paper provide an overview of the risks of major (and minor) complications associated with the administration of anesthesia in obstetrics; but the comments apply only to the more-developed countries. However, in the rest of the world, where the majority of the population lives and where the natality is much higher, maternal (and fetal) morbidity and mortality are still today much higher [90], whether due to anesthesia or not. World Health Organization (WHO), the International Planned Parenthood Federation, and the Population Council show that leading causes of maternal death are:

- severe bleeding (25%)
- infection (15%)
- unsafe abortion (13%)
- eclampsia (12%)
- obstructed labor (8%)
- other direct causes such as ectopic pregnancy, embolism, and anesthesia-related complications (8%)
- Indirect causes such as: anemia, malaria, or heart disease (almost 20%)

In the meantime, this paper recommends that all maternity unit staff should develop:

- a higher level of awareness of potential problems
- early consultant involvement
- more-skilled anesthetic help

in order to decrease the complication rate associated with obstetric anesthesia and analgesia.

All these preventive measures point toward an increase in the number of regional anesthetics when anesthesia or analgesia is indicated, advanced planning, and human resource investment.

References

1. Report on Confidential Enquiries into Maternal Deaths in England and Wales 1972-1974. London, HMSO
2. Report on Confidential Enquiries into Maternal Deaths in the United Kingdom 1994-1996. London, HMSO
3. Hawkins JL, Koonin LM, Palmer SK, Gibbs CP (1997) Anesthesia-related deaths during obstetric delivery in the United States, 1979-1990.Anesthesiology 86:277-284
4. Report on Confidential Enquiries into Maternal Deaths in England and Wales 1978-1980. London, HMSO
5. Report on Confidential Enquiries into Maternal Deaths in the United Kingdom 1988-1990. London, HMSO
6. Parker J, Schiffer MA, Nelson F. (1979) Maternal and perinatal mortality. In: Marx (ed) Clinical management of mother and newborn. Springer, New York Berlin Heidelberg, pp 241-274
7. Chadwick HS, Posner K, Caplan RA, et al (1991) A comparison of obstetric and nonobstetric anesthesia malpractice claims. Anesthesiology 74: 242-249

8. Hawthorne L, Wilson R, Lyons G, et al (1996) Failed intubation revisited: 17 years' experience in a teaching maternity unit. Br J Anaesth 76: 680-684
9. Tsen LC, Pitner R, Camann WR (1998) General anaesthesia for Cesarean section at a tertiary care hospital 1990-1995: indications and implications. Int J Obstet Anesth 7: 147-152
10. Pilkington S, Carli F, Dakin MJ, et al (1995) Increase in Mallampati score during pregnancy. Br J Anaesth 74: 638-642
11. Dresner M, Lyons G (1996) Increase in Mallampati score during labour. Int J Obstet Anesth 5: 214
12. Brown GW (1995) A survey of anaesthesia for Caesarean section. Int J Obstet Anesth 4: 214-218
13. Hawkins JL, Gibbs CP, Orleans M, et al (1997) Obstetric anesthesia work force survey, 1981 versus 1992. Anesthesiology 87: 135 –143
14. Morgan BM, Magni V, Goroszenuik T (1990) Anaesthesia for emergency caesarean section. Br J Obstet Gynaecol 97: 420-424
15. Crosby ET, Cooper RM, Douglas M, et al (1998) The unanticipated difficult airway with recommendations for management. Can J Anaesth 45: 757-776
16. Rainaldi MP, Tazzari PL, Scagliarini G, et al (1998) Blood salvage during caesarean section. Br J Anaesth 80:195-198
17. Potter PS, Waters JH, Burger GA, et al (1999) Application of cell-salvage during Cesarean section. Anesthesiology 90:619-621
18. Chestnut DH, Dewan DM, Redick LF, et al (1989) Anesthetic management for obstetric hysterectomy: a multi institutional study. Anesthesiology 70:607
19. Glosten B, Gianas BS, Chadwick HS, et al (1995) Practical aspects of regional anesthesia for cesarean delivery, failure rates and anesthetic preparation times – an observational study.Anesthesiology 83:A977
20. Riley ET, Cohen SE, Macario A, et al (1995) Spinal versus epidural anesthesia for cesarean section: a comparison of time efficiency, costs, charges and complications. Anesth Analg 80: 709-712
21. Morgan P (1995) Spinal anesthesia in obstetrics. Can J Anaesth 42: 1145-1163
22. Chadwick HS, Posner K, Caplan RA, et al (1991) A comparison of obstetric and nonobstetric anesthesia malpractice claims. Anesthesiology 74: 242-249
23. Edelman JD, Wingard DW (1980) Subdural hematomas after lumbar puncture. Anesthesiology 52: 166-167
24. Reid FA, Thorburn J (1991) Headache after spinal anaesthesia (editorial). Br J Anaesth 67: 674-677
25. Parlow JL, Einarson DW (1991) An unusual cause of delayed postmyelogram headache. Anesthesiology 75: 145-146
26. Endelman JD, Wingard DW (1980) Subdural hematomas after lumbar puncture. Anesthesiology 52: 166-167
27. Loo CC, Irested L (1999) Cauda equina syndrome after spinal anaesthesia with hyperbaric 5% lignocaine: a review of six cases of cauda equina syndrome reported to the Swedish Pharmaceutical Insurance 1993-1997.Acta Anaesthesiol Scand. 43:371-379
28. Wybla SW, Bayhi D, Webre D, Viswanathan S (1992) Bilateral subdural hematomas after dural puncture: delayed diagnosis after false negative computed tomography scan without contrast. Reg Anest. 17:52-53
29. Rasmussen BS, Blom L, Hansen P, Mikkelsen SS (1989) Postspinal headache in young and elderly patients. Anaesthesia 44: 571-573
30. Wiesel S, Tessler MJ, Easdown LJ (1993) Postdural puncture headache: a randomized prospective comparison of the 24 gauge Sprotte and the 27 gauge Quincke needles in young patients. Can J Anaesth 40:607-611
31. Ravindran RS, Viegas OJ, Tasch MD, et al (1981) Bearing down at the time of delivery and the incidence of spinal headache in parturients. Anesth Analg 60: 524-526
32. Halpern S, Preston R (1994) Postdural puncture headache and spinal needle design. Metaanalyses. *Anesthesiology: 81: 1376-1383*

33. Lambert DH, Hurley RJ, Hertwig L, Datta S (1997) Role of needle gauge and tip configuration in the production of lumbar puncture headache. Reg Anesth 22:66-72
34. Lynch J, Krings EJ, Strick K, et al (1991) Use of a 25-gauge Whitacre needle to reduce the incidence of postdural puncture headache. Br J Anaesth 67: 690-693
35. Cooney C, Gallagher H (1991) Spinal needles. Br J Anaesth 67: 360
36. Carrie LES, Collins PD (1991) 29-gauge spinal needles. Br J Anaesth 66: 145-146
37. Lesser P, Bembridge M, Lyons G, MacDonald R (1990) An evaluation of a 30-gauge spinal needle for spinal anaesthesia for caesarean section. Anaesthesia 45: 767-768
38. Norris MC, Leighton BL (1990) Continuous spinal analgesia for labor and delivery does not decrease the incidence and severity of headache after dural puncture. Reg Anesth 15:285
39. Duffy P, Crosby ET (1999) The epidural blood patch. Resolving the controversies Can J Anesth 46: 878-886
40. Patin DJ, Eckstein EC, Harum K, Pallares VS (1993) Anatomic and biomechanical properties of human lumbar dura mater. Anesth Analg 76: 535-540
41. Norris MC, Leighton BL, DeSimone CA (1989) Needle bevel direction and headache after inadvertent dural puncture. Anesthesiology 70: 729-731
42. Richardson MG, Wissler RN (1999) The effects of needle bevel orientation during epidural catheter insertion in laboring parturients. Anesth Analg 88:352–356.
43. Ready LB, Cuplin S, Haschke RH, Nessly M (1989) Spinal needle determinants of rate of transdural fluid leak. Anesth Analg 69: 457-460
44. Aida S, Taga K, Yamakura T, et al (1998) Headache after attempted epidural block: the role of intrathecal air. Anesthesiology 88:76-81
45. Lybecker H, Moller JT, May O, Nielsen HK (1990) Incidence and prediction of postclural puncture headache. A prospective study of 1021 spinal anesthesias. Anesth Analg 70: 389-394
46. Kang SB, Goodnough DE, Lee YK, et al (1992) Comparison of 26- and 27-gauge needles for spinal anesthesia to ambulatory surgery patients. Anesthesiology 76:734-738
47. Seeberger MD, Kaufmann M, Staender S, et al (1996) Repeated dural punctures increase the incidence of postdural puncture headache. Anesth AnaIg 82: 302-305
48. Burke D, Wildsmith JAW (1997) Meningitis after spinal anaesthesia. Br J Anaesth 78: 635-636
49. Camann WR, Murray RS, Mushlin PS, Lambert DH (1990) Effects of oral caffeine on postdural puncture headache. A double-blind, placebo-controlled trial. Anesth Analg 70: 181-184
50. Gormley JB (1960) Treatment of postspinal headache.Anesthesiology 21 :565-66
51. Carrie LES (1993) Postdural puncture headache and extradural blood patch. Br J Anaesth 71: 179
52. Beards SC, Jackson A, Griffiths AG, Horsman EL (1993) Magnetic resonance imaging of extradural blood patches: appearances from 30 min to 18 h. Br J Anaesth 71: 182-188
53. Mandell G, Ramanathan S (1996). Effectiveness of prophylactic blood patches in laboring parturients: a prospective study. Anesth Analg 82:S291
54. Loeser EA, Hill GE, Bennett GM (1978) Time vs success rate for epidural blood patch. Anesthesiology 49 :147 –148
55. Baysinger CL, Menk EJ, Harte E, Middaugh R (1986) The successful treatment of dural puncture headache after failed epidural blood patch. Anesth Analg 65:1242-1244
56. Bart AJ, Wheeler AS (1978) Comparison of epidural saline placement and epidural blood placement in the treatment of post-lumbar puncture headache.Anesthesiology 48:221-223
57. Barrios-Alarcon J, Aldrete JA, Paragas-Tapia D (1989) Relief of post-lumbar puncture headache with epidural Dextran 40: a preliminary report. Reg Anesth 14:78-80
58. Yucel A, Ozyalcin S, Talu Gkey, et al (1999) Intravenous administration of caffeine sodium benzoate for post dural puncture headache. Reg Anesth Pain Med 24:51-54
59. Carp H, Singh PJ, Vahera R, Jayaram A (1994) Effects of the serotonin- receptor agonist sumatriptan on postdural puncture headache: report of six cases. Anesth Analg 79: 180-182
60. Sprigge JS (1999) The use of sumatriptan in the treatment of post dural puncture headache after accidental lumbar puncture complicated a blood patch procedure. Anaesthesia 54:95-96

61. Choi A, Laurito CE, Cunningham FE (1996) Pharmacologic management of postdural puncture headache. Ann Pharmacother 30:831-839
62. Gil F, Garcia-Aguado R, Barcia J, et al (1998) The effect of fibrin glue patch in an vitro model of post dural puncture leakage. Anesth Analg 87:1125-1128
63. Collier BB (1994) Treatment for dural puncture headache. Br J Anaesth 72: 366
64. Atulkumar MK, Foster PA (1997) Adrenocorticotropic hormone infusion as a novel treatment for postdural puncture headache. Reg Anesth 22: 432-434
65. Bromage PR (1997) Neurological complications of subarachnoid and epidural anesthesia. Acta Anaesthesiol Scand 41:439-444
66. Chadwick HS (1996) An analysis of obstetric anesthesia cases The American Society of Anesthesiologists closed claims project database.Int J Obstet Anesth 5:258-263
67. Bademosi O, Osuntokun BO, Van de Werd HJ, Bademosi AK (1980) Obstetric neuropraxia in the Nigerian African. Int J Gynaecol Obstet 17:611-614
68. Ong BY, Cohen MM, Esmail A, et al (1987) Paresthesias and motor dysfunction after labor and delivery. Anesth Analg 66:18-22
69. Babayev M, Bodack MP, Creatura C (1998) Common peroneal neuropathy secondary to squatting during childbirth. Obstet Gynecol 91:830-832
70. Holdcroft A, Gibberd FB, Hargrove R, et al (1995) Neurological complications associated with pregnancy. Br J Anaesth 75:522-526
71. Crawford JS (1985) Some maternal complications of maternal analgesia for labour.Anesthesia 40:1219-1225
72. Ong BY, Cohen MM, Esmail A, et al (1987) Paresthesias and motor dysfunction after labor and delivery. Anesth Analg 66:18-22
73. Holdcroft DE, Hibbard EM (1990) Serious non-fatal complicationsassociated with extradural block in obstetric practice. Br Anaesth 7:41
74. Scott DB, Tunstall ME (1994) Serious complications associated with epidural/spinal blockade in obstetrics: a two-year prospective study. Int J Obstet 4:134-139
75. Holdcroft A, Gibberd FE, Hargrove R, et al (1995) Neurological complications associated with pregnancy. Br J Anaesth 75:522-526
76. Puech MJ, Godkin R,Websater S (1998) Complications of obstetric epidural anesthesia and analgesia of 10995 cases Int J Obstet Anesth 7:5-11
77. Rajakulendran Y, Rahman S. Venkat N (1999) Long-term neurological complication following traumatic damage to the spinal cord with a 25 gauge Whitacre spinal needle. Int J Obstet Anesth 8:62-66
78. Yuen TST, Kua JSW,Tan IKS (1999) Spinal haematoma following epidural anesthesia in a patient with eclampsia. Anesthesia 54:350-354
79. Lao TT, Halpern SH, MacDonald D, et al (1993) Spinal subdural haematoma in a parturient after attempted epidural anesthesia. Can J Anaesth 40:340-345
80. Kindler C, Seeberger M, Siegemund M, Schneider M (1996) Extradural abscess complicating lumbar extradural anesthesia and analgesia in an obstetric patient. Acta Anaesthesiol Scand 40:858-861
81. Mills GH, Howell SJL, Richmond MN (1994) Spinal cord compression immediately following, but unrelated to analgesia. Anesthesia 49:954-956
82. Scott DE, Hibbard EM (1990) Serious non-fatal complications associated with extradural block in obstetric practice. Br Anaesth 7:41
83. Scott DB,Tunstall ME (1994) Serious complications associated with epidural/spinal blockade in obstetrics: a two-year prospective study. Int J Obstet Anesth 4:133-139
84. Paech MJ, Godkin R, Websters (1998) Complications of obstetric epicural analgesia and anaesthesia of 10995 cases. Int J Obstet Anesth 7:5-11
85. Holdcroft A, Gibberd FE, Hargrove R, et al (1995) Neurological complications associated with pregnancy. Br J Anaesth 75:522-526
86. Bader AM, Datta S, Gilbertson L, Kirz L (1992) Regional anesthesia in women with chorioamnionitis. Reg Anesth 17:84-86

87. Panchal S, Arria AM, Labhsetvar SA (2001) Maternal mortality during hospital admission for delivery: a retrospective analysis using a state maintained database.Anesth Analg 93:134-141
88. Endler GC, Mariona FG, Sokol RJ, et al (1988)Anesthesia related maternal mortality in Michigan 1972-84. Am J Obstet Gynecol 159:187-183
89. Rochat RW, Koonin LM, Atrash HK, et al (1988) Maternal mortality in the United States: report from the Maternal Mortality Collaborative. Obstet Gynecol 72-91
90. Centers for Disease Control and Prevention (1998) Maternal Mortality, United States 1982-96 MMWR 47:705-707

The Obstetric Patient in Intensive Care: Causes of Admission and Important Considerations

V.A. ROBSON, J. A. CROWHURST, S.J. BRETT

The critically ill obstetric patient provides a unique clinical challenge to the intensive care physician, in view of the alterations of maternal physiology which occur in pregnancy and the puerperium, the presence of the foetus and the occurrence of diseases and complications specific to pregnancy. Intensive care admission is necessary for a small number of pregnant or postnatal women. This chapter reviews the causes of admission to intensive care (ICU) and some of the critical care issues related to the care of the obstetric patient.

Causes of admission to Intensive Care

In the United Kingdom (UK) maternal mortality is audited by a multidisciplinary committee which compiles and publishes a Confidential Report every three years. These Confidential Enquiries into Maternal Deaths Reports (CEMDs) are widely regarded as the 'gold standard' of maternal mortality reporting in the developed world. The 1994-96 CEMD reported 268 maternal deaths, of which 134 were a direct result of pregnancy and 134 due to a pre-existing condition aggravated by pregnancy. Thirty-six fortuitous deaths were also included and discussed [1]. This revealed a total maternal mortality rate of 12.2 per 100 000 pregnancies in the United Kingdom.

Table 1. Causes of maternal deaths in UK (from CEMD Reports [1, 2, 3])

Cause of death	1988-90	1991-93	1994-96
Thromboembolism	33	35	48
Pregnancy induced hypertension	27	20	20
Haemorrhage	22	15	12
Amniotic fluid embolism	11	10	17
Early pregnancy	24	18	15
Sepsis	7	9	14
Anaesthetic related	4	8	1
Other direct causes	17	13	7
Cardiac problems	18	37	39
Other indirect causes	75	63	95
Total	238	228	268

Table 1 shows the death rates from the main causes of death, collated from the three most recent CEMD reports [1-3]. It can be seen that thromboembolism remains the commonest cause of mortality, followed by pregnancy induced hypertension and haemorrhage. However, only 35% of these patients were treated in an ICU [1]. The remainder were managed in High Dependency Units (HDU), which are increasingly common in UK obstetric units.

There is no similar countrywide audit of maternal morbidity, however several studies have looked at the reasons for admission of obstetric patients to the ICU. These reasons can similarly be divided into *direct* (pregnancy-related), and *indirect* (unrelated to pregnancy).

Table 2. Causes of admission in UK ICUs

Cause of ICU Admission				**Reference**				
	[4]	**[5]**	**[6]**	**[7]**	**[8]**	**[9]**	**[10]**	**[11]**
Pregnancy induced hypertension	13		21	2	80	83	11	101
Haemorrhage	4	3	8	4	23	70	11	111
Sepsis		2	1		1	5	5	15
Pulmonary Embolism						1		
Amniotic fluid embolism				1		2		3
Anaesthesia related	3		1	3	4			
Cardiac disease			1	1	4	7	3	
Pneumonia		2	1					
Respiratory disease					6	18	2	
Other pre-existing medical condition			3				2	
Other	4	2	2		16	28		
Total number of admissions	23	11	39	13	144	210	43	342
Number of Deaths	2	1	2	0	3	7	1	6
Number of deliveries	21 983	11 000	7 148	9 425	19 020	122 850	5 764	unknown
ICU admissions per 1 000 deliveries	1.0	1	5.5	1.4	7.5	1.7	7.5	-

Table 2 shows the number of admissions of parturients to intensive care units and the principal reasons for admission from several UK studies carried out during the 1990's. The number of admissions per 1 000 deliveries ranges from 1.0 to 7.5 in the UK studies, giving an ICU admission rate of 8.2 to 61 admissions per maternal mortality in the Confidential Enquiry. A study of admissions over five years carried out in our ICU at Hammersmith Hospital, which takes patients from the tertiary referral obstetric unit at Queen Charlotte's Hospital, demonstrated 6.4 ICU admissions per 1 000 deliveries [10]. The largest UK data set of obstetric ICU admissions has been collected by the Intensive Care National Audit and Research Centre, which has data from 91 UK ICUs [11]. Of 342 obstetric admissions, 101 were a result of pregnancy induced hypertension and 111 of haemorrhage. Six of these patients died.

Table 3. Deaths of obstetric patients in ICUs

Cause of ICU Admission	References [4]	[5]	[6]	[8]	[10]	[11]	[9]	[13]	[14]	[15]	[16]	[17]	[18]	[19]	[20]
Pregnancy induced hypertension	2		1	1			1	6		1				1	
Haemorrhage							1	5				1			
Sepsis1					1		1	1							
Pulmonary embolism							1	1			1	1			
Amniotic fluid embolism				2											
Fatty liver of pregnancy							1	1							
Cardiac disease							1	2					1		
Pneumonia		1											4	1	
Malignancy			1										2		
Intracranial haemorrhage											1		2		
Overdose								1						1	
Stevens-Johnson														1	
Unknown							1								
Not stated						6		2	4				1		
Total number of deaths	2	1	2	3	1	6	7	22	4	1	3	2	1	0	4
Death rate (percentage of ICU obstetric admissions)	8.6	9.1	5.1	2.1	2.3	1.8	3.3	5.1	6.8	2.2	2.3	3.6	10.4	12.5	7.0

The number of critical care (ICU and HDU) beds in the UK is lower than the number of beds in many other developed countries, thus many cases of severe morbidity are managed outside of ICU. A recent study of severe obstetric morbidity in the South of England identified 12 such cases per 1 000 deliveries [12]. The causes of admission to ICU of those obstetric patients who died in these UK studies and a series of similar studies from other developed countries are shown in Table 3.

The causes of ICU admission, and of death in ICU, are somewhat different from the causes of death reported by the CEMD. Pregnancy induced hypertension and major haemorrhage are the leading cause of admission in all studies. Thromboembolism and amniotic fluid embolism, although major causes of death in the CEMD reports, do not feature as the leading causes of admission to ICU, even of those patients who died. This implies perhaps that these conditions in obstetric patients are either rapidly fatal, or do not usually cause significant morbidity when first diagnosed, or alternatively severity of the illness is recognized when it is too late.

Comparable studies have been carried out in a variety of other developed countries (Table 4).

Table 4. Causes of admission in non-UK ICUs

Cause of ICU admission	**[11]**	**[21]**	**[14]**	**[15]**	**Reference** **[16]**	**[22]**	**[17]**	**[18]**	**[19]**	**[20]**
Country	France	Ireland	Israel	Israel	Canada	Canada	Canada	USA	USA	USA
Pregnancy induced hypertension	114	0	9	15	28	23	14	8	7	22
Haemorrhage	87	7	11	11	34	17	12	8	4	17
Sepsis	19		14	5	13	2	8	3	6	
Pulmonary embolism	29			1			4	2		
Amniotic fluid embolism							2			
Anaesthesia related	6		4	4						
Fatty liver of pregnancy									2	
Cardiac disease	13	3		1	18		2	14	2	
Pneumonia		1		3		1		16	3	26
Respiratory disease	23	1	6		13	2	3	9	1	
Other pre-existing medical condition		3				18				
Suicide attempts	27								2	
Other	27	2	14	6	25	2	12	31	2	
Total number of admissions	435	17	58	46	131	65	55	96	32	172
Number of deaths	22	0	4	1	3	0	2	10	4	12
Number of deliveries		26166		19474	44340		76119			30405
ICU admissions per 1000 deliveries	3.1	0.6		2	3	2.6	0.7		4	5.7

A similar range of ICU admission rates of 0.6 to 5.7 per 1000 deliveries can be seen. The range of conditions requiring ICU admission is also similar, with pregnancy induced hypertension being the commonest reason for admission in most studies. Of note is the increased incidence of pulmonary embolism in the French study [13] and the incidence of pneumonia in all of the USA studies [18-20]. The latter may reflect an increased ICU bed availability and a lower threshold for admission.

The causes of ICU admission have traditionally been divided into three categories (Table 5), however an alternative classification is given in Table 6.

Table 5. Causes of ICU admission

Pregnancy–related	**Pre-existing medical conditions**	**Unrelated to pregnancy**
Thromboembolism	Cardiac disease (congenital, valvular ischaemic)	Trauma
Amniotic fluid embolism	Respiratory disease (e.g., asthma, cystic fibrosis)	Self-harm
Pregnancy induced Hypertension	Diabetes	Sepsis
Obstetric haemorrhage	Neurological disease	
Obstetric sepsis	Renal disease	
Non-obstetric sepsis		

Table 6. Causes of intensive care unit (ICU) admission – alternative classification

Unpredictable	Possibly predictable	Predictable
Amniotic fluid embolism	Pregnancy induced hypertension	Sever cardiac disease (e.g., Eisenmenger's syndrome, pulmonary hypertension)
Thromboembolism	Sepsis	Severe respiratory disease (e.g., chronic respiratory failure, cystic fibrosis)
Massive haemorrhage Anaesthesia-related problems	Massive haemorrhage	Severe multisystem disease
Abruption		

The predictability of some reasons for admission allows for planning of care in advance. Some parturients with severely limited physiological reserve, particularly of the respiratory or cardiovascular systems, may be expected to tolerate the changes of pregnancy and delivery poorly, thus needing intensive care support for any deterioration in their condition. In such predictable cases it is important to involve all the relevant professionals in the planning of their pregnancy care, including obstetricians, anaesthetists, physicians and intensivists, and prenatal multidisciplinary meetings are invaluable. It is likely that increasing numbers of these women will be encountered, as advances in surgical techniques and medical therapy enable more patients with cardiac, respiratory and other life-threatening diseases to reach adulthood. Although the prognosis for some of these women who become pregnant (e.g., Eisenmenger's syndrome) remains poor [23], they may still choose to go ahead with a pregnancy [10]. Moreover, the increasing age of parity is likely to increase the incidence of other conditions such as severe diabetes, obesity and ischaemic heart disease in parturients in the future. In the UK maternal age of primiparity has already increased from approximately 22 years of age to almost 30 years of age in the past decade [1].

However many of the causes of ICU admission are unpredictable before or during pregnancy, thus establishing protocols for dealing with emergencies such as major haemorrhage or maternal cardiac arrest is useful.

Clinical considerations

Most obstetric patients admitted to ICU are postnatal. UK studies report less than 20% of obstetric patients are admitted while pregnant [8-10]. It may be that the haemodynamic changes which occur at delivery cause a deterioration in the woman's condition. Alternatively recognition of the need for ICU transfer may precipitate a decision to deliver the foetus. There may also be a reluctance to move a pregnant woman from the obstetric unit unless absolutely necessary.

The main indications for admission are for cardiorespiratory support and monitoring. A smaller proportion of obstetric ICU patients require ventilation (44% to 61%) [4, 7, 9, 10] than non-obstetric patients. The duration of ICU stay is shorter, with median length of stay 1 to 3 days [8-10] and 35.7% to 56% being discharged in less than 48 hours [4, 7, 9]. Some of these patients, who do not require ventilation, could be managed in a HDU with appropriate support from intensivists [8, 9, 21, 24].

Physiological changes of pregnancy

A series of physiological changes occur during pregnancy and the puerperium which are relevant to the intensivist caring for the obstetric patient. Cardiac output increases by 20% at 10 weeks gestation and by 40% at term [25], with an increase in both heart rate (10-30%) and stroke volume [26]. The systemic vascular resistance falls, accompanied by a decrease in arterial blood pressure to a minimum at 28 weeks. Blood pressure then slowly increases, but remains below pre-pregnancy levels. These changes are greater with multiple pregnancies. Many pregnant women demonstrate a significant fall in blood pressure when supine, due to aorto-caval compression. This can reduce systemic venous return and uterine blood flow, and cause foetal distress. Central venous pressure and pulmonary artery wedge pressure remain unchanged, but cardiac output measured by pulmonary artery catheter increases by about 40% at term [27]. During labour cardiac output increases further, particularly during contractions [28].

Total lung capacity and vital capacity remain unchanged, but there is a two-fold increase in alveolar ventilation at term mainly due to an increase in tidal volume [25]. The anteroposterior and lateral diameters of the thorax increase as the ribs become more horizontal and the diaphragm moves upwards. The functional residual capacity is reduced by up to 20% at term and oxygen consumption increases progressively throughout pregnancy; hence in the apnoeic pregnant patient hypoxia develops more rapidly.

Increased minute ventilation leads to a fall in maternal partial pressure of carbon dioxide to approximately 4 kPa, but the pH remains within the normal range [25] due to compensatory bicarbonate loss. Hence, total body buffering capacity is reduced. However, alkalaemia from hyperventilation and reduced venous return caused by positive pressure ventilation can reduce uterine blood flow. Hyperaemia, oedema and increased friability of airway mucosa can make insertion of endotracheal tubes and nasogastric tubes more difficult and hazardous [26]. Pregnancy is associated with reduced lower esophageal sphincter tone [25], so the obstetric patient is at risk of aspiration of gastric contents whenever airway reflexes are depressed.

The placenta does not act as a barrier to drug transfer. In particular lipophilic, low molecular weight, non protein-bound drugs will readily cross to the foetus. Foetal blood is more acidaemic than maternal, hence basic drugs such as pethidine and bupivacaine achieve higher free concentrations in the foetal circulation than in the maternal circulation, particularly if there is foetal distress [25].

Foetal monitoring

Continuous electronic foetal heart rate monitoring is used to assess foetal well-being, which may influence management decisions particularly in respect of the timing of delivery. A normal foetal heart rate of 120 to 160 beats per minute with a significant degree of beat-to-beat variability is associated with a good outcome. However the specificity for foetal asphyxia of the heart rate patterns is low, and interpretation requires the specific expertise of a midwife or obstetrician. Other assessments of foetal well-being include the ultrasonographic biophysical profile (foetal movements, foetal breathing movements, foetal limb tone, amniotic fluid volume, reactivity to stimuli) and foetal scalp blood sampling for acid-base measurements [26].

Drug therapy

Inotropes

There are few data on the use of inotropic drugs in human pregnancy. From animal studies, ephedrine has been shown to increase maternal blood pressure as well as increase uterine blood flow, thus improving foetal hypoxaemia. However maternal hypotension and inadequate cardiac output will compromise foetal blood supply, so adequate volume replacement and left lateral positioning have an important role in optimizing haemodynamics [26].

Antihypertensives

Patients with pregnancy induced hypertension may require peripheral vasodilators. Hydralazine, nifedipine and methyldopa are the most commonly used agents. All these drugs have the risk of excessive hypotension and reduction in uterine blood flow. Angiotensin converting enzyme inhibitors should not be used, as they are associated with foetal renal dysfunction.

Magnesium sulfate

Magnesium is used as an anticonvulsant to prevent seizures in eclampsia and severe pre-eclampsia. It is given by infusion to maintain serum levels of 2 to 3.5 mmol/L [26]. It potentiates non-depolarizing muscle relaxants, and respiratory depression and cardiac conduction abnormalities have been reported with toxic levels. Parenteral calcium can be administered to reverse these adverse effects.

Tocolytics

Ritodrine, salbutamol or other beta-2-agonists may be used to inhibit uterine contractions to prevent preterm labour or following external cephalic version. These can cause hyperglycaemia, hypokalaemia, sodium and water retention, pulmonary oedema and tachyarrhythmias. Side effects may be seen following discontinuation of these agents. Other tocolytics such as glyceryl trinitrate, magnesium, volatile anaesthetic agents or the oxytocin antagonist atosiban are also used, but their use is usually reserved for acute tocolysis.

Drugs to reduce uterine haemorrhage

Oxytocin, given by bolus and infusion, promotes uterine contraction to reduce post partum uterine haemorrhage. In bolus form it produces tachycardia and hypotension. In large doses it also has an antidiuretic effect and can cause hyponatraemia from water retention. Carboprost (a prostacyclin F_2–analogue) may be given by the intramuscular or the intramyometrial route. Side-effects include hypertension, nausea and vomiting, bronchoconstriction and increased intrapulmonary shunt.

Mechanical ventilation

Tracheal intubation requires a rapid sequence induction of anaesthesia with cricoid pressure because of the risk of acid aspiration. The ventilator should be set bearing in mind the increased alveolar ventilation requirements of the obstetric patient and the expected partial pressure of carbon dioxide of approximately 3.5 to 4 kPa. Both maternal respiratory acidosis and alkalosis are detrimental to the foetus.

Acute respiratory distress syndrome (ARDS) in the pregnant patient poses particular difficulties: permissive hypercapnia is potentially hazardous, as it leads to foetal acidosis; high levels of positive end expiratory pressure (PEEP) may compromise uterine perfusion; and there are no data on the effect of prone positioning on foetal perfusion [29]. No studies have been carried out using nitric oxide in pregnancy, however there are two case reports of its successful use [29].

Cardiopulmonary resuscitation

The usual resuscitation techniques are used, but with early intubation to reduce the risk of aspiration of gastric contents. Beyond 20 weeks gestation a wedge or lateral tilt (15 to 30 degrees) of the pelvis is employed to minimize aorto-caval compression. If spontaneous cardiac output has not been restored in five minutes, then emergency Caesarean section is indicated to improve the chances of survival of both mother and foetus [30, 31]. Advanced life support should continue during the surgery.

Where to look after the critically ill obstetric patient

The critically ill obstetric patients needs the expertise of the intensivist and ICU nurses, experienced in critical care and of the obstetrician, neonatologist and midwife, who have the specialist experience of pregnancy and childbirth. A number of tertiary referral centres in the USA have obstetric ICUs where this expertise is combined [26]; in the UK these patients are managed on general ICUs or on obstetric HDUs.

The CEMD report 1994-96 [1] recommended that every consultant obstetric unit should have an HDU. However in 1997 only 41% of such units had at least one designated high dependency bed [24], and 55% recognized the need for more in their unit. Some obstetric units are isolated geographically from general hospitals. Nineteen percent of consultant obstetric units in the UK do not have a general ICU on their site, necessitating the transfer of a critically ill obstetric patient by ambulance to another hospital [24]. Thirty-one percent have no resident anaesthetist [24].

The general lack of high dependency facilities leads to a number of non-ventilated obstetric patients being looked after on ICUs, who could be cared for in a high dependency environment [8, 9, 21, 24]. However the anaesthetists, midwives and obstetricians caring for these women need adequate training and experience in care of the critically ill patient.

The criteria for admission to ICU include those which apply to the non-pregnant critically ill patient, and in many units more liberal criteria are applied to admit the 'potentially ill' obstetric patient [6]. Such admissions may prevent severe complications due to the rapid onset of certain obstetric emergencies and the relative inexperience of the obstetric staff in caring for critically ill patients. Thus, strict criteria for admission to the ICU cannot be universally applied as much depends on local circumstances.

Maternal mortality in the developed world is rare. On the labour ward maternal safety may be taken for granted, with the focus being on the safety of the foetus or newborn infant and on the psychosocial aspects of childbirth. However maternal *morbidity* is more common, each case of morbidity can be viewed as a mortality 'near-miss'.

The obstetric patient on the ICU presents a unique challenge. The intensivist may be unfamiliar with the physiological norms of pregnancy, and certain disease states are unique to pregnancy.

The presence of the foetus in the critically ill patient may necessitate changes in management strategies. The response to these challenges requires close communication between the health care professionals of the critical care, obstetric and neonatal departments, with early planning wherever possible. There is also an important educational role for the intensivist in teaching the obstetric staff who may increasingly be looking after these patients in obstetric HDUs.

References

1. Department of Heath (1998) Why mothers die. Report on Confidential Enquiries into Maternal Deaths in the United Kingdom 1994-1996. HMSO, London
2. Department of Heath (1996) Report on Confidential Enquiries into Maternal Deaths in the United Kingdom 1991-1993. HMSO, London
3. Department of Heath (1993) Report on Confidential Enquiries into Maternal Deaths in the United Kingdom 1988-1990. HMSO, London
4. Graham SG, Luxton MC (1998) The requirement for intensive care support for the pregnant population. Anaesthesia 44:581-584
5. Hughes RL (1990) The requirement for intensive care support for the pregnant population. Anaesthesia 45:65
6. Yau EHS, Groves PA, Wathen NC et al (1990) The requirement for intensive care support for the pregnant population. Anaesthesia 45:65-66
7. De Mello WF, Restall J (1990) The requirement for intensive care support for the pregnant population. Anaesthesia 44:888
8. Wheatley E, Farkas A, Watson D (1996) Obstetric admissions to an intensive therapy unit. International Journal of Obstetric Anaesthesia 5:221-224
9. Hazelgrove JF, Price C, Pappachan J et al (2001) Multicentre study of obstetric admissions to 14 intensive care units in southern England. Crit Care Med 29:770-775
10. Umo-Etuk J, Lumley J, Holdcroft A (1996) Critically ill parturient women admitted to intensive care: a 5 year review. International Journal of Obstetric Anaesthesia 5:79-84
11. Rowen K, Goldfrad C (2000) Obstetric admissions to the case mix programme. Presentation at Intensive Care Society Spring Meeting 2000 and Personal Communication
12. Waterstone M, Bewley S, Wolfe C (2001) Incidence and predictors of severe obstetric mortality: case control study. BMJ 322:1089-1093
13. Bouvier-Colle M-H, Salanave B, Ancel P Y et al (1996) Obstetric patients treated in intensive care units and maternal mortality. Eur J Obstet Gynecol Reprod Biol 65:121-125
14. Lewinsohn G, Herman A, Leonov Y et al (1994) Critically ill obstetrical patients: Outcome and predictability. Crit Care Med 22: 1412-1414
15. Cohen J, Singer P, Kogan A, et al (2000) Course and outcome of obstetric patients in a general intensive care unit. Acta Obstet Gynecol Scand 79:846-850
16. Mahutte NG, Murphy-Kaulbeck L, Le Q, et al (1999) Obstetric Admissions to the Intensive Care Unit. Obstet Gynecol 94:263-266
17. Baskett TF, Sternadel J (1998) Maternal intensive care and near-miss mortality in obstetrics. Br J Obstet Gynaecol 105:981-984
18. El-Solh AA, Grant BJB (1996) A comparison of Severity of Illness Scoring for Critically Ill Obstetric Patients. Chest 110:1299-1304
19. Kilpatrick SJ, Matthay MA (1992) Obstetric Patients Requiring Critical Care. Chest 101:1407-1412
20. Hogg B, Hauth JC (2000) Intensive Care Unit Utilization During Pregnancy. Obstet Gynecol 95:62S
21. Ryan M, Hamilton V, Bowen M et al (2000) The role of a high-dependency unit in a regional obstetric hospital. Anaesthesia 55:1155-1158
22. Lapinsky SE, Kruczynski K, Seaward GR et al (1997) Critical care management of the obstetric patient. Can J Anaesth 44:325-329

23. Yentis SM, Steer PJ, Plaat F (1998) Eisenmenger's syndrome in pregnancy: maternal and fetal mortality in the 1990's. Br J Obstet Gynaecol 105: 921-922
24. Cordingley JJ, Rubin AP (1997) A survey of facilities for high risk women in consultant obstetric units. International Journal of Obstetric Anaesthesia 6:156-160
25. Thorburn J, Reid J (1996) Physiology of pregnancy and the placenta. In Prys-Roberts C, Brown BR (ed) International Practice of Anaesthesia. Butterworth Heinemann, Oxford
26. Lapinsky SE, Kruczynski K, Slutsky AS (1995) Critical Care in the Pregnant Patient. Am J Respir Crit Care Med 152:427-455
27. Clark SL, Cotton DB, Lee W et al (1989) Central hemodynamic assessment of normal term pregnancy. Am J Obstet Gynecol 161:1439-1442
28. Robson SC, Dunlop W, Boys RJ et al (1987) Cardiac output during labour. BMJ 295:1169-1171
29. Campbell LA, Klocke RA (2001) Implications for the Pregnant Patient. Am J Respir Crit Care Med 163:1051-1054
30. Resuscitation Council (UK) and European Resuscitation Council (2000) Advanced Life Support Manual 4th edition. Resuscitation Council (UK) and European Resuscitation Council, London
31. Marx G (1982) Cardiopulmonary resuscitation of the late pregnant woman. Anesthesiology 58:156

High Dependancy Unit in the Obstetric Department

I. SMILOV, I. TRAYANOV, I. KOVACHEV

The critically ill pregnant woman represents a unique challenge to the clinician. The patient's disease, as well as any potential therapy, simultaneously affects two individuals with vastly different physiologies.

The high dependency unit (HDU) in the obstetric department is area where maximum personnel and technologic support are available to the patient, who require more intensive observation and treatment. It would not normally accept patients requiring mechanical ventilation, but could manage those receiving invasive monitoring. Not every pregnant woman requires or benefits from the HDU. However, the support and interventions practicable in the HDU are absolutely essential to the survival of certain patients.

Principles of invasive haemodynamic monitoring in pregnancy

An understanding of cardiovascular changes associated with normal and abnormal pregnancy is essential for the treatment of pregnant women and allows management for some individual cases, based on the fundamental assumptions about maternal physiology. Additional information is required when the mother is severely ill and when the baseline haemodynamic functioning is abnormal. Under most circumstances in pregnancy, women are able to regulate their haemodynamic condition without interference. In circumstances where intervention is necessary, the appropriate therapeutic modality can frequently be chosen with reference to the clinical settings and clinical signs.

Indications

Indications for use of invasive haemodynamic monitoring in pregnant women can be classified into the following categories [1]:

- Severe oliguria. Urine output less than 30 ml/hr for 3 hours in the face of other parameters suggesting an adequate intravascular volume. Most often this indication is seen in severe preeclamptics whose oliguria continues despite attempts at conservative fluid resuscitation [2].

- Significant maternal cardiac disease (NYHA Classes III and IV). The narrow therapeutic window requires invasive monitoring to maintain appropriate hydration during labour, anaesthesia and potential haemorrhage [3].
- Impaired maternal oxygenation associated with pulmonary oedema.
- Conditions, such as septic shock, in which vasoactive agents are required to support blood pressure and cardiac output.

Principles of noninvasive haemodynamic monitoring in pregnancy

Noninvasive haemodynamic monitoring traditionally has been limited to the measurement of the heart rate, blood pressure, and orthostatic changes in blood pressure. However, in critically patients, sufficient data frequently are unavailable to make necessary clinical decisions. Application of invasive haemodynamic monitoring requires an experienced team and may have a potential risk to the patient. Furthermore, invasive haemodynamic monitoring is not always warranted in patients with mild cardiovascular compromise in relation to the potential risk.

M-mode echocardiography and real-time ultrasound are well-established means of cardiac evaluation and are used to generate static and moving images. Doppler ultrasound, in contrast, can be used to generate qualitative and quantitative information related to blood flow and velocities and can provide measurement of some parameters usually evaluated with invasive haemodynamic techniques. In complicated pregnancies, the method has been used to describe changes associated with pheochromocytoma [4], antihypertensive therapy [5], structural cardiac diseases, postpartum haemorrhage [6] and preeclampsia [7].

HDU management of pregnant patients with cardiac diseases

Patients with cardiac diseases in post vaginal delivery and post caesarean section period

1. General considerations

- Basic risk factors increase with cardiac disease and maternal physiologies during pregnancy and after delivery.

- Perioperative general evaluation which includes labour and delivery.
- Laboratory studies such as complete blood cell count, electrolyte and blood gas analysis, glucose, creatinine and blood urea nitrogen (BUN) and liver function tests.
- Non-invasive studies (ECG; chest x-ray and echocardiography).
- Cardiac consultation and obstetrics consultation.
- Bacterial endocarditis prophylaxis. Strict aseptic technique. Antibiotics.
- Abnormal haemostasis.
- Cyanotic patients.
- Monitoring.
- Drugs and drug effects.
- Side effects (from anaesthesia, from delivery and from cardiac disease).
- Standards (national and international) for safety in obstetrics and obstetrics anaesthesia.
- You can use epidural analgesia for postoperative pain relief with extreme caution, arterial blood pressure should stay stable. Non-steroidal anti-inflammatory drugs (NSAIDs) or opioids are recommended in this case.

2. Aortic stenosis or idiopathic hypertrophic subaortic stenosis and post delivery intensive care

Aortic stenosis is the only valvular lesion that is directly associated with the risk of postoperative ischaemia, myocardial infarction (MI) and postoperative maternal death.

3. Aortic regurgitation and post delivery intensive care

4. Mitral stenosis and post delivery intensive care

5. Mitral regurgitation or mitral valve prolapse and post delivery intensive care

6. Congenital heart disease and post delivery intensive care

7. Other heart diseases in pregnancy and post delivery intensive care

- Primary pulmonary hypertension.
- Hypertensive disorders.
- Cardiomyopathy of pregnancy.
- Dissecting aneurysm of the aorta.
- Pericarditis.
- Coronary artery disease.

- Cardiac dysrythmias.
- Cardiac transplantation.

HDU management of the pregnant diabetic patient

Between 3 and 7% of all pregnancies are accompanied by diabetes. Gestational Diabetes Mellitus (GDM) represents nearly 90% of all pregnancies complicated by diabetes [8]. Type 1 diabetes is found in 4% of those pregnancies. The rest of them are complicated by type 2 diabetes. Caesarean section is performed in 30 to 77.4% of diabetic pregnancies depending on the type of diabetes and the population studied [9].

The latter is one of the reasons for the high number of diabetic parturients admitted to the HDU. Criteria for admission to the HDU and indications for intubation and mechanical ventilation are similar for diabetic parturients and non-pregnant patients. Diabetic ketoacidosis is the most frequent indication for HDU admission of a pregnant diabetic patient.

Diabetic ketoacidosis

Diabetic ketoacidosis (DKA) is a complication of diabetes and is an emergency with an extremely high risk of foetal mortality. Foetal loss rates have been reported in excess of 50% [10]. Today, this complication is rarely a cause of maternal death. Maternal loss rates are 1% or less, but no substantial reduction in the maternal mortality rate has occurred in the past 30 years [11]. Perinatal mortality is slightly higher in diabetic women than the general population.

Treatment of DKA

The treatment of DKA involves rehydratation, restoration of electrolyte homeostasis, and normalization of serum glucose with appropriate doses of insulin. The management protocol of diabetic ketoacidosis in pregnancy includes:

- Rapid but careful history and physical examination with special attention to: patency of airway, mental status, cardiovascular and renal status, source of infection, and state of hydration.
- Initial biochemical evaluation should consist of immediate assessment of blood ketones, blood glucose (finger stick) and urine ketones, including immediate order for plasma glucose, blood gases and pH, serum elec-

trolytes, BUN, amylase, and a complete blood count. Chest film, ECG, and appropriate bacterial cultures are also to be obtained if indicated.

- As soon as the initial chemistries are drawn, 1 L of normal saline is given in the first hour, with a subsequent infusion of 0.45% sodium chloride 200-700 ml/h. Total fluid must not exceed 5 L within 8 hours.
- With the confirmation of diagnosis of diabetic ketoacidosis, 0.4 U of regular insulin / kg body weight is given (half as i.v. push and half as s.c.). In comatose patients or ICU admissions, 7-10 U of insulin is given per hour as a continuous infusion.
- Plasma glucose is determined hourly and electrolytes and blood gases are recorded every 2-4 hours. If plasma glucose does not fall by 10% in the first hour, an initial priming dose of insulin is repeated or the rate of insulin infusion is doubled.
- After satisfactory glucose decrement, 7 U of regular insulin is given per hour as either i.m. or s.c. intermittent injection or as i.v. infusion until plasma glucose reaches 11 mmol/L (200 mg/dl).
- As soon as plasma glucose reaches 11 mmol/L, 5% glucose is glucose in 0.45% saline if sodium is > 140 mEq/L or 5% glucose is used in 0.9% saline if sodium is < 140 mEq/L. A rate of 100-300 ml/h is used depending on the state of hydration. Insulin 10 U/2h s.c. is given until diabetic ketoacidosis is controlled (defined as plasma glucose < mmol/L, HCO_3 > 15 mEq/L, and pH >7.3, and serum ketone negative at 1:2 dilution).
- If initial potassium is < 3.5 mEq/L, potassium supplements should be provided at the rate of 40 mEq/L with the initial insulin therapy (1/3 as KPO_4 and 2/3 as KCl). Potassium is given at a rate of 20 –30 mEq per liter after the first liter of solution if potassium > 3.5 but < 5.5 mEq/L, and urinary output is adequate. Potassium is not given if potassium > 5.5 mEq/L. With abnormal potassium, serum potassium is repeated every 1-2 hours.
- Na bicarbonate is given for a pH > 7.0, but 44 mEq of $NaHCO_3$ is given for a pH > 6.9. For a pH < 6.9, 88 mEq of $NaHCO_3$ is given. Each 44 mEq of $NaHCO_3$ is to be run for 30 min with 15 mEq of KCl.
- The above is repeated every 2 hours until pH > 7.0.
- Ancillary measures include: stomach aspiration in unconscious patient; O_2 therapy for PO_2 < 80 mm Hg; plasma expander for consistent hypotension and antibiotic therapy, as needed.
- Precipitating factors should be monitored as well as the patient's clinical condition with frequent management.

The underlying cause of DKA should not be neglected. Correction of the metabolic derangement can only be successful if the underlying cause is treated. A thorough search for infection should be made.

The foetus should be carefully monitored if it has attained a potentially viable gestation age. Delivery of a compromised foetus should be delayed unless the mother is metabolically stable. Correction of the maternal deficiencies generally rapidly adjusts the metabolic deficits of the foetus as well.

HDU management of obstetric haemorrhage

Haemorrhagic shock is a disparity between the circulating blood volume and the capacity of the vascular bed as a result of blood loss.

Common causes of obstetric haemorrhage

1. Antepartum and intrapartum
- Placental abruption
- Placenta previa
- Uterine rupture

2. Postpartum
- Retained placenta
- Uterine atony
- Uterine rupture
- Genital tract trauma
- Coagulopathy

Goals of therapy
- Systolic pressure 90 mmHg
- Urine output 25 ml/h
- Normal mental status
- Eliminate source of haemorrhage
- Avoid overzealous volume replacement

Preeclampsia

The postoperative management of the preeclamptic patients is an important clinical challenge. The provision of anaesthesia and analgesia for normal and operative delivery and postoperative care of these mothers provide a particular clinical challenge requiring considerable skill and experience on the part of the anaesthetist.

I. General considerations

1. Respiratory system. Pulmonary oedema occurs most frequently after operative and non-operative delivery. Laryngeal oedema may worsen during the operative procedure and cause airway embarrassment that requires reintubation a few minutes after extubation.
2. Cardiovascular system. There are increases in the systemic vascular resistance, the left ventricular stroke work index, and the left ventricular diastolic dysfunction. There is a poor correlation between the central venous pressure (CVP) and pulmonary capillary wedge pressure (PCWP). Hypertension must be treated. Antihypertensive therapy should be continued as long as clinically indicated.
3. Central nervous system. Headaches, hyperreflexia, visual disturbances and convulsions can be present. Convulsions (compared with enchephalopathy) are not directly related to the elevation in blood pressure. Convulsions must be controlled. Anticonvulsant medication is given as long as the patient remains symptomatic.
4. Kidneys. Progress to acute renal failure is common, especially in cases with hypotension or severe proteinuria.
5. Liver. There is reduced enzyme activity. Hemolysis, elevated liver enzymes, low platelets (HELLP) syndrome and hepatic rupture is a rare, but serious complication.
6. Coagulation. Some patients have thrombocytopenia and in severe cases platelet counts may fall rapidly. These cases may develop the HELLP syndrome and the disseminated intravascular coagulation (DIC) syndrome.

II. Management of preeclamptic patients in ICU. Multi-disciplinary management of these patients

1. Monitoring.
2. Reduction of maternal complications.

- Management of cardiovascular function.
  - Control of hypertension (Hydralazine, Dehydralazine, beta-blockers, Nifedipine, continuous infusion of Nitroprusside or Nitroglycerine).
  - Intravenous fluid therapy(red blood cells, platelets concentrate, fresh-frozen plasma, Albumin and crystalloids). Control of fluid balance.
- Management of convulsions (Magnesium sulphate, Benzodiazepines, Barbiturates, Phenytoin). There is no clarity in the literature in regards to the best drugs for eclamptic convulsion.
- Treatment of oliguria.

- Intravenous fluid therapy.
- Nonosmotic diuretics.

- Management of respiratory function. Oxygen therapy.
- Management of coagulation abnormalities.
- Pain relief. Good quality postoperative analgesia can ease the management of these cases.

References

1. Clarck SL, Horenstein JM, Phelan JP (1985) Experience with the pulmonary artery catheter in obstetrics and gynecology. Am J Obstet Gynecol 152:374
2. Clarck SL, Greenspoon JS, Aldah CD, et al (1986) Severe preeclampsia with persistent oliguria. Management of hemodynamic subsets. Am J Obstet Gynecol 154:490
3. Benedetti TJ, Cotton DB, Read JC, et al (1980) Hemodynamic observations in severe preeclampsia with a flow-directed pulmonary artery catheter. Am J Obstet Gynecol 136:465
4. Cooms A, Easterling T, Schmucker B (1989) Hemodynamic observations during paroxismal hypertension with pheochromocytoma in pregnancy. Obstet Gynecol 74:439
5. Easterling T, Benedetti T, Schmucker B (1989) Antihypertensive therapy in pregnancy directed by noninvasive hemodynamic monitoring. Am J Perinatol 6:86
6. Robson S, Boys R, Hunter S (1989) Maternal hemodynamics after normal delivery and delivery complicated by postpartum hemorrhage. Obstet Gynecol 74:234-239
7. Easterling T, Watts D, Schmucker B (1987) Determination of cardiac output during pregnancy: validation of Doppler technique and clinical observations in preeclampsia. 69:845
8. Kitabchi AE, Wall BM (1995) Diabetic ketoacidosis. Med Clin North Am 79:9
9. Multicenter survey of diabetic pregnancy in France (1991) Gestation and Diabetes in France Study Group Diabetes Care 14: 994-1000
10. American Diabetes Association (2001): Clinical Practice Recommendations. Diabetes Care 24: 5-10
11. Gunton JE, McElduff A, Sulway M, et al Outcome of pregnancies complicated by pre-gestational diabetes mellitus. Aust N Z Obstet Gynaecol 2000; 40(1): 38-43

Obstetric Anaesthesia and Maternal Morbidity and Mortality

I.F. RUSSELL

Obstetric Anaesthesia may result in both maternal *mortality* and *morbidity* but, while maternal death is a clear and unambiguous end point, morbidity is more difficult to define, ranging as it does, from minor temporary complaints (e.g. sore throat, local tissue bruising) to major permanent pathology (e.g. neuropathy, paralysis). This chapter will examine the factors underlying the changes in anaesthetic related maternal mortality and morbidity over the past 50 years.

Maternal death

With the introduction of the triennial *Confidential Enquiries into Maternal Deaths* in England and Wales (CEMD) in 1952 [1] and the later reports in the series [2-15] the contribution of anaesthesia to maternal deaths became more widely understood. Comparison of the anaesthetic causes of death in the first CEMD report [1] with the later reports reveals the importance of such reports in influencing subsequent practice. In the first reports [1-2] deaths were recorded in association with operator anaesthetists, general anaesthesia outside hospital (e.g. in the patient's home or in small maternity hospitals) and inhalational anaesthesia (e.g. ether, chloroform, cyclopropane, trilene). A significant cause of maternal mortality in the early reports [1-3] was general anaesthesia for forceps delivery (25 of the 49 deaths in the 1952-54 report [1]) and as a consequence obstetricians were encouraged to make greater use of local anaesthesia – pudendal block and perineal infiltration.

The knowledge that general anaesthesia for forceps deliveries was a major cause of maternal deaths stimulated changes in practice: by 1967-69 [6] there were only 2 forceps related deaths and this was at a time before epidural anaesthesia could have made any real impact. More recently, epidural or spinal anaesthesia has become widely used for forceps delivery. By the 1970's deaths associated with forceps deliveries were down to single figures and by the late

1980's they had virtually disappeared [7-12]. The last reported anaesthetic death associated with forceps delivery was in the 1998-90 CEMD report when a woman refused to have an epidural anaesthetic for a proposed forceps delivery and regurgitated a large quantity of gastric contents at induction of general anaesthesia [13]. Today, in our own unit, there would have to be an unusual combination of circumstance before anyone would contemplate using general anaesthesia for a forceps delivery and perusal of the Department of Health data for the UK indicates that only around 1% of instrumental deliveries receive general anaesthesia [16].

Since intubation of the trachea was rarely practised at the time of the first CEMD report [1] there were no deaths from failed intubation but 32 of the 49 deaths were due to aspiration of gastric contents. In the first report [1] there were 5 deaths related to the use of thiopentone and muscle relaxant and this combination was "recognized as a definite risk" but whether intubation was attempted in these women is not clear since at this time muscle relaxants were often used as part of "lissive anaesthesia" without intubation. The changes in the basic anaesthetic technique for Caesarean section gradually become obvious over the years as comments regarding intubation are included in the reports. While no mention of intubation is made in the first report [1] the author of the second report [2] indicates with surprise "that in 10 cases, including 3 Caesarean sections, tracheal intubation does not appear to have been planned." In the 1961-63 report [4] comments on intubation are made more forcefully - "Failure to intubate the trachea seems to be the commonest fault," "Failure to intubate the trachea as a planned procedure was the principal avoidable factor" - and cricoid pressure receives its first mention. Thus, it would appear that intubation of a pregnant patient had now become the expected standard of care and in the 1964-66 report [5] it is noted that "Failure to intubate the trachea as a planned procedure did not occur." However, deaths where mothers were not intubated continued to be reported in the 1967-69 [6] and 1970-72 [7] reports. The CEMD reports [1-15] show clearly how the emphasis on problems changes with time. As intubation became the norm comments began to appear on the poor application (or non application) of cricoid pressure, the lack of antacid prophylaxis, and the misuse of drugs, particularly muscle relaxants and their reversal agents.

In the first CEMD report [1] anaesthesia was responsible for 3.5% (49) of the 1 410 reported maternal deaths but, by the late 1960's the number of anaesthetic related maternal deaths was still 50 while maternal deaths from other causes had declined significantly – to 455 [6]. Thus, anaesthesia became the third most common cause of maternal mortality, accounting for some 11% of the total maternal deaths. Virtually all the anaesthetic deaths were in association with general anaesthesia and the most important factor causing death was a problem with the airway patency: either *failed intubation* and/or *aspiration* of gastric contents. As indicated above, there were other problems also related to general anaesthesia such as misuse of drugs, poor post-op care and post extubation difficulties. All these complications of general anaesthesia led to the view that, if possible general anaesthesia should be avoided: "There is of course only one certain way of avoiding pulmonary aspiration (death) during general anaesthesia and that is the substitution of an appropriate form of regional anaesthesia" [17]. Anaesthesia remained the third most common cause of maternal death until the mid 1980's when it slipped to 8th or 9th of the nine listed causes of maternal death [12-15].

From the mid 1970's there has been a steady increase in the proportion of Caesarean sections performed under regional anaesthesia and this has been associated with a steady reduction in anaesthetic related maternal mortality. The association of increasing use of regional anaesthesia and declining maternal mortality provoked intense argument as to the exact contribution made by regional anaesthesia to the reduction in maternal mortality and a debate was organized: "general anaesthesia is contraindicated for Caesarean section where regional anaesthesia is possible" (Controversies in Obstetric Anaesthesia, Queen Charlotte's and Chelsea Hospital, London, 1993). Within the obstetric anaesthetic community views were split. At one extreme was the view that deaths in association with regional anaesthesia were rare because regional anaesthesia was inherently safer than general anaesthesia. At the other extreme was a belief that deaths were rare with regional anaesthesia because it was very likely that, despite appearances, regional anaesthesia for Caesarean section was hardly used in the UK: it was suggested that the widespread use of regional anaesthesia was only an impression created by a few atypical high profile anaesthetists "talking it up" and that there was no evidence to demonstrate that regional anaesthesia was used widely in the UK. The fact that there was no evidence to support either of these views was the stimulus for the two national studies of obstetric anaesthesia [18, 19].

The controversies debate and the results of the surveys [18, 19] led the author to investigate, in some detail, the changes in anaesthetic maternal mortality in relation to anaesthetic practice. In order to do this it was necessary to obtain some further background data on regional anaesthesia for the era before detailed records were available. Epidural analgesia for labour was introduced into the UK in the late 1960's following the Fourth World Congress of Anaesthesiologists held in London in 1968 [20]. However, as comments by the leading UK obstetric anaesthetists of the day reveal, at this time epidural anaesthesia was scarcely used for Caesarean section. Tunstall, when describing the management of a labouring woman with an epidural states "If Caesarean section is required we normally give a standard GA" [21]. Similarly, Crawford stated "The route into the epidural space can be used to provide anaesthesia for the operation (Caesarean section) although we do not ourselves use this technique" [22]. Moir, stated "I am rather less enthusiastic with epidural analgesia for Caesarean section" and his data supported this reticence with only 33 out of 1 800 epidurals being used for caesarean section [23].

From around 1950 until the late 1980's spinal anaesthesia was scarcely used in obstetrics, indeed many considered the use of spinal anaesthesia be contra-indicated for obstetric use [24, 25]. While Macdonald [24] felt "Deliberate dural puncture has a limited place in the obstetric unit," Crawford was much more forthright and stated "The choice of spinal anaesthesia for Caesarean section is to be condemned. I do not wish to, indeed I am determined not to, play Russian Roulette with a patient's life" [25]. However, Russell [26] argued strongly for the use of spinal anaesthesia pointing out the limitations and drawbacks to epidural anaesthesia as espoused by Carrie [27] and Abouleish [28] : "Spinal anaesthesia is used by anaesthetists who know the limitations of epidural analgesia and the advantages to be gained by using a spinal" [27]: "Epidural analgesia, a potentially dangerous technique, has been overused. The substitution of spinal for epidural analgesia, especially for caesarean section, is not only preferable for the foetus, but safer for the mother" [28]. From these historical comments it is reasonable to assume that few Caesarean sections were performed under regional anaesthesia until around the mid 1970's.

The National surveys [18, 19] showed a declining use of general anaesthesia and an increase in the use of regional anaesthesia, particularly spinal anaesthesia. Now spinal anaesthesia is the most common anaesthetic for Caesarean section in the UK [19]. At first glance, the reduction in anaesthetic related maternal mortality appears to have paralleled the reduction in the use of general anaesthesia (Fig. 1), reinforcing the belief of a direct association between the reducing maternal mortality and the declining use of general anaesthesia. However, this oversimplifies the matter. While the percentage use of general anaesthesia has indeed declined dramatically, over this same time span there has been a significant increase in the number of Caesarean sections performed. Figure 2 illustrates the relationship between the declining number of anaesthetic related maternal deaths, the number of Caesarean sections conducted under general anaesthesia, the number of Caesarean sections under regional anaesthesia and the total number of Caesarean sections performed. Figure 2 demonstrates that roughly the same number of general anaesthetics were given in the early 1970's (when 100% of cases received general anaesthesia) as in the early 1990's (when only around 40% - 45% received general anaesthesia). Yet despite similar numbers of general anaesthetics the number of direct anaesthetic deaths

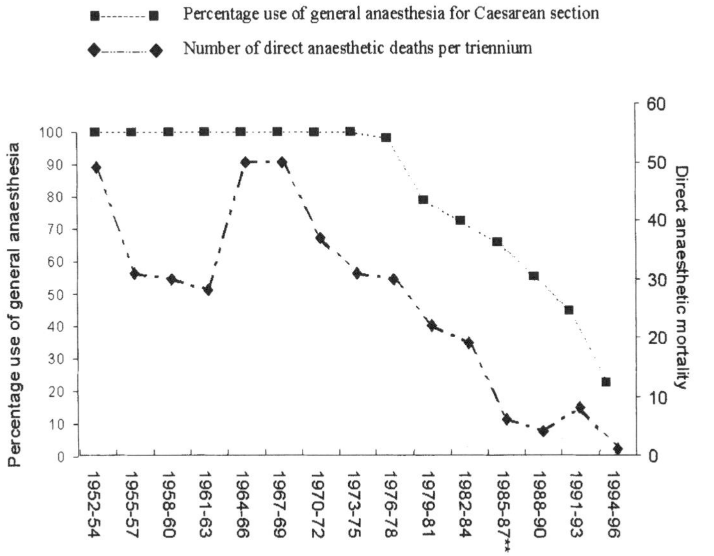

Fig.1. Comparison of direct anaesthetic maternal mortality with the percentage use of general anaesthesia for Caesarean section.
**1985-87 was the first time data were collected for the whole of the United Kingdom. Before 1985 the data refers to England and Wales only.
Data for these graphs were extracted or calculated from references [1-16, 18-25, 29-33]

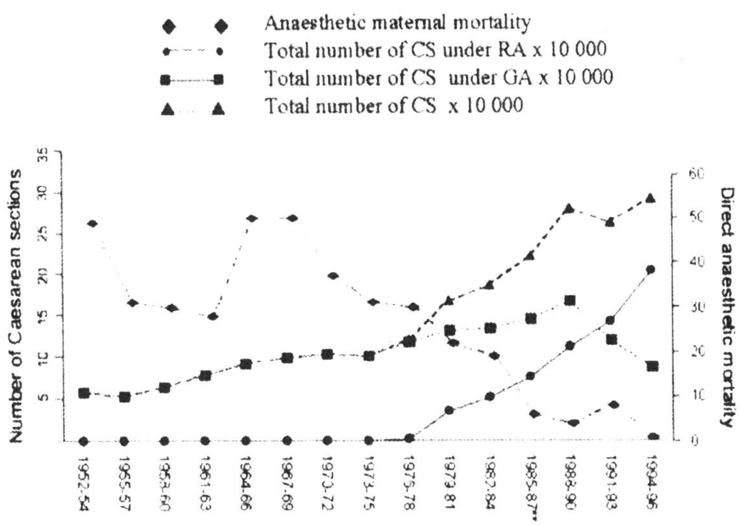

Fig. 2. Graphical representation of the change with time of the number of Caesarean sections performed, the number of caesarean sections performed under general anaesthesia, and the number of caesarean sections performed under regional anaesthesia. The direct anaesthetic maternal mortality is also plotted to enable a comparison with the number of general anaesthetics administered.
**1985-87 was the first time data were collected for the whole of the United Kingdom. Before 1985 the data refers to England and Wales only.
Data for these graphs were extracted or calculated from references [1-16, 18-25, 29-33]

was different: 37 compared with 8 [7, 14]. This difference is even more dramatic if the 1960's are compared with the 1990's.

For most of the period covered by the CEMDs [1-15] there has been no reduction in the actual number of general anaesthetics given, indeed there has been a steady increase in general anaesthetic numbers, reaching a peak around the late 1980's. Despite this the direct anaesthetic related maternal mortality had declined to single figures. In the 1994-96 CEMD report [15] there were around 87 000 Caesarean sections conducted under general anaesthesia with no direct deaths due to general anaesthesia compared to the 59 000 Caesarean sections under general anaesthesia recorded in the 1952-54 report with 24 deaths (the other 25 deaths were associated with an unknown number of general anaesthetics for forceps deliveries) [1].

Therefore, it would appear that the reduction in anaesthetic related maternal mortality may be related to factors other than simply a greater use of regional anaesthesia for Caesarean section. In the first Triennial report [1] it is stated in the anaesthetic chapter –"this series of cases clearly demonstrated the difficulties and risks of obstetric anaesthesia and emphasizes the need for special skills and experience. It would appear that an anaesthetist experienced in obstetric work should be available at night, when most of these cases so often occur, as well as by day." Similar pleas are made throughout most of the reports. In 1964-66 report [5] we can read "There is a need for more general realization that patients with obstetric emergencies are gravely at risk and need the knowledge and skill of an experienced anaesthetist" and in the 1970-72 report [7] it was pointed out that of the 26 cases with an avoidable anaesthetic factor, 22 involved junior staff – thus suggesting the need for "better supervision or the use of more experienced anaesthetists." In the 1982-84 report [11] the reduction in anaesthetic related maternal deaths is noted and it was felt that this was probably due to the "growing awareness over this period that obstetric anaesthesia cannot safely be left to unsupervised beginners in the speciality." However, the comment was also made that many of the deaths still "reflected the administrative failure of leaving inexperienced junior anaesthetists to care for patients who required the most skilled attention" [11]. In the 1991-93 report [14] we are reminded that "Lack of consultant (anaesthetist) involvement is a recurring problem which must be solved" as "trainee or locum anaesthetists failed to appreciate the severity of the patient's condition." In the most recent report 1994-96 [15] with only a single direct anaesthetic death [related to substandard care of a combined spinal-epidural anaestesia (CSE)] it is pointed out that the great improvement since the last report is a "tribute to those responsible for provision of obstetric anaesthesia services." Because of the very low number of anaesthetic related maternal deaths in this report [15] there was a significant change in its presentation and format: maternal deaths were included "where the standard of anaesthetic care was satisfactory but the case may prove useful for trainee anaesthetists."

With the continued emphasis on improving the experience of anaesthetists involved in obstetric anaesthesia it seems most likely that changes in obstetric anaesthesia staffing and standards have been the main reason for the decline in anaesthetic maternal mortality. Over the past 20 years there has been a great expansion of specialist obstetric anaesthetic posts and also several sets of guidelines have been produced to aim at raising the standards of obstetric anaesthesia [34-37]. In addition there have been changes in the training of junior anaesthetists such that they must have at least 12 months experience and then an appropriate period of obstetric anaesthesia training before they can work on a labour ward without close supervision ward. These documents [34-37] and the changes in junior training have assisted obstetric anaesthetists in driving forward improvements in the both the training and supervision of junior anaesthetists, introducing 24 hour resident anaesthetic cover often dedicated solely to obstetrics, introducing modern anaesthetic equipment with comprehensive anaesthetic monitoring, introducing trained assistants for the anaesthetist in the maternity hospital, introducing proper recovery facilities, participating in multidisciplinary antenatal clinics for patients with complex medical pathologies or specific anaesthetic problems and setting out clear plans for the management of these patients, encouraging the closure of small units where provision of adequate standards of care is difficult to cover, and encouraging the incorporation of isolated units onto centralized sites. The above is exemplified by the changes within my own hospital group. I was appointed 21 years ago as the first consultant in Hull with a specialist obstetric anaesthesia training. At that time our two stand-alone isolated maternity units were responsible for some 6 000 deliveries per annum and one of these units had no resident anaesthetic cover at all. Now we are about to move into a single centralized unit and we have 5 specialist consultant obstetric anaesthetists with trainee anaesthetists resident 24 hours per day, 7 days per week. Throughout the UK other hospitals have followed a similar pattern. It is likely that these hard fought changes have been the real reasons for the raised standards of obstetric anaesthesia so that anaesthetic trainees no longer provide care for pregnant women in an unsupported environment.

Neurological damage

Today, with a very low anaesthetic related maternal mortality, over 75% of

Caesarean sections being performed under some form of regional anaesthesia [19, 32] and 31% of women receiving epidural analgesia for labour [33] the emphasis has changed from mortality to morbidity. As indicated in the introduction morbidity is difficult to define and even more difficult to audit on a national basis [38]. There is no formal definition of what might constitute "significant morbidity." One suggestion is that "severe morbidity" would leave a patient with permanent damage or that the majority of patients suffering "severe morbidity" would have spent some time in an intensive care unit [38]. While such patients would undoubtedly have suffered "severe morbidity" such definitions would exclude some serious complications of regional anaesthesia which usually result in no morbidity but, if not correctly managed, could result in morbidity or mortality. These are the life threatening side effects of regional anaesthesia (e.g., the accidental intravenous injection of an "epidural dose" of local anaesthetic, total spinal anaesthesia, and post dural puncture headache). Many surveys have been performed in an attempt to estimate the morbidity associated with obstetric anaesthesia, particularly with regional anaesthesia and these have been recently reviewed [39]. Today, the most worrisome source of long term morbidity in obstetric anaesthetic practice is nerve or spinal cord damage. This may arise as a result of direct trauma from needles or catheters, toxicity due to chemical contaminants or preservatives added to drug ampoules, infection (either iatrogenic or disseminated leading to meningitis or abscess formation), or vascular accidents (anterior spinal artery syndrome, haematoma). These anaesthetic related causes of neurological problems must be differentiated from obstetric causes (e.g., damage to the lumbar plexus, femoral nerve or obturator nerve by the foetal head or obstetric forceps) and patient related causes (e.g., prolapsed intervertebral disc, spinal stenosis, vascular anomaly, tumours, or syrinx of the spinal cord) [39, 40].

It would appear [39] that the risk of serious neurological morbidity to any individual woman is low but because of the potentially large numbers of regional anaesthetics performed a significant number of women could be at risk. In the author's unit some 55% of women receive epidural analgesia for labour and over 95% of all Caesarean sections are carried out with a regional technique – this results in us performing some 3 000 or more obstetric regional anaesthesia/analgesia procedures per annum. Nationally, the Caesarean section rate is currently around 22% [33] and the RA rate for Caesarean sections is in excess of 75% [19, 32]. The average epidural rate for labour is in the region of 31% [33]. Thus, a rough estimate based on 600 000 deliveries per annum [16] suggests that over 250 000 obstetric regional anaesthesia procedures are performed in the UK per annum.

The surveys reviewed by Loo et al. [39] indicate an incidence of reversible neuropathy of up to 0.35% with a few cases of more serious or permanent neurological morbidity occurring once or twice per 100 000 cases (e.g. epidural abscess, anterior spinal artery syndrome, meningitis). Spinal haematoma seems to be an extremely rare complication after obstetric regional anaesthesia [39, 40] but subdural haematoma is well recognized as a complication of accidental dural puncture and post dural puncture headache.

In terms of avoiding direct neurological damage from needles or catheters three recent related publications deserve detailed scrutiny and serious consideration by all anaesthetists, not only obstetric anaesthetists. These papers suggest that a change of practice may be required when performing spinal or CSE anaesthetics. Broadbent et al. [41] demonstrated unequivocally that anaesthetists are unable to identify reliably the lumbar interspaces. In particular, when L3/4 was the interspace to be identified this was correct in only 15% of the cases. The most worrisome aspect of this inability to identify L3/4 was that all the *errors of identification* were made in a cranial direction: L3/4 was wrongly identified one space higher in 53%, two spaces higher in 28%, three spaces higher in 2%, and four spaces higher in 1% (e.g., in these latter cases T11/12 was actually identified as L3/4). The findings of this study [41] stimulated an editorial [42] and link in with a number of case reports [43, 44]. Reynolds [43] describes 7 medico-legal cases involving damage to the conus of the spinal cord, all caused by spinal needles-either single shot spinals or CSE and, in the same journal issue, Parry [44] describes two cases of conus damage due to CSE. In nearly all the cases [43, 44] magnetic resonance imaging (MRI) scans indicated the conus damage at a higher level than that recorded by the anaesthetist – in some cases as high as T10-T12 thus lending further support to the findings of Braodbent et al. [41]. While the epidural space may be approached with relative safety along the whole length of the spinal canal, once the dura is breached it is a very different matter. Above the tip of the conus the space between the dura and the spinal cord is minimal and needles penetrating the dura can easily impinge on the spinal cord.

The problem of identifying an appropriate interspace is twofold: Tuffier's line joining the iliac crests does not cross the lumbar spine at a constant level, but may vary from as low as L5/S1 up to L3/4 [43] and, at the same time, the conus of the spinal cord may terminate anywhere between the lower border of the body of L1 and the lower body of L1 [43]. In addition, there is some evidence that in women a greater proportion of spinal cords (43%) may extend to L2 compared to men (27%) [45]. Reynolds [42] believes that today's anaesthetists may have forgotten the lessons of the past and makes the plea that since Tuffier's line never overlaps with the conus of the cord in normal individuals spinal needles should not be inserted above this level [46].

Post dural puncture headache

With an incidence varying from 0.4% to 4% [47, 48] post dural puncture headache (PDPH) is one of the most common causes of post natal morbidity. PDPH or its treatment can result in significant morbidity. As well as the typical "spinal" headache, the low spinal fluid pressure after dural puncture may cause symptoms from virtually every cranial nerve [39, 40]. The most common cranial nerves affected are the 8th cranial nerve (vestibulocochlear nerve - with changes in hearing, clicking in the ears or tinnitus which may sometimes be permanent) and the 6th cranial nerve (Abducens – causing weakness or paralysis of the affected lateral rectus muscle). Usually a blood patch will cure the problem but sometimes the blood patch can also affect the cranial nerves [40]. Long term headache lasting for years and cases of subdural haematoma causing death have been described following mismanaged/untreated PDPH [49]. A problem of modern obstetric practice with early hospital discharge (e.g., 6 hours post delivery) is that women may go home with an unrecognized dural puncture: around a third of dural punctures are not recognized at the time of epidural insertion and only become evident when PDPH ensues [47]. Thus unless these early discharge women who have had an epidural are given clear instructions they may suffer very severe headaches at home which are not recognized for what they are. These women may then receive quite inadequate or inappropriate treatment from their family doctor and eventually be referred to neurology services where invasive and non invasive diagnostic procedures are performed! PDPH is best prevented by meticulous regional anaesthetic technique: for spinal anaesthesia this would entail the use of small (£ 24 gauge) atraumatic (pencil point) needles and for epidurals this most probably means avoiding the use of air as a loss of resistance medium and avoiding rotation of the epidural needle once the epidural space has been entered. There is debate about the immediate management of a dural tap with an epidural needle – insert the catheter into the spinal fluid or remove the needle and start all over again [50]. Logically, inserting the epidural catheter into the spinal fluid and using it as a spinal catheter is the simplest and most expedient treatment. This avoids any further trauma to the mother and, in particular, avoids the 10% risk of a second dural tap [51, 52]; it ensures rapid pain relief and provides the capability of almost instant anaesthesia for any eventuality; there is some evidence that using the epidural catheter in the subarachnoid space may significantly reduce the severity of the headache and the need for a blood patch [53-55]. On the other hand, bearing in mind the conus damage discussed above, there are those who feel threading a catheter into the subarachoid space is fraught with danger. Review of the literature does not lend support to this belief: the excess of neurological problems seen in association with spinal catheters appears to be related to damage from the needles used to insert those catheters.

Recently it has been suggested that a high regional block may be "the failed intubation of the new millennium" [56]. The authors [56] produce evidence to show that, in strict numerical terms, there is roughly the same number of total spinals (from spinal and epidural anaesthesia) as there is of failed intubations with GA. Because of the smaller number of general anaesthetics performed compared to regional anaesthetics the incidence is very different: recent publications suggest failed intubation may occur in between 1 in 250 to 1 in 885 general anaesthetic cases [56] while the risk of a total spinal is around 1 in 3 300 regional anaesthetic cases [56]. However, it must be made clear that in terms of morbidity, a total spinal has a much lower risk than a failed intubation. Since the management of a total spinal usually requires intubation of the airway and artificial ventilation, in theory, only those total spinals which are also associated with a failure to intubate are at risk. This risk can be easily calculated as the failed intubation risk multiplied by the total spinal risk – this indicates a risk of between 1: 825 00 and 1:2 900 000 cases.

However, this is an underestimate of the real risk of a regional anaesthetic case also suffering a failed intubation. The most common reason for a woman who has a regional anaesthetic to require endotracheal intubation is a failed block which requires the induction of general anaesthesia. In a large survey of over 60 000 Caesarean sections 3% of the regional anaesthetics required conversion to general anaesthesia [19]. Thus the real risk of an attempted regional anaesthetic case requiring to be intubated is the product of the total spinal rate, the failed regional anaesthetic rate at Caesarean section, and the failed intubation rate. Since the risk of a total spinal is very small (0.03%) the most significant factor affecting the need for intubation of a regional anaesthetic case is the failure rate for that regional anaesthetic technique. The survey by Shibli & Russell [19] revealed a wide difference among units in their regional anaesthesia failure rates: while the median rate of block failure requiring conversion to GA was 3%, the range among the units surveyed was from zero at one extreme to 88% at the other. Thus, it would appear that to reduce the potential for maternal morbidity there is a need for units to examine the factors underlying a high regional anaesthetic failure rate.

Although the combined risk of regional anaesthesia failing and then intubation failing with a subsequent general anaesthetic is low, it is, nevertheless, a real risk and maternal deaths following such a scenario are described [11, 12]. The "reverse" of the above scenario may also lead to maternal death. A case is described where general anaesthesia was attempted but intubation failed, the patient was awakened safely but total spinal with respiratory arrest occurred following attempted epidural anaesthesia [12]. This latter case led to much debate as to which regional anaesthetic technique is safest following a failed intubation.

Another potential source of morbidity in modern obstetric anaesthetic practice is respiratory depression from intrathecal or epidural narcotics. Such respiratory depression, which has been described after virtually all epidural and intrathecal narcotic drugs [57-63], has been reviewed in detail [64] and may be more likely when CSE is used. All the above cases [57-63] can be classified as early onset respiratory depression and none resulted in long term morbidity since the patients were under the direct supervision of the anaesthetist at the time of the respiratory depression. Late onset respiratory depression is the most feared complication and much has been written about it but it is extremely uncommon in the young obstetric patient population [64]. Furthermore, it is felt that any nurse trained and allowed to administer parenteral narcotics should have the necessary skills to monitor patients after intraspinal narcotics. Parenteral narcotics can produce as much, if not more, respiratory depression as intraspinal narcotics [64].

Long term backache is another source of morbidity for the pregnant woman. A series of publications based on a retrospectively obtained data set [65, 66] purported to show that backache and a multitude of other symptoms were more common in women who had epidural analgesia as compared to women who did not receive epidural analgesia. The papers received widespread publicity in the national press and brought the issue of backache and epidural analgesia into the public eye. Unfortunately, the press never publicized the articles critical of these papers. This subject is discussed in depth by Russell et al. [67, 68] and their conclusion was that "pregnant women may be reassured that there is no prospective evidence linking backache with a particular type of pain relief in labour."

Conclusions

This short chapter has highlighted the changes in anaesthetic mortality over the last 50 years. The importance of obtaining adequate information with which to interpret the reasons for the decline in maternal mortality is emphasised. The valuable lessons provided by the CEMD reports [1-15] are still important today and are of relevance to anyone striving to develop or improve an obstetric anaesthesia service.

References

1. Ministry of Health Reports on Public Health and Medical Subjects 97. Report on Confidential Enquiries into Maternal Deaths in England and Wales 1952-54. London, Her Majesty's Stationery Office 1957
2. Ministry of Health Reports on Public Health and Medical Subjects 103. Report on Confidential Enquiries into Maternal Deaths in England and Wales 1955-57. London, Her Majesty's Stationery Office 1960
3. Ministry of Health Reports on Public Health and Medical Subjects 108. Report on Confidential Enquiries into Maternal Deaths in England and Wales 1958-60. London, Her Majesty's Stationery Office 1963
4. Ministry of Health Reports on Public Health and Medical Subjects 115. Report on Confidential Enquiries into Maternal Deaths in England and Wales 1961-63. London, Her Majesty's Stationery Office 1966
5. Department of Health and Social Security Report on Public Health and Medical Subjects 119. Report on Confidential Enquiries into Maternal Deaths in England and Wales 1964-66. London, Her Majesty's Stationery Office 1969
6. Department of Health and Social Security Report on Health and Social Subjects 1. Report on Confidential Enquiries into Maternal Deaths in England and Wales 1967-69. London, Her Majesty's Stationery Office 1972
7. Department of Health and Social Security Report on Health and Social Subjects 11. Report on Confidential Enquiries into Maternal Deaths in England and Wales 1970-72. London, Her Majesty's Stationery Office 1975
8. Department of Health and Social Security Report on Health and Social Subjects 14. Report on Confidential Enquiries into Maternal Deaths in England and Wales 1973-75. London, Her Majesty's Stationery Office 1979
9. Department of Health and Social Security Report on Health and Social Subjects 26. Report on Confidential Enquiries into Maternal Deaths in England and Wales 1976-78. London, Her Majesty's Stationery Office 1982
10. Department of Health and Social Security Report on Health and Social Subjects 29. Report on Confidential Enquiries into Maternal Deaths in England and Wales 1979-81. London, Her Majesty's Stationery Office 1986
11. Department of Health Report on Health and Social Subjects 34. Report on Confidential Enquiries into Maternal Deaths in England and Wales 1982 - 84. London, HMSO 1989
12. Department of Health, Welsh Office, Scottish Home and Health Department, Department of Health and Social Services, Northern Ireland. Report on Confidential Enquiries into Maternal Deaths in the United Kingdom 1985-87. London, HMSO 1991
13. Department of Health, Welsh Office, Scottish Office Home and Health Department, Department of Health and Social Security, Northern Ireland Report on Confidential Enquiries into Maternal Deaths in the United Kingdom 1988-1990. London, HMSO 1994
14. Department of Health, Welsh Office, Scottish Office Home and Health Department, Department of Health and Social Services, Northern Ireland Report on Confidential Enquiries into Maternal Deaths in the United Kingdom 1991-1993. London, HMSO 1996
15. Department of Health, Welsh Office, Scottish Office Department of Health, Department of Health and Social Services, Northern Ireland. Why Mothers Die. Report on Confidential Enquiries into Maternal Deaths in the United Kingdom 1994-1996. London, The Stationery Office 1998
16. NHS Maternity Statistics, England:1995-96 to 1997-98 http://www.doh.gov.uk/public/sb0114.htm.
17. Moir DD (1980) General Anaesthesia. In: Moir DD (ed) Obstetric Anaesthesia and Analgesia, Bailière Tindall, London, pp 145
18. Brown GW, Russell IF (1995) A survey of anaesthesia for Caesarean section. Int J Obstet Anesth 4:214-218

19. Shibli KU, Russell IF (2000) A survey of anaesthetic techniques used for Caesarean section in the UK in 1997. Int J Obstet Anesth 9:160-167
20. Crawford JS (1972) Foreword. In: Doughty A (ed) Proceedings of the Symposium on Epidural Analgesia in Obstetrics, HK Lewis & Co ltd, London, pp 3-4
21. Tunstall ME (1972) in Doughty A (ed) Proceedings of the Symposium on Epidural Analgesia in Obstetrics, HK Lewis & Co ltd, London pp 65
22. Crawford JS (1972) in Doughty A (ed) Proceedings of the Symposium on Epidural Analgesia in Obstetrics, HK Lewis & Co ltd, London pp 90
23. Moir DD (1972) in Doughty A (ed) Proceedings of the Symposium on Epidural Analgesia in Obstetrics, HK Lewis & Co ltd, London pp 73 & 77
24. Macdonald R, Lyons G (1983) Epidural blood patch. Anaesthesia 38: 1230
25. Crawford JS (1990) Spinal is better than epidural anaesthesia for elective Caesarean section - Arguments against. In: Morgan B (ed) Controversies in Obstetric Anaesthesia, Number 1, Edward Arnold, London, pp 12-19
26. Russell IF (1990) Spinal is better than epidural anaesthesia for elective Caesarean section - Arguments for. In: Morgan B (ed) Controversies in Obstetric Anaesthesia, Number 1, Edward Arnold, London, pp 1-11
27. Carrie LES (1980) Spinal Analgesia - an alternative route. In: Doughty D (ed) Epidural Analgesia in Obstetrics: a second symposium. Llyod-Luke, London, pp 179-182
28. Abouleish E, Bourke D (1984) Concerning the use and abuse of test doses for epidural anesthesia. Anesthesiology 61:344-345
29. Chamberlain G, Gunn P (eds) (1987) Birthplace: Report of the confidential enquiries into facilities available at the place of birth, conducted by the National Birthday Trust. Wright, Chichester
30. Chamberlain G, Wraight A, Steer P (eds) (1993) Pain and its relief in childbirth. The results of a national survey conducted by the National Birthday Trust. Churchill Livingstone, Edinburgh London Madrid Melbourne New York Tokyo.
31. NHS Maternity Statistics, England: 1989-90 to 1994-95. Department of Health Statistical Bulletin 1997/28
32. Khor LJH, Jeskins G, Cooper GM et al (2000) National obstetric anaesthetic pactice in the UK 1997/1998. Anaesthesia 55: 1168-1172
33. Dr Foster (2001) The Good Birth Guide. The Sunday Times Magazine July 15. (www.drfoster.co.uk)
34. Anaesthetic Services for Obstetrics - a Plan for the future: with special reference to the smaller obstetric unit (1987). The Association of Anaesthetists of Great Britain and Ireland (9 Bedford Square, London, WC1B 3RA) and the Obstetric Anaesthetists Association (PO Box 3219, London, SW13 9XR) e-mail: secretariat@oaa-anaes.ac.uk *(http://www.oaa-anaes.ac.uk).*
35. Recommended minimum standards for Obstetric Anaesthesia Services (1995) (Obstetric Anaesthetists Association, PO Box 3219, London, SW13 9XR) e-mail: secretariat@oaa-anaes.ac.uk. *(http://www.oaa-anaes.ac.uk).*
36. Guidelines for Obstetric Anaesthesia Services (1998) The Association of Anaesthetists of Great Britain and Ireland (9 Bedford Square, London, WC1B 3RA) and The Obstetric Anaesthetists Association (PO Box 3219, London, SW13 9XR) e-mail: secretariat@oaa-anaes.ac.uk *(http://www.oaa-anaes.ac.uk).*
37. The OAA Training Module (1998) The Obstetric Anaesthetists Association (PO Box 3219, London, SW13 9XR) e-mail: secretariat@oaa-anaes.ac.uk.
38. Harmer M (1997) Maternal Mortality - is it still relevant? Anaesthesia 52:99-100
39. Loo CC, Dahlgren G, Irested L (2000) Review. Neurological complications of obstetric regional anaesthesia. Int J Obstet Anesth 9:99-124
40. Russell IF (1997) Postpartum neurological problems. in Russell IF, Lyons G (eds) Clinical Problems in Obstetric Anaesthesia. Chapman & Hall Medical, London Weinheim New York Tokyo Melbourne Madras pp 149-160.

41. Broadbent CR, Maxwell WB, Ferrie R et al (2000) Ability of anaesthetists to identify a marked lumbar interspace. Anaesthesia 55:1122-1126
42. Reynolds F (2000) Logic in the safe practice of spinal anaesthesia. Anaesthesia 55;1045-1046
43. Reynolds F (2001) Damage to the conus medullaris following spinal anaesthesia. Anaesthesia 56;238-247
44. Parry H (2001) Spinal cord damage. Anaesthesia 56:290
45. Thomson A (1894) Fifth annual report of the committee of collective investigation of the Anatomical Society of Great Britain and Ireland for the year 1893-94. Journal of the Anatomy and Physiology 29:35-60
46. Hogan QH (1994) Tuffier's line: the normal distribution of anatomic parameters. Anesth Analg 78:194-195
47. Gleeson CM, Reynolds F (1998) Accidental dural puncture rates in UK obstetric practice Int J Obstet Anesth 7:242-246
48. Paech M, Banks S, Gurrin L (2001) An audit of accidental dural punctures during epidural insertion of a Tuohy needle in obstetric patients. Int J Obstet Anesth 10:162-167
49. Reynolds F (1993) Dural puncture and headache: Avoid the first but treat the second. Br Med J 306; 874-876
50. Russell IF (2001) In the event of accidental dural puncture by an epidural needle in labour, the catheter should be passed into the sub-arachnoid space. Controversies in Obstetric Anaesthesia, Obstetric Anaesthetists Association, London.
51. Norris MC, Leighton B. Continuous spinal anesthesia after unintentional dural puncture in parturients. Reg Anesth 1990; 15: 85-287
52. Rutter S, Shields F, Broadbent et al (2001) Management of accidental dural puncture in labour with an intrathecal catheter: an analysis of 10 years experience. Int J Obstet Anesth 10:177-181
53. Cohen S, Daitch JS, Goldiner PL (1989). An alternative method for management of accidental dural puncture for labor and delivery. Anesthesiology 70:164-165
54. Samaan A, Russell IF (1993) Management of accidental dural punctures with subarachnoid catheters. Anaesthesia 48:451
55. Segal S, Lawrence CT, Datta S (1999) Intrathecal catheter insertion following unintentional dural puncture reduces the requirement for epidural Blood Patch. Anesthesiology Part 4 Supplement, A69
56. Yentis S, Dob DP (2001) High Regional block - the failed intubation of the new millennium. Int J Obst Anesth 10:159-161
57. Brockway MS, Noble DW, Sharwood-Smith GH et al (1990), Profound respiratory depression after extradural fentanyl. Br J Anaesth 64:243-245
58. Noble DW, Morrison LM, Brockway MS et al (1991). Adrenaline, fentanyl, or adrenaline and fentanyl as adjuncts to bupivacaine for extradural anaesthesia in elective Caesarean section. Br J Anaesth 66:645-650
59. Myint Y, Bailey PW, Milne BR (1993) Cardiorespiratory arrest following combined spinal epidural anaesthesia for Caesarean section. Anaesthesia 48:684-686
60. Hays RL, Palmer CM (1994) Respiratory depression after intrathecal sufentanil during labour. Anesthesiology 81: 11-512
61. Hughes SC (1997) Respiratory depression following intraspinal narcotics: expect it! Int J Obstet Anesth 6:145-146
62. Jaffee JB, Drease GE, Kelly T et al (1997) Severe respiratory depression in the obstetric patient after intrathecal meperidine or sufentanil. Int J Obstet Anesth 6:182-184
63. Ferguson S, Brighouse D, Valentine S (1997) An unusual complication following combined spinal-epidural anaesthesia for Caesarean section. Int J Obstet Anesth 6:190-193
64. Hughes SC (1992) Intraspinal opiates in obstetrics. In Shnider S M, Levinson G (eds) Anesthesia for Obstetrics 3rd Ed , Lippincott Williams and Wilkins Philadelphia pp 157 - 191
65. MacArthur C, Lewis M, Knox EG et al (1990) Epidural analgesia and long term backache after childbirth. Br Med J 301:9-12

66. MacArthur C, Lewis M, Knox EG (1992) Investigation of long term problems after obstetric epidural anaesthesia. Br Med J 304:1279-1282
67. Russell R, Reynolds F (1995) Long term effects of epidural analgesia. In Bogod DG (ed) Obstetric Anaesthesia. Ballière's Clinical Anaesthesiology December Ballière Tindall London Vol 9 (no. 4); 607–622.
68. Russell R, Dundas R, Reynolds F (1996) Long term backache after childbirth: prospective search for causative factors Br Med J 312:1384-1388

Disseminated Intravascular Coagulation in the Obstetric Patient

S. Mangione, A. Giarratano

Disseminated intravascular coagulation (DIC) has been suggested to be a syndrome rather than a disease. This syndrome is often connected to a systemic pathology and is always secondary to an underlying disease. DIC is characterised by a systemic activation of coagulation system, with the generation and deposition of fibrin and microvascular thrombi in various organs. It is a systemic thrombohaemorrhagic disorder associated with a well-defined clinical situation, laboratory evidence of procoagulant activation, fibrinolytic activation, inhibitor consumption and biochemical evidence of end-organ dysfunction [1, 2, 3].

Recently it has been demonstrated that coagulation disorders are related to the inflammatory response found in systemic disorders sepsis and obstetric diseases. Clinical conditions frequently associated with DIC are summarized in Table 1.

Table 1. Clinical conditions frequently associated with DIC

"Acute" DIC	*"Chronic" DIC*
Sepsis	Autoimmune disease
Gram negative	Renal vascular disorders
Gram positive	Hematologic disorders
Obstetric diseases	Inflammatory disorders
Intravascular hemolysis	
Hemolytic trasfusion reactions	
Massive trasfusions	
Vascular disorders	
Viremias	
Severe candidemia	
Hematologic malignancy	
Burns	
Crush syndrome	
Politrauma	
Acute liver disease	
Pancreatitis	

Incidence

There is a significant number of clinical reports about the incidence of DIC in sepsis. Some of these studies show a difference in the incidence of DIC in Gram + or Gram – sepsis [4] . Moreover a recent report [5] shows that there are no significant differences in the incidence of DIC based on different pathogenesis. It is impossible to state an incidence correlated to a specific pathology, but it is very interesting notice that there is a positive correlation between the occurrence of DIC and the severity of the APACHE II, SAPS II scores in the critically ill patients.

Pathogenesis

In the last 20 years extensive efforts have been dedicated to the exploration of the coagulation system. This is particularly true if we consider the actual knowledge of the procoagulant cascade and the antithrombotic mechanism.

Surely a central role for the activation of blood coagulation is produced by the tissue factor and its pathway inhibitor (TFPI). The thrombin generation in these conditions is associated with a dysfunction of the inhibitory mechanism. The elevated levels of PAI-1 can be measured by the consequent impairment of fibrinolysis. DIC occurs when the following are recorded: 1) a massive activation of procoagulant cascade; 2) a suppression of natural anticoagulant pathways; 3) the inactivation of the fibrinolytic system [5]. In the past years a strict correlation between the coagulation cascade and the inflammatory response defined as SIRS has been observed.

Figure 1 shows the correlation between the coagulation cascade and the

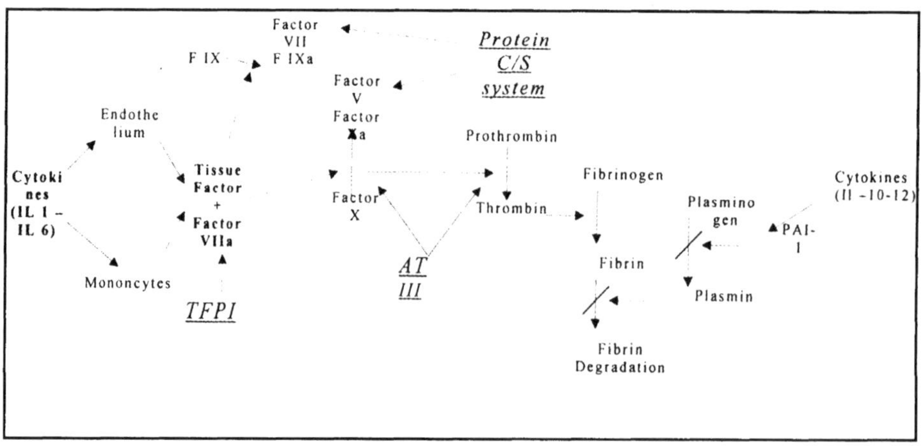

Fig. 1. Coagulation, inflammatory response and natural inhibitors

inflammatory response which is frequently seen in sepsis. An important role in the modulation of the coagulation system is developed by the simultaneous activity of the natural inhibitors of TFPI, Antithrombin (AT III) and Protein C (PC/S). Recently it has been shown that these inhibitors have a specific "anti-inflammatory activity" mediated by thrombin or other factors (Fig. 2) [6].

Many authors have supported the double functions for AT III and PC, and recent reports confirm this hypothesis [7, 8].

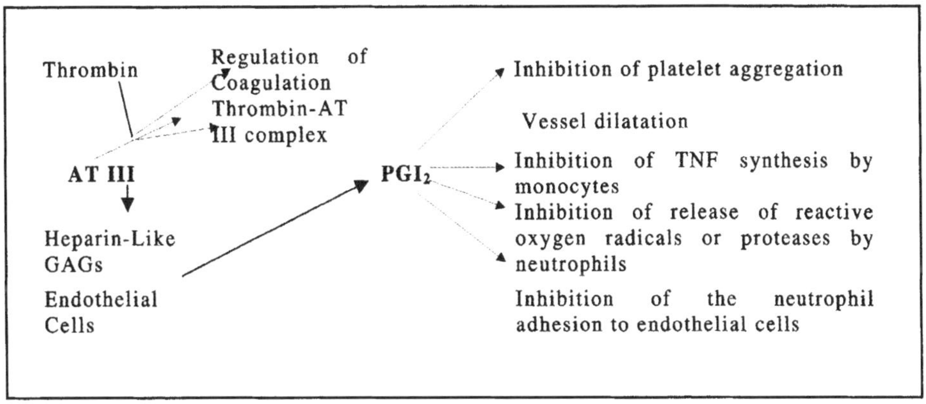

Fig. 2. Antithrombin III (AT III) and antinflammatory actions

DIC and obstetric diseases

A condition of chronic intravasal coagulation is normal during pregnancy and is strictly correlated to the natural evolution of pregnancy (Table 2)

Table 2. Pregnancy and chronic compensated intravasal coagulation. (personal data)

	NO PREGNANCY (median) I III	PREGNACY TRIMESTER (median)	PREGNANCY TRIMESTER (median)
FIBRINOGEN (g/L)	2.90	3.33	4.63
FACTOR II %	106	125	115
PLATELETS (n x 1,000)	230	215	180
AT III %	98	90	85
PROTEIN C %	95	95	90
TAT (mcg/1)	0.9	6.2	13.5

During pregnancy blood coagulation homeostasis may be affected by both acquired and congenital alterations.

In this context, pregnancy and/or altered evolution of pregnancy during peripartum may cause significant alterations of the blood coagulation homeostasis. The most known and dangerous blood coagulation alteration is DIC, which frequently causes an acute status of high grade maternal and foetal mortality. Preeclampsia is one of the most important obstetric syndromes of morbidity and mortality [9, 10, 11]. Recently, several authors have recently studied the pathogenesis of this syndrome during pregnancy discovering new diagnostic and therapeutic strategies [12, 13].

Redman and his co-workers [12] affirm that preeclampsia is a part of a more generalized intravascular inflammatory reaction involving intravascular leukocytes as well as the clotting and complement systems. There is supporting evidence that confirms this condition and in a prior study we have found significant differences between the inflammatory cytokines network recorded in mild and severe preeclampsia compared with normal [14] pregnancy. This condition is monitored with an organ dysfunction score system, and is associated to the severity of clinical preeclampsia as well as a significant decrease in AT III and PC levels (functional activity)[15].

Table 3. Obstetric conditions frequently associated with DIC

Pre-eclampsia – HELLP syndrome
Septic abortion
Abruptio placnta – Placentaprevia
Dead fetus syndrome
Amniotic fluid embolism
Post-partum haemorrhage
Puerperal thrombosis
Natural Inhibitor Familial Deficiency (AT III – Protein C)
Recurrent pregnancy loss (LAC +)

Based on these findings we have focused our attention on the observation that some obstetric diseases are frequently associated with coagulation abnormalities.

The diseases involved in this phenomenon (Preeclampsia and also Lupus Anti-Coagulant (LAC) + recurrent pregnancy loss) are characterized by an endothelium disease in which a variety of systems (coagulation, complement, cytokines) have a determining role during the genesis and evolution.

Our hypothesis assumes to validate the relevance of the control of the coagulation cascade and also modulates the abnormal inflammatory response registered in severe preeclampsia. This response may cause a multiple organ dysfunction associated with DIC [16].

The "anti-inflammatory effects" of the natural coagulation inhibitors of AT III and Protein C assume a different therapeutic action not only on the coagulative status but also on the related SIRS.

However it is probable that additional unknown factors, or additional known factors without completely known activities, are certainly involved in the evolution of both clinic and blood coagulation status in the high risk obstetric patient. This concept is also supported by the fact that the complex blood coagulation system is related to both the complement system and the cytokine network.

Diagnostic criteria

The laboratory manifestations in a patient with suspected DIC vary. Patients differ in the intensity of the DIC as well as the features of the underlying disease.

Acute, massive activation of DIC produces abnormalities reflecting a thrombin generation consisting of: (a) thombocytopenia, (b) prolonged PT and PTT (c) reduced plasma fibrinogen concentration, (d) high levels fibrin monomers, fibrinopeptide A, prothrombin activation peptides, and thrombin-antithrombin III (T-AT) complexes. Elevated levels of D-dimer reflect the generation of plasmin (Fig. 3) [17].

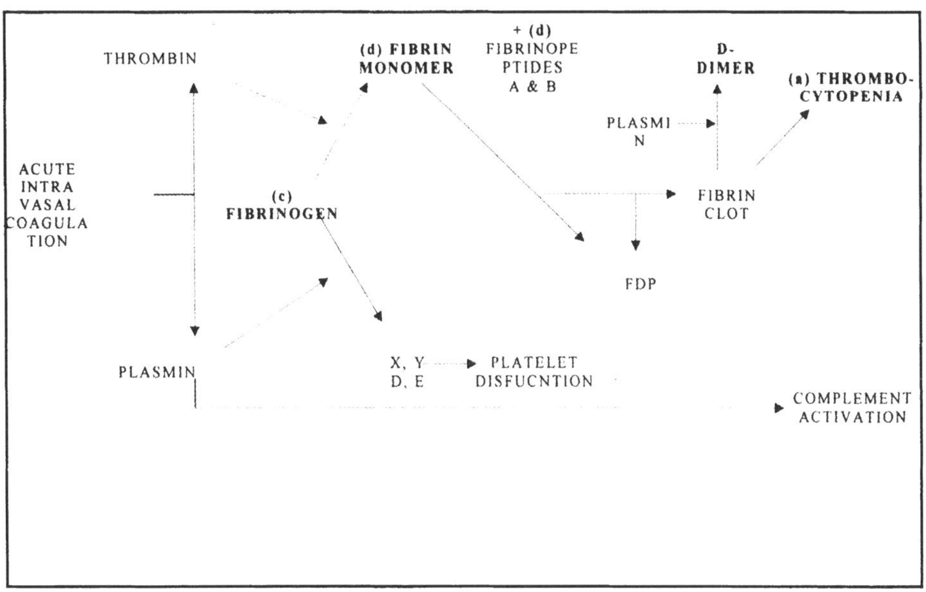

Fig. 3. Markers of procoagulant anf fibrinolytic systems

The most significant laboratory tests od DIS are listed in Table 4.

During clinical practice we have reported that a precocious decrease of AT III and Protein C associated with a positive D-dimer has a good sensitivity and specificity to predict an incoming acute intravasal coagulation. This happens 12-48 hours before the reduction of platelets and is an adequate treatment the onset of DIC.

Table 4. The most significant laboratory tests in disseminated intravascular coagulation

D-dimer
AT III
Fibrinopeptide A
Platelet factor 4
FDP
Platelet count
Protein C
Fibrinogen
Prothrombin time
Activated PTT

Monitoring and treatment

In the last years we have prepared a protocol for the monitoring and treatment of DIC at our Obstetric and General Intensive Care Unit (ICU).

To monitor blood coagulation during a normal pregnancy we suggest that AT III levels and Protein C levels should be recorded after the 26th week and the D-dimer should be recorded after the 30th week. In the pathologic pregnancies this monitoring is performed weekly and includes a TAT complex (for the presence of procoagulant activation), and FDP (for the presence of fibrinolytic status). LDH and fibrinonectin are also used as markers for organ and endothelial dysfunction in preeclampsia.

The first step of treatment is to remove the aetiology of obstetric disease. General principles for the treatment of the procoagulant condition and the inhibitor consumption are listed in Table 5.

In conclusion it is very important for us to underline that these general principles have to be applied under clinical conditions with consultation from Obstetricians and the laboratory specialists.

Future studies of natural coagulation inhibitors of AT III and Thrombomodulin- Protein C system, may change the therapeutic approach to some of these diseases and the clinical evolution of the correlated coagulation abnormalities [18, 19, 20].

Table 5. Treatment protocols in the obstetric patient

FIRST APPROACH
• A T III concentrates to the purpose to maintain range over 100%
• Use heparin only after the correction of A T III deficiency and if strictly necessary
GENERAL APPROACH (DIC)
• Fresh Frozen Plasma (from 10 to 20 ml/kg)
•• A T III at high doses (3000 - 4000 IU /day)
•• FIBRINOGEN only if under 0.25 g/lt
• Platelets if number under 70,000
•• NO PPSB
•• HEPARIN to low doses only after the correction A T III deficiency and in a sure absence of haemorrhage

References

1. Bick LR (1995) Disseminated intravascular coagulation: objective criteria for clinical and laboratory diagnosis and assessment of therapeutic response. Clin. Appl. Thromb. Hemostas. 1:3-23
2. Bick LR, Murano G (1994) Physiology of hemostasis Clin Lab Med 14:677-708.
3. Brozovic M (1987) Disseminated intravascular coagulation. In: Haemostasis and Thrombosis Churchill-Livingstone, pp: 535-541 -
4. Corrigan JJ (1968) Changes in the blood coagulation system associated with septicaemia. N Engl J med 279:851-856
5. Bick LR (1998) Pathophysiology of DIC Sem Thromb Hemostas 24:3-18
6. Okaijma K, Uchiba M (1998) The anti-inflammatory properties of AtIII : new therapeutic implications in severe sepsis. Sem Thromb Hemostas 24:3-18
7. Horie S, Ishi H, Kazama M (1990) Heparin-like glycosoaminoglican is a receptor for AtIII dependent but not for thrombin-dependent prostacyclin production in human endothelial cells. Thromb Res 59:895
8. Hoffman M, Cooper ST (1995) Thrombin enhances monocyte secretion of tumor necrosis factor and interleukin-1 by two distinct mechanism. Blood Cells Molec Dis 21:156-167
9. Gore M, Eldon S, Trofatter KF et al (1987) Pregnancy induced changes in the fibrinolytic balance evidence for defective release of tissue plasminogen activator and increased levels of the fast-acting tissue plasminogen activator inhibitor .Am J Obst Gynecol 156:674-680.
10. Paternoster DM, Stella A, Simioni P, et al (1996) Fibronectin and antithrombin as markers of preeclampsia in pregnancy Europ J Obst Gyn Reprod Biol, 70: 33-39
11. Reister F, Heil W, Rath W (1997) Coagulation disorders in Obstetrics. Biom Progr 10:62-67.
12. Redman CWG, Sacks GP, Sargent IL. (1999) Preeclampsia: an excessive maternal inflammatory response to pregnancy Am J Obstet Gynecol 180:499-506
13. Mangione S, Giarratano A, Leone I, Mangione D (1996) Monitoraggio e trattamento delle coagulopatie in ostetricia ad alto rischio. Min Anes 62:623-626.
14. Gilabert J, Fernandez JA, Espana F, et al (1988) Physiological coagulation inhibitors (protein C, protein S and antithrombin III) in severe preeclamptic states and in users of oral contraceptives. Thromb. Res. 49: 319-329.
15. Giarratano A, Cuccio G, Mangione S (2000) Effects of AT III treatment (high doses) in severe pre-eclampsia and HELLP syndrome with alterations of coagulation inhibitors and inflammatory markers: a preliminary report. Crit Care 4:s17
16. Gando S, Kameue T, Nanzaki S, Nakanishi Y (1995) Cytochines, soluble thrombomodulin and

disseminated intravascular coagulation in patients with systemic inflammatory response syndrome. Thromb Res 80:519-526
17. Stormorken H (1979) Interrelationship between coagulation, the fibrinolytic and the kallikrein and kinin system .Scandin J Hematol 34:24-27
18. Maki M, Takao K, Terao T, et al (2000) Atithrombin therapy for severe preeclampsia: results of a double-blind , randomized, placebo-controlled trial . Thromb Hemost; 84:583-90
19. Esmon CT (2001) The normal role of activated Protein C in maintaining homeostasis and its relevance to critical illness . Crit care 5:S7-12.
20. Giarratano A, Capogna G, Celleno D, et al (2000) A new approach in the treatment of severe preeclampsia and HELLP syndrome using high doses of Antithrombin III.26s3:S321-417

Cardiopulmonary Resuscitation in the Parturient

J. DOUGLAS

Cardiopulmonary arrest in the parturient is a relatively rare event but it has potentially serious consequences for the mother and her foetus. Causes in the pregnant patient are similar to those in the non-pregnant patient but embolism (pulmonary thromboembolism, amniotic fluid embolism, air), trauma and haemorrhage are more common events in contrast to the non-pregnant patient where cardiac disease is more common [1] (Table 1). As the age of women bearing children increases, ischaemic cardiac disease may become a more prominent causal factor.

Table 1. Aetiology of cardiopulmonary arrest in pregnancy

1. Ventilation perfusion mismatch: embolism (air, amniotic fluid, thrombus)
2. Haemorrhage: placental pathology (previa, abruptio), uterine hypotonia, uterine inversion, ruptured aneurysm (splenic, aortic), genital lacerations
3. Trauma
4. Cardiac: pre-existing conditions (congenital, acquired, arrhythmia, myocardial infarction)
5. Iatrogenic: regional anaesthesia – local anaesthetic toxicity, high block, unopposed vagal activity; general anaesthesia - failed intubation, pulmonary aspiration of gastric contents; other – magnesium sulphate
6. Pulmonary: pneumothorax, severe asthma
7. Miscellaneous: sepsis, metabolic, cerebral (including eclampsia, subarachnoid haemorrhage)

The physiological changes of pregnancy have an important impact on cardiopulmonary arrest and its management. Of these the most significant are the increase in cardiac output, increase in oxygen consumption, decrease in functional residual capacity and aortocaval compression. Because of the increase in blood volume signs and symptoms of acute blood loss may appear late. Decreased functional residual capacity and increased oxygen consumption cause desaturation to occur earlier in pregnant than in non-pregnant patients. After 20 weeks gestation the uterus compresses the aorta and inferior vena cava affecting venous return when the woman is supine. The decreased venous return causes a decrease in cardiac output and until aortocaval compression is relieved it may be difficult or impossible to resuscitate the pregnant patient.[2] Other changes of importance are the increased propensity to arrhythmias during pregnancy and the anatomical changes to the airway that increase the risk of difficult intubation.

Importance of aortocaval compression

Marx (1982) reported on five women who suffered cardiac arrest during inadvertent intravascular injection of 0.75% bupivacaine [2]. In three of these women the infant was delivered "with dispatch" and the mothers all survived with no sequelae. In the other two women delivery was delayed and the women had permanent neurologic damage. Marx pointed out that aortocaval compression may limit the effectiveness of cardiac massage and delivery of the infant improves maternal circulation. Numerous case reports confirm the benefits of early Caesarean section in improving maternal outcome [3-7].

Causes of cardiopulmonary arrest in the pregnant woman

Because of the increase in coagulation factors the pregnant patient is prone to develop thromboembolic disease. In the most recent Confidential Enquiries into Maternal Deaths in the United Kingdom [8] thromboembolic disease was the number one cause of maternal death with a rate of 21.8/million maternities. Sudden cardiopulmonary collapse and/or death may be the initial presentation.

Amniotic fluid embolism (AFE), a condition peculiar to pregnancy, occurs in 1 in 8 000 to 1 in 80 000 pregnancies and is accompanied by a high mortality rate. The diagnosis is usually made on clinical grounds with cardiopulmonary collapse being the presenting feature in most cases. In an analysis of the United States national registry for AFE, Clark et al. [9] reported that 87% of the patients in the series suffered cardiopulmonary arrest. The overall maternal mortality in this series was 61% but only 15% survived neurologically intact.

Haemorrhage also may lead to cardiac arrest. Because of increased blood volume, heart rate and cardiac output hypovolemia is often unrecognized until significant blood loss has occurred. Haemorrhage may be concealed, particularly with placental abruption. Causes of haemorrhage specific to pregnancy include placental abruption, placenta previa, uterine hypotonia and genital tract lacerations. Rare causes of haemorrhage are rupture of major vessels, such as the ascending aorta or splenic artery, which have been weakened by the hormones of pregnancy.

Although myocardial infarction is rare during pregnancy it is attended by a high mortality rate[10]. The symptoms of myocardial infarction may be misinterpreted as gastroesophageal reflux, a common complaint during pregnancy. Myocardial infarction and cardiac arrest can occur following administration of ergonovine [11].

Magnesium sulphate is commonly used to treat premature labour and for prophylaxis in preventing eclampsia. Levels beyond therapeutic range can lead to cardiac and respiratory arrest.

Anaesthesia related causes

Hypoxia and anoxia secondary to airway problems (difficult or failed intubation, pulmonary aspiration of gastric contents) are the most common causes of anaesthetic-related cardiopulmonary arrest and maternal mortality during general anaesthesia [8, 12].

Unexpected cardiac arrest can also occur under spinal and epidural anaesthesia. Cardiac arrest is often secondary to the accidental intravenous injection of a local anaesthetic [13] or an unexpectedly high block, but it may occur independently. Attention was drawn to this by Caplan et al. [14] who reported on 14 cases of sudden cardiac arrest in healthy, non-pregnant patients undergoing spinal anaesthesia. Although resuscitation began promptly neurologic outcome was poor. In several cases epinephrine was given late in the resuscitation. The authors recommended the administration of epinephrine early in cases of sudden bradycardia and a full resuscitation dose of epinephrine to be given when cardiac arrest is recognized. It is postulated that these arrests are secondary to unopposed vagal stimulation in the presence of cardiac sympathetic blockade.

Large studies of regional anaesthesia in parturients indicate that unexpected cardiac arrest is a rare complication [15-19] (Table 2). There are a few case reports of cardiac arrest under spinal or epidural anaesthesia in parturients [20-23]. Two prospective studies of complications associated with spinal anaesthesia for Caesarean section reported no cardiac arrests but the incidence of bradycardia (rate 2 bpm) ranged from 2.1% to 6.7% [24, 25].

Table 2. Serious complications of regional anaesthesia in the parturient

Author	Block type	Number of blocks	High blocks	Cardiac arrest	Local anaesthetic toxicity
Scott	E, S	122,989	21	2	2
Paech	E	10,995	8	0	4
Sinclair	E,S	?	22	1	5
Scott	E	506,00	20	3	20
Crawford	E	27,057			

E=Epidural, S=Spinal

Resuscitation

The principles of resuscitation are similar to those for any cardiopulmonary arrest, namely ventilation, cardiac massage, appropriate medications, treatment of underlying cause and defibrillation, where appropriate (Table 3). The resuscitation algorithms should be followed as for non-pregnant patients. Cardioversion and adenosine have been used successfully to treat arrhythmias during pregnancy [26].

Table 3. Principles of Resuscitation

1. Avoid aortocaval compression after 20 weeks gestation
2. Oxygenation – desaturation occurs rapidly
3. Endotracheal intubation – to protect the airway
4. In late gestation if resuscitation unsuccessful after 3-5 minutes, deliver the foetus
5. Use tracheal route or intravenous sites in the upper body to administer fluids and medications
6. Determine aetiology during resuscitation and treat specifically (e.g., haemorrhage)

Some specific pregnancy considerations are the need to rapidly secure the airway and supply 100% oxygen as oxygen consumption and risk of pulmonary aspiration of gastric contents are increased in the parturient. If the pregnancy is greater than 20 weeks gestation, left uterine displacement has to be provided during resuscitation. Rees and Willis [27] have devised the Cardiff wedge that enables closed cardiac massage at a tilt of 27 degrees. Goodwin and Pearce [28] suggest using a human wedge with the patient supported against the knees of an individual not involved in the resuscitation. The most recent Guidelines for resuscitation [29] suggest using the angled backs of several chairs and the angled thighs of several rescuers to maintain the lateral position during cardiac compressions in the pregnant woman. The accompanying figure shows the woman in the full lateral position. In the authors opinion it would be difficult to deliver effective chest compressions in the full lateral position. If resuscitative measures are not successful within 3-5 minutes Caesarean delivery should be done to improve venous return [3-7]. In this situation delivery of the foetus is being done for maternal reasons, but it will also improve the outcome for the infant [4]. Some recommend open cardiac massage if resuscitation is not successful in 15 minutes.

Other considerations include using the tracheal route or upper arm to administer intravenous medications. The femoral route should not be used as aortocaval compression or ongoing haemorrhage from the uterus may interfere with drugs getting to the central circulation. With spinal/epidural induced arrest early administration of epinephrine is essential.

In summary the common causes of maternal cardiac arrest differ from those in the non-pregnant population. As initial resuscitation is undertaken the differential diagnosis should be considered and appropriate specific therapy initiated. Important points for resuscitation include the use of left uterine displacement in any pregnancy greater than 20 weeks gestation and if resuscitation is not achieved in 3-5 minutes then immediate delivery is indicated to facilitate maternal resuscitation. Pulseless electrical activity is common and may indicate inadequate left uterine displacement or concealed haemorrhage.

References

1. Dildy GA, Clark SL (1995) Cardiac arrest during pregnancy. Obstet Gynecol Clin N Am.;22:303-314
2. Marx GF (1982) Cardiopulmonary resuscitation of late-pregnant women. (letter). Anesthesiology;56:156
3. Cardosi RJ, Porter KB (1998) Cesarean delivery of twins during maternal cardiopulmonary arrest. Obstet Gynecol 92:695-697
4. Katz VL, Dotters DJ, Droegemueller W (1986) Perimortem Cesarean delivery. Obstet Gynecol 68:571-576
5. Parker J, Balis N, Chester S et al (1996) Cardiopulmonary arrest in pregnancy: successful resuscitation of mother and infant following immediate Caesarean section in labour ward. Aust NZ J Obstet Gynaecol 36:207-210
6. Lindsay SL, Hanson GC (1987) Cardiac arrest in near-term pregnancy. Anaesthesia 42:1074-1077
7. O'Connor RL, Sevarino FB (1994) Cardiopulmonary arrest in the pregnant patient: A report of a successful resuscitation. J Clin Anesth 6:66-68
8. Lewis G, Drife J (eds.) (1998) Why Mothers Die. Report on Confidential Enquiries into Maternal Deaths in the United Kingdom 1994-1996. HMSO
9. Clark SL, Hankins GDV, Dudley DA et al (1995) Amniotic fluid embolism: analysis of the national registry. Am J Obstet Gynecol 172:1158-1169
10. Bembridge M, Lyons G (1988) Myocardial infarction in the third trimester of pregnancy. Anaesthesia 43:202-204
11. Tsui BCH, Stewart B, Fitzmaurice A et al (2001) Cardiac arrest and myocardial infarction induced by postpartum intravenous ergonovine administration. Anesthesiology 94:363-364
12. Hawkins JL, Koonin LM, Palmer SK et al (1997) Anesthesia-related deaths during obstetric delivery in the United States, 1979-1990. Anesthesiology 86:277-284
13. Albright GA (1979) Cardiac arrest following regional anesthesia with etidocaine or bupivacaine. (editorial) Anesthesiology 51:285-287
14. Caplan RA, Ward RJ, Posner K et al (1988) Unexpected cardiac arrest during spinal anesthesia: a closed claims analysis of predisposing factors. Anesthesiology 68:5-11
15. Scott DB, Tunstall ME (1995) Serious complications associated with epidural/spinal blockade in obstetrics: a two-year prospective study. International Journal of Obstetric Anesthesia 4:133-139
16. Paech MJ, Godkin R, Webster S (1998) Complications of obstetric epidural analgesia and anaesthesia: a prospective analysis of 10 995 cases. International Journal of Obstetric Anesthesia 7:5-11
17. Sinclair M, Simmons S, Cyna A (1999) Incidents in obstetric anaesthesia and analgesia: an analysis of 5 000 AIMS reports. Anaesth Intensive Care 27:275-281
18. Scott DB, Hibbard BM (1990) Serious non-fatal complications associated with extradural block in obstetric practice. Br J Anaesth 64:537-541

19. Crawford JS (1985) Some maternal complications of epidural analgesia for labour. Anaesthesia 40:1219-1225
20. Sjoberg F, Gupta A, Bengtsson M (1993) Cardiac arrest during Caesarean section. International Journal of Obstetric Anesthesia 2:174-176
21. Hawthorne L, Lyons G (1997) Cardiac arrest complicating spinal anaesthesia for Caesarean section. International Journal of Obstetetric Anesthesia 6:126-129
22. Matta BF, Magee P (1992) Wenckebach type heart block following spinal anaesthesia for Caesarean section. Can J Anaesth 39:1067-1068
23. Thrush DN, Downs JB (1999) Vagotonia and cardiac arrest during spinal anesthesia. Anesthesiology 91:1171-1173
24. Juhani TP, Hannele H (1993) Complications during spinal anesthesia for Cesarean delivery: a clinical report of one year's experience. Reg Anesth 18:128-131
25. Shen C-L, Ho Y-Y, Hung Y-C et al (2000) Arrhythmias during spinal anesthesia for Cesarean section. Can J Anesth 47:393-397
26. Joglar JA, Page RL (1999) Treatment of cardiac arrhythmias during pregnancy. Safety considerations. Drug Safety 20:85-94
27. Rees GAD, Willis BA (1988) Resuscitation in late pregnancy. Anaesthesia 43:347-349
28. Goodwin APL, Pearce AJ (1992) The human wedge. A manoeuvre to relieve aortocaval compression during resuscitation in late pregnancy. Anaesthesia 47:433-434
29. Anonymous (2000) Part 8: Advanced challenges in resuscitation Section 3: Special challenges in ECC 3F: Cardiac arrest associated with pregnancy. Resuscitation 46:293-295

Cardiopulmonary Resuscitation in the Newborn

D. TREVISANUTO, F. ZACCHELLO

The transition from foetal to extrauterine life is characterized by a series of unique physiologic events: (1) on the alveolar side, the lungs change from a fluid-filled to an air-filled situation, and (2) on the vascular side, pulmonary blood flow increases dramatically, and extrapulmonary shunts (foramen ovale and ductus arteriosus) the initial reverse direction and subsequently close. Such physiologic considerations represent the basis for resuscitative interventions in the newborn. For initial lung expansion, fluid-filled alveoli may require higher ventilation pressure than commonly used in rescue breathing during infancy (ventilation). Physical expansion of the lungs and an increase in alveolar oxygen tension both mediate the decrease in pulmonary vascular resistance and result in an increase in pulmonary blood flow after birth (perfusion). The main goals of resuscitative interventions consist of assuring an adequate ventilation and, consequently, an adequate perfusion during the transition from prenatal to postnatal life. However, it is important to remember that some developmental situations (i.e. prematurity) and/or specific diseases (i.e. meconium aspiration syndrome) may significantly influence pulmonary pathology and resuscitation physiology in the neonate [1].

Although certain physiologic features are unique to the newborn at birth, others are common to infants throughout the neonatal period (28 days of life), and into the first months of life.

International guidelines for neonatal resuscitation were recently published [2]. These new recommendations derive from a systematic process of evaluated evidence proposed by members of the American Academy of Pediatrics, the Pediatric Working Group of the International Liaison Committee on Resuscitation (ILCOR), and the American Heart Association. The strength of evidence for each proposed guideline was classified on the basis of the level of evidence, the study design, and the quality of the methodology. From this integration process a class of recommendation was given for each proposed guideline ranging from interventions considered "always acceptable, proven safe, definitely useful" (class I) to practices defined as "unacceptable, no documented benefit, may be harmful" (class III).

Although there are several controversies in neonatal resuscitation, International Guidelines 2000, endorsed by a group of experts in the field of resuscitation, represent the most effective practices for neonatal resuscitation, based upon current research, knowledge, and experience.

The "philosophical approach" to neonatal resuscitation indicated by the new guidelines suggest that "the actions are dictated an integrated evaluation rather than by evaluation of a single vital sign, followed by action on the result, and then evaluation of the next sign (sequential action)". At the initial evaluation, if the term infant that is breathing or crying, the skin colour is pink, and the muscle tone is good he or she can remain with the mother to receive routine care (warmth, clearing the airway, drying) [2].

Although neonatal resuscitation remains divided into *4 categories of action (basic steps, ventilation, chest compressions, medications and fluid),* the algorithm for resuscitation of the newly born infant is partially changed [2] (Fig. 1). In particular, International Guidelines 2000 propose several changes with respect to the previous neonatal resuscitation guidelines (1992) [2, 3]:

1. Meconium aspiration syndrome;
2. Temperature;
3. Oxygenation and ventilation;
4. Chest compressions;
5. Medications, volume expansion, and vascular access;
6. Ethics.

Meconium aspiration syndrome

Meconium aspiration syndrome is a frequent event in the delivery room [4]. In presence of meconium-stained infants, the previous guidelines suggested to perform (a) a suction of the nose, mouth, and posterior pharynx before delivery of the body, (b) a direct laryngoscopy immediately after birth for suctioning of residual meconium from the hypopharynx, and (c) intubation/suction of the trachea [3]. However, several papers demonstrated that tracheal suctioning of the vigorous infant with meconium-stained fluid does not improve outcome and may cause complications [4, 5]. The "new" guidelines suggest that intubation of the trachea in meconium-stained infants has to be limited to patients with *"absent or depressed respiration, decreased muscle tone, or heart rate d bpm"* [2]. The same recommendations were previously reported in the ILCOR advisory statement [6].

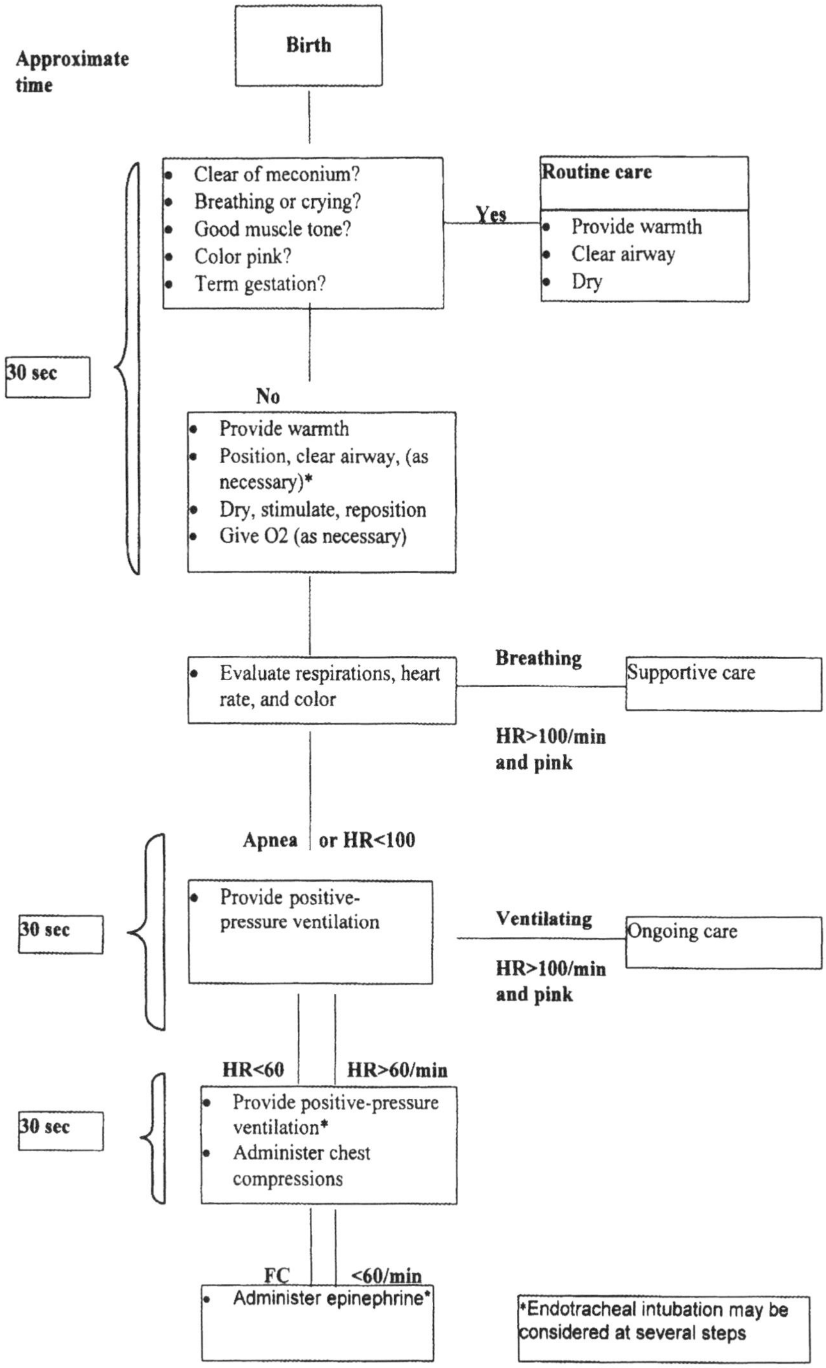

Fig. 1. Algorithm for resuscitation of the newly born infant

Temperature

It is essential to keep the infant warm by preventing heat loss from evaporation and radiation, in particular the preterm and severely asphyxiated babies [7]. The guidelines 2000 advise *to avoid hyperthermia* because it is associated with perinatal respiratory depression [8]. In animal and human studies, *selective or cerebral hypothermia* demonstrated a prevention of brain damage. Controlled human studies are needed to recommend this therapy for routine care in delivery room [9, 10].

Oxygenation and ventilation

Recent clinical studies demonstrated that asphyxiated neonates can be resuscitated with room air as efficiently as pure *oxygen*, confirming previous experimental studies in which a damage by oxygen therapy was reported [11-14]. These data, however, are not sufficient to change the classical recommendations that advise *to use 100% oxygen during assisted ventilation.* If oxygen is not available, the guidelines 2000 suggest to perform assisted ventilation using room air [2]. *Laryngeal mask airway* is becoming accepted as a form of airway management by nursing and medical staff in adult resuscitation, and it has been suggested that it may have a role in neonatal resuscitation [15, 16]. Recently Gandini and Brimacombe reported positive results using the laryngeal mask airway in 104 consecutive normal and lowbirth weight infants needing neonatal resuscitation [17]. However, perspective randomized trials are needed to demonstrate whether or not there is a role for laryngeal mask airway in neonatal resuscitation and whether that role is an alternative to bag and mask ventilation or tracheal intubation. International Guidelines 2000 include the laryngeal mask airway in Class Indeterminate ("preliminary research stage with promising results, but insufficiently available"). They outline that the laryngeal mask airway "may be an effective alternative for establishing an airway during resuscitation of the newly born infant, particularly if bag-mask ventilation is ineffective or attempts at tracheal intubation have failed" [2]. At present, there is an ongoing study to evaluate the use of the laryngeal mask airway in our Region (43000 birth/year).

Even if as a Class Indeterminate, the new recommendations report the possibility to recur to the exhaled CO_2 detection for confirmation of tracheal tube placement, particularly when clinical evaluation is equivocal [2].

Chest compressions

Perlman and Risser demonstrated that chest compressions are a rare evenience in neonatal resuscitation. In fact, only 39 (0.12%) of 30 839 infants were administered chest compression and/or epinephrine as part of cardiopulmonary resuscitation in the delivery room [18]. The new guidelines have changed two recommendations for the external cardiac massage in regards to the technique and the depth of compression [2]. *Two thumb compression* is the preferred method for external cardiac massage in the newborn infant. Chest compressions by this technique generate higher arterial and coronary perfusion pressure than the two finger method [19, 20]. The aim should be to produce three chest compressions for every lung inflation (3/1). The *depth of compression has to be a third of the anterior-posterior diameter of the chest*, differently from the previous recommendations that suggested an absolute depth (1.3 - 1.9 cm) [2].

Medications, volume expansion, and vascular access

Drug administration is indicated when the heart rate remains less than 60 bpm after a minimum of 30 seconds of adequate 100% oxygen ventilation and external cardiac massage [2]. This indication has changed with respect to the previous guidelines that suggested administration of drugs in presence of heart rate less than 80 bpm despite adequate ventilation and chest compressions [3]. However, this is a rare case in the neonatal resuscitation [18]. In fact, the cause of "arrest" is different in neonates with respect to adults. The terminal rhythm in adults usually results from coronary artery disease and subsequent acute myocardial ischaemia. In neonates, the terminal rhythm derives from hypoxia [1]. For this reason the most important step for correcting neonatal cardiac arrest or bradycardia is through adequate ventilation [1-3]. Because a recent meta-analysis found an increased mortality in adult critically ill patients treated with human albumin [21], the International Guidelines 2000 *do not support the use of albumin-containing solutions for initial volume expansion* [2]. In hypovolemic infants, the fluid of choice for volume expansion is an isotonic crystalloid solution such as normal saline or Ringer's lactate. O-negative red blood cells may be administrated when replacement of large-volume blood loss is required. The most rapidly accessible routes for drug administration are the trachea and the umbilical vein. Peripheral sites may be adequate for venous access, but may be difficult to cannulate and are time consuming. *Intraosseus access* can be considered for medication administration if the umbilical vein or other direct venous accesses are not quickly available [2].

Ethics

A part of the International Guidelines 2000 is dedicated to the ethical aspects of the neonatal resuscitation [2]. "Recommendations" are reported for situations in which *non-initiation* of resuscitation (confirmed gestational age less than 23 weeks, or birth weight less than 400 g, anencephaly, or confirmed trisomy 13 or 18) or *discontinuation* (cardiorespiratory arrest lasting more than 15 minutes) may be appropriate. However, local discussions to formulate guidelines which take in account local resources and follow-up data are recommended. Recently, in our Institution guidelines for extremely low birth weight infant resuscitation were discussed and reported in a local protocol.

Personnel

All of those involved in delivery, including physicians, nurses and anaesthesiologists, must have the knowledge and the skills needed to perform neonatal resuscitation [1-3].

On the basis of the classical NRP guidelines for neonatal resuscitation, we examined the personnel practice in the delivery rooms of 3 regional Centres at different levels (level I, II, III) [22]. From January 1st to December 31st of 1994, we studied 3 492 neonates. The results are reported in Table 1.

Table 1. Number (%) of resuscitated neonates and therapeutic intervention (oxygen supplementation and/or face mask ventilation; chest compressions; drugs) in the 3 Centres of different level. (Modified from Trevisanuto D et al Ped. Med. Chir. [Med. Surg. Ped.], 1997; 19: 77-80)

Centre	Level I	Level II	Level III
Resuscitated neonates	11 (5.6%)	83 (4.6)	213 (14%)
Oxygen/face mask ventilation	9 (81.8%)	62 (74.6 %)	27 (12.6%)
Endotracheal intubation	2 (18.2%)	21 (25.4%)	189 (87.4%)
Chest compressions	6 (54.5%) (3%)*	19 (22.8%) (1%)	0
Epinephrine	0	0	1
Volume expanders	0	0	0
Sodium bicarbonate	0	2	4
Naloxone	0	0	1
Atropine	0	0	1
Isoprenaline	0	0	1

*Percentage of all neonates

These data demonstrate significant differences in neonatal resuscitation practice of the 3 Regional Centres. Theoretical and practical recommendations for correct neonatal resuscitation have to be implemented

Since 1996, the Department of Paediatrics at Padua University has held 2 day courses on neonatal resuscitation. The courses are taught by experienced neonatologists and are based on a NRP training program from an education manual endorsed by the American Heart Association and the American Academy of Pediatrics. We evaluated the gained knowledge of the paediatric residents following participation throughout the course. A written test consisting of 80 questions that were derived from a standard test of the American Heart Association Neonatal Resuscitation Manual was administered to 25 paediatric residents before, at the end, and 6 months after the NRP course.

The questions were evenly divided into the four major steps of the neonatal resuscitation: 1) initial step of resuscitation; 2) ventilation, including bag mask ventilation and endotracheal intubation; 3) chest compression; and 4) administration of medications and fluids. The participants took the test examination under standardized conditions, strictly supervised, and were requested to complete the test within 45 minutes. The questions included multiple choice, fill in, and true/false questions. The grading of the test, performed by neonatologist instructors, was objective and carried out according to the standard instructions of the Instructor's Manual for Neonatal Resuscitation.

The scores for the pretest, posttest, and follow-up test were analysed using

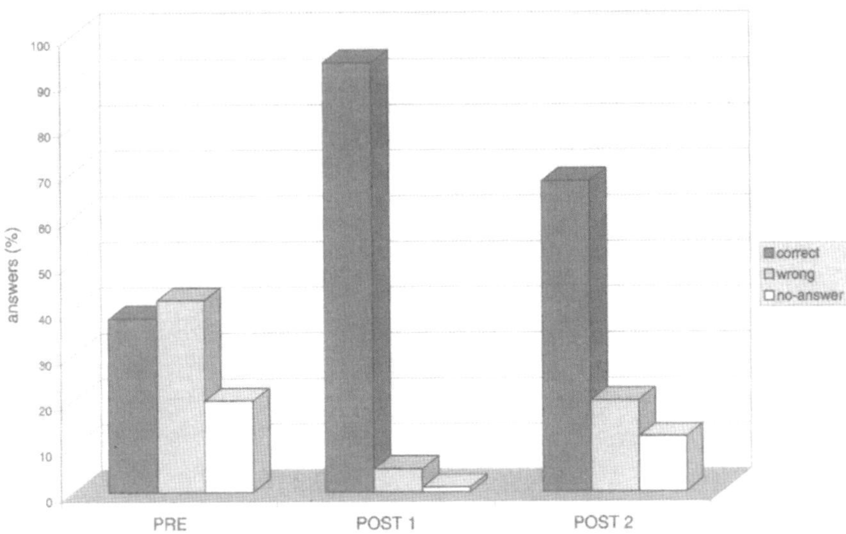

Fig. 2. Percentage of answers (correct, wrong, no answer) before (PRE), immediately after (POST

univariate repeated measures of analysis of variants (ANOVAs). Results are reported as percentages of right answers. (Fig. 2.)

Our study demonstrates that, although the structure on NRP was originally designed for the US health care system, it seems to work in an Italian health care context. The knowledge gained by paediatric residents participating in the NRP course is very high, but is not retained over time [23].

Similar to American and Canadian experiences, these data suggest that a refresher course may be needed prior to the end of the usual 2-year certification period of NRP providers [1-3].

Conclusions

Newborn resuscitation is one of the most frequent procedures carried out in medicine. Planned attendance by personnel skilled in advanced neonatal resuscitation at every delivery is essential for effective resuscitation. Standardization of clear guidelines and implementation of simple resuscitative techniques can significantly improve our intervention. However, further research will open new concepts for ameliorating our knowledge on this interesting field.

References

1. Bloom RS (1997) Delivery room resuscitation of the newborn. In: Neonatal-perinatal medicine. Diseases of the fetus and infant. (eds) RJ. Mosby Ed., pp 376-403
2. Anonymous (2000) International guidelines for neonatal resuscitation: an excerpt from the guidelines 2000 for cardiopulmonary resuscitation and emergency cardiovascular care: international consensus on science. Pediatrics 106:1-16
3. Bloom RS, Cropley C (1992) Textbook of neonatal resuscitation. American Heart Association and Elk Grove, IL: American Academy of Pediatrics. Ed. Chameides L. Dallas, TX
4. Wiswell TE, Tuggle Jm, Turner BS (1990) Meconium aspiration syndrome: have we made a difference ? Pediatrics 85:715-721
5. Wiswell TE (2000) Meconium in the Delivery Room Trial Group: delivery room management of the apparently vigorous meconium-stained neonate: results of the multicenter collaborative trial. Pediatrics 105:1-7
6. Kattwinkel J, Niermeyer S, Nadkarni V et al (1999) ILCOR advisory statement: resuscitation of the newly born infant. Pediatrics 103:1-13
7. Narendran V, Hoath SB (1999) Thermal management of the low birth weight infant: a cornerstone of neonatology. J Pediatr 134:529-531
8. Lieberman E, Lang J, Richardson DK, Frigoletto FD, Heffner LJ, Cohen A (2000) Intrapartum maternal fever and neonatal outcome. Pediatrics 105:8-13
9. Vannucci RC, Perlman JM (1997) Interventions for perinatal hypoxic-ischemic encephalopathy. Pediatrics 100:1004-1014
10. Gunn AJ, Gluckman PD, Gunn TR (1998) Selective head cooling in newborn infants after perinatal asphyxia: a safety study. Pediatrics 102:885-892

11. Feet BA, Bruun NC, Hellstrom-Westas et al (1998) Early cerebral metabolic and electrophysiological recovery during controlled hypoxemic resuscitation in piglets. J Appl Physiol 84:1208-1211
12. Medbo S, Yu X-Q, Berger KJ et al (1997) Pulmonary circulation and plasma - endothelin-1 (P-ET-1) during hypoxia and reoxygenation with 21% and 100% O_2 in piglets. Pediatr Res 42:307-311
13. Saugstad OD, Rootwelt T, Aalen O (1998) Resuscitation of asphyxiated newborn infants with room air or oxygen: an international controlled trial. The Resair 2 study. Pediatrics 102:E1
14. Vento M, Asensi M, Sastre J, Garcia-Sala F, Pallardo FV, Vina J (2001) Resuscitation with room air instead of 100% oxygen prevents oxidative stress in moderately asphyxiated term neonates. Pediatrics 107:641-647
15. Pennant JH, White PF (1993) The laryngeal mask airway. Its uses in anesthesiology. Anesthesiology 79:144-163
16. Paterson SJ, Byrne PJ, Molesky MG, Seal RF, Finucane BT (1994) Neonatal resuscitation using the laryngeal mask airway. Anesthesiology 80:1248-1253
17. Gandini D, Brimacombe JR (1999) Neonatal resuscitation with the laryngeal mask airway in normal and low birth weight infants. Anesth Analg 89:642-643
18. Perlman JM, Risser R (1995) Cardiopulmonary resuscitation in the delivery room: associated clinical events. Arch Pediatr Adolesc 149:20-25
19. Slywka B, Whitelaw C, Goldsmith L (1998) Comparison of the two-finger vs the two-thumb method of chest compressions. Acad Emerg Med 5:397
20. Houri PK, Frank LR, Menegazzi JJ, Taylor R (1997) A randomized controlled trial of two-thumb vs two-finger chest compression in a swine infant model of cardiac arrest. Prehosp Emerg Care 1:65-67
21. Cochrane Injuries Group Albumin Reviewers (1998) Human albumin administration in critically ill patients: systematic review of randomized controlled trials. BMJ 317:235-240
22. Trevisanuto D, Ferrarese P, Cantarutti F et al (1997) Neonatal resuscitation in delivery room: the experience in 3 Veneto's Centres. Med. Surg. Ped. 19:77-80.
23. Trevisanuto D, Ferrarese P, Cavicchioli P et al (1998) Valutazione dell'efficacia di un corso di rianimazione neonatale in sala parto durante il corso di specializzazione in Pediatria. Atti del Congresso della Società Italiana di Neonatologia, 22-24 ottobre, Rimini. Development Physiopathol and Clinics 8 (Suppl):219-220

Legal and Ethical Implications of Obstetric Anaesthesia

J. DOUGLAS

There are many legal and ethical questions that confront the obstetric anaesthetist. There is an integral relationship between law and ethics such that the law makes mandatory what the health care profession considers ethical. Although obstetric anaesthetists are concerned about the possibility of litigation one has to consider the underlying ethical principles and base one's conduct on those principles. The four guiding prima facie principles in making any ethical decision are autonomy (individual choice), beneficence (do good, prevent harm, remove harm), non-maleficence (do no harm) and justice (treat like cases alike, be fair) [1].

Informed Consent for Labour Analgesia

The law of informed consent helps ensure that the ethical principle of autonomy is respected. Although the law may vary slightly from country to country there are some basic ethical and usually legal requirements for informed consent [2]. The requirements for informed consent are: it must be given voluntarily; the patient must have capacity (ability to understand); the consent must be specific with respect to the individual doing the procedure and to the procedure; and lastly, there is the requirement of disclosure of risks and benefits of the procedure (Table 1).

Table 1. Requirements for informed Consent

1. Voluntary agreement
2. Capacity
3. Consents to specific procedure and to physician performing it
4. Is advised of and understands the risk and benefits of the procedure

In summary the individual giving consent must understand what they are being asked to do and their agreement must be voluntary. Therefore, good communication between the physician and the woman is essential.

People often use the term competence or capability rather than capacity. Essentially the three terms have the same meaning: the ability of an individual to make an informed decision. Treatment without consent could result in an action for battery [3]. Battery is touching someone without their consent. Even if there is no injury to the patient, in law damages may be awarded. Alternatively, if injury occurs and the consent was not informed then it is considered negligence.

Negligence is a legal term that implies that harm was done to a patient because the physician did not follow standard practice. In order to establish negligence in countries which practice "common law", such as Canada, the UK and the US, there has to be injury and evidence that the injury occurred as a direct result of the physician's breach of duty (failing to do the medical procedure at a requisite level of skill). For a claim of negligence to be successful the patient must be able to show: 1) the physician owed a duty of care to the patient; 2) the physician failed to meet the standard of care required of him or her under the circumstances; 3) the patient must have suffered injury; and 4) the physician's conduct must have caused the injury [3].

Caplan [4] explored the database of the Closed Claims Project in the US to determine the impact of informed consent (or lack thereof) on anaesthesia liability. He reported that informed consent was rarely a liability issue but examination of the records often revealed that the consenting process was inappropriate in 21% of the claims, appropriate in 42% of the claims and could not be assessed in 37% of the claims. Where consent was a factor in a lawsuit, it involved failure to follow the patient request or the patient was not informed of a specific complication or there was an unexpected change in the conduct of anaesthesia. The only obstetric case mentioned involved consent for an epidural during labour but no details were provided.

In 1988 Knapp [5] reviewed the Lexis database in the US and found three legal cases based on adequacy of consent given during labour. In all three cases the anaesthetist was not found liable. The courts cited three factors supporting the physician having obtained informed consent. The factors were information had been given to the patient, the patient did not object to the procedure and the patient co-operated during the procedure.

One of the questions which continues to confront the obstetric anaesthetist is "How do I obtain informed consent from a patient who is in pain and who may not be competent after receiving opioid analgesia?" In some hospitals anaesthetists are not allowed to approach patients in early labour to disclose the risks and benefits of epidural analgesia. Printed information about the types of analgesia available at the hospital are often provided antenatally but patients sometimes are unwilling to consider an epidural until confronted with pain that is unrelieved by other forms of analgesia. Additionally, women may not remember what is contained in the pamphlet [6]. If a woman does not give her consent for an epidural prior to labor and requests it during pain one has to question whether the requirements for informed consent are fulfilled. In particular, does she understand the risks and benefits of the procedure and will she retain that information.

Some women enter hospital with a birth plan that includes the specific statement that they do not want to have an epidural, no matter how much pain they are having. Some anaesthetists may consider the birth plan an advance directive and not provide an epidural. In an editorial Scott [7] stated that she felt it unethical to withhold pain relief from a distressed woman and questioned whether it was even possible for the woman to make an informed decision prior to labour without first experiencing the pain of labour. In other words, how can the woman know that she will not need the pain relief provided by the epidural until she knows how much pain she will have during labour. The choice of providing an epidural under those circumstances is the responsibility of the attending anaesthetist, but the author agrees with Scott that the ethical response is to provide pain relief using the most effective method, namely an epidural.

Another question often asked is "How much information should be provided?" In Canada and the US the standard is not based on what the physician thinks the patient needs to know, but on what a reasonable patient, under that patient's circumstances, would be expected to know before making an informed decision [3, 8]. This usually amounts to full disclosure of the most significant risks, including paralysis and death.

Pattee and colleagues [9] surveyed 60 postpartum women who had an epidural for labour. These women wanted all complications discussed prior to giving consent, especially those associated with the highest morbidity and mortality. Thirty-seven of these women had received an opioid prior to the consent process but they were as satisfied with the consent process as those who had not received an opioid. Women also indicated that the discomfort of labour did not interfere with their ability to understand the information being provided.

A postal survey of obstetric anaesthetists in the US and UK found that American anaesthetists were more likely to obtain a separate written consent (47% vs. 22%) and discuss more risks and benefits of the epidural analgesia (52% vs. 15% $p<0.001$) [10]. The majority in both groups reported that some form of written information was provided to the women antenatally. A signed written consent is not an informed consent unless the risks and benefits have been disclosed and the woman is given the opportunity to ask questions.

In 1995 members of the Obstetric Anaesthetists' Association were questioned regarding the information that they would provide to a woman prior to anaesthesia for caesarean section [11]. Most felt that revealing full information was inappropriate and indicated that they would slant the information to the woman to suggest the type of anaesthesia the anaesthetist would recommend. In other words, if the anaesthetist felt a regional was most appropriate they would slant the discussion of risks and benefits to favour regional anaesthesia. The consent obtained under these circumstances is not informed and may be invalid if injury results.

Gerancher et al. [12] examined the ability of a woman to recall the pre-anaesthesia discussion with her anaesthetist. Information regarding epidural analgesia was provided to 113 women either verbally or verbally and written. The verbal group had a brief interview covering 10 points from a checklist. The other group had the same interview but then was given an informed consent form that detailed the 10 points. The investigator and the patient reviewed the form simultaneously then it was signed by both and the woman given a copy. Questions were answered for both groups. The recall of information was tested 5-7 months later. There was a statistically higher recall score in the women provided with verbal plus written information (median of 90 vs 80 out of a possible total score of 100 points). Seventy-six women considered the consenting process helpful but six found a written consent process alarming and two said they were unable to give informed consent. These results are similar to those from studies of recall among ambulatory surgical patients, implying that women in labour are as able to provide consent as patients about to undergo surgery. However, Affleck et al. [13] suggested that the amount of recall may be dependent on the number of risks presented and that a physician does not need to enumerate every risk.

Swan et al. [14] found that attendance at an antenatal epidural information class improved recall of information about possible complications of epidural analgesia. These authors recommend the next-of-kin to be present during the consenting process during labour.

Other important consent issues

Blood products

As anaesthetists are usually the physicians administering blood in the operating room another area of concern is consent for blood products. Because of the risks of transfusion, as well as for religious reasons, many women now refuse blood products. This presents the anaesthetist with an ethical dilemma, especially in situations where the woman's life is at risk from massive haemorrhage. The respect for autonomy dictates that her wishes are honoured but the principles of beneficence and non-maleficence would suggest blood to be administered. In most countries the courts have upheld the woman's decision to refuse blood and the physician who elects to administer blood may find themselves sued for battery.

Obstetric Anaesthesia Research

An additional challenge for the obstetric anaesthetist is obtaining consent for obstetric anaesthesia research, especially during labour. Dorantes et al. [15] postulated that a research anaesthetist may have difficulty obtaining consent from a woman in labour because there has been no previous contact with the woman, the woman may be concerned about the effect of the research protocol on the foetus and she may be in pain at the time of recruitment. To verify the validity of these concerns they asked parturients, who had either agreed or refused to participate in a study of epidural analgesia for labour, to complete a questionnaire. This questionnaire was designed to determine the reasons for their consent or refusal. Not surprisingly the most important reason why they failed to consent to the study was their pain or discomfort at the time. Women who consented did so based on their understanding of the importance of the study and the potential benefit of the research to other women. Only one patient felt pressure to consent.

In a related area, namely ambulatory and day of admission of surgical patients, Mingus et al. [16] found that patients felt capable of making a decision on the day of surgery regarding research participation. This should be reassuring to the anaesthetist doing studies on Caesarean section patients.

Rights of foetus versus rights of mother

As obstetric anaesthetists are frequently named in litigation regarding a poor obstetric outcome it is important to recognize issues related to the rights of the foetus versus those of the mother. Lescale et al. [17] surveyed 372 consecutive patients undergoing non-elective Caesarean delivery to see what conflicts existed between the patient and her physician regarding consent for the procedure. A small number (8.7%) felt that they did not have adequate input in the decision making process. They recommended that all women facing a non-elective caesarean delivery should have more details with respect to the risk of the procedure. In the UK a ruling in 1997 [18] upheld the principle that a physician cannot perform a Caesarean section or other obstetric interventions on mentally competent women without their consent. Prior to this ruling, the anaesthetist could have been asked to provide anaesthesia to a woman who had not consented to the operative procedure.

Reasons for litigation

When are anaesthetists most likely to be sued or involved in litigation? A review of obstetric anaesthesia cases from the American Society of Anesthesioloists (ASA) closed claims project database revealed that maternal death and newborn brain damage were the most common injuries [19]. Although maternal death was associated more commonly with general anaesthesia newborn morbidity and mortality were not specific to any type of anaesthetic. Backache, headache, maternal nerve damage and pain during anaesthesia were predominantly associated with regional anaesthesia.

Awareness during general anaesthesia for Caesarean section is another reason for possible litigation [20]. Lyons et al. [21] found that only one of 28 patients with awareness sought legal advice. Awareness associated with pain may be more of an impetus for legal redress.

Avoidance of litigation

It is not always possible to avoid litigation. However there are steps that one can take to decrease the chances of being sued. The most important of these is to ensure that every effort is made to obtain informed consent through discussion of the risks and benefits of the procedure, allowing the woman time to ask questions. Written material or a consultation prior to the need for the procedure, such as epidural analgesia, also enhances the consenting process. All discussion should be documented. This may mean having the patient sign a written informed consent form, but one will be negligent unless the woman has the opportunity to learn about the risks of the procedure and to ask questions. If an unexpected event should occur (e.g., an inadvertent dural puncture), discuss it with the woman and see her in follow-up. Again, visits should be documented. Good communication often avoids later problems. Treat the woman and her family with respect.

References

1. Beauchamp TL, Childress JF (1994) Principles of Biomedical Ethics. Oxford University Press, New York, p 38
2. Cotler M, Katz R (1994) Consent. In: Scott WE, Vickers MD, Draper H (ed) Ethical Issues in Anaesthesia. Butterworth-Heinemann Ltd, Oxford, pp 33-49
3. Battaglia JM (1996) Medical malpractice claims in the US legal system. International Journal of Obstetric Anesthesia 5:254-257
4. Caplan RA (2000) Informed consent: Patterns of liability from the ASA Closed Claims project. American Society of Anesthesiologists Newsletter. 64:7-9

5. Knapp RM (1990) Legal view of informed consent for anesthesia during labor (letter). Anesthesiology 72:211
6. Rolbin S, Unger R, Hew E et al (1989) Obstetric anaesthesia: informed consent. (letter). Can J Anaesth 36:253
7. Scott WE (1996) Ethics in obstetric anaesthesia (Editorial) Anaesthesia 51:717-718
8. Slusarenko P, Noble WH (1985) Epidural anaesthesia: concerns regarding informed consent. (letter) Can Anaesth Soc J 32:681-682
9. Pattee C, Ballantyne M, Milne B (1997) Epidural analgesia for labour and delivery: informed consent issues. Can J Anaesth 44:918-923
10. Bush DJ (1995) A comparison of informed consent for obstetric anaesthesia in the USA and the UK. International Journal of Obstetric Anesthesia 4:1-6
11. Lanigan C, Reynolds F (1995) Risk information supplied by obstetric anaesthetists in Britain and Ireland to mothers awaiting elective Caesarean section. International Journal of Obstetric Anesthesia 4:7-13
12. Gerancher JC, Grice SC, Dewan DM et al (2000) An evaluation of informed consent prior to epidural analgesia for labor and delivery. International Journal of Obstetric Anesthesia 9: 168-173
13. Affleck PJ, Waisel DB, Cusick JM et al (1998) Recall of risks following labor epidural analgesia. J Clin Anesth 10:141-144
14. Swan HD, Borshoff DC (1994) Informed consent-recall of risk information following epidural analgesia in labour. Anaesth Intensive Care 22:139-141
15. Dorantes DM, Tait AR, Naughton NN (2000) Informed consent for obstetric anesthesia research: factors that influence parturients' decisions to participate. Anesth Analg 91:369-373
16. Mingus ML, Levitan SA, Bradford CN, Eisenkraft JB (1996) Surgical patients' attitudes regarding participation in clinical anesthesia research. Anesth Analg 82:332-337
17. Lescale KB, Inglis SR, Eddleman KA et al (1996) Conflicts between physicians and patients in non-elective Caesarean delivery: incidence and the adequacy of informed consent. Am J Perinatol 13:171-176
18. Dyer C (1997) Appeal court rules against compulsory Caesarean section. BMJ 324:993
19. Chadwick HS (1996) An analysis of obstetric anesthesia cases from the American Society of Anesthesiologists closed claims project database. International Journal of Obstetric Anesthesia 5:258-263
20. Anonymous (1979) On being aware. (Editorial) Br J Anaesth 51:711-712
21. Lyons G, Macdonald R (1991) Awareness during Caesarean section. Anaesthesia 46:62-64

IN MEMORIAM

In 2001, good news and dramatic events alternated. Some of the latter were to affect deeply the sensitivity and very essence of civil society. The tragedy which has recently involved mankind has left deep wounds. The question is whether these wounds will ever heal and the world forget. Another sorrow in this sad and gloomy 2001 is the recent death of colleagues, teachers and friends Prof. Antonio Brienza and Prof. Gian Paolo Novelli. Both Brienza and Novelli shone in their commitment and dedication to Perioperative Medicine and Critical Care. Their work was always an example to others, including their sometimes ostentatious emphasis on the centrality of the patient. Their ability of clinical synthesis and pioneering experience in supporting a young discipline made it possible for Brienza and Novelli to acquire a correct teaching and training methodology for new students. This was accompanied by an increase in their attention for clinical research, not for its own sake but with the objective of improving patients' lives. Both have the merit of having created a School enlivened by the industrious activity of many young enthusiastic students and collaborators. Brienza and Novelli believed firmly in the importance of their own mission and obtained prestigious international acknowledgements. They represented the Italian scientific community at various levels. Their loss was a shock to us all. It is not the objective of this short note to dwell upon the professional and cultural heritage that Prof Antonio Brienza and Prof. Gian Paolo Novelli left to future generations. There will be other opportunities to remember that. Antonio and Gian Paolo, on behalf of Italian Anaesthesiology, thank you so much.

Prof. Antonino Gullo
Trieste, 16th November 2001

INDEX

A

B

D

E

F

J

K

L

M

P

Q

R

S

T

W

X

Z

Finito di stampare nel novembre 2001
dalla Stella Arti Grafiche s.r.l. - Trieste

Printed by Printforce, the Netherlands